TEXT BOOK OF HUMAN OSTEOLOGY
VOLUME 1

STRUCTURE AND SCIENCE OF THE HUMAN SKELETON

Dr. Kavita Ramanathan

ALLIED HEALTH PRESS

Text book of Human Osteology Volume 1

Structure and Science of the Human Skeleton

Author: **Dr. Kavita Ramanathan**

Allied Health Press
4164 Lakeshore Road
Burlington ON L7L 1A4
Canada
www.alliedhealthpress.com
Email: orders@arclereducation.com

ISBN: 978-1-77956-768-0

ABOUT THE AUTHOR

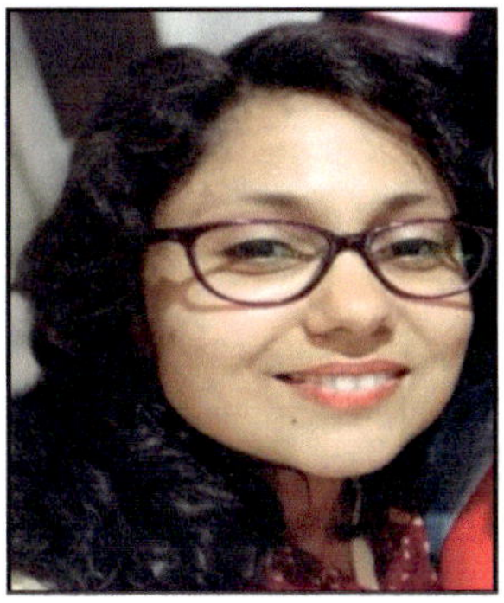

Dr Kavita Ramanathan is an accomplished medical professional with experience working through the length and breadth of India. With 16+ years in clinical and anatomic pathology, she understands the normal and abnormal functioning of the human body in depth. Also, she held positions in the senior management for 8+ years and designed business strategies. She successfully helped organisations attain profitability while maintaining quality and service standards. Additionally, during the COVID-19 pandemic, she contributed significantly by aligning operations to support government initiatives. She earned her undergraduate and graduate medical degrees from reputed institutions under the University of Mumbai, India, and she also holds an MBA in Finance. Dr Kavita volunteers with a non-profit organisation where she tutors students from low-income schools for over two decades. Post-pandemic, she quit her corporate job to pursue her passion of teaching and writing. Currently, she tutors high school and university students in biology, psychology, and medical sciences. Additionally, she authors books, articles, and blogs on topics related to health and well-being. Her strong academic background, enriched with a vast and varied experience, shapes her into a mature and sensible professional.

Brief Table of Contents

Getting Started with This Book

Chapter Openers

A list of Chapter Outline is presented providing a brief Introduction to what will be covered in the chapter.

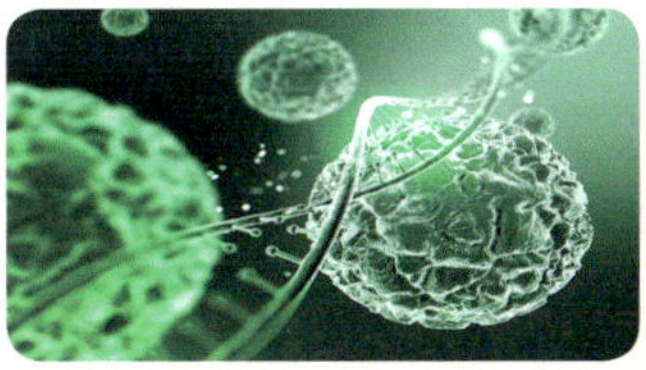

Introduction

Often referred to as the science of life, biology is a broad field of study aimed at comprehending the several kinds of life on Earth, from tiny creatures to sophisticated multicellular entities. Comprising several subfields, including molecular biology, ecology, and evolutionary biology, each of which advances our knowledge of living systems, this field clarifies the mechanisms controlling life events, including development, reproduction, and interaction with the surroundings, which is the central goal of biology. Moreover, biology fills in the void between the natural sciences and medicine by offering a necessary understanding of health, illness, and the interactions between organisms and their environments. Dealing with urgent global issues such as climate change, biodiversity loss, and new diseases depends on an awareness of these complex biological interactions, therefore highlighting the critical part biology plays in modern civilization. Fundamentally, biology explores and tests ideas about the living world using the scientific method. Through methodical observation and experimentation,

LEARNING OBJECTIVES

After studying this chapter, you will be able to:

1. Discuss the scientific method in biology;
2. Explain the cell theory;
3. Discuss the genetics and heredity;
4. Evolution and natural selection;
5. Focus on ecology and ecosystems;
6. Learn about human biology;
7. Evaluate the plant biology;
8. Explain the microbiology;
9. Focus on current trends in biology.

1.1. The Scientific Method in Biology

Learning Outcome

1. Describe the steps of the scientific method;
2. Focus on hypothesis formation;
3. Learn about experimental design.

Learning Outcomes

The beginning of each section of every chapter contains a set of Learning Outcomes that inform students of concepts they should understand. These outcomes help students understand what they should be able to do if they have mastered the material in that section.

Test Your Knowledge

Throughout each chapter, Test Your Knowledge cues you to note which topics have been covered and to self-test your understanding of the material presented.

Test Your Knowledge

1. Explain why correlation does not imply causation in scientific experiments.
2. How does the scientific method help reduce the influence of personal opinions in research?

Chapter Summary

The Summary Section appear at the end of each chapter and summarize main concepts covered throughout the chapter. These points provide key concepts in an engaging and meaningful way.

Summary

The investigation of biological principles highlights the importance of a comprehensive view of life by reflecting the intricate interactions that occur within living systems. The complexity of biology goes beyond individual species or systems, as this essay highlights; it also includes the interactions that mold ecosystems and affect biodiversity. Researchers can conduct in-depth analyses of metabolomic data using sophisticated technologies like MetaboAnalyst, which offer insights into the molecular mechanisms underlying these interactions. As demonstrated by the developments in MetaboAnalyst, for example, the integration of diverse omics data promotes a thorough understanding of metabolic pathways and helps identify important biological markers necessary for research on development and disease (Chong et al., 2018). Additionally, the phenomenon of ecological invasions is a key component of biological research and a vital field of study. The introduction of non-native species into unfamiliar habitats has significant ramifications and calls for multidisciplinary management strategies. Examining the origins and effects of these biological incursions, invasion science has become a crucial field that highlights the need to comprehend ecological dynamics and community interactions. As interest in biological invasions increases, new findings are emerging that put conventional ecological theories and practices to the test. The importance of incorporating various scientific viewpoints is shown by this developing discipline, which also highlights how invasive species shape ecosystems and advances our knowledge of ecological resilience (David et al., 2013). When taken as a whole, these discoveries from invasion science and metabolomics highlight the value of multidisciplinary biology research. Fostering cross-disciplinary collaboration and utilizing technological breakthroughs to improve our comprehension of intricate biological interactions are crucial as we look to the future of biological research. In addition to deepening our understanding of the complexities of life, this method lays the groundwork for tackling urgent environmental issues. Future studies can ensure the continued relevance of biology in a world that is constantly changing by acknowledging the interconnection of biological systems and opening the door to creative solutions that support sustainability and biodiversity conservation. We might imagine a thorough comprehension of life that serves both academia and society at large through ongoing investigation and integration of scientific knowledge.

Knowledge Assessment

The chapter includes material designed to review and reinforce each content. It includes Critical Thinking Questions to help test of your understanding of information presented in the chapter and Short answer Questions to review your understanding of the key concepts presented in the chapter.

Critical Thinking Questions

1. **Who is known as the "Father of Modern Biology"?**
   a. Aristotle
   b. Charles Darwin
   c. Gregor Mendel
   d. Louis Pasteur
2. **What is the basic unit of life?**
   a. Atom
   b. Molecule
   c. Cell
   d. Organism
3. **Which branch of biology studies the interaction of organisms with their environment?**
   a. Genetics
   b. Ecology
   c. Physiology
   d. Botany
4. **Which macromolecule is the main source of energy for living organisms?**
   a. Proteins
   b. Lipids
   c. Carbohydrates
   d. Nucleic acids
5. **DNA is primarily responsible for which function in living organisms?**
   a. Energy production
   b. Protein synthesis
   c. Storing genetic information
   d. Regulating body temperature

Short Answer Questions

1. What is biology, and why is it important to study biology?
2. What are the three main domains of life, and how are they different from one another?
3. Define homeostasis and give an example of how it works in living organisms.
4. What is the cell theory, and why is it fundamental to biology?
5. How do autotrophs and heterotrophs differ in the way they obtain energy?
6. What is the scientific method, and how is it applied in biological research?
7. Discuss how biology helps address global challenges such as climate change, disease, and food security.
8. Explain the levels of biological organization from the smallest unit to the largest. Provide examples at each level.
9. Describe the relationship between structure and function in biology, giving specific examples from cells or organs.
10. How has the discovery of genetics shaped our understanding of inheritance and variation among organisms?

Supplementary Materials

Key Terms: A list of key terms is given for quick reference

KEY TERMS FROM THIS CHAPTER

Annotation enrichment analysis	Biological structure	Cell
Cell theory	Cellular structure	Ecology
Ecosystems	Genetics	Human biology
Microbiology	Natural selection	Organism
Plant biology		

Further Resources: Recommendations for additional readings, websites, and multimedia resources.

References

1. Argelaguet, R., Velten, B., Arnol, D., Dietrich, S., Zenz, T., Marioni, J. C., Buettner, F., et al. (2018). Multi-omics factor analysis—A framework for unsupervised integration of multi-omics data sets. *Molecular Systems Biology, 14.* https://doi.org/10.15252/msb.20178124.
2. Bacher, S., Blackburn, T. M., Essl, F., & Genovesi, P. (2017). *Socio-Economic Impact Classification of Alien Taxa (SEICAT).* https://core.ac.uk/download/286567949.pdf (accessed on 8th March 2025).
3. Barnett, R., Brace, S., Cucchi, T., & Dobney, K. (2013). *Divergent Evolutionary Processes Associated with Colonization of Offshore Islands.* https://core.ac.uk/download/20664364.pdf (accessed on 8th March 2025).

Detailed Table of Contents

CHAPTER 9

The Pelvic Girdle and Lower Limb in Human Osteology 273

CHAPTER 10

The Hands and Feet in Human Osteology 305

CHAPTER 11

Skeletal Variation and Identification in Human Osteology 339

CHAPTER 12

Laboratory and Field Methods in Osteology 373

Index 405

LIST OF FIGURES

PREFACE

The human skeleton has been both a chronicle of our evolutionary past and a manual for daily life for ages. Its study reveals the support and shape behind every movement, the protection for the vital organs, and the record left by growth and adaptation. From the first moments of life to the final years of life, bones respond to mechanical, metabolic, and environmental stressors. An understanding of how bone forms, is remodeled, and ages illuminates fracture healing, developmental abnormalities, and congenital disorders. A comprehensive knowledge of bone form and function is also based in varied fields such as clinical anatomy, physical anthropology, and reconstructive surgery.

Aside from its mechanical role, the skeleton harbors evidence of past health, disease, and lifestyle. Archaeologists' excavations typically center around skeletal remains to reconstruct the lives of individuals and populations in the past. Forensic anthropologists make decisions regarding identity, age estimation, and cause of death based on subtle bone morphological differences. Radiographic assessment of bone structure and density is applied to inform clinical diagnosis of osteoporosis and metabolic bone disease in the hospital. This subject falls at the boundary between basic science and application and encourages a systems perspective of how living tissue records genetic programming and external forces over time.

Textbook of Human Osteology – Volume 1 provides a detailed introduction to the human skeleton, with basic theory supplemented by descriptive anatomy. It begins with the introduction of concepts in bone biology and development and then takes students through each major region of the skeleton. Text is supplemented by detailed illustrations, pointing out landmarks and relationships. Either employed in a classroom, laboratory, or clinical library reference, this book establishes the vocabulary and building blocks for additional osteology and allied health study.

Chapters in this book are designed to take readers step by step from foundational principles to practical application in the examination of the human skeleton.

- Chapter 1 provides historical background and general definitions of human osteology, tracing early anatomical studies, milestones in the unveiling of bone science, and the development of present-day terminology. Briefly reviewing landmark studies and developments in osteological methods, the chapter gives readers a clear vocabulary and background for further research.
- Chapter 2 covers bone cells, matrix composition, and hierarchical microstructure-to-whole-bone architecture. It addresses osteoblasts' functions, osteocytes' functions, and osteoclasts' functions in bone formation and bone resorption, the composition

of the organic and mineral phases, and illustrates how microscopic structural components such as lamellae and Haversian systems contribute to the strength and toughness of whole bones.

- Chapter 3 examines growth patterns of skeletal development, ossification centers, and timing differences. It outlines endochondral and intramembranous mechanisms of ossification, emphasizes the appearance and epiphyseal fusion of plates, and discusses factors—genetic, nutritional, and mechanical—that influence growth patterns and lead to normal or abnormal proportions of the skeleton.
- Regional anatomy comes next. The bones of the neurocranium are described in Chapter 4, each unit and landmark of the cranial vault being described. The viscerocranium is dealt with in Chapter 5, with the facial bones, their articulations, and characteristic surface features laid out for identification and reconstruction.
- Chapter 6 discusses vertebral anatomy and alignment through the spinal column, describing cervical, thoracic, lumbar, sacral, and coccygeal segments. It shows normal and variant configurations of vertebrae, explains patterns of curvature, and discusses the clinical significance of alignment deviations.
- In Chapter 7, the ribs and sternum are covered, as are thoracic cage mechanics. This chapter describes how the ribs are attached, how the ribs, vertebrae, and sternum are articulated, and how the costal cartilage assists in respiratory movements.
- Chapter 8 describes the shoulder girdle and upper limb bones, scapular and clavicular anatomy, humerus, radius, and ulna, and their corresponding articulations. It is interested in functional morphology, including range of motion and muscle attachments. Chapter 9 deals with the pelvic girdle and lower limb, the hip bones, femur, tibia, and fibula, and their joint surfaces, commenting on sex and population variation.
- Chapter 10 deals with the small bones of the feet and hands, and it explains carpals, tarsals, metapodials, and phalanges. It provides naming conventions, variants, and their utility in archaeological and forensic contexts.
- Chapter 11 deals with bone form variations, sex determination, and variations between populations. It explains metric and non-metric methods for analyzing skeletal features, statistical procedures for sex and ancestry estimation, and how to handle mixed or unknown cases.
- Finally, Chapter 12 outlines standard laboratory and fieldwork techniques for measurement, recording, and conservation of skeletal remains. It covers excavation equipment, cleaning equipment, measuring instruments, photography, and digital recording procedures to ensure correct data and long-term preservation.

Together, these chapters constitute a complete manual of human osteology, from cellular processes to regional anatomy and practical methodological practice.

This book is intended for advanced undergraduate and graduate students in anthropology, archaeology, forensic science, and anatomy, as well as medical and dental trainees who require a broad understanding of skeletal form. It will also be helpful to researchers, laboratory technicians, and clinicians who need a detailed reference on bone biology, structure, and regional anatomy.

INTRODUCTION TO HUMAN OSTEOLOGY

1

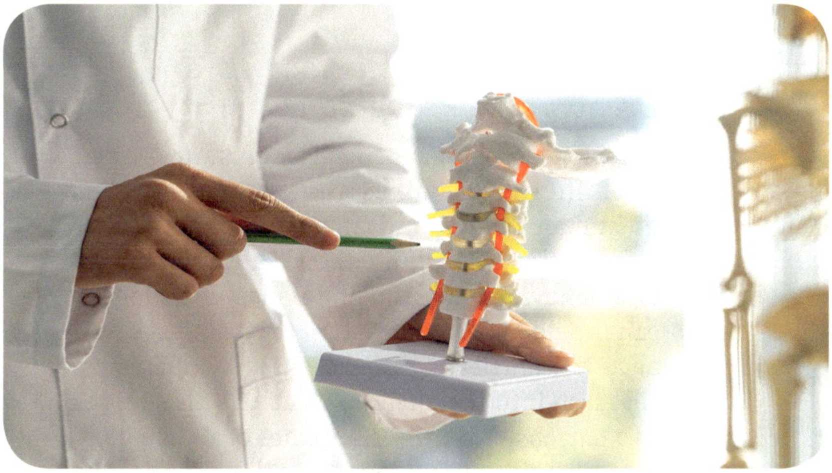

Introduction

Osteology, the scientific study of bones, is a crucial part of biological anthropology and forensic science. It is the identification, classification, and analysis of the human skeleton, which are critical to understanding many aspects of human biology, health, and evolution. The significance of osteology extends beyond basic anatomical study; it's a galvanizing force in fields such as criminology and archaeology, where skeletal remains provide priceless insights into ancient populations, migration, and demographic shifts. Osteology also enables medical applications, allowing clinicians to assess bone health and diagnose conditions such as osteoporosis and arthritis. Thus, knowledge of osteology not only contributes to academic expertise but also has practical applications in preserving human history and improving health outcomes. The ability to identify and analyze skeletal remains is a must for forensic science, and osteology helps determine the age, sex, ancestry, and health status of a person, which can prove useful in criminal prosecution. For instance, the ability to recognize

LEARNING OBJECTIVES

After studying this chapter, you will be able to:

1. Describe the historical evolution of osteology
2. Discuss human skeletal anatomy
3. Understand bone physiology and structure
4. Identify osteological analysis methods
5. Identify osteological indicators of health and disease
6. Evaluate ethical problems in osteological research

dissimilarities in various skeletal features is critical in cases of unidentified human remains, allowing police to recognize individuals and provide closure for families of missing persons. The practicality of the topic underscores the need for rigorous osteology training, as emphasized by current educational studies. Results indicate that those taught by experiential hands-on learning perform well in basic skills, e.g., bone identification, directly translating to effective learning outcomes. Experiential, touch-oriented learning in education strengthens the connection between osteological information and its applicability in real-world scenarios, thereby enhancing the discipline's relevance. Moreover, osteology is gaining significance in anthropological research, shedding light on human adaptation and evolution.

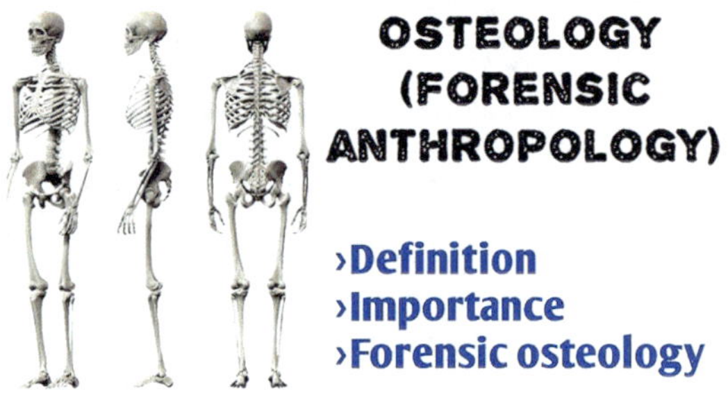

Figure 1.1. The scientific study of bones, encompasses a crucial aspect of biological anthropology and forensic science.

Source: https://i.ytimg.com/vi/WoWoo0czMgU/hq720.jpg?sqp=-oaymwEhCK4FEIIDSFryq4qpAxMIARUAAAAAGAElAADIQj0AgKJD&rs=AOn4CLBkJPCZjmU362hEUKxz4tll8nI_3w.

Through the examination of remains, osteologists can understand diet patterns, medical conditions, and adaptations to the environment of early humans. Not only does this improve our understanding of human history, but also how pressures to evolve have changed the shape of the human skeletal system through time. The investigation of patterns of bone decay and burial practices, which is the focus of archaeological study, also brings osteology back into contact with broader questions of cultural practice and social dynamics. Thus, the value of osteology extends beyond anatomical knowledge but to its comprehensive worth in interrogating the intersection of biology and culture, and its applicability to contemporary and ancient human life, bridging past and present narratives in our pursuit to understand humankind (Figure 1.1).

Explanation of Osteology as a Branch of Anthropology

Osteology, a major subspecialty of anthropology, scientifically examines the skeletal remains of human beings and ancestors to demystify information regarding their culture, biology, and behaviors. By studying bones, osteologists can provide vital information regarding age, sex, ancestry, and health status of the individuals. This research into the skeletal structure also serves as a liaison among the disciplines of archaeology, forensic science, and bioarchaeology, facilitating a more comprehensive understanding of ancient societies. By opening the door to osteology, anthropologists not only discover historical data but also uncover contemporary implications for human evolution and adaptation. These findings are significant for understanding the roles of culture and environmental factors in shaping bone formation across different populations, thereby providing a general account of human ancestry. The procedures employed during osteological studies vary, but most commonly involve qualitative and quantitative methods to derive information from bones. Techniques such as metric analysis of bone measurements and morphological assessments are fundamental, as they allow researchers to determine population differences and track changes over time. Improvements in statistical modeling, including Generalized Estimating Equations (GEE), have enhanced the analytical framework in bioarchaeology, for example, by addressing scalar problems that may arise when studying joint diseases like osteoarthritis. For instance, applications of GEE in the analysis of elbow joint disease in prehistoric populations have identified specific activity and lifestyle patterns, thereby deepening our understanding of how social practice is reflected in skeletal well-being. Attention at this methodological level is significant in fine-tuning validity and richness of outcomes in human osteology to allow for more sophisticated comprehension of past populations and their morbidity. Osteology is also a vital resource in forensic anthropology, aiding in identifying remains in legal contexts. Forensic osteologists aim at breaking down skeletal evidence in an attempt to establish age at death, developmental anomalies, and potential trauma, which are fundamental components of criminal investigations.

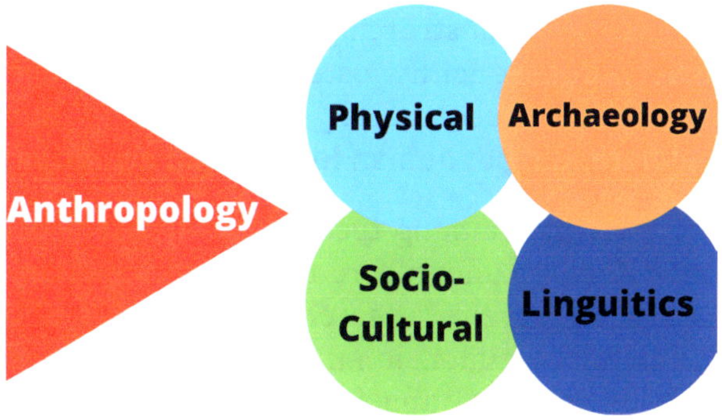

Figure 1.2. A critical subspecialty within anthropology.

Source: https://www.anthromania.com/wp-content/uploads/2021/06/physical-1.png.

Studies contrasting the comparative efficacy of evidence recovery by searchers at varying levels of experience demonstrate how much training and experience can pay off in forensic results. This not only reinforces the importance of sound methodology, but also the broader consequences for the legal justice system, where skeletal analysis can make or break a case. The intersection of osteology and forensic science emphasizes the discipline's practical application while confirming its importance to anthropological inquiry since it not only illuminates segments of human lives but also leaves a trace of social conditions and past events (Figure 1.2).

Significance of Studying Human Bones in Understanding Human Evolution

Human osteology is an essential field of study in the context of human evolution due to the fact that the skeletal system represents an evolutionary history of our species' former adaptation as well as survival strategies. By examining bone shape and density, researchers can understand the way of life and health of our ancestors. For instance, variations in bone structure, such as the development of sturdy femurs in early hominins, have implications for bipedal gait and locomotor efficiency. Besides, fossilized bones provide significant information regarding the diet, mobility, and environments of early human individuals. Such anatomical information enables scientists to make hypotheses related to how pressures of evolution affected not only physical characteristics but survival-necessitated behaviors. Hence, human osteology is central to constructing a narrative of human ancestry, bridging the gap between modern humans and their ancestors. With the incorporation of high-tech imaging devices such as CT, the science of human osteology has been revolutionized, enabling greater accuracy in the study of bone characteristics. These advances enormously enhance our understanding of human evolution by permitting three-dimensional reconstruction of skeletal remains so that detailed comparisons may be made between species. Architectural designs in cancellous bone of hominin taxa, for example, reveal biomechanical adaptations and demonstrate how body shape resolves into function across environments. Studies employing such methodology not only enhance our knowledge of human skeletal evolution but also trace functional adaptation across the centuries, illustrating how our ancestors coped with environmental pressures. The integration of technology into bone analysis, therefore, facilitates greater comprehension of the evolutionary processes that created the modern human, enhancing human origins research. Also, the history of human bones is more concerned with morphology than with social and cultural values of human evolution. The remains themselves reveal how early humans adapted to their environments, formed societies, and engaged in activities such as tool use and communal living. By examining the impact these behaviors have had on bone development, scientists can infer lifestyle changes driven by significant transformations in human history. For instance, wear patterns on bones and teeth reveal dietary changes brought about by agriculture. These findings demonstrate the interrelatedness of biological and cultural evolution, and how social and environmental factors shape our human species. Consequently, the study of human bones not only informs us about body evolution but also deepens our understanding of the broader context in which those changes occurred.

Applications of Osteology in Forensic Science and Archaeology

The use of osteology in forensic science significantly enhances the ability to identify human remains and identify the circumstances of death. Forensic anthropologists use osteological methods to analyze skeletal remains in various situations, including crime scenes and mass casualty incidents. By examining bone morphology, forensic experts can establish biological profiles, which include age, sex, ancestry, and estimates of stature. This is useful information to law enforcement agencies when they work with unidentified remains and is applied in legal cases such as homicide investigations and mass casualty events. The synergy of osteology and modern technology, such as three-dimensional scanning and facial recognition, has enhanced forensic identification protocols. Through these advancements, forensic anthropologists can produce valid reconstructions of decedents, leading to higher identification rates and aiding victims' families in obtaining closure. For archaeology, the applications of osteology go beyond identification since it is a vital means for learning about past human behavior and cultural traditions. Analysis of skeletons can enable scientists to obtain information regarding diet, health, and even the social structure of groups of people residing during different eras in history. For instance, isotopic analysis of bone content can tell us what ancient humans consumed, what they ate, and whether there was trade. Further, osteological analysis can detect traces of disease and injury, providing a window into the lives and ailments of previous societies. These factors enhance individuals within archaeological sites, but also to reconstructing larger narratives of society. Consequently, osteological knowledge contributes substantially to enriching our understanding of human history and evolution.

The synergies among technology, archaeology, and osteology underscore the interdisciplinary nature of current research. For example, the use of three-dimensional scanning combined with osteological analysis has enabled more complete documentation of the skeletal remains and artifacts found at archaeological sites. The method has been applied to create digital repositories that facilitate the study of both osteological and archaeological material, preserving even the minutest details for future studies. Such breakthroughs also enable cross-disciplinary studies and the integration of knowledge from history, anthropology, and even computer science. As scientists seek these integrations, the applications of osteology will expand, to the advantage of forensic investigation as well as archaeological interpretation. Through the crossing of these disciplines, we are in a stronger position to learn about human remains and what they represent in our common past, as exemplified in projects involving 3D scanning technology, as discussed in Anderson et al. (2012) (Figure 1.3).

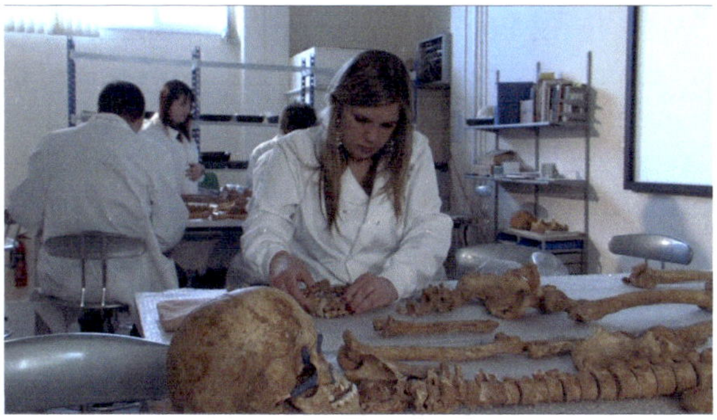

Figure 1.3. Applications of osteology in forensic science and archaeology.

Source: https://external-content.duckduckgo.com/iu/?u=https%3A%2F%2Fi.ytimg.com%2Fvi%2F92u2seWMYqM%2Fmaxresdefault.jpg&f=1&nofb=1&ipt=a9a2880cebb10a488a2b4ede51fbe51caace0c2a6deb2aa4e9cce271e904a819.

1.1. Historical Development of Osteology

Learning Outcome

1. Early studies and contributions of ancient civilizations
2. Key osteology historians and what they learned
3. Technique and technology developments in bone analysis

The scientific field of osteology, which deals with the study of bones, has a rich historical development depending on various scientific and cultural developments. The earliest ideas about the structure and function of bones date back to ancient civilizations, such as the Egyptians and Greeks, who made basic anatomical observations. It wasn't until the Renaissance, characterized by renewed interest in the human body, that osteology emerged as a distinct field. Innovators such as Andreas Vesalius dethroned prevailing anatomical assumptions, focusing on direct observation and dissection. This shift laid the groundwork for further investigation in human and comparative osteology, which would eventually play a significant role in explaining human evolution and development as observed through the advancement of bioarchaeology. The addition of osteology to the broader field of bioarchaeology has significantly expanded our knowledge of past societies. By studying skeletal remains, scientists have uncovered vital information about the health, diet, and social organization of ancient people. For example, the use of sophisticated statistical techniques has sharpened the interpretation of osteoarchaeological evidence, enabling more subtle insights into conditions such as osteoarthritis (OA). The use of Generalized Estimating Equations (GEE) to counter complexity in the data is a modern approach that enhances the quality of osteological studies, yielding firm interpretations from skeletal information. With further growth in osteology, the ability to marry statistical analysis with bioarchaeological outcomes will shed further light on human well-being and lifestyle over the ages, testifying to the field's relevance within today's scientific framework (Bass et al., 2019). As osteology matures, it becomes increasingly convergent with many other disciplines, including genetics, archaeology, and anthropology, to create a multidisciplinary system for learning human history. Examination of skeletal features not only aids in reconstructing the individual's life history but also provides information on larger-scale evolutionary trends within the Hominidae family. Recent findings, such as those to erectoid hominids of Sarstedt, place a focus on meticulous osteological scrutiny to uncover the physiological adaptability of our clade (Czarnetzki et al., 2012). Such integration between osteology and molecular biology and cultural anthropology can be seen as evidence of the field's capacity for engaging with discussions on human adaptation and diversity. With every step forward in research techniques, the past expansion of osteology will undoubtedly cast valuable light on the complex tapestry of human existence and evolution.

1.1.1. Early Studies and Contributions From Ancient Civilizations

Ancient cultures' contributions to human osteology are seminal, as they laid the earliest foundations for the study of human bony structures and pathologies. Archaeological findings reveal that early researchers carefully measured skeletal remains, often attributing them to particular cultural practices, diseases, and social class. The analysis of the Van Castle Mound, for instance, identifies significant information from 328 skeletons dating to the Medieval period, with multiple instances of trauma recorded. Such an analysis reveals stress patterns for day-to-day life, occupation, and dietary habits. The understanding of the fact that specific skeletal trauma was prevalent due to labor-intensive processes not only informs us about the ancient lifestyles but is also an introduction to modern-day paleopathological analysis. Such initial work emphasizes the intricate nature of the association between physical status and environmental factors, the essence of current osteological studies. Ancient societies also contributed to understanding pathological states of the skeleton. Studies have focused on various conditions, ranging from trauma through infection and degenerative disease, typically drawing inferences from burial contexts and burial practice. As a case in point, the study of Van Castle Mound's cases of trauma can show how some categories of injury, such as depression fractures and post-fractural infection, can reveal information about past social roles and healthcare. The osteological evidence reinforces physical stresses undergone by populations and unmasks the effects of hard work and nutrition on bone health. Such past information is echoed in present research strategies, which employ comparable analysis and explanation to establish the skeletal impact of biomechanical stress, a continuity of investigation from prehistoric to contemporary osteological studies. Ancient techniques for studying the skeleton remain pivotal in organizing modern paleopathology. As scientists progress on the shoulders of past scientists, techniques are ever-refined to assess skeletons' conditions more accurately. Following the methods called for by Verano and Ortner, current research focuses on the meticulous recording of ailments such as osteoarthritis and entheses to better understand the biological consequences of physical work in ancient societies. The focus on a small-data strategy in modern osteological studies reflects ancient practices, as it emphasizes well-preserved specimens and combines age and sex to enable comprehensive analysis. Notably, this continuous dialogue not only pays respect to contributions made by ancient cultures but also drives the development of human osteology to a more sophisticated understanding of changes in the skeleton linked to biological and cultural factors, thereby creating a bridge between the past and present in osteology (Figure 1.4).

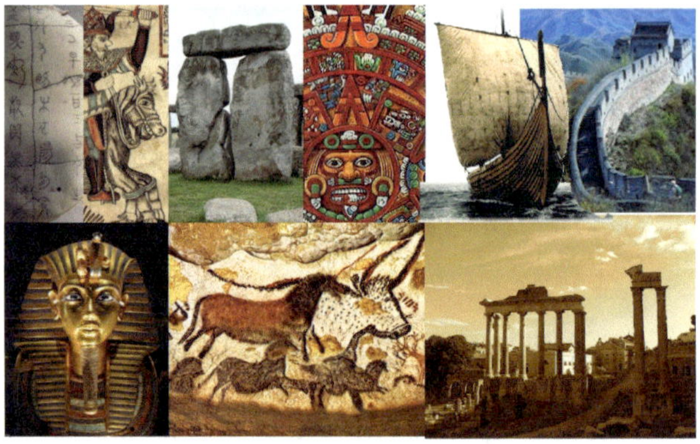

Figure 1.4. Early studies and contributions from ancient civilizations.

Source: https://external-content.duckduckgo.com/iu/?u=https%3A%2F%2Fo.quizlet.com%2F3xm-XxhRonpKyEnElqZK1Q_b.jpg&f=1&nofb=1&ipt=a6c4c09f02e4390dd79f3c0f285157216aad44450acb4f12dcf09b77b5d9defa.

1.1.2. Key Figures in the History of Osteology and Their Discoveries

The osteology, or the study of bones, has evolved mainly with the assistance of many great names from the past. One of them is the Italian anatomist Giovanni Battista Morgagni, whose work in the 18th century laid the foundations of modern anatomical pathology. Morgagni's careful dissections and observations opened up the understanding of the correlation between bone changes and diseases, finally making us wiser about osteology both as a science and as a medical application. His pioneering work, De Sedibus et Causis Morborum, not only spearheaded the anatomical study but also pointed towards the significance of bone integrity and structure in determining medical illness. Morgagni's legacy endures, with current osteological research still referencing his original method, demonstrating the enduring impact of his work in the field. In recent years, discoveries about ancient human remains have continued to contribute to the evolution of osteology, as can be seen with archaeological digs like those at Marcahuamachuco and Cerro Amaru. Scholars who conducted these excavations recovered skeletal remains exhibiting complex taphonomic modification, evidence of varied burial practices adopted by past societies. The remains of a young adult woman whose stature was above average were recovered with proof of postmortem bone modification to support dismemberment, which is a demonstration of sacrificial behaviors deeply embedded in the cultural environment (Spigelski et al., 2009). This application of osteological analysis not only sheds light on individual health and lifestyle but also reflects general social trends among ancient populations, emphasizing the interrelation between cultural behavior and the physical record in skeletal populations. Developments in osteological research are further brought to the fore by the discoveries surrounding the burial of an individual known as Ava. She was excavated from a cist at Achavanich, and she was found with many artifacts, including a Beaker and flint tools, that provided information on how she lived and died (Barnes et al., 2018). The detailed analyses conducted between 2014 and 2017 provided comprehensive information on her diet, genetic profile, and body build, all derived through novel approaches in osteology. The integration of the skeletal and archaeological records underscores the interdisciplinary nature of modern osteological inquiry, in which genetic and isotopic analyses come together to provide a comprehensive portrait of past humans. These results not only enrich our history of human biological existence but also reaffirm the ongoing utility of osteology in unearthing the nuances of human experience over time.

1.1.3. Evolution of Techniques and Technologies in Bone Analysis

Bone analysis technology and technique have seen significant progress in the past, particularly the advent of modern imaging. The bone analysis was performed based on naked-eye observation and basic measurements, which, although necessary at the time, were inadequate for highlighting subtle structural features. As more research was conducted, procedures to examine bone morphology started adopting newer techniques such as radiography and computed tomography (CT), which allowed for more extensive studies of the deeper bone morphology without destructive sampling. With CT scans, researchers could produce three-dimensional models from skeletal remains, providing more detailed information on external and internal bone morphology. This advance not only reinforces our grasp of osteological attributes but also assists in making informed interpretations of functional morphology in extinct groups, underlining the value of technological advancement in human osteology. Furthermore, the union of computer-aided reconstruction techniques has transformed how scientists research bone mechanics and pathology. These technologies enable researchers to explore how bones respond to various factors, such as stress and strain, which are crucial to understanding their biomechanics. An example is the study of the mammalian jaw adductor musculature, in which advances in imaging technology have revealed seminal insights into evolutionary changes. By using CT imaging to reconstruct the musculoskeletal framework in non-mammalian and mammalian specimens, researchers can compare anatomical characteristics in species and throughout eras. Comparative analysis of this type provides critical information that informs hypotheses about evolutionary adaptation and the functional capabilities of ancient species. The careful incorporation of these findings indicates ongoing evolution of technique within the framework of human osteology, furthering the interrelation of technological advancements and our evolving understanding of skeletal biology. Finally, the collaborative nature of recent research is a testament to the imperative of interdisciplinary collaboration in the examination of bones. The effectiveness of large-scale investigations depends on combining resources and expertise, and on sampling materials from various organizations, as seen in work carried out by numerous state museums and universities. The collective project is particularly evident in archaeological and paleontological contexts, where joint access to collections optimizes the diversity of research outcomes. For instance, scientists can now capitalize on global collaborations that provide access to exotic specimens, thereby enhancing our understanding of skeletal variation and evolution across populations. The effective combination of technology, collaboration, and knowledge sharing is a demonstration of the progress in developing osteology in a manner that guarantees research contributes significantly to the overall debate regarding human evolutionary history and biological diversity, as demonstrated by the accomplishments documented in research facilitated through research grants and institutional collaboration (Abdala et al., 2016; Cooper et al., 2013) (Figure 1.5).

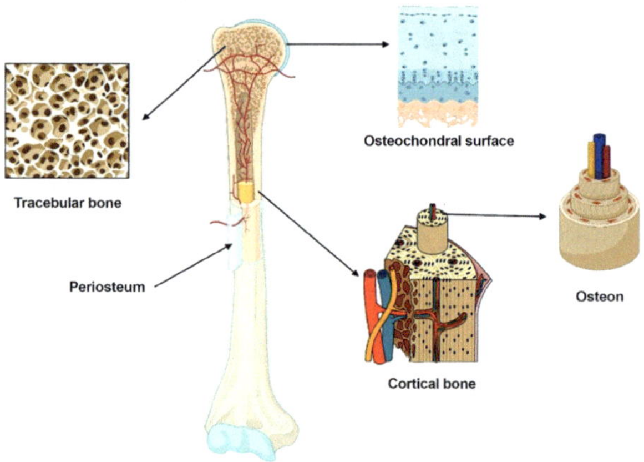

Figure 1.5. Evolution of techniques and technologies in bone analysis.

Source: https://www.mdpi.com/jfb/jfb-16-00168/article_deploy/html/images/jfb-16-00168-g001.png.

Test Your Knowledge

1. How did early studies of bones in ancient civilizations contribute to the development of osteology?
2. Who are the key historians or scholars in osteology, and what important knowledge did they contribute?

1.2. Anatomy of the Human Skeleton

Learning Outcome

1. Overview of the appendicular and axial skeleton
2. Principal bones and their roles
3. Differences in human skeletal anatomy among populations

The anatomy of the human skeleton is a central part of human osteology, a field that encompasses the physical make-up and the biological functions of bones. Made up of 206 discrete bones in an adult human, this system supports the body, assists in movement, and protects sensitive organs. All bones fall into one of two broad categories: the axial skeleton, the skull, vertebral column, and rib cage, and the appendicular skeleton, the limbs and girdles. This categorization helps to comprehend the individual functions of different skeletal components in movement and defense, ultimately uncovering the interrelatedness of form and function. A comprehensive investigation of these categories, therefore, informs not just anatomical understanding but also helps toward explanations of evolutionary refinement over time, in keeping with broader themes within anthropology and medical science. The anatomy of the human skeleton makes a significant contribution in forensic examination to enrich the process of identifying remains, particularly decomposed and fractured bones. For instance, the foot's morphology has been of interest in recent literature, as it plays a critical role in human identification in forensic analysis. More specifically, the lower limbs, often retrieved individually, present unique challenges and opportunities in ascertaining one's biological profile. Understanding how varied skeletal structures aid in skeletal identification underscores the necessity of integrated research, especially given the presentation of public cases of dismemberment or extensive decomposition that do justice to the challenge forensic practitioners face. Emphasizing anatomical detail of the lower limbs and feet can continue to improve identification methods, therefore demonstrating the practical applications of osteological research beyond teaching (Barrett et al., 2014). Furthermore, pediatric osteology provides insight into the anatomical differences present in developing skeletons, emphasizing demographic and health influences during human growth.

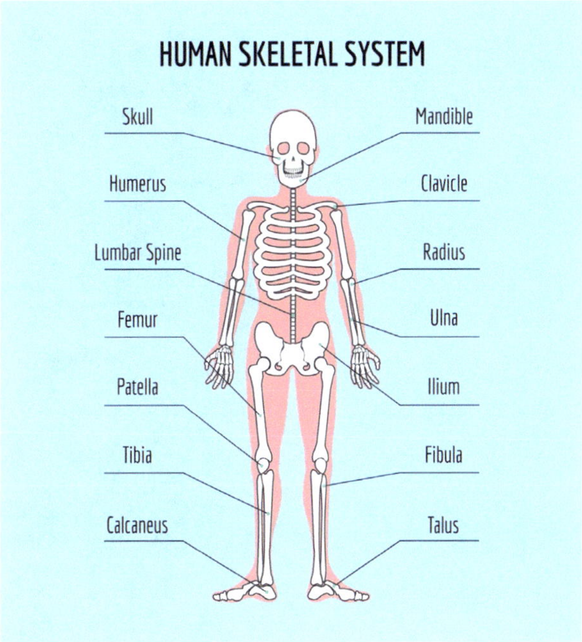

Figure 1.6. The anatomy of the human skeleton.

Source: https://external-content.duckduckgo.com/iu/?u=https%3A%2F%2Fi.pinimg.com%2Foriginals%2Fc4%2F87%2F5a%2Fc4875ab68cea344277113f6a91b0cb85.jpg&f=1&nofb=1&ipt=8d30d9609bc6d1eb2d5fa6fc6c51749c46175bc7391684996273923 9eac467b3.

Analysis of skeletal remains, such as those recovered from archaeological sites like the Tyson site, reveals the conditions affecting subadults. Skeletal analysis can tell us about growth patterns, health crises, and even cultural rituals such as cranial modification. These findings chronicle not only the anatomy of children and babies but also the social behavior and environmental pressure that may have influenced their health. By studying various characteristics of these skeletons, scientists continue to build a more comprehensive picture of human osteology and contribute to knowledge of human history and biological variation (Dockall et al., 1994) (Figure 1.6).

1.2.1. Overview of the Axial and Appendicular Skeleton

The axial skeleton is one of the two significant components of the human skeleton and is made up of 80 bones that form the body's center axis. It includes the skull, vertebral column, rib cage, and sternum and has crucial functions of protection, support, and attachment. The skull, for instance, encloses and safeguards the brain and provides support for sensory organs and sites for attachment of facial expression muscles.

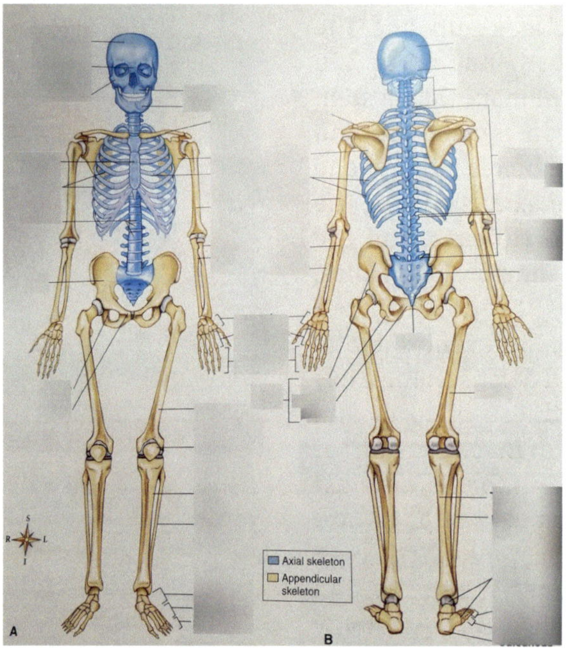

Figure 1.7. The axial skeleton represents one of the two primary divisions of the human skeleton.

Source: https://o.quizlet.com/tRoyU1vbUMKLEKUA.7OqcA_b.png.

The vertebral column supports the head and trunk and encloses the spinal cord, providing structural support and flexibility. Similarly, the rib cage protects vital thoracic organs and enables the lungs to expand and contract during respiration. The axial skeleton diversity parallels the intricate function of human anatomy and physiology in offering a supportive point of departure towards osteological studies and clinical implications in clinical practices. However, the appendicular skeleton comprises limb bones and their girdles and consists of 126 bones. The appendicular skeleton is very specialized for movement and interaction with the world. The upper limbs, including humerus, radius, and ulna, are adapted to all-around motion and handling of objects, facilitated by the shoulder girdle constituted by clavicle and scapula. In the lower limb, the femur, tibia, and fibula provide structural support to weight-bearing functions such as walking and running. The pelvic girdle, composed of the ilium, ischium, and pubis, serves a dual function: providing stability and support and protecting the reproductive and digestive organs. The appendicular skeletons' form and operation reinforce its evolutionary role in providing support to enhanced locomotion and also facilitating physical movements necessary for survival and reproduction. It is essential to understand how the axial and appendicular skeletons relate to possess a thorough understanding of human osteology. The two parts complement one another in structural support, protection, and movement. As an illustration, the axial skeleton supports the body's center while the appendicular skeleton enables dynamic movement, illustrating a complementary relationship that is necessary for simple activities like standing and complex movements like running or throwing. Moreover, several features of the two skeletons, such as limb bones and vertebrae, give insight into evolutionary adaptation over time. Comparative study of the skeletal structures within various species shows much information about functional morphology, enabling more understanding of anatomical variation and homoplasy in the vertebrate lineage, as revealed by comparative studies in osteological literature (Taylor et al., 2013; Paretsis et al., 2020;) (Figure 1.7).

1.2.2. Major Bones and Their Functions

The human skeletal system comprises 206 major bones, each with unique roles that are important for an organism's survival and overall health. Of these, the long bones, such as the femur and humerus, play critical roles in locomotion and support. The femur, the longest bone in the body, supports weight and joins the hip joint to the knee, and facilitates bipedal walking. The humerus of the upper arm, on the other hand, enables diverse arm motion through its ball-and-socket joint at the shoulder, which significantly supports dexterous and strength-requiring work. All these bones are involved in hematopoiesis, as bone marrow in them produces blood cells, thereby pointing to the multifunctional role of major bones in human physiology. The vertebral column, a part of the axial skeleton, is composed of vertebrae that protect the spinal cord and provide structural support for the body. The column consists of 33 vertebrae, divided into cervical, thoracic, lumbar, sacral, and coccygeal regions, each with distinctive shapes and functions. The cervical vertebrae support the head and facilitate its movement, whereas the lumbar vertebrae counteract weight loads from the upper body and accommodate flexion and extension.

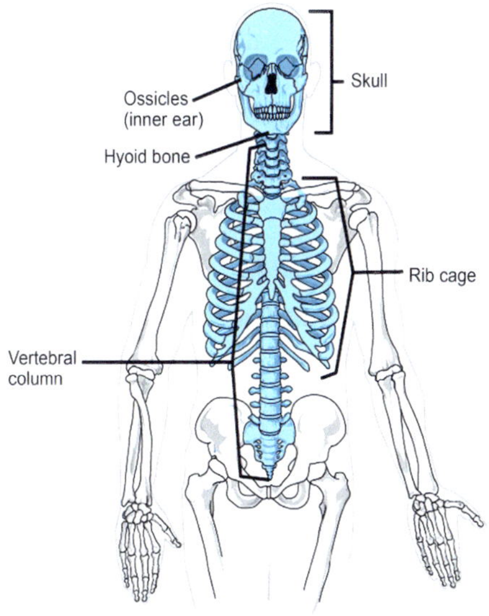

Figure 1.8. The human skeletal system.

Source: https://external-content.duckduckgo.com/iu/?u=https%3A%2F%2Fs3-us-west-2.amazonaws.com%2Fcourses-images%2Fwp-content%2Fuploads%2Fsites%2F1223%2F2017%2F02%2F07233902%2FFigure_38_01_04.jpg&f=1&nofb=1&ipt=2cacc32d5019ab6d8b19316b4123e7de4d1231e03b1f0dc108cd107638a13c55.

The sacrum, formed by fused vertebrae, connects the spine to the pelvis and facilitates pelvic function and stability. Also, the shock and weight are absorbed by the vertebral bodies through the intervertebral discs, providing spinal flexibility during human movement without compromising the spine, thus bearing witness to the sophisticated design of the skeletal system. However, another vital category of big bones are the flat bones, which include the skull, sternum, and ribs. The primary role of these bones is protection, encasing vital organs such as the brain, heart, and lungs. The flat skull bones consist of fused plates that protect and cover the brain and also serve as attachment points for neck movement and facial expression muscles.

Similarly, the ribs form a protective chamber around the thoracic cavity, allowing air to enter and exit during respiration. The sternum, located centrally in the chest, acts as an anchor for the ribs, providing structural support and protecting the body organs. In combination, these flat bones are an example of an evolutionary adaptation that enhances protection and support throughout the human osteological system, demonstrating how various skeletal components work synergistically to support the overall functioning of the body (Figure 1.8).

1.2.3. Variations in Human Skeletal Structure Across Populations

Calculating human skeletal variation between populations reveals much regarding health, diet, and environmental adaptation. Skeletal morphology reflects the intricate interaction between genetic predisposition and lifestyle factors, including diet, activity levels, and even socioeconomic status. By studying these variations, scientists can construct a narrative of human adaptation across geographic localities. For instance, populations under chronic physical stress may exhibit robust skeletal adaptations in response to environmental demands. Adaptation function of this kind shows how the human skeleton is not only a structural frame but also a dynamic record of previous lifestyles and patterns of health. In addition, such studies contribute to a broader picture of human evolution by explaining the selective pressures that have led to the diversification of skeletal attributes across cultures and geographical regions. The study of dental enamel microstructure offers a unique window into the effects of past health and environmental factors on bone growth. This has been shown in recent research to be applicable to fetal-maternal health throughout pregnancy, as well as postnatal individual health. For example, analysis of premolar and molar enamel structure provides valuable insight into the stress experienced during critical growth periods.

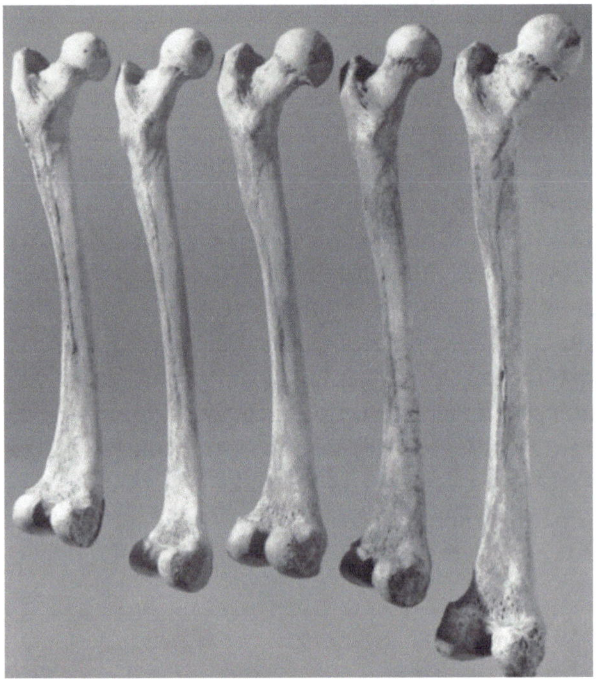

Figure 1.9. Variations in human skeletal structure across populations.

Source: https://ars.els-cdn.com/content/image/3-s2.0-B9780120884674500077-f04-03-9780120884674.jpg.

This research has broader implications than individual health, since these measurements can be used to establish population health baselines, particularly in pre-industrial groups. As has been appreciated in studies of ancient groups, analysis of enamel microstructure can provide essential data for understanding past health trends and the demographic transition, thereby enhancing our understanding of human adaptation to varied ecological regimes (Bondioli et al., 2017). Furthermore, broadening the analytical scope to incorporate information from skeletal remains across multiple localities allows scientists to document changes in health and in environmental influences on bone growth over time. Skeletal evidence can provide critical insights into the living situations and dietary habits of various populations, unraveling the impact of environmental factors on the health of human beings. Trends observed in such analyses usually mirror major socio-cultural shifts that reverberate across generations, affecting anything from mobility patterns to social structure. Notably, the health disparities research does not merely call for an appreciation of osteological data but also asks pertinent questions about how these health states have emerged alongside human activity and environmental alteration. Finally, integrating these outcomes yields a more comprehensive picture of human adaptation and resilience to diverse environmental stressors (Steckel, 2025) (Figure 1.9).

Test Your Knowledge

1. What are the main components of the axial and appendicular skeleton in the human body?
2. How does human skeletal anatomy vary among different populations?

1.3. Bone Composition and Physiology

Learning Outcome

1. Variation in human skeletal morphology between groups
2. Structures of bone tissue and types of bones
3. Contribution of mineral and organic materials to the integrity of bones

The human bone structure is a complex interplay of organic and inorganic materials, whose combined properties confer toughness and strength. Collagen makes up approximately 90% of the organic fraction and is a structural protein that provides tensile resistance and flexibility, while the inorganic matrix is primarily hydroxyapatite, a calcium phosphate mineral. The unique composite structure allows bones to withstand various mechanical stresses during daily activities. Significantly, the hierarchical organization of bone—from collagen fiber patterns at the microscopic level to bone macroscopic architecture—has a significant control over its own mechanics. A better understanding of the structure is key to understanding disease conditions such as osteogenesis imperfecta, where alterations in collagen production affect bone weakness and increase fracture susceptibility. Hence, the intricate properties of bone composition highlight its adaptive nature in the human skeleton and its importance in maintaining overall skeletal integrity (Albert et al., 2013). In addition to its composition, bone physiology possesses a dynamic mechanism of bone formation and remodeling that is crucial for skeletal well-being. Osteocytes, osteoblasts, and osteoclasts, the three bone cells responsible for regulating bone remodeling and adapting to varying mechanical loads, are the primary modulators of the process. Bone formation is the role of osteoblasts, which secrete collagen and other organic components, while bone resorption is caused by osteoclasts, which dissolve the mineralized matrix. This adaptive dynamic remodeling process ensures the maximum bone density and form to resist mechanical stress. For instance, an investigation of microstructural differences across bone regions has established that mechanical environments regulate cancellous bone structure and, consequently, influence bone strength. Such physiological flexibility attests to the importance of mechanical load for ensuring bone stability throughout the range of human life (Abourachid et al., 2018). Bone physiology, in particular, is not merely a question of mechanical adaptation but also one of intricate hormonal regulation of both bone formation and resorption. Other hormones, such as parathyroid hormone, calcitonin, and estrogen, also have a marked effect on bone cell activity. Parathyroid hormone, for instance, enhances osteoclast activity and thus bone resorption, whereas calcitonin increases osteoblast activity and decreases resorption. This hormonal balance is crucial, particularly in aging, when diminished estrogen levels in postmenopausal women may contribute to excessive bone resorption and an increased risk of osteoporosis. As knowledge of hormonal regulation of bone physiology grows, it becomes increasingly evident how indispensable it is for protecting skeletal health and preventing degenerative bone disease. This interconnectedness between hormonal balance and bone turnover underscores the need for further investigation in human osteology, particularly regarding the prevention of bone-related pathologies (Albert et al., 2013) (Figure 1.10).

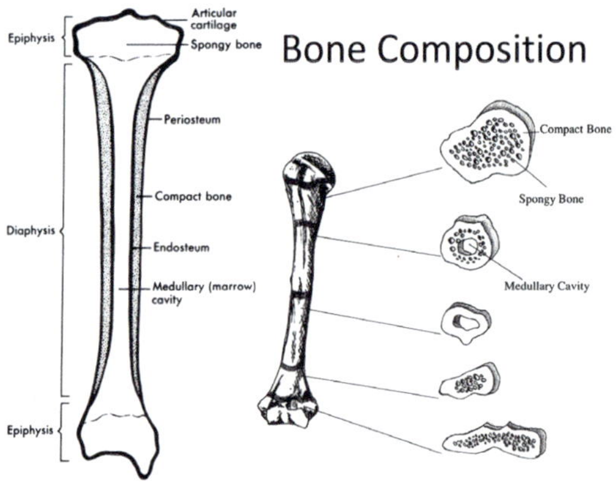

Figure 1.10. Bone composition and physiology.

Source: https://external-content.duckduckgo.com/iu/?u=https%3A%2F%2Fimage1.slideserve.com%2F2023881%2Fslide1-l.jpg&f=1&nofb=1&ipt=63d2911d28012297ece0c706c8a0c18a124b69893ff27a8a4c3f3e228a1e7738.

1.3.1. Types of Bone Tissue and Their Characteristics

Several specific bone tissue types make up the human skeleton, each with its own specialized functions required for the maintenance of general skeletal health. The two primary types of bone are cortical (compact) bone and cancellous (spongy) bone. Cortical bone is dense and forms the outer covering of bones, providing strength and support in weight-bearing structures. It is composed of

Haversian systems, or closely clustered osteons, which give it rigidity and strength. Cancellous bone, however, is composed of a honeycomb-like porous network that is flexible but reduces the overall bone weight. This bone has a key function in providing the space for bone marrow in which blood cells develop, and plays a critical function in transferring forces experienced by the skeleton in movements and activities. In addition to cortical and cancellous bones, bone tissue is further categorized into primary and secondary bones based on developmental stages and remodeling cycles. Primary bone, or woven bone, is the initial bone that is formed during fetal development and fracture healing. It contains disorganized collagen fibers and lower mineralization, rendering it less mechanically robust than secondary bone. Primary bone is replaced by highly organized secondary bone, with a clearly defined lamellar structure, after remodeling occurs. Secondary bone shows greater mechanical strength and is a measure of the adaptive capacity of the skeletal system to various environmental stresses and functional demands. Each of these differences is significant for understanding the dynamic nature of bone tissue under changing physiological and pathological conditions. Another vital characteristic of bone tissue is its histological complexity, reflecting its diverse functional demands. Various cell types are involved in bone formation and repair, including osteoblasts, osteocytes, and osteoclasts. Osteoblasts produce new bone matrix, while osteocytes, which form from osteoblasts, maintain bone tissue and sense mechanical stresses, initiating required modifications. Osteoclasts resorb bone to maintain bone remodeling and calcium homeostasis. This balance of cell types emphasizes the dynamic equilibrium between bone formation and resorption and reveals that bone is a dynamic tissue constantly adapting to the body's needs. Histological research, including that of supraspinous ossified rods in sauropod dinosaurs, elucidates evolutionary processes in bone structure and function, affirming the necessity of understanding bone characteristics in both modern and past contexts (Abdalla et al., 2015; Barrett et al., 2014).

1.3.2. The Role of Minerals and Organic Components in Bone Health

The intricate structure and function of bones rely largely on both organic and mineral compounds, which are essential for overall bone health. Minerals, particularly calcium and phosphorus, constitute the primary inorganic component of bone tissue and play essential roles in providing strength and stiffness. Calcium, for instance, is essential in bone mineralization and is also a central signaling molecule that plays a role in a variety of physiological processes. The subtle harmony between these minerals is vital; deficiency or excess can cause conditions such as osteoporosis or osteomalacia, underscoring the need for an adequate mineral supply to maintain skeletal integrity. Moreover, their interaction with organic materials like collagen not only contributes to the mechanical strength of bone but also helps in the practical storage and mobilization of nutrients necessary in the body, which is indicative of their cooperative function in bone health. In addition to their mineral content, organic bone components, particularly collagen, provide the ideal form for bone structure and strength. Collagen fibers contribute tensile strength, which is critical to the bones' ability to resist the daily forces to which they are subjected. Type I collagen, the most abundant form found in bones, is credited with the toughness and flexibility of the skeletal system. Organic components, such as proteoglycans and glycoproteins, play a critical role in regulating mineralization and cell recruitment during bone remodeling. Upkeep of a perfect balance between inorganic and organic constituents is a condition precedent to effective bone regeneration. Upsets in balance can lead to defective bone formation and weakened fracture resistance, all the more reason for employing an all-inclusive approach to bone health, embracing mineral as well as organic modalities in prevention and treatment. Subsequent studies on the relationship between immune function and bone health broadened understanding of how organic substances and minerals affect bone stability. Osteoimmunology, a new and developing area of research, explores the connection between the immune system and bone metabolism. Chronic inflammation-induced oxidative stress has an adverse effect on bone remodeling and results in bone loss, particularly in diseases such as osteoporosis (Élisa Choukroun et al., 2024). Furthermore, therapeutic applications of the natural compounds found in Traditional Chinese Medicine (TCM) have evolved into an adjunct strategy in bone management. Certain phytochemicals, such as resveratrol and ginsenoside, have been shown to promote osteoporosis by balancing osteoblast and osteoclast function and enhancing the significance of organic and mineral interactions in the skeletal structure (Zhou et al., 2023). This interdisciplinary perspective highlights the need for combined approaches to ensure bone health and prevent related disorders (Figure 1.11).

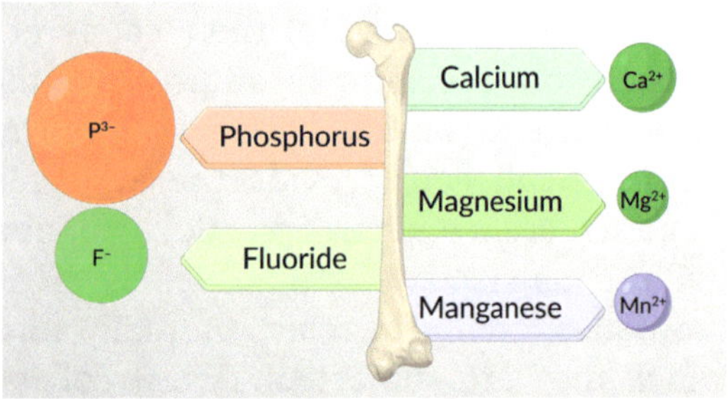

Figure 1.11. The role of minerals and organic components in bone health.

Source: https://www.jove.com/files/media/science-education/science-education-thumbs/14021.jpg.

1.3.3. Bone Remodeling and the Impact of Age and Lifestyle

Bone remodeling is a dynamic, continuous physiological process that balances bone formation and resorption, with significant effects that vary with age and lifestyle. Throughout life, bone undergoes a cycle of remodeling, with osteoclasts resorbing bone and osteoblasts forming new bone tissue. With progressive aging, particularly after menopause in females, bone resorption comes to outstrip formation, leading to decreased bone density and an increased risk of osteoporosis and fractures. Hormonal changes, physical inactivity, and alterations in nutrient absorption brought about by aging all contribute to having negative impacts on the bones. A proper understanding of such mechanisms is essential; hence, examining interventions that could reverse or halt bone loss associated with aging is a significant area of study in human osteology and bone health. Apart from this, lifestyle also plays a significant role in bone remodeling, with physical exercise, nutrition, and health significantly impacting. Regularly exercising weight-bearing strengthens the bone and stimulates osteoblast activity, resulting in bone development. On the other hand, physical inactivity can lead to muscle atrophy and a loss of bone density. Consuming nutrients, especially vitamin D and calcium, plays a vital role in maintaining bone health because these nutrients support bone mineralization and structural integrity. Inappropriate use through food may increase bone loss with aging and the risk of fractures. Some research indicates that an imbalance between the oxidants and antioxidants, or oxidative stress, may also affect bone quality and regeneration. Thus, quantification of lifestyle variables is crucial in planning interventions for effective bone management. Finally, communication between bone remodeling and the immune system cannot be overlooked, as conditions of chronic inflammation can have a dramatic effect on bone. The emerging field of osteoimmunology highlights intricate communication between the immune and skeletal systems, which illustrates that inflammatory events may lead to abnormal bone formation and increased resorption. Diseases like periodontitis and peri-implantitis, which have their basis in immune dysregulation, demonstrate the effects of inflammation on bone. Bone management, therefore, needs to include measures that will improve immune function, possibly preventing oxidative stress and ensuring efficient healing and regeneration. With a growing understanding of bone remodeling and its modulation by aging, lifestyle, and immune processes, it is essential to develop holistic, multidisciplinary approaches to maintaining skeletal health at all phases of life, drawing upon the principal themes discussed in human osteology.

Test Your Knowledge

1. What factors contribute to variation in human skeletal morphology?
2. How do mineral and organic components work together to maintain bone strength and integrity?

1.4. Methods of Osteological Analysis

Learning Outcome

1. Bone identification and classificatory methods
2. Radiographic and imaging technologies employed in osteology
3. Biomechanical analysis of bones

The methods of osteological analysis comprise a range of techniques by which scholars can gain valid interpretations from bones. The methods range from mere visual assessments and macroscopic examination, in which bone morphology can be highly informative about an individual's age, sex, and ancestry. Metric methods are used to supplement the analysis, in which skeletal components are measured precisely to obtain biological variables and population characteristics. For instance, the lengths and widths of long bones can provide information about stature and standards of living. Combining these methods offers a comprehensive approach, offering a foundation for the study of skeletal biology and life history, and contributing to broader anthropological and archaeological issues about human variation and adaptation. During recent decades, there has been an increasing role of technical progress on osteological analysis, particularly through the application of imaging techniques such as computed tomography (CT) and digital reconstruction. These allow a non-destructive approach to the examination of inner bone structure, providing insight into the evolution of the musculoskeletal system and the biomechanics of skeletal samples. For example, Abdala et al. (2016) describe how the development of three-dimensional models through these imaging technologies has revolutionized synapsid jaw adductor musculature understanding. Advanced imaging enables scientists to observe detailed anatomical interactions and trace evolutionary development in skeletal anatomy. This has significant implications for reconstructing functional adaptations and interpreting the mammalian evolutionary record, underscoring the contribution that modern technology now makes to osteological research. Furthermore, osteological analysis is also challenged by the problems posed by differential preservation conditions, especially in cremation assemblages. The analysis of cremated remains is a significantly methodologically challenging process since fragmentation and disruption of bone structure pose a problem. Kurila et al. (2015) emphasize the potential biases that can develop in macroscopic analysis, pointing to the risks of underrepresentation of population groups such as infants and preschool children. The intricacy of sexing and aging cremated human remains adds a further complexity to osteological analysis, necessitating advanced methodologies to achieve reliable demographic profiles. These issues emphasize the importance of developing standardized procedures and interdisciplinary approaches in bioarchaeology to ensure that analyses are rigorous and consistent in interpreting the skeletal remains across diverse burial practices (Figure 1.12).

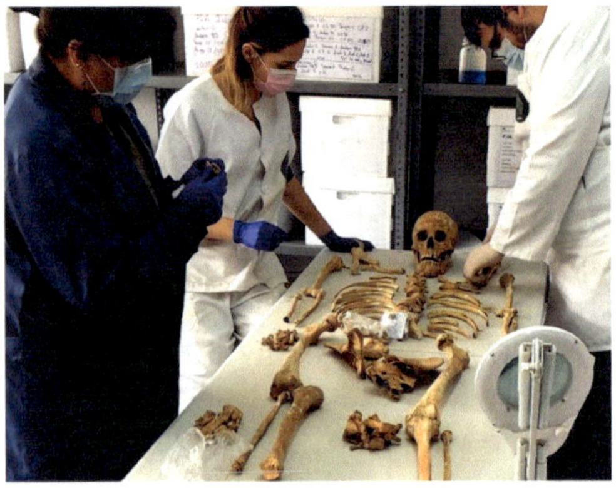

Figure 1.12. The methods of osteological analysis.

Source: https://www.archaeological.org/wp-content/uploads/2022/01/2g_Advanced-Osteological-Bioarchaeological-Techniques-Inca-Peru-1.jpg.

1.4.1. Techniques for Bone Identification and Classification

The field of human osteology involves a range of bone identification and classification methods that are of both forensic and archaeological importance. The prominent one is the study of the morphological characteristics of bones in terms of size, shape, and surface topography, which have an important role to play in differentiating human bones from the bones of other animals. For instance, the analysis of specific characteristics, such as the pelvic structure and cranial features, allows practitioners to construct a biological profile that includes sex, age, and ancestry. Biological profiling is crucial because it informs the identification step when dealing with fractured or decomposed remains, thereby maximizing the likelihood of accurate conclusions regarding the individual's identity. Furthermore, the ability to interpret a single bone can be extremely useful, making accurate classification techniques important in osteological studies (Barrett et al., 2014). Improved imaging techniques also play a crucial role in bone classification and recognition, exceptionally when traditional methods may not provide the same level of results. Imaging modalities such as computed tomography (CT) and magnetic resonance imaging (MRI) provide precise three-dimensional models of skeletal specimens, enabling non-invasive work. These imaging modalities improve the visualization of structures that are difficult to examine with standard visual inspection and help reconstruct the individual bones in a manner difficult to achieve using traditional visual inspection. In forensic contexts, they may also be employed to expose internal structures and pathologies that may provide further clues to identification, thereby improving the general understanding of the available remains. The use of these new techniques in conjunction constitutes a leap forward for human osteology, both in terms of accuracy and validity of bone classifying procedures (Abdala et al., 2016). Osteologists, anthropologists, and forensic scientists need to work together to develop improved methods of identifying and classifying bones. Interdisciplinary work enables the exchange of methodologies and results that enrich knowledge of human remains. For example, when remains are broken up and recovered from crime scenes or archaeological sites, integrating classical osteological approaches with advanced technologies can provide more comprehensive interpretations. Moreover, ongoing research and documentation of the discipline contribute to an ever-growing database of evidence that helps detect skeletal variations and anomalies that are meaningfully significant for the identification of remains. The coming together of these emerging techniques through cross-fertilization of expertise helps in building best practices that enhance accuracy in the identification of human bones and address the real need for innovation within an increasingly dynamic field that continuously resolves new problems and complexities (Barrett et al., 2014).

1.4.2. Radiographic and Imaging Technologies in Osteology

The advancement of radiographic and imaging technologies has significantly transformed the practice of osteology, facilitating research and clinical practice. Techniques such as X-ray, CT, and MRI allow detailed visualizations of the skeletal system without invasive procedures. These techniques not only permit the detection of skeletal remains in forensic examinations but also facilitate the assessment of pathological bone conditions. For instance, osteological examination based on X-ray images may identify fractures, joint disease, and disease markers and assist in giving a comprehensive evaluation of bone condition. Moreover, creating three-dimensional reconstructions of CT scans significantly contributes to the field of skeletal anatomy, and researchers can study subtle anatomical variations that may be pivotal for identifying human remains or analyzing evolutionary patterns. The integration of sophisticated imaging technologies has also pushed the study of single skeletal elements and, hence, greater knowledge of their functional morphology. For example, CT imaging-based research has illuminated the patella, the largest sesamoid bone in the human skeleton, revealing its biomechanical roles as a joint leverage amplifier and tendon stabilizer. Research indicates that, while a typical mature morphology is common to most species, tremendous diversity characterizes the development and morphology of the patella among reptiles, suggesting a complex evolutionary history. Such findings suggest how technology for imaging and osteological research engages, such that results through the radiographic process may indeed influence studies in the evolutionary adaptation of the bony component.

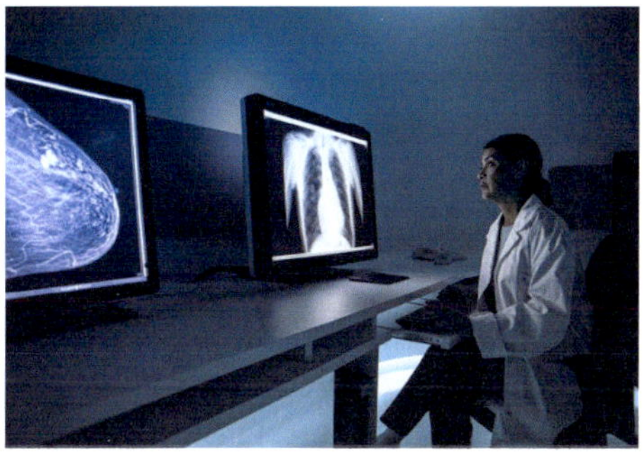

Figure 1.13. Radiographic and imaging technologies in osteology.

Source: https://www.biharparamedical.org/wp-content/uploads/2024/05/Bachelor-in-Radiology-and-Imaging-Technology-BRIT.jpg.

Therefore, imaging technologies are not only used for diagnostics but also as critical tools in the discovery of the evolutionary history of bony structures. In forensic anthropology, the use of radiographic technologies plays a central role in the process of human remains identification. The challenge posed by identifying broken or decomposed skeletal components can be greatly alleviated by using imaging methods that reveal extensive anatomical detail. As noted in recent forensic literature, effective identification often hinges on widespread knowledge of anatomical variance among individuals, which can be investigated entirely by imaging. This is such a requirement in cases where dismemberment or extreme decomposition has caused trouble in earlier evaluation. By providing insights into the biological profile of skeletal remains, imaging modalities such as CT and MRI enhance forensic examination accuracy and aid legal investigation. As forensic practitioners continue to advance these techniques, radiographic tools become increasingly prominent to facilitate practical application and to authenticate investigations in human osteology (Barrett et al., 2014; Benjamin et al., 2016) (Figure 1.13).

1.4.3. Biomechanical Analysis of Skeletal Remains

The biomechanical analysis of skeletal remains is a significant methodological approach in human osteology that enables researchers to infer the lifestyles and activities of ancient individuals. By analyzing the various aspects of bone morphology, it is possible to deduce the functional adaptations of bones in response to specific biomechanical demands. This is particularly helpful in determining patterns of physical activity, pathology, and general health. For instance, comparative studies of joint surfaces can identify the presence of osteoarthritis, which certain forms of movement or work can cause (Bass et al., 2019). The application of biomechanics principles facilitates an improved understanding of how environmental pressures and social practices influenced human bone development during evolution, furthering the comprehension of evolutionary biology and anthropological science. In addition, biomechanical assessment enables the determination of hand dominance and dexterity patterns in remains, with crucial implications for understanding the cognitive and cultural facets of ancient human populations. For example, studies of the postcranial skeleton and dentition can provide evidence of handedness, as seen in Neandertal Regourdou 1. A thorough evaluation of upper-limb asymmetries can reveal patterns of manual lateralization, demonstrating not only practiced skills but also cognitive features related to tool use and language (Bondioli et al., 2012). These revelations extend beyond basic physical examination, presenting a challenge for scientists to establish links among skeletal morphology and complex cultural rituals that governed human communities. Hand mechanics in prehistoric settings highlight the intricate relationships among biomechanics, technology, and social conduct. Beyond assisting to provide insight into individual lives, biomechanical interpretation of skeletal remains also continues to narrate larger stories of anthropology about population health and coping mechanisms. By applying advanced statistical techniques, e.g., Generalized Estimating Equations (GEE), researchers can address scalar issues in bioarchaeological analysis, thereby making data analysis more efficient (Bass et al., 2019). These techniques enable the analysis of multiple articular surfaces and their associated pathologies, thereby facilitating the interpretation of skeletal remains across different demographic groups. This holistic approach promotes a better appreciation of how populations developed in relation to their surroundings, emphasizing the interdependent nature of biomechanics, health, and way of life in shaping the human experience over time. Finally, the field of biomechanics not only enriches our understanding of physical anthropology but also provides insights into the social and cultural processes of ancient cultures.

Test Your Knowledge

1. How are radiographic and imaging technologies used in osteological analysis?
2. What is the role of biomechanical analysis in understanding bone structure and function?

1.5. Osteological Indicators of Health and Disease

Learning Outcome

1. Shared skeletal markers of nutritional insufficiencies
2. Evidence of trauma and its relevance to lifestyle
3. Signs of infectious diseases in ancient populations through osteology

Osteology provides essential information on ancient patterns of health and disease, assisting researchers in gaining insights into the lives of ancient peoples. By analyzing skeletal remains, it is possible to identify signs of various pathologies that indicate a person's overall health status at different stages of life. For instance, lesions in the bones can indicate infectious diseases, malnutrition, or chronic diseases that have left traces on the osseous skeleton. Additionally, observation of growth patterns such as Harris lines can inform scientists about stress or malnutrition during years of growth. This insight extends our understanding of how environmental and social circumstances affected the health of individuals and, by extension, contributes to a broader narrative on population wellbeing and vulnerability in historical populations. The concentration on particular demographic groups adds more to understanding disparities in health from an osteological perspective. Research, including the study of medieval girls' and young women's skeletal remains, offers fascinating insights into the existence of this group, routinely unrepresented in the historical record. Analysis of over 300 skeletal remains yielded valuable data on these groups' health, growth, and mortality, revealing that gender, socio-economic status, and childcare practices have implications in medieval society. These findings highlight osteology's ability to bypass historical biases in written records, enabling, somehow or another, a more comprehensive study of health across gender and age groups. By uncovering the lives and health status of subjects who have traditionally been bypassed, osteology fosters greater insight into the formation of society and its impact on health. Moreover, osteological analysis across different archaeological contexts also advances knowledge of disease and health. For example, the excavation of human remains at a burial site on Saaremaa Island, Estonia, offered an opportunity to investigate unconventional burial behavior during the late 7th to early 8th centuries. The skeletons, consisting of the skeletal remains of seven men, had distinctive features that differed from local burial patterns, such as a total absence of commonly found animal remains. This deviation in burial patterns reflects cultural attitudes towards death and health rituals. Additionally, when combined with archaeological data, these skeletons can determine patterns of health associated with cultural practices, climate, and environmental interactions. This again highlights osteology's vital contribution to untangling the multifaceted weave of human health and social organization across the past, offering a holistic framework for understanding illness and health in earlier populations (Figure 1.14).

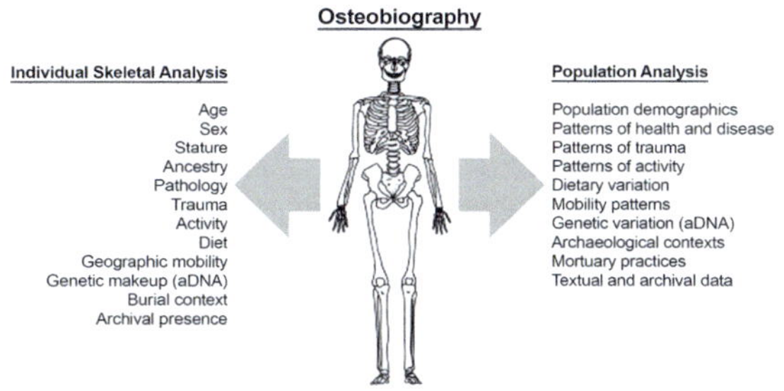

Figure 1.14. Osteological indicators of health and disease.

Source: https://ars.els-cdn.com/content/image/3-s2.0-B9780323907996000331-f00033-01-9780323907996.jpg.

1.5.1. Common Skeletal Markers of Nutritional Deficiencies

may provide important information about previous nutritional deficiencies that affected individuals. Such studies, although not specific indicators of stress, are commonly used in osteological research to assess non-specific markers of stress, including enamel hypoplasia and dental caries. Enamel hypoplasia, characterized by atypical enamel development, usually occurs due to prolonged periods of nutritional inadequacy during critical developmental stages. Similarly, the prevalence of some skeletal lesions, such as porotic hyperostosis and cribra orbitalia, can be attributed to iron-deficiency anemia or other nutritional deficiencies. By analyzing these markers, scientists can reconstruct the dietary patterns and health status of individuals and groups over time and reveal the broader social significance of malnutrition across contexts. In studies examining skeletal remains from ancient cemeteries, such as the Acacia Park Cemetery, these dietary deficiencies are evident in aggregate data on skeletal indicators. For example, commingled human bone can be used to discern demographic profiles and prevailing general health patterns among populations living in specific environments.

Using biological profiling techniques, such as age-at-death estimation and analysis of skeletal markers, the degree of nutritional stressors over time can be quantified. The relationship between the skeletal markers and the way of life of communities to a great extent facilitates the interpretations of how food cultures and environmental factors affected individuals' general health, especially in pre-industrial societies. Besides, the skeletal frailty index (SFI) is a crucial tool used to assess the impact of nutrition deficiency on individuals from archaeological samples, like medieval Poland. SFI integrates various skeletal and dental indicators of stressors and therefore quantifies the frailty individuals experienced throughout their lives.

The study of the Kałdus site shows significant differences in age- and sex-adjusted skeletal frailty scores, suggesting that environmental health, social status, and ethical concerns may have exacerbated these deficits (Tuggle et al., 2021). The frequency of skeletal signs of stress is so great that it indicates that the individuals in these groups suffered from severe nutritional hardship, telling a compelling history of nutrition dynamics, health, and the state of society in the past, and being a significant area of research towards an overall understanding of human osteology (Figure 1.15).

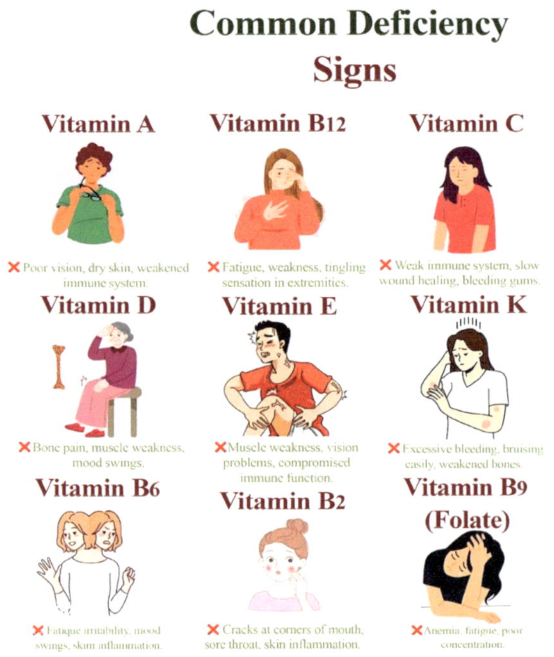

Figure 1.15. Common skeletal markers of nutritional deficiencies.

Source: https://p16-sign-sg.lemon8cdn.com/tos-maliva-v-ac5634-us/ocsH8BfXETIAXt2C65opEJiiFNAsAzbnBlgdB4~tplv-sdweummd6v-text-logo-v1:QGNvdXJ0bmV5Y2h1cmNod2VsbA==:q75.jpeg?lk3s=c7f08e79&source=lemon8_seo&x-expires=1753012800&x-signature=oqdoEkhrnmB%2B37kc79wV2%2BEIT4Q%3D.

1.5.2. Evidence of Trauma and Its Implications for Lifestyle

Knowledge of trauma as expressed in human skeletal remains is instrumental in determining the lifestyle of ancient people. Through osteological analysis, several traumas are revealed that are indicative of daily activities, social roles, and environmental stress. The presence of osteoarthritis (OA) in skeletal samples, for instance, can indicate habitual movements or hard labor performed by individuals. Better techniques, such as Generalized Estimating Equations (GEE), enable researchers to assess the prevalence and distribution of OA better, thus correlating articular surfaces and presenting a total view of joint health. This degree of analysis is crucial for understanding how lifestyle-associated physical stresses can contribute to degenerative diseases in the long term and thereby connect biomechanical stressors with the health of people living in specific cultures and conditions (Bass et al., 2019). Trauma can also vary significantly with the nature of activities people have undertaken during their lifetime, as evidenced by some pathologies found in the skeletal remains. For example, a male case from the Late Iron Age displays a series of lifestyle markers, such as cranial fractures and skeletal deformities that may be representative of a horse-riding lifestyle. The presence of enthesopathies at the proximal femur, one of those associated with horse riders, illustrates how certain occupations may lead to consistent injuries and long-term degenerative alterations. The case demonstrates the intersection of physical health and workplace hazards, providing core data for recasting issues faced by people based on their lifestyles and the health of their environments (Khudaverdyan et al., 2017). Additionally, exploring the impact of trauma transcends the person and extends to public understandings of lifestyle and health. Knowledge of the prevalence of specific injuries, such as fractures and degenerative illnesses, enables researchers to make inferences about activity, conflict, play, and community norms, including work. Evidence of pervasive fractures can suggest a society with a lot of physical violence or hazardous environments, as occurred in the case of the subject whose clavicle fracture most likely stemmed from falls or blunt trauma. They are utilized to inform not just the bodily hardship of these lifestyles but the cultural and social structures that impacted people's experiences and survival. More broadly, the study of trauma and its impact is important for reconstructing the complex narratives of human experience in ancient societies, thereby enriching our understanding of human osteology (Khudaverdyan et al., 2017).

1.5.3. Osteological Signs of Infectious Diseases in Historical Populations

The analysis of osteological signs of infectious disease in ancient populations provides vital insights into the dynamics of ancient societies' health. Pathologies apparent on skeletal remains, e.g., deformity or lesions, typically signal infectious diseases like leprosy, syphilis, and tuberculosis that significantly influenced the demographics of the populations. By studying skeletal markers, researchers can determine the prevalence and impact of such diseases, thereby reconstructing the lives and health conditions of ancient people. Such analyses contribute to a broader image of how infectious diseases influenced the demographic structure, morbidity patterns, and even socio-economic conditions over time, thereby situating current concerns about health as an extension of past tendencies. Their integration is critical, since it facilitates the monitoring of evolution and environmental pressures acting upon human health throughout the past. In the world of ongoing research, novel techniques in forensic anthropology and human osteology have enhanced our capacity to unravel the complex tales inscribed in human bones. Science that focuses on osteological trauma allows scientists to make inferences about the prevalence of infectious illness and associated wounds, to gain insight into the daily lives of populations from the past. By looking at environmental and occupational exposures, researchers can ascertain how various socio-economic groups managed the burden of disease, thereby exposing inequalities in access to health care and living standards. These findings show that class and wealth significantly influenced susceptibility to infections and overall health outcomes. Through the synthesis of a detailed study of remains, the lives of individuals and populations are made real, narrating the entwining of health, illness, and socio-economic organization in the past (Lloyd et al., 2018). Furthermore, applying health indices from osteological records brings into perspective disease patterns and their relevance to human adaptation to changing environments over centuries. Comparing skeletal data from a range of localities allows an evaluation of how infectious diseases thrived across diverse ecological contexts, revealing complex interactions between people and the environment. Notably, population migration into less favorable ecological settings is correlated with emerging health emergencies, suggesting an adaptive but ultimately detrimental response. The interpretation of these skeletal signs is far from speculative; it enhances current understanding of health disparities and the chronic influence of disease on human populations. This broader perspective ultimately strengthens the case for recognizing historical epidemiological trends as organic components of current public health discourse, especially in light of long-standing global disease challenges (Steckel, 2025) (Figure 1.16).

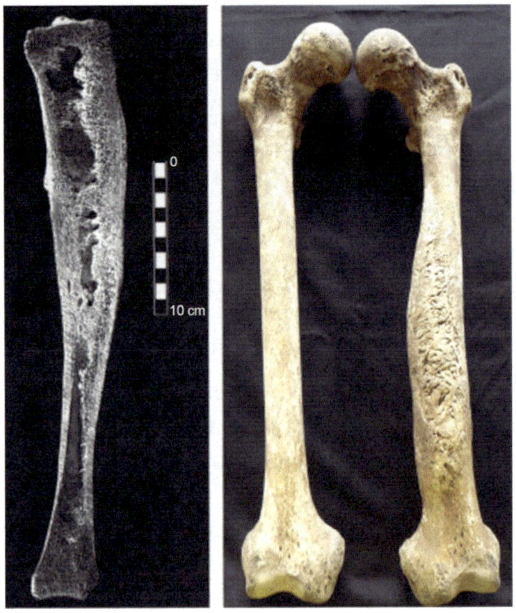

Figure 1.16. Osteological signs of infectious diseases in historical populations.

Source: https://ars.els-cdn.com/content/image/3-s2.0-B9780128097380000107-f10-30-9780128097380.jpg.

Test Your Knowledge

1. What skeletal markers indicate nutritional deficiencies in osteological remains?
2. How can signs of infectious diseases be identified in ancient populations through osteological analysis?

1.6. Ethical Considerations in Osteological Research

Learning Outcome

1. The worth of consent and respect for human remains
2. Cultural sensitivities to the examination of bones
3. Legal precedents governing the excavation and analysis of skeletal remains

Ethics in osteological research play a highly critical function in maintaining the integrity of the field on the one hand and the protection of human remains' dignity on the other. Researchers conducting research in the field of human skeletal materials must operate in sensitive moral contexts that include consent, reburial, and the representation of marginalized groups. The treatment of human remains also reflects broader social attitudes, particularly towards indigenous and ancestral communities. Such communities may view the excavation and analysis of bones as a desecration of their culture rather than science. This requires an ethical approach in which scientists collaborate with such communities so that their intentions regarding how to treat and repatriate remains are respected. Ultimately, the ethical basis that guides osteological research must tip in favor of the pursuit of knowledge, while balancing it with respect and tact shown to the dead and their descendants. Moreover, procedures employed in osteological research must conform to ethical principles that take into account the well-being of participants in educational settings. With recent developments in distance learning, particularly during the COVID-19 pandemic, the importance of haptic learning, in which touch is central, has emerged. The study demonstrated that students who participated in remote osteology lectures using take-home plastic model skeletons performed as well as their peers in traditional labs in bone identification proficiency (Gamble et al., 2024). But ethical aspects extend beyond pedagogical outcomes; they encompass educators' responsibility to ensure equal access to educational materials. Providing all students, regardless of their condition, with quality osteological learning reinforces the ethical commitment to inclusivity and respect within the academic community. Osteological research is also defined by a delicate balance between innovation and ethical practice, particularly in developing methods and materials for research.

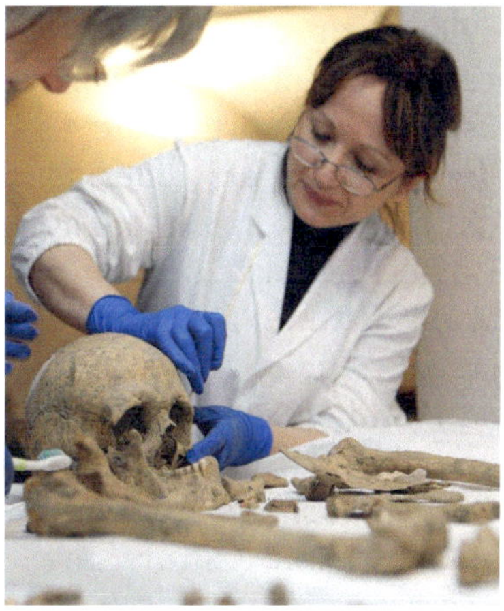

Figure 1.17. Ethical considerations in osteological research.

Source: https://archaeobiomics.com/wp-content/uploads/2023/05/RB2-1-932x1030.jpg.

As recent studies show, the use of biological materials—such as collagen membranes in bone-healing research—requires careful ethical scrutiny to avoid animal rights violations and ensure that the practice meets industry standards (Angelis et al., 2017). This necessitates transparency and ethical surveillance in the research process. Professionals must conduct critical ethical assessments to protect the integrity of their methods and anticipate the ethical issues arising from their work. By identifying and applying these ethical issues, osteological scientists can facilitate a culture of integrity, responsibility, and respect for human remains and research methodology (Figure 1.17).

1.6.1. The Importance of Consent and Respect for Human Remains

In human osteology, respect for and consent regarding human remains are ethical cornerstones that govern not only research practices but also teaching procedures. Working with human remains has extremely high moral implications through respect for the dead and their individual or cultural narratives. The importance of obtaining transparent consent from donors or their representatives cannot be overstated; it ensures an honoring of human beings both in life and in death. The upholding of ethical principles around consent ensures that we avoid continuing injustices from the past and respect people's cultural traditions about death and burial. Lastly, recognition of the humanity of whose remains are being analyzed is imperative to establishing a responsible academic culture that respects ethical integrity as much as scientific inquiry. Respecting human remains is also extended to the treatment of materials in academic environments. As curricula increasingly adopt diverse learning modalities, it is increasingly necessary to emphasize the ethical component of these practices. For instance, employing state-of-the-art technologies such as 3D imaging, as tested in research examining their efficacy relative to more traditional methods, raises issues regarding the respectful presentation of bony structures. Such technologies can radically enhance learning opportunities and make osteology more accessible and engaging for learners. However, in the absence of due consideration for the ethical connotations present, it is quite easy to commodify human remains. As professionals, it is our duty to ensure that students are educated to handle human osteology with due deference, so that every skeletal item represents a singular tale worthy of dignity and respect (Schulz et al., 2022). More importantly, the consequences of respect and consent for human remains extend beyond the lab and classroom. The interdisciplinarity of osteological studies ensures that findings have a significant impact on other fields, such as anthropology, forensic science, and medicine. The researchers thus have to take extra care to ensure they handle human remains ethically, so that their findings enhance knowledge without interfering with cultural sensitivities. This is particularly true when the use is forensic, in which case the human remains may be used in criminal investigations. Consent is particularly relevant here, as the affected families may find public representation of the remains upsetting. Thus, developing a culture that encourages ethical values in the practice of human osteology investigation is needed to guarantee not only scientific progress but also social dignity about the identity and history of the individuals represented (Tynes et al., 2014).

1.6.2. Cultural Sensitivities Surrounding the Study of Bones

The study of human bones, though grounded in science, always appears to converge strongly with matters of culture. Particularly so when considering the impact of analyzing human remains of indigenous peoples. Such remains are often highly culturally and spiritually meaningful, being representative of ancestors and holding narratives. Dealing with such remains has the potential to create an impression of disrespect and desecration among descendant communities, especially if they imagine that their ancestors are being treated as specimens for scientific interest. Osteologists, therefore, need to navigate these subtleties with a clear ethical sensitivity so that they echo cultural perceptions and honor them. In doing this, they are part of a larger vision of human osteology that goes beyond merely strict anatomical investigation, incorporating socio-cultural paradigms into the narrative of human bones. They are second;

the shifting status of museums and institutions receiving human remains is yet another topic of cultural sensitivity regarding osteological investigation. Furthermore, museums have been collecting and exhibiting human bones for a very long time, often without regard for descendant communities. However, as evidenced by current practice, there is a paradigm shift aimed at the ethical imperatives that inform the management and display of such remains. Best practice now favors an inclusive policy that accommodates the wishes and beliefs of individuals in relation to the remains. Continuing controversy over the care and handling of human remains in museums underscores the need for greater accountability and cultural sensitivity. By fostering collaborative relationships with indigenous people and adhering to standardized procedures, osteologists can minimize the potential for cultural insensitivity and create a less disrespectful scholarly environment (Page et al., 2011).

Furthermore, the implications of research findings extend beyond the academic community and affect public attitudes toward cultural heritage and the dead. The portrayal of bones in scientific publications and museum displays can also directly impact society's beliefs about cultural heritage, with the likely tendency to reinforce stereotypes and myths. Researchers thus must be careful about the stories that they convey through their studies. Presentation of results must not just be anatomical or evolutionary significance, but also consider cultural contexts and ancestral connections. By emphasizing an inclusive approach that respects the cultures of human bones, osteologists can be helpful in the discourse on human diversity and history. In this way, the study of bones extends beyond the boundaries of science, instead being an interface of scholarship and cultural sensibilities, enhancing the subject of human osteology (Hogan et al., 2014) (Figure 1.18).

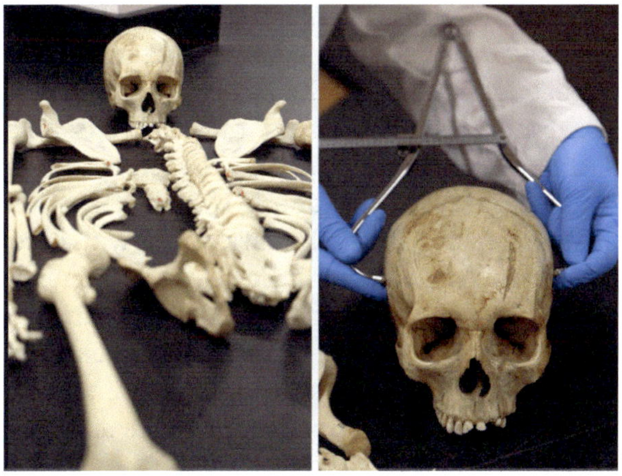

Figure 1.18. Cultural sensitivities surrounding the study of bones.

Source: https://textbooks.whatcom.edu/tracesarchaeology/wp-content/uploads/sites/60/2021/12/Bioarchaeology-Fig3.png.

1.6.3. Legal Frameworks Governing the Excavation and Analysis of Skeletal Remains

Legal frameworks governing the excavation and analysis of skeletal remains are a central aspect of the science of human osteology, as they define the ethical and procedural guidelines in which scientists must operate. These regulations are often determined by factors such as cultural heritage law, indigenous peoples' rights, and legislation on human remains. In the US, federal law, like the Native American Graves Protection and Repatriation Act (NAGPRA), requires consultation with the Native American population and includes provisions on repatriating ancient remains. State law may also offer varying degrees of protection, such as prohibitions on illegal digs and the creation of legal processes for excavation. By respecting these paradigms, osteologists can responsibly address bone remains without transgressing against the dead and also the cultural context to which they originally belonged. Ethical concerns in human osteology cannot be overstated, given that scientists at times must address issues that compromise the harmony between scientific inquiry and respect for the dead. Ethical principles guide researchers in considering the repercussions of their studies on humans, especially when exhuming graves. An example is that excavation of ancient bones should be carried out with care, taking into consideration the scientific benefits and avoiding any offense to descendants or related cultural groups. As may be understood in the field of paleopathology, awareness of disease among past populations relies as much on biological data as on recognition of the sociocultural problems involved in working with human remains (Grauer et al., 2022). This ethical approach incorporates the life histories of individuals whose remains are analyzed, with the ethical duty of honoring their stories in pursuing a greater understanding of health and disease in ancient populations (Zahn-Hiepler et al., 2019). Legal and ethical approaches also intersect in the proper documentation and analysis of skeletal remains. Researchers are obliged to maintain proper records that report pertinent information on contextual and biographical aspects of the remains. These involve precise documentation of burial practices, age, gender, and buried artifacts, which are significant for interpreting the social and cultural values of earlier societies. Alternatively, compliance with legal and ethical requirements promotes transparency and accountability in human osteology. With advancing technology, scientists need to stay alert to refine legislation that considers emerging techniques without undermining human dignity. Through proper application of these paradigms, scholars can contribute to the human skeletal biology knowledge pool and honor the complex history embedded in each excavation and analysis.

Test Your Knowledge

1. Why are consent and respect essential when handling and studying human skeletal remains in osteological research?
2. What legal precedents regulate the excavation and analysis of skeletal remains?

SUMMARY

Human osteology provides essential data on the anatomical and evolutionary foundation of human skeletal development. Understanding the complexities of bone morphology and its population variations reveals not only physical adaptations that facilitate survival but also the evolutionary paths taken by our ancestors. The intricate interaction between form and function of the skeleton highlights how adaptations have impacted locomotor patterns and other bodily behaviors. Thus, human osteology provides a window into the broader history of human evolution for both biological and anthropological inquiry. By continually expanding on the anatomical data represented in the human skeleton, particularly with comparative studies with hominoid taxa, the role of evolutionary forces in shaping our skeletal morphology is underscored once again. The results on wrist morphology, for example, help clarify the intricacies of functional adaptations that have arisen in response to environmental pressures. This evolutionary mosaicism, as indicated in several anatomical units, implies that skeletal elements are under several selective pressures and that such pressures can bring about varied morphological results. Research on the evolution of the wrist bone in hominoids reiterates the notion that more than one evolutionary pathway can persist and that each can make an independent contribution to forelimb functional adaptation across diverse species, including humans (Barros et al., 2013). The investigation of locomotor adaptations among archosaurs, specifically the shift between quadrupedal and bipedal modes of locomotion, underscores the role of biomechanical assessment in osteological research. Through combined ranges of motion and muscle activity, researchers have a deeper understanding of the nature of the association between some anatomical variations and locomotor economy and ecological niches. The opposing locomotor extremes within Archosauria disclose the dynamic relationship between anatomical morphology and functional capacity, and how lifestyle and behavior have been drastically altered through evolutionary adaptation. Lastly, these advanced interactions between form and function in the human skeleton emphasize the significance of human osteology not just for understanding our own kind, but also for piecing together the broader evolutionary history of vertebrate life (Allen et al., 2017).

Human osteology is at the center of numerous fields, including anthropology, medicine, and forensic science. Bone analysis enables researchers to reconstruct historical ways of life, assess health conditions, and even infer the mode of death. Not only are human bones required to provide structural support, but they can also serve as a repository of historical and biological information. Using osteological analysis, experts can establish age, sex, and ancestry, providing immense information about population dynamics and trends in health over the years. In addition, intricate bone development and evolution in humans are of utmost significance for understanding the evolutionary mechanisms and biomechanical processes that have shaped present-day human physiology. Osteology of human beings is of central significance to clinical medicine, aside from its relevance to anthropology. Understanding the human skeleton is essential for diagnosing and managing a range of medical conditions, such as osteoporosis and fractures. Understanding bone architecture and composition assists health professionals in setting appropriate treatment plans and surgical techniques. Advancements in imaging and diagnostic technologies, such as computed tomography, have also enabled non-surgical methods for visualizing and assessing bone structures. This technology also enables further assessment of bone quality and health, closing the gap between knowledge of skeletal biology and clinical practice. Also, human osteology extends its application into forensic science. Skeletal analysis can provide helpful information in criminal investigations, including victim identification or reconstructing the events surrounding their death. Osteological knowledge is used by forensic anthropologists to estimate time since death, trauma, and ancestry, thereby helping in legal cases. With the emergence of sophisticated methods in osteological analysis, including isotopic studies and advanced imaging techniques, the field continues to evolve, providing deeper insights into both ancient populations and contemporary issues. The intersection of human osteology with forensic applications exemplifies its multifaceted importance in understanding human history and addressing modern societal challenges.

KEY TERMS FROM THIS CHAPTER

- Appendicular Skeleton
- Articular Surface
- Axial Skeleton
- Bone Marrow
- Bone Morphology
- Cartilage
- Compact Bone
- Diaphysis
- Endosteum
- Epiphysis
- Foramen
- Haversian System (Osteon)
- Joint
- Ligament

CRITICAL THINKING QUESTIONS

1. Which of the following is not a function of bones?
   a. Support
   b. Hematopoiesis
   c. Hormone production
   d. Respiration

2. Which of the following bones is part of the axial skeleton?
   a. Humerus
   b. Femur
   c. Sternum
   d. Tibia

3. Into which category does the femur belong?
   a. Flat bone
   b. Short bone
   c. Irregular bone
   d. Long bone

4. Which of the minerals listed is found most frequently in bones?
   a. Magnesium
   b. Potassium
   c. Calcium
   d. Sodium

5. What is the compact bone structural unit called?
   a. Osteocyte
   b. Osteon
   c. Trabecula
   d. Lacuna

Short Answer Questions

1. Define osteology and its importance in the study of human anatomy.
2. What are the major divisions of the human skeleton?
3. Distinguish between compact and spongy bone.
4. Define "ossification" and describe the difference between intramembranous and endochondral ossification.
5. Describe the similarities and differences among true ribs, false ribs, and floating ribs.

Answers to Critical Thinking Questions

1. (d); 2. (c); 3. (d); 4. (c); 5. (b)

REFERENCES

1. Bishop, P. J., Hocknull, S. A., Clemente, C. J., Hutchinson, J. R., Farke, A. A., Beck, B. R., Barrett, R. S., & Lloyd, D. G. (2018). Cancellous bone and theropod dinosaur locomotion. Part I—an examination of cancellous bone architecture in the hindlimb bones of theropods. *PeerJ*, *6*, e5778. https://doi.org/10.7717/peerj.5778Abdala, A., Abdala, A., Adams, A., Allin, E. F., Allin, C., Anthwal, N., Barghusen, H., et al. (2016). Morphological evolution of the mammalian jaw adductor complex. https://core.ac.uk/download/151161615.pdf (accessed on 18th July 2025).
2. Abdalla, O., Abdel Meguid, E. M., Barreto, C., Bonaparte, J. F., Bonaparte, J. F., Campos, D., Casal, G. A., et al. (2015). Histological evidence for a supraspinous ligament in sauropod dinosaurs. https://core.ac.uk/download/159287253.pdf (accessed on 18th July 2025).
3. Abourachid, A., Alexander, R. M., Allen, P. W., Allmendinger, C., Attene, F., Bakker, R. T., et al. (2018). Cancellous bone and theropod dinosaur locomotion. Part III—Inferring posture and locomotor biomechanics in extinct theropods, and its evolution on the line to birds. https://core.ac.uk/download/161818791.pdf (accessed on 18th July 2025).
4. Adlam, R., Arnold, R. M., Arnold, R., Bachmann, S., Baraybar, J., Burns, K., Carter, A., et al. (2014). A preliminary examination of differential decomposition patterns in mass graves. https://core.ac.uk/download/1441337.pdf (accessed on 18th July 2025).
5. Ahmed, F., & Maisano, J. (2017). ToScA North America (6–8 June 2017, The University of Texas, Austin, TX) Program. https://core.ac.uk/download/211334283.pdf (accessed on 18th July 2025).
6. Albert, C., Busse, B., Harris, G. F., Jameson, C., et al. (2013). 3D micron-scale imaging of the cortical bone canal network in human osteogenesis imperfecta (OI). https://core.ac.uk/download/213084385.pdf (accessed on 18th July 2025).
7. Allen, V., Hutchinson, J. R., Otero, A., Pol, D., et al. (2017). Forelimb muscle and joint actions in Archosauria: Insights from *Crocodylus johnstoni* (Pseudosuchia) and *Mussaurus patagonicus* (Sauropodomorpha). https://core.ac.uk/download/141887609.pdf (accessed on 18th July 2025).
8. Allmäe, R. (2011). Human bones in Salme I boat-grave, the island of Saaremaa; Estonia. https://core.ac.uk/download/25069068.pdf (accessed on 18th July 2025).
9. Anderson, M., Davy-Jow, S., Lorenz, K., Schofield, D., et al. (2012). Roman portraiture and biometric identification. https://core.ac.uk/download/33573163.pdf (accessed on 18th July 2025).
10. Barnes, I., Booth, T., Boyle, A., Brace, S., et al. (2018). 'Ava': A Beaker-associated woman from a cist at Achavanich, Highland, and the story of her (re-) discovery and subsequent study. https://core.ac.uk/download/227987273.pdf (accessed on 18th July 2025).
11. Barrett, B., Bidmos, M. A., Bidmos, F. A., Bidmos, R. A., Bilge, M., British Broadcasting Corporation, British Broadcasting Corporation, et al. (2014). The foot in forensic human identification–A review. https://core.ac.uk/download/30660095.pdf (accessed on 18th July 2025).
12. Barros, A. P., Kivell, T. L., & Smaers, J. B. (2013). Different evolutionary pathways underlie the morphology of wrist bones in hominoids. https://core.ac.uk/download/30704900.pdf (accessed on 18th July 2025).

13. Basibuyuk, G. O., Basoglu, O., Erkman, A. C., Kaya, T., et al. (2016). Cranial and post-cranial traumatic injury patterns in Van Castle Mound medieval population. https://core.ac.uk/download/84612475.pdf (accessed on 18th July 2025).

14. Bass, W. M., Brothwell, D. R., Buikstra, J. E., Dieppe, P., Felson, D., Gagnon, C. M., Gagnon, C. M., et al. (2019). Evaluating elbow osteoarthritis within the prehistoric Tiwanaku state using generalized estimating equations (GEE). https://core.ac.uk/download/323311271.pdf (accessed on 18th July 2025).

15. Becker, S. K. (2019). Osteoarthritis, entheses, and long bone cross-sectional geometry in the Andes: Usage, history, and future directions. https://core.ac.uk/download/323311202.pdf (accessed on 18th July 2025).

16. Benjamin, M., Camp, C. L., Castanet, J., Cope, E. D., Gauthier, J. A., Haines, R. W., Haines, R. W., et al. (2016). Anatomy, morphology, and evolution of the patella in squamate lizards and tuatara (*Sphenodon punctatus*). https://core.ac.uk/download/36779107.pdf (accessed on 18th July 2025).

17. Bondioli, L., Coppa, A., Dean, C., et al. (2017). New regression formula to estimate the prenatal crown formation time of human deciduous central incisors derived from a Roman imperial sample (Velia, Salerno, Italy, I-II cent. CE). https://core.ac.uk/download/98348292.pdf (accessed on 18th July 2025).

18. Bondioli, L., Fiore, I., Frayer, D. W., Guatelli-Steinberg, D., et al. (2012). Hand to mouth in a Neandertal: Right-handedness in Regourdou 1. https://core.ac.uk/download/14525571.pdf (accessed on 18th July 2025).

19. Choukroun, É., Parnot, M., Surmenian, J., Gruber, R., Cohen, N., Davido, N., Simonpieri, A., et al. (2024). Bone formation and maintenance in oral surgery: The decisive role of the immune system—A narrative review of mechanisms and solutions. *Bioengineering, 11*(191), 191. https://doi.org/10.3390/bioengineering11020191 (accessed on 18th July 2025).

20. Cooper, A., Evin, A., Scheu, A., Ursing, B. M., Edwards, C. J., Koutsogiannouli, E. A., Lee, E. J., et al. (2013). Use of domesticated pigs by Mesolithic hunter-gatherers in northwestern Europe. https://core.ac.uk/download/19506510.pdf (accessed on 18th July 2025).

21. Czarnetzki, A., von Rautenfeld, D., & Samii, M. (2012). The phylogenetic principles of MMA: A hypothetical biostratigraphy model. https://core.ac.uk/download/pdf/1569968.pdf (accessed on 18th July 2025).

22. De Angelis, F., Di Carlo, S., Guarnieri, R., Mencio, F., et al. (2017). Bone healing in extraction sockets covered with collagen membrane alone or associated with porcine-derived bone graft: A comparative histological and histomorphometry analysis. https://core.ac.uk/download/153371256.pdf (accessed on 18th July 2025).

23. Dockall, H. D. (1994). Human skeletal remains from the Tyson site (41SY92). https://core.ac.uk/download/215496487.pdf (accessed on 18th July 2025).

24. Gamble, J. A., & Gilmour, R. J. (2024). Bones at home supporting haptic learning and universal design beyond the biological anthropology laboratory. https://core.ac.uk/download/644028705.pdf (accessed on 18th July 2025).

25. Grauer, A. (2022). Introduction. https://core.ac.uk/download/614446076.pdf (accessed on 18th July 2025).

26. Hogan, L. (2014). Maturing temporal bones as non-neural sites for transforming the speech signal during language development. https://core.ac.uk/download/151574121.pdf (accessed on 18th July 2025).

27. Khudaverdyan, A. Y., Khachatryan, H. H., & Eganyan, L. G. (2017). The human skeleton from the late Iron Age burial of Shirakavan (Armenia): A case study. https://core.ac.uk/download/212454402.pdf (accessed on 18th July 2025).

28. Kurila, L. (2015). Cremation as limitation? A paleo demographic inquiry into the accuracy of macroscopic analysis of cremated human remains based on an East Lithuanian sample. https://core.ac.uk/download/43658404.pdf (accessed on 18th July 2025).

29. Lewis, M., Shapland, F., & Watts, R. (2015). The lives and deaths of young medieval women: The osteological evidence. https://core.ac.uk/download/42153597.pdf (accessed on 18th July 2025).

30. Lloyd, B. M. (2018). Forensic anthropology, paleopathology, and the creation of osteobiographies. https://core.ac.uk/download/229540736.pdf (accessed on 18th July 2025).

31. Narayan, E. (2023). Animal Science Annual Volume 2023. *Veterinary Medicine and Science*. https://doi.org/10.5772/intechopen.113979 (accessed on 18th July 2025).

32. Page, K. M. (2011). The significance of human remains in museum collections: Implications for collections management. https://core.ac.uk/download/230662014.pdf (accessed on 18th July 2025).

33. Paretsis, N. F., Pizzutto, C. S., Rosenfield, D. A., Yanai, L., et al. (2020). Osteologia bruta e radiografia digital da capivara comum (*Hydrochoerus hydrochaeris*), Carl Linnaeus, 1766 para aplicação científica e clínica. https://core.ac.uk/download/386148848.pdf (accessed on 18th July 2025).

34. Schulz, E. (2022). Teaching pedagogy of online vs in-person learning: Relative to osteology. https://core.ac.uk/download/533927336.pdf (accessed on 18th July 2025).

35. Spigelski, S. A. (2009). Mysteries of the dead: A taphonomic analysis of the skeletal remains from the Peruvian Highland sites of Marcahuamachuco and Cerro Amaru. https://core.ac.uk/download/621602011.pdf (accessed on 18th July 2025).

36. Steckel, R. H. (2025). The best of times, the worst of times: Health and nutrition in pre-Columbian America. https://core.ac.uk/download/pdf/6646131.pdf (accessed on 18th July 2025).

37. Studebaker-Reed, M. S. E. (2018). The impact of training and experience on the recovery of evidence in outdoor forensic scenes: Implications for human remains recovery. https://open.bu.edu/bitstream/2144/31280/5/StudebakerReed_bu_0017N_13567.pdf (accessed on 18th July 2025).

38. Taylor, M. P., & Wedel, M. J. (2012). Why sauropods had long necks; and why giraffes have short necks. https://core.ac.uk/download/29026739.pdf (accessed on 18th July 2025).

39. Taylor, M. P., & Wedel, M. J. (2013). Caudal pneumaticity and pneumatic hiatuses in the sauropod dinosaurs *Giraffatitan* and *Apatosaurus*. https://core.ac.uk/download/29026919.pdf (accessed on 18th July 2025).

40. Tuggle, A. C., Crews, D. E., & Marklein, K. E. (2021). Skeletal frailty at Kałdus, a medieval Poland early Piast dynasty cemetery. https://core.ac.uk/download/395403577.pdf (accessed on 18th July 2025).

41. Tynes, J. F. (2014). A mixed methods investigation of post-secondary students' long bone anatomy knowledge retention through constructivism and the works of Vesalius. https://core.ac.uk/download/217397093.pdf (accessed on 18th July 2025).

42. Winter, R. M. (2016). Analysis of a commingled skeletal sample from Acacia Park Memorial Cemetery. https://core.ac.uk/download/230810544.pdf (accessed on 18th July 2025).

43. Zahn-Hiepler, S. (2019). Tracing life histories through biological manifestations in a 19th-20th century Midwestern poor farm: Asymmetry, robusticity, and adaptive response at the Milwaukee Poor Farm. https://core.ac.uk/download/270048025.pdf (accessed on 18th July 2025).

44. Zhou, C., Shen, S., Zhang, M., Luo, H., Zhang, Y., Wu, C., Zeng, L., et al. (2023). Mechanisms of action and synergetic formulas of plant-based natural compounds from traditional Chinese medicine for managing osteoporosis: A literature review. *Frontiers in Medicine, 10*. https://doi.org/10.3389/fmed.2023.1235081.

BONE BIOLOGY AND STRUCTURE IN HUMAN OSTEOLOGY

2

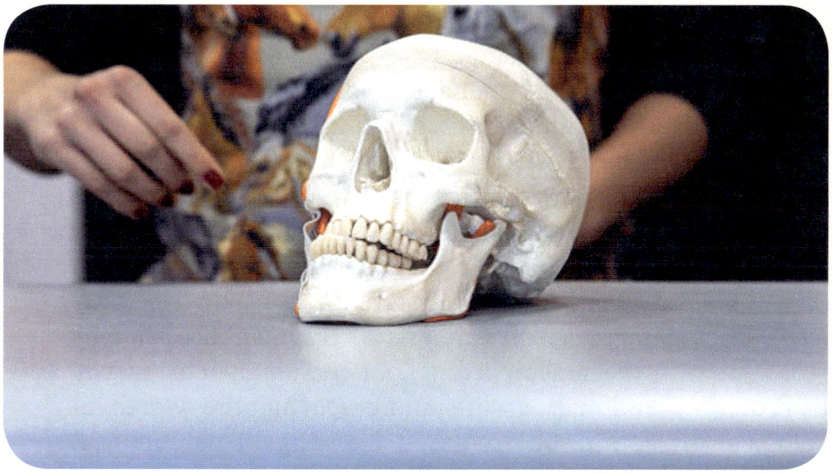

LEARNING OBJECTIVES

After studying this chapter, you will be able to:

1. Discuss bone structure and composition
2. Explain that bone types are classified based on their structure and function
3. Emphasize bone growth and development
4. Learn the process of bone remodeling
5. Understand bone health and diseases
6. Discuss diagnostic methods used in osteology

Introduction

Understanding the structure and biology of bone is crucial in osteology, particularly when dealing with human skeletal systems. Bone is not only a structural system but also a physiologically active tissue involved in processes of mineral homeostasis and metabolic interactions. The complexity of bone biology, with its macroscopic and microscopic features, allows profound insight into an individual's health, development, and evolutionary past. By investigating aspects of trabecular or cancellous bone, which is notoriously porous, it is possible to estimate not only the mechanical properties of bones but also their evolutionary adaptation to locomotor modes. This understanding of bone biology forms the basis for a further discussion of how architectural design within different vertebrate lineages can shed light on locomotor biomechanics and their evolution across species. Comparative analysis of cancellous bone, particularly in humans and other vertebrates, has been intriguing for its ability to inform on biomechanical function and adaptability. Recent studies have now well established that cancellous bone architecture is responsive to mechanical environments and loading conditions, as demonstrated by extensive methodologies such as computed tomographic imaging. Fine-grained analysis of theropod dinosaurs, for instance, shows that these architectural patterns can be associated with specific locomotor strategies, thereby allowing a rich appreciation of evolutionary adaptation. The value of these findings lies not only in the level of our knowledge of extinct animals but also in the illustration of the principles that govern the structural integrity and function of human bones. Applying these lessons in comparative osteology to human disease, scientists can gain a greater appreciation for the complex interplay of genetics, environment, and motion in the development of bone structure. In addition, bone mechanics studies enable basic advances in clinical and evolutionary biological research. By linking bone architecture to biomechanical functions, current studies can apply finite element modeling techniques to simulate and predict bone deformation across various physiological scenarios. The use was illustrated in research on theropod dinosaurs, in which typical modes of cancellous bone architecture served as the basis for hypotheses regarding limb postures and muscle support strategies. These same questions not only illuminate the morphologic change behind avian species but also signal critical continuity in biomechanical principles critical to human osteology. Ultimately, the study of bone structure and biology bridges evolutionary theory with clinical application, thereby lending legitimacy to the value of osteological study for understanding both past and current skeletal wellness.

Definition of Osteology

To define osteology, one should consider its position within the broader discipline of biological anthropology, as well as its emphasis on bone study. Osteology is a scientific inquiry that centers on the form, function, and development of bones as part of understanding human biology and pathology. This specialty also has several branches, including developmental, comparative, and forensic osteology, which together contribute to building a complex model of skeletal systems. The importance of osteology is further heightened in human osteology, where it aids in identifying not only anatomical features but also in assessing age, sex, and health from skeletons. This wide-ranging understanding leads to uses ranging from anthropology to medicine, showing the essential role osteology plays in bridging gaps between disciplines and enhancing our understanding of human evolution and health. An essential aspect of osteology is its methodology, which includes both qualitative and quantitative techniques for analyzing skeletal remains. Osteology often requires hands-on experience to grasp the intricacies of bone identification and feature analysis. For instance, the analysis of fragmentary remains can shed important light on human demography and way of life, underscoring the worth of haptic, object-based learning in osteological education. Recent research highlights the importance of take-home materials, such as plastic model skeletons, in addressing the challenges posed by distance education during crises like the COVID-19 pandemic. Research results grounded in evaluating remote-learning approaches indicate that students can achieve learning objectives equivalent to those of traditional face-to-face approaches, validating the merit of pedagogical practices adapted to contemporary learning environments (Gamble et al., 2024). The evolutionary value of osteology extends beyond human contexts and spans comparative research across species, offering insights into the biomechanics and adaptations of skeletal systems. Studies in cancellous bone architecture in non-avian theropods are cases in point for how osteological principles can enhance our knowledge of locomotion and behavior in extinct species. Such studies can recognize significant patterns in the skeletons of various taxa and allow scientists to extrapolate biomechanical traits related to locomotion and adaptation to lifestyle. Through bone structure examination in a variety of species, osteology contributes to a more intricate knowledge of evolutionary correlations and ecological tactics through time. This intersection of history and current osteological inquiry highlights the field's continued relevance, both in being used to apply to paleontological information as well as to inform the methods used in modern human biology that have implications for medicine and health (Aamodt et al., 2018) (Figure 2.1).

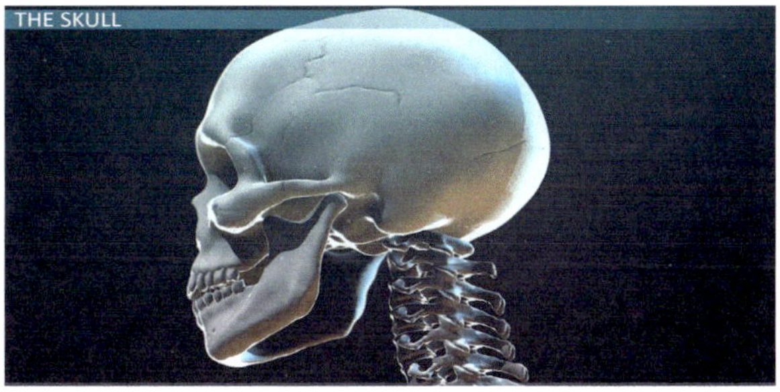

Figure 2.1. To understand the concept of osteology.

Source: https://external-content.duckduckgo.com/iu/?u=https%3A%2F%2Fstudy.com%2Fcimages%2Fvideopreview%2F0yx5svp8pp.jpg&f=1&nofb=1&ipt=78f7351405fb05b4a9dbacee9073f8f0195702ac14724b67cd76e847627860a6.

Importance of Studying Bone Biology

Bone biology plays an important role in the study of not only human anatomy but also how conditions and diseases affect skeletal integrity. Analyzing bone structure and function allows researchers to determine important information about the life cycle of bones and how regenerative processes occur through remodeling and repair. As an example of this concept, recognizing the cellular composition of bones, including their osteoblasts, osteoclasts, and osteocytes, lays the foundation for comprehending diseases such as osteoporosis and osteogenesis imperfecta. These diseases result in catastrophic morbidity in the form of fragility fractures with a disproportionate burden on older adults. Recognizing the biology of bone also has practical application and therapeutic implications for patient care in clinical orthopedics and geriatrics. Hence, systematic study of bone biology not only forms the core of biological inquiry but also of developing health sciences. In the study of bone's mechanical properties, bone biology also plays an important role across many areas, such as biomechanics and bioengineering. Bone is an adaptive tissue that responds to mechanical loading, and its architecture reflects these adaptations, which are revealed by techniques such as computed tomography. For instance, analysis of cancellous bone architecture and variations across species is highly enlightening regarding locomotor biomechanics and overall skeletal health. As outlined in research on theropod dinosaurs, cancellous bone architecture can be compared between extinct and living organisms to illustrate evolutionary modifications that facilitate movement and survival (Aamodt et al., 2018). Integrating findings from comparative anatomy, researchers can create more robust models that inform hypotheses on human movement and injury mitigation, underscoring the fundamental importance of examining bone biology in relation to mechanical function (Aamodt et al., 2018). The importance of bone biology extends beyond familiarity with human anatomy; its broader applications lie in evolutionary biology and paleontology. Data derived from ongoing research on bones has the potential to be applied to interpreting the structures of extinct animals on a biological basis and, as such, deepen our understanding of evolutionary adaptation through geologic time. The anatomic and functional analysis of bone structure provides insight into the behaviors and lifestyles of these species as revealed by the differences in architectural patterns of cancellous bone between dinosaurs and birds. Comparative studies provide information on the processes of adaptation that created the diverse forms of life found today. As highlighted by imaging technologies and data analysis in research institutions such as the University of Texas, ongoing discoveries in bone biology continue to illuminate past and present biological mysteries (Ahmed et al., 2017). This mutual interest deepens our appreciation of life's complexity, establishing a valuable bridge between paleontology and modern medicine.

2.1. Composition of Bone

Learning Outcome

1. Organic bone constituents;
2. Inorganic bone constituents;
3. Collagen role in bone structure.

Bone composition is a complex interaction of organic and inorganic compounds working together towards bone mechanical strength and biological functions. Hydroxyapatite is the primary inorganic compound, a calcium phosphate mineral, that imparts stiffness and structural integrity. Approximately 60% to 70% of bone weight is mineral with a crystalline structure, which contributes to bone's stiffness. This is supported by organic matter, in the form of collagen fibers, which make up approximately 30% of bone composition. These fibers provide tensile strength and elasticity, allowing bones to absorb stress without fracturing. This organic matrix is critical, as it not only influences mechanical properties but also cellular functions, such as bone metabolism regulation. This delicate balance between the inorganic and organic components is required in preserving the integrity of bones throughout life. Bone also has specific structural features that are crucial to its function and strength. Spongy bone or cancellous bone is a porous, lattice-like bone structure that offers lightweight strength as well as housing for bone marrow. This form is typically found at the distal ends of long bones and in vertebrae, offering greater surface area for metabolic function while minimizing weight. Cortical bone, or dense outer bone, provides the strength and support necessary for weight-bearing activity, resisting bending and compressive loading. A system with both forms optimally engineered for strength and function is formed by integrating them. The physiological composition of these bone types includes various cells—osteocytes, osteoblasts, and osteoclasts—that maintain bones in good health by regulating bone modeling and remodeling processes, as the latter refers to the dynamic nature of bone exposed to mechanical loading and metabolic needs. Additionally, understanding bone composition entails exploring its pathological significance, as in osteogenesis imperfecta (OI).

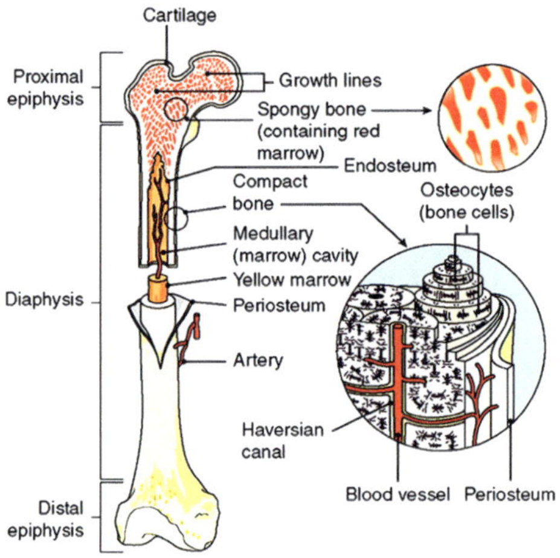

Figure 2.2. The composition of bone.

Source: https://external-content.duckduckgo.com/iu/?u=http%3A%2F%2Fbrianrmz.weebly.com%2Fuploads%2F6%2F4%2F8%2F6%2F64862207%2F_8857912_orig.png&f=1&nofb=1&ipt=c4f729552644ce20fb7506db512e9e8c37599d2036444854b46b2d90a6d6ee44.

OI is characterized by increased bone weakness with collagen composition defects and an altered hierarchical structure of bone that severely compromises its mechanical properties. Research into microstructural parameters of compromised OI bone has revealed significant differences in cortical porosity and canal diameter compared with healthy controls, which further compromises it to fracture. These results show that variations in bone composition directly influence biomechanical strength and resistance. Ongoing research in bone biology not only elucidates the complexities of healthy bone composition but also explains the variations that lead to disorders, underscoring why this discipline is important in the field of human osteology and in developing effective treatments for bone-related diseases (Albert et al., 2013) (Figure 2.2).

2.1.1. Organic Components of Bone

The organic content of bone plays a critical role in its overall structure and function, contributing to its strength and resilience. Composed primarily of collagen fibers, organic content represents about one-third of the bone matrix. Collagen provides tensile strength, enabling bones to resist twisting and stretching forces. In addition to collagen, osteopontin and osteocalcin are two significant non-collagenous proteins that facilitate the attachment of minerals to the collagen scaffold and play key roles in the mineralization process. The organic matrix not only serves as a structural element but also as a critical medium for bone remodeling and repair, which underlines the dynamic nature of skeletal tissue. These organic components should be comprehended to unlock the intricacies of bone growth and homeostasis, thereby influencing the field of human osteology and its applications in forensic medicine and clinical practice. Additionally, the organic matrix of bone supports cellular processes necessary for maintaining its integrity. Within the matrix, various cell types are deposited, including osteoblasts, osteocytes, and osteoclasts, each contributing uniquely to bone metabolism. Osteoblasts accomplish bone building through the synthesis of organic matrix and starting mineralization. Bone resorption is carried out by osteoclasts, maintaining a balance critical to bone homeostasis. Remodeling occurs continuously in response to mechanical stress and hormonal signals, reflecting the adaptive nature of bone. The interaction of these bone cell constituents underscores the role of the organic material in maintaining bone solidity throughout life. Any change of their functions, consequently, leads to such diseases as osteoporosis, underscoring the need for research in this area.

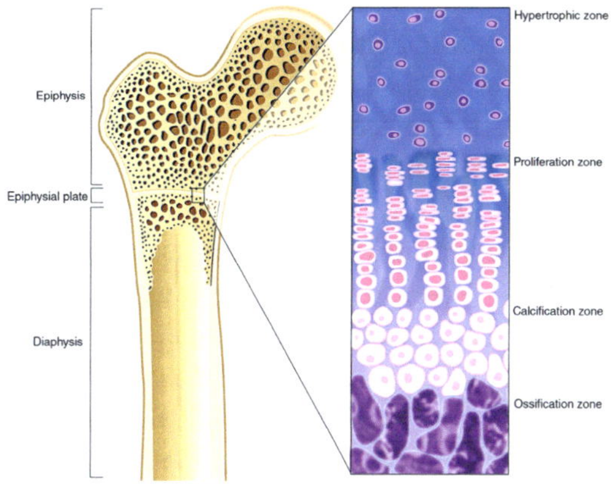

Figure 2.3. The organic components of bone.

Source: https://external-content.duckduckgo.com/iu/?u=https%3A%2F%2Fmir-s3-cdn-cf.behance.net%2Fproject_modules%2F1400%2F2f46f856305337.59a88fbef33d3.png&f=1&nofb=1&ipt=fb3130a4ea373e689f9e57e8bfa3b360dcb56d56312ffcc0d0cfbdda1e1a48d1.

When dealing with forensic anthropology, analysis of organic bone content is pivotal to the determination of the circumstances in which skeletal remains have ended up. Bone fracture features provide insight into the timing and nature of trauma, particularly perimortem, ante mortem, and postmortem situations. Some aspects, such as layered disruption and crushed edges, can point towards perimortem trauma where bone is fresh and retains some characteristic of living bone that can yield information regarding the forces experienced at injury (Dalmases et al., 2017). Besides, such knowledge is used to formulate a story about the life and death of individuals and the conditions they experienced. Thus, studies of the organic components of bone not only enhance our understanding of biological processes but also strengthen forensic techniques and connect biology with the legal system in human osteology (Figure 2.3).

2.1.2. Inorganic Components of Bone

It is the inorganic bone structure that determines the bone's structure and function in the human skeleton. Primarily composed of hydroxyapatite, a crystalline substance made of calcium phosphate and minor minerals, bone is rigid yet flexible. This mineralization helps bones resist compressive stresses, allowing them to support the weight of the body and facilitate movement. Further, trace elements like magnesium and fluoride play a role in the biological activity and resistance of bone tissue. Equilibrium among these inorganic components is crucial as it affects not just the bone's mechanical properties but also its storage capacity for minerals and contribution to metabolic processes that support overall health (Brun et al., 2016). Histological examination has revealed significant species differences in bone inorganic content, driven by adaptations to universal environmental stresses and by functional needs. Variation in the size and composition of human vs. non-human hydroxyapatite crystals, for instance, attests to evolutionary significance concerning movement and load-bearing functions. These findings provide a backdrop for interpreting the impact that structural variation can have on bone resilience under varying conditions, e.g., taphonomic processes such as thermal alteration, which can erode the identification and classification of skeletal evidence (Brouchoud et al., 2016). The recognition of species-based variation underscores the need for careful inspection in forensic and anthropological contexts, particularly when attempting to define the origin and biological context of skeletal evidence. Furthermore, the interaction between bones' inorganic structures and their biological functions emphasizes its functional role to metabolic activity rather than mere support. Bones are dynamic reservoirs of minerals for physiological function, releasing phosphorus and calcium into the circulation whenever required to maintain homeostasis. This biochemical function is one that is illustrated under conditions of stress or dietary deficiency, where the release of these minerals can be utilized to control physiological events. Thus, the inorganic content of bone not only confers physical properties but also underlies key characteristics of total-body metabolism and health. Hence, it is all the more important to understand the intricacy of these components to realize their significance in osteological research as well as clinical application in bone illness, as well as in health (Brun et al., 2016).

2.1.3. Role of Collagen in Bone Structure

The role of collagen in bone is critical, as this protein forms the primary organic matrix, providing tensile strength and structural integrity. Collagen in bone is primarily type I, which organizes into a hierarchical pattern that forms a scaffold for mineral deposition. This scaffolding is integral to the mechanical properties of bones, including stiffness and elasticity. The organization of collagen fiber complexes influences force transmission through bone and, in turn, affects resistance to fracture. Collagen network pathology can impair mechanical function, underscoring the importance of collagen for musculoskeletal health. Knowledge of the physical properties of collagen and their influence on bone structure provides insight into many disorders and conditions that weaken skeletal integrity, including osteogenesis imperfecta, in which defects in collagen result in greater bone fragility and structural instability (Albert et al., 2013). Further, collagen's interaction with mineral components, mainly hydroxyapatite, is an important factor in characterizing bone quality. The mineralization process, in which the phosphate and calcium ions precipitate within the collagen matrix, is essential to maintain bone strength. As described in recent literature reviews, mineralization of collagen fibers reinforces the bone's load-bearing capacity and thus makes it resistant to fractures (Amling et al., 2019). Levels of mineralization can vary with age and health, affecting not only bone structure but also its mechanical properties.

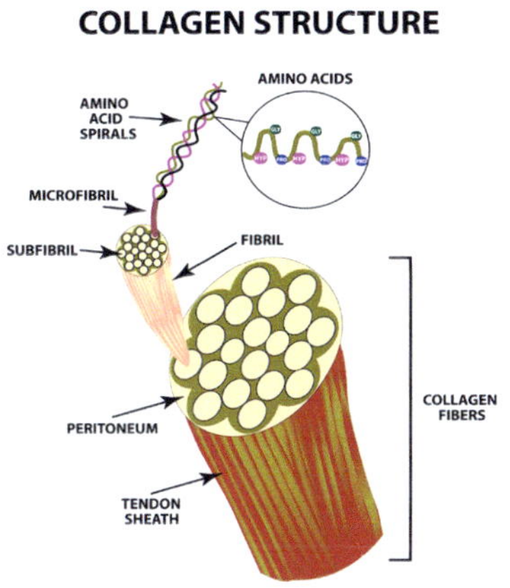

Figure 2.4. The role of collagen in bone structure.

Source: https://external-content.duckduckgo.com/iu/?u=https%3A%2F%2Fcdn1.vectorstock.com%2Fi%2F1000x1000%2F10%2F05%2Fcollagen-structure-infographics-vector-23021005.jpg&f=1&nofb=1&ipt=37c51c6717bea4fc5c30917781241d7581e76f1e88c55dd3cb550eae8913d433.

Bone formation, from a largely woven composition in youth to a much better-organized lamellar structure in adulthood, can be taken as an indication of improved collagen orientation and mineralization as age progresses. These alterations play an important role in the resistance of bone to mechanical load, with pediatric relevance. In juvenile ages, when bone remodeling is occurring, collagen fiber direction and packing are more accurately determined. This development is associated with the acquisition of mechanical resistance; studies show that children between 2 and 14 years old exhibit a remarkable enhancement of bone stiffness and strength, hand in hand with improved collagen architecture and mineralization (Amling et al., 2019). Such adaptations are critical for maintaining skeletal integrity in the face of growth spurts and physical demands. The collagen matrix not only supports necessary mineralization but also provides a responsive framework that can change under varying mechanical loads, further preventing fractures. Thus, collagen's role is not passive; it actively participates in the physiological changes in bone structure that occur during development, and its significance in bone biology and human osteology is underscored (Figure 2.4).

Test Your Knowledge

1. What are the main organic constituents of bone tissue?
2. What role does collagen play in maintaining bone structure and strength?

2.2. Types of Bone

Learning Outcome

1. Features of cortical bone
2. Features of cancellous (trabecular) bone
3. Functional variations among bone types

Bone types in human osteology are classified based on structure and function, both of which are of extreme significance for the overall biomechanics of the skeleton. The main types are long bones, short bones, flat bones, irregular bones, and sesamoid bones. Long bones, including the femur and humerus, have a long shape and are crucial for locomotion and support. In contrast, short bones—those found in the wrist—are stabilizing and facilitate a variety of movements. Flat bones, including the sternum and cranial bones, are mainly for protection and attachment points for muscles. Irregular bones, such as vertebrae, have varying shapes that are suitable to their respective body functions. Lastly, sesamoid bones, e.g., the patella, develop in tendons and provide mechanical advantages in movement. The microstructural composition of bones varies significantly across different bones and reflects their respective functional specializations. For instance, the very dense Haversian bone present in some sauropod dinosaurs, as cited in recent research, demonstrates how bone adjusts to mechanical stress in complex ways. Such histological features are crucial for understanding how different types of bone are used for different physiological purposes. Dense bone is found in the long bones of the human body and is responsible for bearing weight and providing rigidity, whereas in short and flat bones only spongy bone is present, which provides a light structure with toughness and shock resistance. In this differentiation of bone architecture, not only do their mechanical characteristics change, but they also exert an overall influence on the body's metabolic processes, showing the deep involvement of both structural and functional processes in bone. In forensic use, the different bone types play a crucial role in identifying and analyzing human remains. Identification of skeletal remains can give valuable information about the age, sex, ancestry, and some life history of the subject regardless of the decomposition stage. Interestingly, foot bones and lower limbs have been reported in forensic contexts because they are frequently recovered as broken fragments from various environments, including beaches. Despite this, a surprising lack of extensive literature on the foot within forensic human identification has been reported in recent studies. This knowledge of the foot bones, along with their diversity, provides crucial information for forensic experts to reconstruct biological profiles, eventually enhancing the accuracy and effectiveness of the processes of identifying human remains in osteological studies (Barrett et al., 2014) (Figure 2.5).

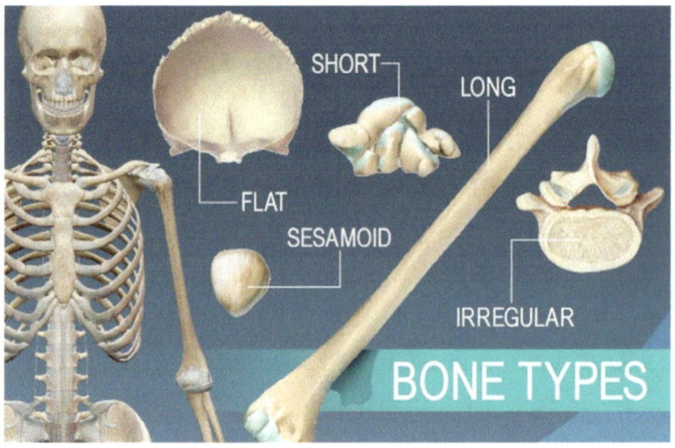

Figure 2.5. The bone types are classified based on their structure and function.

Source: https://external-content.duckduckgo.com/iu/?u=https%3A%2F%2Fwww.visiblebody.com%2Fhs-fs%2Fhub%2F189659%2Ffile-2122072719-jpg%2FLearn_Articles%2FSkeleton_System%2FSet_1_Bone_Types%2F1-Five-Types-Of-Bones-1232W.jpg&f=1&nofb=1&ipt=557379e9dcd5b9e3789e90c10ab670ea40ae61d85f5047dbf7c33dfffbcc1571.

2.2.1. Cortical Bone Characteristics

The external layer of the skeletal system, cortical bone, is what provides the body's structural support and mechanical stability. Its structured and compact nature makes the cortical bones' principal function that of providing strength and encasing inner tissues. Cortical bone has a densely mineralized matrix composed primarily of calcium phosphate, organized into functional units known as osteons. This intricate architecture provides for load distribution and resistance to torsion and bending. Microstructural alterations, such as increased porosity or changes in canal diameter, have been shown by studies to have a marked influence on bone's mechanical properties, leading to an enhanced risk of fracture. These highlight the importance of being aware of cortical bone morphology while evaluating overall skeletal health and human osteology biomechanics. Research has shown that the character of cortical bone may vary significantly across populations and ages. For instance, osteogenesis imperfecta (OI), a collagen biosynthesis defect with a genetic basis, has been shown to remodel the 3D structure and composition of cortical bone components in significant ways. Higher cortical porosity and wider canals were observed in children with OI than in controls in a comparative study. These are structural alterations that compromise the mechanical strength of the bone; hence, patients with OI are at higher risk for fractures. The quest for such characteristics not only has implications for the explanation of individual pathologies but also for the fine-tuning of methodology employed in the clinical assessment, such as the utilization of sophisticated imaging techniques to evaluate bone quality and density across various populations, thus reemphasizing the necessity of an individualized approach in managing bone health (Albert et al., 2013). Second, the ability of cortical bone to be plastic in response to mechanical loading renders it a key consideration in osteological health across the life-course. The dynamic control of the remodeling process, through the balance between osteoblast and osteoclast activity, allows for the bone to adapt to fluctuating mechanical loads. This plasticity is observed in individuals subjected to repetitive physical exercise, in which greater loading can be linked to more dense, robust cortical bone formation through increased periosteal and endosteal apposition. Conversely, long-term immobilization or disuse can lead to bone density loss, underscoring the central role of mechanical stimuli in skeletal health. The hierarchical nature of bone demonstrates not just the biological significance of cortical bone but also the evolutionary significance of cortical bone in the support of locomotion and motor functions, and its properties are associated with broader implications in human disease and biology (Aamodt et al., 2018) (Figure 2.6).

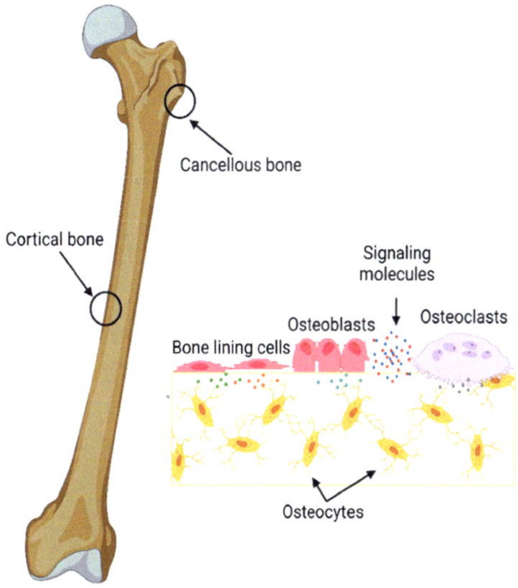

Figure 2.6. Cortical bone characteristics.

Source: https://external-content.duckduckgo.com/iu/?u=https%3A%2F%2Fwww.researchgate.net%2Fpublication%2F370953643%2Ffigure%2Ffig1%2FAS%3A11431281160713976%401684833589897%2FBone-includes-both-cortical-and-trabecular-bone-In-the-cellular-area-bone-comprises.png&f=1&nofb=1&ipt=95b874e66c5bdb90ca27db4d7093054f159e5c45192aa0fdbcc1978609c24351.

2.2.2. Cancellous (Trabecular) Bone Characteristics

The cancellous bone, or trabecular bone, is a vascular and less dense bone that plays a very crucial role in general skeletal function. Its spongy structure is predominantly located at the ends of the long bones, at the vertebrae, and in the ribs, conferring both strength and lightness. Unlike its counterpart, cortical bone, the cancellous bone's intricate network of trabeculae provides for the best loading distribution and internal stability. The spatial organization of cancellous bone makes it resilient to mechanical stress while minimizing its weight, which is vital for human osteological mobility and equilibrium. Of particular interest is that the cancellous bone structure is dynamically responsive to varying mechanical loads and physiological needs, reflecting its responsiveness to varied activities and functions, and further underscoring its significance in both normal and high-impact physical situations. The cancellous bone's functional characteristics are intimately interrelated with its structure. Experiments involving high-technology imaging techniques have shown that these trabecular structures vary across many species, including humans and extinct tetrapods such as theropod dinosaurs. For example, cancellous bone architecture in certain theropods is comparable to that in humans and reflects similar adaptive mechanisms for locomotor biomechanics (Aamodt et al., 2018). The trabecular network, besides supporting vertical loading, also resists varied forces during locomotion, such as flexion and compression. Apart from this, some orientations and patterns of trabecular bone can shed light on the mechanics of movement, which can be significant for the behavior and locomotion of modern and ancient species. This correlation between bone structure and function underscores the importance of comparing cancellous bone architecture within the context of biomechanics and evolutionary adaptation. Cancellous bone functionality and integrity are top concerns for skeletal integrity as a whole, particularly in aging or in conditions such as osteoporosis. The balance of bone formation and bone resorption in cancellous bone is quite significant in order to maintain the strength of the skeleton. In osteogenesis imperfecta, for instance, mutations are known to cause significant alterations in trabecular parameters, such as reduced bone volume and defective osteoblast function, as reflected in studies showing typical histological features in patients (Alsaedi et al., 2017). These lead to increased fracture risk and compromised mobility. In addition, its increased sensitivity to treatment interventions, such as bisphosphonate therapy, is an indicator of its greater potential for restoration and bone density control. Identification of the properties and responses of cancellous bone thus has significant implications for clinical interventions and for health sciences in bone management.

2.2.3. Differences in Function Between Bone Types

The diversity of bones in the human skeleton reflects their varied functional purposes, required for overall skeletal stability and locomotion. Compact and spongy (or cancellous) bone are the two significant types of bone, each with a specific function. Compact bone, being a complex and dense tissue, forms the exterior surface of all bones, adding strength and support. It is of most significance where there is maximum mechanical stress, such as in the shafts of long bones. Spongy bone, however, which is most frequently at the ends of long bones and in the interior of flat bones, possesses a porous structure that allows it to support bone marrow and produce blood cells. This structural divergence is significant as it not only influences the mechanical function of bones but also their biological functions within the skeleton. The differences in bone types are not only limited to structure but also to their individual biological functions. Compact bone primarily facilitates the biomechanical stability of the skeleton and serves as a reservoir for calcium and phosphorus for metabolic functions. This role is complemented by the spongy character of spongy bone that effectively supports hematopoiesis, the formation of blood cells in the red marrow, as well as the absorption of shock due to its elastic lattice-like structure. Spongy bone also plays a role in storing and releasing minerals and is of great importance to the body's capacity to maintain mineral homeostasis. The two-functionality of bone types exhibits a remarkable adaptation process that balances structural stability with metabolic requirements and, conversely, the complexity of bone biology and function. Furthermore, pathological conditions may profoundly affect the functional differences among bone types, revealing their respective vulnerabilities. Such diseases, for instance, include osteogenesis imperfecta (OI) that can weaken the mechanical stability of compact bone and spongy bone and result in increased susceptibility to fracture and brittleness. Research in OI has established certain microstructural changes in cortical bone, such as an increase in cortical porosity and altered properties of the canal network which directly affect its strength and toughness (Albert et al., 2013). The research suggests the correlation between the structure of the bone and its mechanical properties, and how deviations in one form of bone can cascade and cause effects on the functioning of the entire skeletal system. Understanding these functional differences among bones provides significant context for the treatment of various bone-related conditions and for the development of osteological research (Abzhanov et al., 2019) (Figure 2.7).

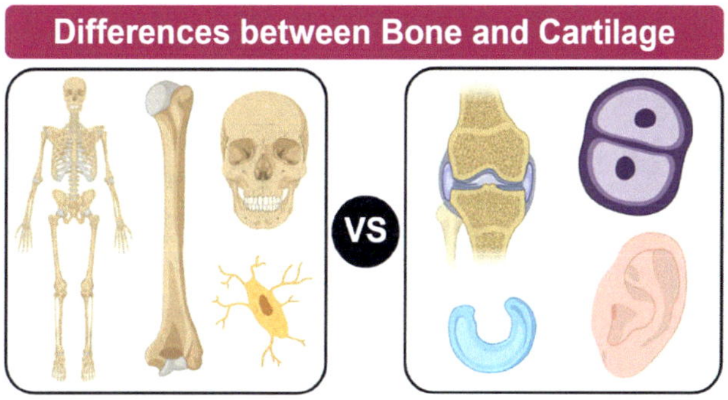

Figure 2.7. Differences in function between bone types.

Source: https://external-content.duckduckgo.com/iu/?u=https%3A%2F%2Fmicrobenotes.com%2Fwp-content%2Fuploads%2F2020%2F07%2FDifferences-between-Bone-and-Cartilage-Bone-vs-Cartilage.jpeg&f=1&nofb=1&ipt=b2733144349cc138ef2ec17a9655ca4fb8509fcf25b9c02dc022e84db2ef67d4.

Test Your Knowledge

1. What are the key features of cancellous (trabecular) bone?
2. How do different types of bone vary in structure and function?

2.3. Bone Development and Growth

Learning Outcome

1. Intramembranous ossification;
2. Endochondral ossification;
3. Factors influencing bone growth.

Bone growth and development are fundamental processes that determine the overall structure and strength of the human skeletal system. This intricate process begins even during embryonic development, when mesenchymal cells differentiate into osteoblasts that help form new bone. The basic bone structure is formed through intramembranous and endochondral ossification. Intramembranous ossification is characteristic of flat bones, such as the skull, whereas endochondral ossification occurs more frequently in long bones, where hyaline cartilage serves as the precursor to bone. Such processes are tightly regulated by multiple signaling pathways, including growth factors and hormones, that guide bone remodeling and maturation throughout a person's life. Bone growth occurs continuously in the body; processes of resorption and deposition continue to run all the time, balancing bone composition and density. Osteoclasts, the bone-resorbing cells, are central to the bone remodeling process by breaking down old or damaged bone. This is counter-balanced by the activity of osteoblasts, which lay down new bone. This dynamic system not only enables the skeleton to adapt to mechanical stresses but also repairs micro-damage from everyday use. In addition, genetic, environmental, and lifestyle factors have an important influence on bone development and growth. It is very important to maintain adequate calcium and vitamin D intake because they are essential for optimal bone mineralization and overall skeletal stability at every stage of life. The interactions between environmental and genetic determinants result in a wide spectrum of phenotypes in bone density and quality. For instance, genetic differences in genes involved in bone remodeling can lead to varying susceptibility to osteoporosis and other diseases. Modern imaging techniques and gene research have revealed that the complexity of bone biology can aid the identification of markers of bone health. Understanding these paradigms has clinical implications in healthcare settings, where interventions aimed at conserving bone stock can maximize skeletal health and reduce the incidence of fractures, especially in high-risk individuals. As research in osteology continues, integrating novel studies will be critical for informing directions for conserving healthy bone stock in human populations, including experimental designs for biomechanical testing and regenerative medicine as potential areas of focus.

2.3.1. Intramembranous Ossification

Intramembranous ossification is a simple process of bone formation that primarily involves the direct conversion of mesenchymal tissue to bone with no intermediate step of cartilage formation. The process is critical during the formation of flat bones such as those of the skull and clavicles. In this process, mesenchymal cells become osteoblasts, the bone-forming cells. These osteoblasts then create an organic matrix that continues to mineralize and form bone. The role of cranial neural crest mesenchyme in this points to the specific cellular interactions and signaling pathways responsible for bone morphology and structure, as with other overarching developmental processes within other vertebrates that favor adaptation and evolution over time (Abzhanov et al., 2019). The importance of intramembranous ossification lies not only in its role in structural development but also in revealing directions for the study of developmental anomalies and adaptive adaptation. The mechanism by which bone structure forms rapidly can be controlled by multiple mechanical and biochemical factors during development. Understanding these influences is crucial not only in the context of healthy osteogenesis but also in the study of cases in which these processes may fail, leading to defects or disease. Examination of these deviations helps us better understand both the evolutionary record of the origin of skeletal forms and the potential clinical manifestations of developmental abnormalities, toward an integrated comprehension of bone health in man and the animal kingdom (Lewis et al., 2017). Studying intramembranous ossification is important in modern osteology. This insight enables one to value the potential of processes during embryonic development to inform current practice in regenerative medicine and orthopedic therapy.

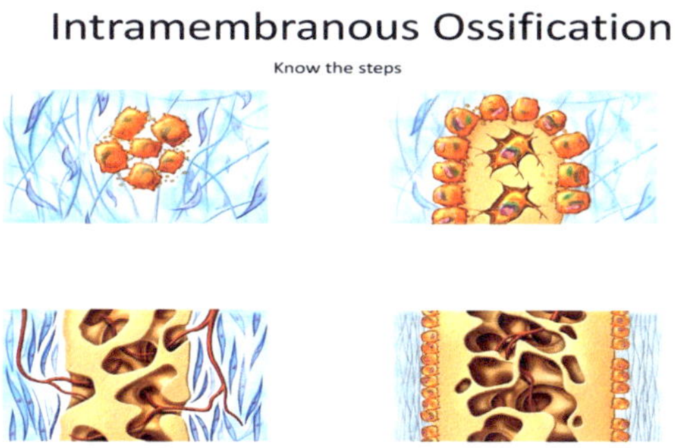

Figure 2.8. Intramembranous ossification.

Source: https://external-content.duckduckgo.com/iu/?u=https%3A%2F%2Fo.quizlet.com%2FAnJrOoxFzXSYZ0wdDkV2Kg_b.jpg&f=1&nofb=1&ipt=2fe014cc9c7bac00c18b5e3fa25d95ea1fe87716846af6972c4b1af3c36cdb22.

For instance, knowledge acquired through this type of ossification can guide strategies for repairing and reconstructing bones in the clinic. In addition, by making inferences between ancient and modern skeletal populations, the examination of intramembranous ossification can be used to investigate conditions in fetal paleopathology, providing insight into the maternal-fetal interactions that contribute to skeletal pathology across generations (Lewis et al., 2017). An understanding of the process thus provides society with a multifaceted view of both the evolution of skeletal structures and their relevance to human health (Figure 2.8).

2.3.2. Endochondral Ossification

Endochondral ossification is a vital process in the formation of the skeleton, particularly long bones and other skeletal structures. This complex biological process begins with a hyaline cartilage model that serves as a template for the development of bone tissue. During fetal development, the cartilage undergoes a series of transformations, including hypertrophy and mineralization, followed by invasion by blood vessels and osteoprogenitor cells. These cells further differentiate into osteoblasts that lay down the bone matrix, thereby mediating the transformation process from cartilage to bone. All this is not just a reflection of the dynamic nature of the skeletal development process but also accounts for the need for tissue remodeling as an integral part of bone biology, so that the nascent skeletal system can dynamically respond to functional loads and mechanical stresses imposed during ontogeny (Inthasan et al., 2017). During ongoing endochondral ossification, the growth plates are particularly crucial, as they regulate longitudinal bone growth. Growth plates occur in the ends of long bones and consist of hypertrophic and proliferating zones of chondrocytes that enable bones to increase in length. The epiphyseal plate has zones that enable the continuous process of cartilage formation and replacement with bone, the balance between cartilage and bone deposition being critical for normal skeletal maturation. In addition, derangements in the process can lead to growth disorders, underscoring the importance of understanding endochondral ossification not only in normal physiology but also in disease states. Here, the intricate regulation of chondrocyte activity demonstrates the subtle interaction between development and growth in human osteology

(Benjamin et al., 2016). Beyond its primary role in bone development, endochondral ossification plays a vital role in fracture repair and bone remodeling. The recruitment of chondrocytes to areas of injury allows for primary cartilage formation, which is subsequently replaced by bone through endochondral ossification. This is the body's exceptional ability to heal and adapt, further demonstrating the value of studying bone biology in detail. Differences in endochondral ossification rates can also provide clinicians with information about healing and potential complications of skeletal injury. Therefore, ongoing research into the processes responsible for this form of ossification has important implications for both treatment and the development of biomaterials aimed at facilitating bone healing, with exciting possibilities for future studies within the field of human osteology (Inthasan et al., 2017) (Figure 2.9).

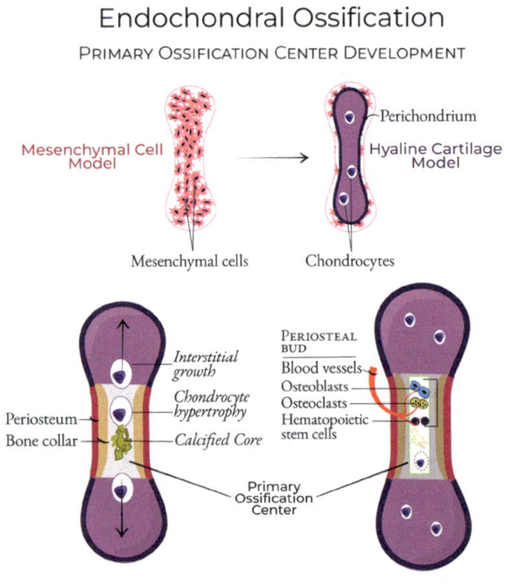

Figure 2.9. Endochondral ossification represents a vital process in skeletal development.

Source: https://d1j63owfs0b5j3.cloudfront.net/term/images/endochondral-ossification-diagram-9545.jpg.

2.3.3. Factors Influencing Bone Growth

The process of bone growth, an intricate ballet of biological and environmental pressures, is imperative for the best skeletal development. Genetic factors undoubtedly are dominant, dictating the ability to grow and the ultimate shape and size of bones. Variations in genes for growth hormone and bone content can produce radically different outcomes in skeletal structure. Furthermore, there is hormonal regulation; growth hormone, thyroid hormone, and sex steroids, for instance, interact synergistically to propel the activity of osteoblasts—osteogenesis cells. Thus, understanding genetics and hormonal interaction is enlightening in its description of the complexity of bone biology, particularly as researchers endeavor to treat growth pathology or abnormal osteological development. Mechanical loading is also a crucial parameter that significantly influences bone growth and architecture. The transfer of mechanical forces during weight-bearing exercises induces osteogenic activity, enhancing bone strength and density. This action is provided by Wolff's Law, which describes that bone remodels itself according to the loads it sustains. The mechanical effects on cancellous bone architecture have been extensively reported, describing its biomechanical milieu sensitivity. The different cancellous architectures observed in theropod dinosaurs provide a window through which to infer locomotor biomechanics and adaptations, as well as how environmental conditions affect bone growth and bone health. Describing these mechanical effects may present new windows of understanding in the therapy and prevention of osteoporotic disease. Nutritional factors are a core influence on bone growth and development, particularly during critical periods such as childhood and adolescence. Adequate intake of essential nutrients such as calcium, vitamin D, and protein is necessary for efficient bone development. Calcium is directly involved in the mineralization process, whereas vitamin D increases the absorption of calcium and phosphate from the gut. These deficiencies can lead to abnormal bone growth, rendering the subject more susceptible to deformity and fractures. Fetal paleopathology has explained these associations, proving the influence of maternal nutrition on fetal bone development (Lewis et al., 2017). Moreover, current evidence emphasizes the importance of dietary patterns throughout life and indicates that an appropriate diet not only supports early bone development but also plays a significant role in maintaining bone health in older age (Figure 2.10).

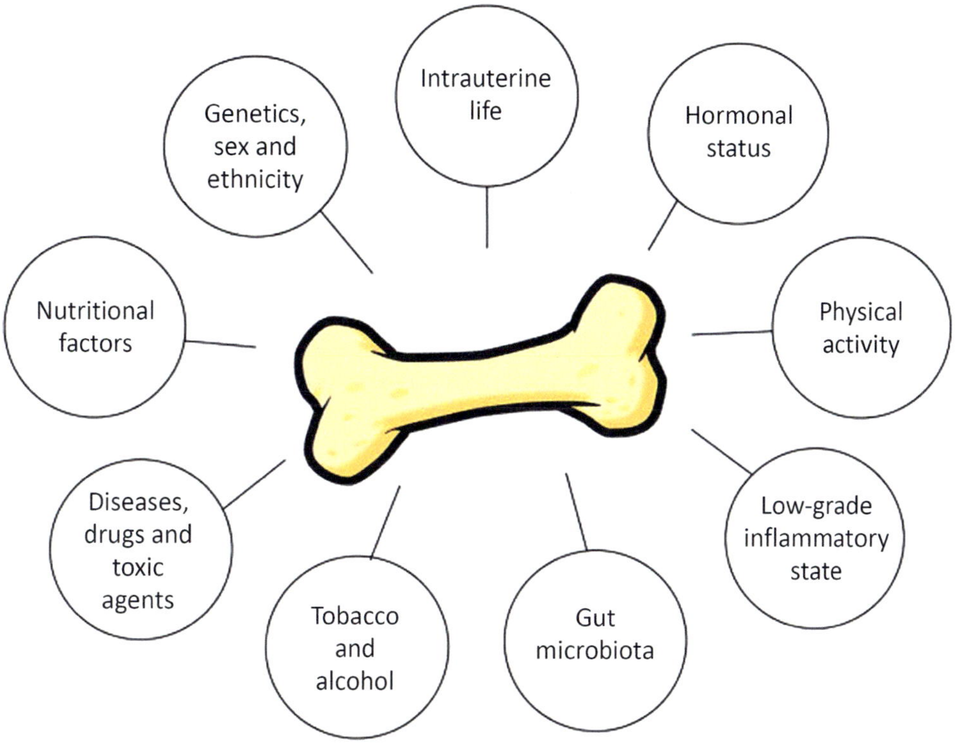

Figure 2.10. The process of bone growth, an intricate ballet of biological and environmental influences.

Source: https://external-content.duckduckgo.com/iu/?u=https%3A%2F%2Fwww.researchgate.net%2Fprofile%2FPilar-Codoner-Franch%2Fpublication%2F327913924%2Ffigure%2Ffig1%2FAS%3A747315405021184%401555185285905%2FFactors-influencing-bone-formation-during-childhood-and-adolescence.jpg&f=1&nofb=1&ipt=0be9d3191dfdf5a29f85d9f6e2dcfd7b680b3d1a470469551c966545ff3bbe23.

Test Your Knowledge

1. What is intramembranous ossification and where does it occur in the human body?
2. What factors influence bone development and growth?

2.4. Bone Remodeling

Learning Outcome

1. The process of bone resorption
2. The process of bone formation
3. Role of osteoblasts and osteoclasts

Bone remodeling is a continuous physiological process vital to maintaining bone health throughout a person's lifespan. This complex process is made possible by the synergistic co-operation of osteoclasts and osteoblasts, respectively, which resorb existing bone tissue and form new bone tissue. Remodeling is stimulated by a range of stimuli, including mechanical stress, hormonal changes, and nutritional influences. Interestingly, bone remodeling enables bones to adapt to loads and strains, thereby achieving maximal structural integrity under physical stress. In response to stress, trabecular and cortical regions adapt by modifying their structure to enhance strength and resistance to fracture, highlighting the dynamic nature of bone as a living tissue. The significance of effective bone remodeling is also underscored by modifications in cancellous bone morphology observed in living and extinct organisms, as documented in recent research on theropod dinosaurs. This chapter shows that cancellous bone is highly responsive to its mechanical environment, reflecting the biomechanical loads acting on these skeletal elements. By studying the three-dimensional features of cancellous bone, researchers have begun comparing the architectural designs of certain theropods with those of the human skeleton. For example, specific architectural features associated with locomotion indicate that non-avian theropods possess cancellous bone features required for effective motion. This appreciation adds depth to how other groups of animals have rearranged their skeletons over evolutionary time, demonstrating the importance of remodeling in locomotor biomechanics. In human osteology, bone quality is paramount, as it affects both strength and fracture susceptibility. Processes such as disease or ageing significantly influence bone remodeling, inducing significant changes in microstructure and mechanical properties. Longitudinal research, for instance, has shown that cortical bone's mechanical resistance is intensified considerably in childhood, indicating essential remodeling that renders weaker woven bone to become stronger lamellar bone. This remodeling is associated with increased mineralization and collagen alignment, which reinforce the structural characteristics of bones and make them more resistant to fracture. Recognition of such remodeling-associated changes not only informs clinical management of bone health but also acknowledges the intricate interplay between bone biology and the mechanical load placed on the skeleton, as elucidated by studies in both modern and ancient populations (Amling et al., 2019) (Figure 2.11).

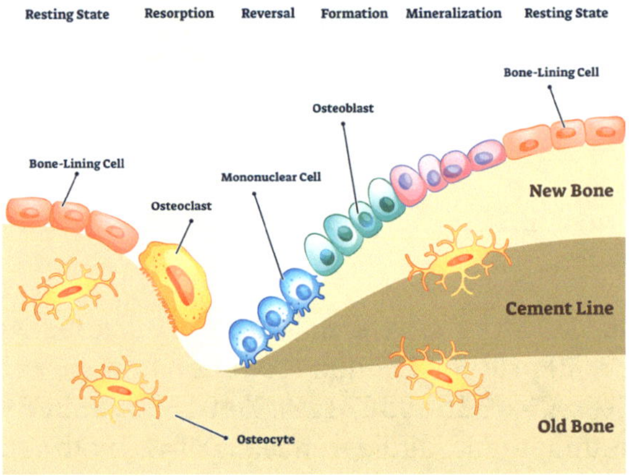

Figure 2.11. Bone remodeling is a continuous physiological process.

Source: https://external-content.duckduckgo.com/iu/?u=https%3A%2F%2Fbiogennix.com%2Fwp-content%2Fuploads%2F2022%2F08%2FBone-Remodeling-v2-1536x1184.png&f=1&nofb=1&ipt=bf35e1aff6a35a48e00a0a1546ccd922afefab10e741b6f02a0be4dbedf682c2.

2.4.1. The Process of Bone Resorption

The process of bone resorption is a key aspect of bone biology that ensures skeletal integrity and calcium homeostasis in the human body. It is a dynamic process in which bone tissue is degraded by professional cells known as osteoclasts, which are derived from monocyte precursors. Bone is destroyed by osteoclasts through the secretion of acids and enzymes that degrade the mineralized matrix, leading to the release of calcium and phosphate into the bloodstream. Not only is osteoclast activity important for normal bone remodeling, but it is also to satisfy metabolic requirements by equilibrating new bone formation by osteoblasts. In addition, dysregulation of bone resorption is involved in pathologies such as osteoporosis, in which resorption exceeds formation, making bones less dense and increasing the risk of fracture, thereby stimulating interest in the biology of this phenomenon in human osteology. A complex interplay of hormones regulates bone resorption and signal transduction pathways. Parathyroid hormone (PTH), calcitonin, and other cytokines are some of the influences that regulate osteoclast activity and, consequently, bone resorption. For example, PTH stimulates osteoclastogenesis by activating receptor activator of nuclear factor kappa-B ligand (RANKL) expression in osteoblasts, leading to binding of RANK on osteoclast precursors and their differentiation into active osteoclasts. Calcitonin, conversely, suppresses osteoclast activity, functioning as an antagonist to PTH action. Knowledge of these regulatory mechanisms provides insight into how disturbances in hormone levels result in disorders of bone density. Furthermore, current studies encompass a broader range of biological cues, and there is a need for an integrative strategy in bone science, especially given the inclusion of skeletal trauma and mechanisms of repair, as discussed in recent anthropological articles on skeletal aging and health status (Buckberry et al., 2015). Examining bone resorption not just illuminates the workings of standard physiological mechanisms but has significant implications for clinical intervention and practice. For instance, therapeutic interventions targeting osteoclast function, such as bisphosphonates, play a crucial role in the management of osteoporosis by preventing bone resorption and maintaining bone density. In addition, new information regarding the osteoclast microenvironment, such as the impact of mechanical tension and inflammatory mediators, is promising avenues for enhanced bone regeneration in the clinic. By exploring the cellular and molecular underpinnings of bone resorption, researchers are well positioned to develop treatments that ensure maximal bone repair while minimizing complications caused by overt resorption. These strategies can be of immense benefit in treating bone loss due to aging, underscoring the need for individualized intervention based on bone biology and structural differences (Abdalla et al., 2015).

2.4.2. The Process of Bone Formation

Bone formation, or ossification, is a multi-step process of cellular interaction, most notably through intramembranous and endochondral ossification. Intramembranous ossification is primarily seen in flat bones such as the skull and clavicles, where mesenchymal stem cells undergo direct differentiation into osteoblasts. Osteoblasts generate osteoid, which mineralizes to form bone matrix. Endochondral ossification, however, has a precursor cartilage model that will eventually be replaced by bone. This process is required for long bone development and consists of the initial establishment of a cartilage template that calcifies, allowing the invasion of blood vessels and the sequential deposition of bone by osteoblasts. Both of these steps are necessary for the growth and development of the skeletal system to provide proper structure and function to an organism throughout its lifetime. Through bone development, dynamic osteoblast, osteoclast, and osteocyte regulation is critical for the preservation of bone homeostasis and health. Osteoblasts contribute to the synthesis and mineralization of bone matrix, while osteoclasts cause bone resorption for the continuation of bone tissue remodeling. Osteocytes, which become ensconced within the bone matrix, act as mechanosensors that can modulate osteoblast and osteoclast activities in line with mechanical load and stress. This resorption-formation equilibrium is indispensable to skeletal remodeling to accommodate physical stresses, as exemplified in athletes under mounting stress, which results in bone density build-up. Osteocytes are therefore central not only in maintenance but also in signaling the call for bone formation or resorption, thereby influencing the overall structure and solidity of the skeletal apparatus. The structural properties of the bone tissue, including strength and density, are heavily influenced by processes of ossification and remodeling. Histological studies have shown that bones are composed of Haversian systems that ensure the efficient distribution of nutrients and the removal of waste products, thereby optimizing the usefulness of the bone as both structural support and living tissue. Microstructural observations among various kinds of bones within vertebrates provide insight into evolutionary advancements of skeletal structures by ossification processes. Abdalla et al. (2015), for instance, document how the ossified structures of extinct organisms exhibit various types of bone tissue and their adaptive significance, while Abdala et al. (2016) link the evolutionary developments of the structure of bones to jaw growth within mammals. These analyses increase our understanding of bone biology and reveal to us the evolutionary pressures that have molded skeletal form, processes, and functions in all species (Figure 2.12).

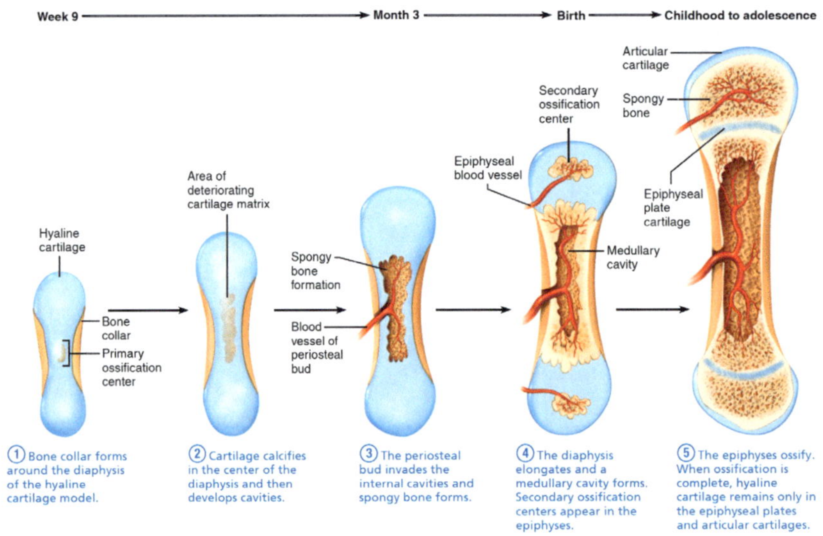

Figure 2.12. The process of bone formation.

Source: https://external-content.duckduckgo.com/iu/?u=https%3A%2F%2Fi.pinimg.com%2Foriginals%2F66%2F3c%2Fd1%2F663cd15a7d765e9b88a1686aefb9b97e.png&f=1&nofb=1&ipt=89153b4787a633078a201255565a48ff4b4c721f1f8a1e9e70b57743d676aece.

2.4.3. Role of Osteoblasts and Osteoclasts

The interplay between osteoclasts and osteoblasts in a complementary manner is the foundation to the maintenance and regulation of bone health, an expression of the law of bone remodeling in human osteology. The cells responsible for bone formation, osteoblasts, are involved in the synthesis and mineralization of bone matrix and therefore play a central role in skeletal structure. They secrete osteoid, an unmineralized bone matrix, which causes the deposition of calcium phosphate to form mature bone. In addition, osteoblast differentiation is tailored by several molecular signals, like the Wnt pathway, that account for the complexity of bone development and repair mechanisms. As emphasized in the current literature, imbalances in the osteoblastic process are responsible for several bone diseases, underscoring the critical role of these cells in sustaining the skeleton's resilience and adaptability (Chyczewski et al., 2012). In contrast, osteoclasts play the bone-resorbing role, integral to the remodeling process as they resorb bone tissue in order to ensure mineral homeostasis and allow the release of calcium into the blood.

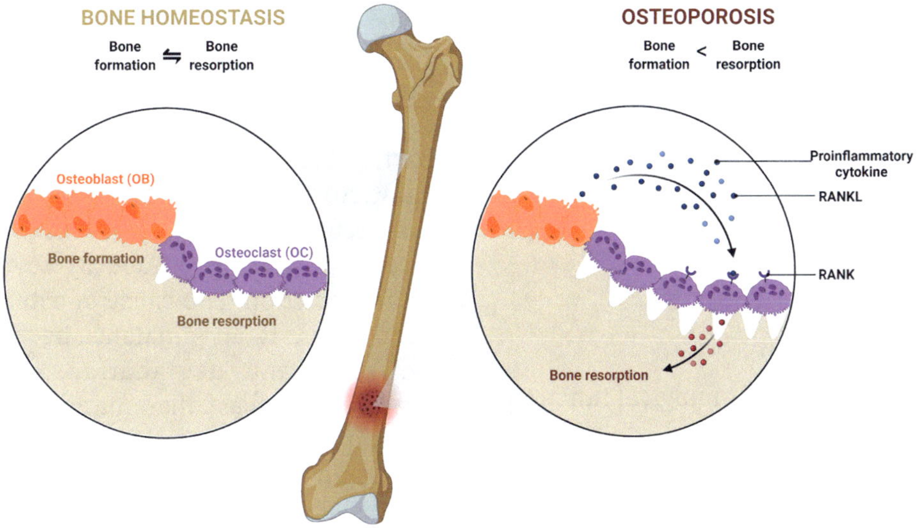

Figure 2.13. The dynamic interplay between osteoblasts and osteoclasts.

Source: https://external-content.duckduckgo.com/iu/?u=https%3A%2F%2Fwww.frontiersin.org%2Ffiles%2FArticles%2F687037%2Ffimmu-12-687037-HTML%2Fimage_m%2Ffimmu-12-687037-g001.jpg&f=1&nofb=1&ipt=fce8b950d712ca0605751704f550d4cda1212cd7dd70e2e63913269b3a2009fd.

They function by releasing acids and proteolytic enzymes to dissolve bone minerals and break down the collagenous matrix. The balance between osteoblastic activity and osteoclastic resorption is optimally regulated, and failure of this interaction is said to give rise to bone disorders such as osteoporosis, characterized by sharply declining bone density. Further, communication between these two cell types is mediated by RANK/RANKL/OPG signaling pathways, which are important for controlling osteoclast formation. Clarification of these processes is important, because they enable new therapeutic strategies to combat bone density diseases (Chyczewski et al., 2012). Experiments on osteoblast-osteoclast interactions have led to an understanding of specific pathological conditions, such as osteogenesis imperfecta (OI), a genetic disorder characterized by brittle bones. For OI type XIV, studies have shown that mutations in the TMEM38B gene alter calcium flux, significantly suppressing osteoblast differentiation and decreasing the number of osteoclasts, thereby impacting bone health and integrity. These facts place special importance on the central role that osteoblasts and osteoclasts have not just in physiological processes but also in the development of some diseases of the bones. By understanding these cellular dynamics more fully, researchers can explore targeted treatments aimed at optimizing bone formation and resorption and bringing new hope to individuals affected by bone disorders (Figure 2.13).

Test Your Knowledge

1. What is bone resorption in the process of bone remodeling?
2. What roles do osteoblasts and osteoclasts play in bone remodeling?

2.5. Bone Health and Diseases

Learning Outcome

1. Common bone disorders (e.g., osteoporosis)
2. Nutrition's impact on bone health
3. Physical activity's role in bone density

The intricate structure and biological functions of bones play critical roles in maintaining skeletal integrity and influencing the pathogenesis of many bone diseases. Bone health is characterized by a balance between bone formation and resorption, which is primarily regulated by osteoblasts and osteoclasts, respectively. Disruption of this balance can lead to degenerative diseases such as osteoporosis, in which increased resorption reduces bone density and increases fracture risk. It is important to recognize such processes, since they become viable for designing efficient prevention and treatment strategies. As an illustration, exercise that loads the bones, along with sufficient calcium and vitamin D, are pillars for robust bone health and mitigating the effects of bone loss due to aging. Furthermore, ongoing research continues to uncover novel pathways in bone metabolism, with new therapeutic modalities in the pipeline for bone diseases. Osteoarthritis is the most prevalent degenerative joint disease, particularly in older adults. Osteoarthritis is characterized by cartilage breakdown and the resulting deformity of the bone, and the disease is often preceded by severe pain and loss of function. The cause of osteoarthritis has been traced to an imbalance between cartilage synthesis and degradation, aggravated by processes such as inflammation and mechanical loading. New research shows cytokines and other biomarkers play a key role in the onset of this disease and, therefore, have potential as therapeutic targets. Understanding the underlying biological processes in osteoarthritis, as well as aiding diagnosis through imaging techniques such as X-rays, also enhances our ability to develop effective treatments aimed at preserving joint health and function over the long term (Inchai et al., 2017). In addition to common degenerative illnesses such as osteoarthritis, bone health studies include lesser-known areas of research. One of them is fetal paleopathology—a field that examines fetal skeletons in archaeological contexts. Such research is important for unearthing knowledge on maternal health and the dangerous conditions under which most pregnancies occurred in the past. Such skeletal evidence is often hard to interpret due to preservation issues and the inherent difficulties of the identification of various lesions in small bones. Despite these difficulties, fetal paleopathology is highly promising for advancing our understanding of historical health patterns and their implications for bone health today. Investigating such conditions at birth or early in life might disentangle key correlations between fetal and maternal health, thereby informing modern practice and policy for prenatal care (Lewis et al., 2017). Through an integrative approach, studies of bone disease and bone health broaden our perspective on human osteology and the complexities of skeletal health across the life course (Figure 2.14).

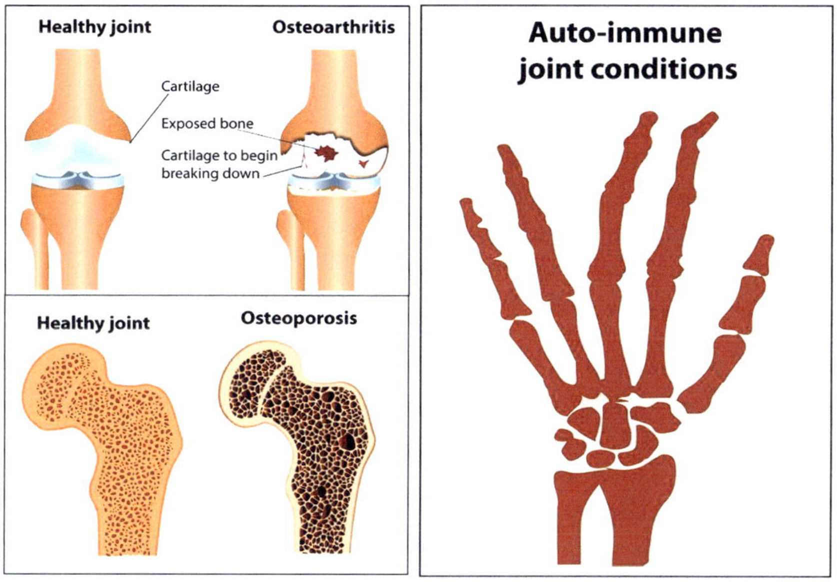

Figure 2.14. The intricate structure and biological functions of bones are critical to maintaining overall skeletal health.

Source: https://external-content.duckduckgo.com/iu/?u=https%3A%2F%2Fnizonamarineproducts.com%2Fwp-content%2Fuploads%2F2020%2F10%2Fosteoarthritis-2.jpg&f=1&nofb=1&ipt=311586c690d66e7351af6f91b03e4b1fe27313488e46b45fb965880746aab5fd.

2.5.1. Common Bone Diseases (e.g., Osteoporosis)

The intricate structure and biology of bones, vital to human biology, can be seriously affected by several bone diseases, the most prevalent being osteoporosis. Osteoporosis affects mostly post-menopausal women and elderly adults, characterized by reduced bone density that leads to an increased risk of fractures. This metabolic disorder is not merely an age-related phenomenon, but rather a result of complex interactions among genetic, hormonal, and environmental factors. The ongoing bone remodeling process, in which old bone is resorbed and replaced with new bone, becomes increasingly disrupted as factors such as reduced activity and hormonal changes impair osteoblast and osteoclast function. Understanding these complexities is crucial for developing targeted preventive and therapeutic treatments against osteoporotic fractures, thereby enhancing the quality of life in osteoporosis and shedding light on universal implications for bone health (Chyczewski et al., 2012). Evidence shows that osteoporosis lies in suboptimal bone mass and structural deterioration, leading to increased fragility. The disease typically has an insidious onset, in that it is hard to pick up early and needs extensive screening of risk factors, including diet, lifestyle choices, and genetic predisposition. For instance, proper intake of calcium and vitamin D is crucial for maintaining bone health, while an inactive lifestyle is also associated with significant bone density loss. Studies of cellular mechanisms of bone remodeling reveal that osteocytes, anchored in the bone matrix, function as sensors that respond to mechanical loading, mediating between bone resorption and formation. Physical immobilization or inactivity thus has long-term effects on bone integrity and health, reflecting the need for an integrated lifelong strategy for bone preservation (Chyczewski et al., 2012).

An integral aspect of treating osteoporosis and other bone disorders is understanding the importance of historical and epidemiological context. Understanding how individuals have conceived of osteoporosis throughout history sheds light on its etiology of multiple causes and on the value of interdisciplinarity in research. Paleopathological studies reveal that bone loss has historically been associated with age and lifestyle, providing insights into the disease's prevalence in the past and its applicability to today's populations. With the world's population trend shifting toward an aging population, osteoporosis will become ever more burdensome, thereby highlighting the necessity for better prevention, diagnosis, and treatment methods. Recognizing osteoporosis as a heterogeneous disease, influenced by extrinsic and intrinsic factors, underscores its heterogeneity and the need for further research to improve management and understanding of bone status throughout life (Curate et al., 2014) (Figure 2.15).

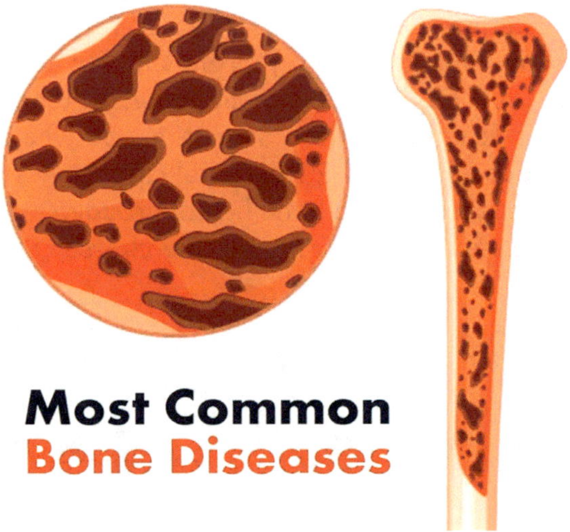

Figure 2.15. Common bone diseases (e.g., osteoporosis).

Source: https://external-content.duckduckgo.com/iu/?u=https%3A%2F%2Fi.ytimg.com%2Fvi%2FpURdRraZi1g%2Fmaxresdefault.jpg&f=1&nofb=1&ipt=25bd3fc55b8ab34cce1dca75f967f4b58d46f93f76403ad41f3c01a7e01424dd.

2.5.2. Impact of Nutrition on Bone Health

Nutrition plays a fundamental role in providing optimal bone health, influencing the structural coherence and functional capacity of bones throughout life. Functional nutrients such as calcium and vitamin D are critical; calcium is the primary mineral found in bones, while vitamin D helps its absorption. Poor intake of these foods can lead to lower bone density and increased risk of fractures, particularly in susceptible populations such as children and the elderly. Also, dietary protein, phosphorus, and magnesium intake contribute to the mineralization process and to the overall health of the skeletal system. This nutrition-nutrient interaction underscores the importance of a balanced diet not only for the prevention of bone disease but also for the promotion of lifetime musculoskeletal well-being, symbolic of the complex processes involved in bone biology and structure in human osteology. In addition to proposing essential nutrients, the context and sequence of nutrient intake can potentially affect bone remodeling mechanisms. For example, research has demonstrated that regular intake of calcium-containing foods enhances the ongoing turnover of bone tissue - an activity crucial for preserving bone strength and structure. This ongoing remodeling is maintained through a range of signaling pathways, such as the Wnt pathway, which integrates nutritional factors and mechanical load to maximize bone formation and resorption. Such a disorder in this homeostasis can lead to conditions like osteoporosis, characterized by spongy bones and an increased risk of fractures. These kinds of interactions are important to identify to formulate efficient public health policy to support bone health across different age groups, emphasizing the importance of nutrition for ensuring the functional aspects of bone biology (Chyczewski et al., 2012). Furthermore, socioeconomic status strongly influences nutritional status, thereby affecting bone health in populations. Historical research, for instance, in the post-medieval London setting, has shown a strong correlation between poverty and weakened maternal and infant skeletal structures. The interplay between poor diet, environmental factors, and health inequalities totally reshapes growth patterns and bone development in vulnerable groups. Evidence indicates that mothers with chronic dietary deficiencies are at a higher risk of giving birth to children with compromised bone structure, an outcome with long-term consequences on their bone health (Aufderheide et al., 2019). This forms the argument for joint health policies that incorporate not only nutritional intake but also broader social determinants of diet quality, thereby underscoring the role of nutrition in bone health and structure (Aufderheide et al., 2019).

2.5.3. Role of Physical Activity in Maintaining Bone Density

Maintenance of bone density throughout the life course contributes to overall skeletal health, and particularly as age advances and individuals become more susceptible to bone diseases such as osteoporosis. Physical activity is one of the main pathways by which bone density is regulated. The plasticity of bone tissue responds to mechanical stress; thus, when subjected to the stresses induced during weight-bearing exercise, bone remodeling is initiated. Remodeling involves both bone resorption and formation, which help sustain, or even increase, bone density. Cyclic resistance exercise and high-impact sport participation is able to enhance this adaptive response by allowing for greater bone mass accumulation, especially during youth and early adulthood. These results emphasize the protective function of physical activity, confirming its key role in the maintenance of skeletal health throughout the course of human life.

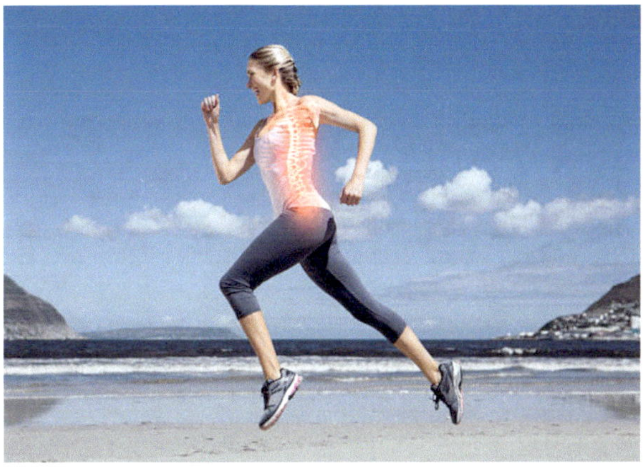

Figure 2.16. Role of physical activity in maintaining bone density.

Source: https://oaidocs.com/wp-content/uploads/2023/03/istockphoto-479572586-612x612-1.jpg.

Evidentiary research also supports the hypothesis that some types of physical activity can have differential effects on different skeletal locations.

For instance, histomorphometric analyses reveal that dynamic loading influences the microstructure of bones, such as the humerus, to a greater extent than static loading, as evidenced in medieval English children engaged in varying levels of manual labor. This implies that more active participation in physical activity leads to more robust bone microstructures, which ultimately provide benefits regarding bone density and strength. The different patterns observed between groups suggest that the quantity and form of physical activity may not only determine gross bone morphology, but also the fine organization of microstructural elements, such as osteons, necessary for the function of the bone. Beyond mere mechanical adaptation, the implications of these findings extend towards a highly evolved interaction among genetics, environmental forces, and lifestyle. Research indicates that children participating in more intense physical activities exhibit higher secondary osteon density and diameter, signifying more biomechanical loading. Surprisingly, though, development of these microstructural properties also varies according to social status and previous work patterns, as revealed in studies across different regions of England. The connection between physical activity and bone density is thus underscored by both biological and sociocultural forces, underscoring the importance of interdisciplinary approaches in demystifying bone health. By encouraging consistent physical activity across the lifespan, society can leverage these discoveries to counter the age-related reduction in bone density, thereby improving skeletal health outcomes for future generations (Figure 2.16).

Test Your Knowledge

1. What are the common bone disorders such as osteoporosis, and how do they affect bone health?
2. How does regular physical activity influence bone density and strength?

2.6. Diagnostic Techniques in Osteology

Learning Outcome

1. X-rays and their relevance
2. MRI and CT scans are employed in bone assessment
3. Bone density testing techniques

Osteology has made significant advances with the application of many diagnostic techniques that enhance our understanding of bone biology and structure. Some of the most important techniques include imaging modalities, such as high-resolution X-ray computed tomography (CT). This technique allows scientists to visualize the fine interior structure of bones in a non-invasive manner, enabling them to take precise measurements of bone quality and density. The University of Texas High-Resolution X-ray CT Facility is an example par excellence in this regard, as it provides state-of-the-art imaging technology that is absolutely critical across academic and research fields. Through the use of multimodal imaging techniques, osteologists can recognize not only macroscopic bone structures but also subtle differences in structure associated with different mechanical environments, thereby advancing understanding of bone pathology and adaptability in ancient and contemporary populations (Ahmed et al., 2017). Another significant diagnostic technique in osteology is cancellous bone analysis, which provides vital insights into mechanical and locomotor processes. Research indicates that cancellous bone is very responsive to its prevailing mechanical environment and, therefore, a superior marker for gauging locomotion in extinct organisms, such as theropod dinosaurs. Researchers are able to infer the biomechanics associated with different postures and movements by analyzing the architectural patterns in cancellous bone. For instance, refined biomechanical modeling has validated correlations between specific cancellous patterns and non-avian theropod postural adaptations, providing insight into how such animals moved and lived in their environment.

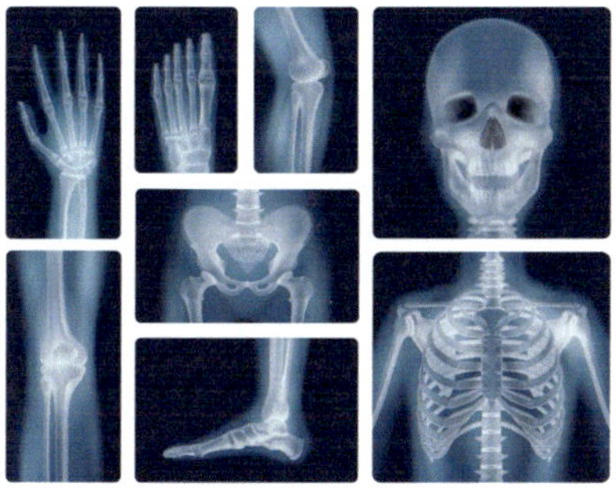

Figure 2.17. The realm of osteology has witnessed significant advancements through the implementation of various diagnostic techniques.

Source: https://www.intakelearn.com/wp-content/uploads/2023/12/6883253_29690-1024x791.webp.

These studies use finite element analysis to align principal stresses with the cancellous bone fabric, thereby offering a holistic understanding of the evolutionary formation of bone structure and its functional implications (Abourachid et al., 2018). Lastly, comparing diagnostic techniques with comparative species studies deepens insight into evolutionary processes in osteology. Techniques like electron microscopy further clarify bone microstructure, allowing scholars to compare extant species' bone quality with that of their extinct kin. Such a comparative approach not only accounts for evolutionary adaptations but also enables clinical practice to advance. As advances continue to be made in understanding how different mechanical environments impact bone form and health, the medical field benefits, enabling more effective bone disease treatments. The continued advancement of diagnostic techniques underscores the importance of interdisciplinary research in osteology, underscoring the need for scientific disciplines to collaborate to deconstruct the intricacies of bone biology and its evolutionary pathways (Ahmed et al., 2017) (Figure 2.17).

2.6.1. X-rays and Their Significance

X-rays in osteology are an important tool for diagnosis that extends beyond imaging to provide more profound understanding of bone biology and morphology. These dynamic electromagnetic waves enable imaging of bone strength and integrity and the detection of conditions such as fractures, lesions, and other bone disorders. The non-invasive nature of X-ray imaging is beneficial in clinical and laboratory settings, as it allows the study of bone characteristics without requiring surgery. Furthermore, X-rays can reveal structural complexities, which are essential to understanding the mechanical properties of bones, and can be utilized to construct treatment protocols for numerous skeletal disease entities, thus vastly enhancing patient care. Besides their clinical utility, X-rays also play an essential role in advancing our existing knowledge of bone biology through research applications. For instance, access to micro-computed tomography (microCT) has revolutionized bone microstructure analysis, enabling scientists to measure cortical porosity and canal connections in bone tissue. These are pivotal for understanding how intricate bone architecture expresses itself in mechanical strength and resilience. Recent studies employing X-ray imaging have demonstrated considerable variability in the above-mentioned parameters between patients with disease and healthy subjects, and the role of X-rays in elucidating the correlation between structural variability and biomechanical function has been emphasized (Albert et al., 2013). Such accurate information on biological variations is pivotal in developing individualized therapeutic plans for subjects with skeletal diseases. Besides, the significance of X-rays extends to veterinary and comparative bone research, advancing overall understanding of bone health in other animals. For instance, using X-ray microCT, local bone thickness and organization have been mapped at various developmental stages in domestic guinea pig studies, illustrating the alterations that occur throughout their lifespan. These findings inform us not only about species-specific fracture patterns and healing, but also about bone adaptation in different physiological regimes (Ahn et al., 2014). Comparing these findings across species allows scientists to make comparisons and draw parallels that further inform our understanding of human osteology and bone biology. Collectively, the application of X-ray technology across both clinical and research contexts makes it a significant contribution to the broader field of bone health and skeletal anatomy.

2.6.2. Magnetic Resonance Imaging (MRI) and Computed Tomography (CT) Scans in Bone Analysis

In the analysis of bone biology and structure within human osteology, the application of advanced imaging technologies like MRI and CT scans is instrumental. These modalities offer never-before-seen information about the complex bone architecture, and so anatomical as well as pathological evaluation becomes feasible. MRI is unique in that it can provide high-resolution images without ionizing radiation, making it the method of choice for assessing soft tissue structures around bones, such as cartilage and ligaments. With bone marrow edema and lesion visualization, MRI allows clinicians to identify osteomyelitis and tumors better than traditional imaging techniques. On the other hand, CT scans excel in the production of high-resolution cross-sectional bone images for assessment of bone density, fractures, and three-dimensional anatomical relationships. The precision that CT imaging provides advantages not just for pre-surgical planning but also for post-operative evaluation to follow bone healing and integration.

CT imaging has been a gold mine for anatomical research, enabling us to better understand the mechanobiological properties of bones, particularly in complex joint geometries. For instance, advances in high-resolution CT technology, such as those at the University of Texas High-Resolution X-ray CT Facility, have opened new horizons for both medical practice and scientific research in bone biology (Ahmed et al., 2017). Coupling MRI with CT scans in the field of human osteology not only enhances clinical practice but also widens educational dissemination and research capacity.

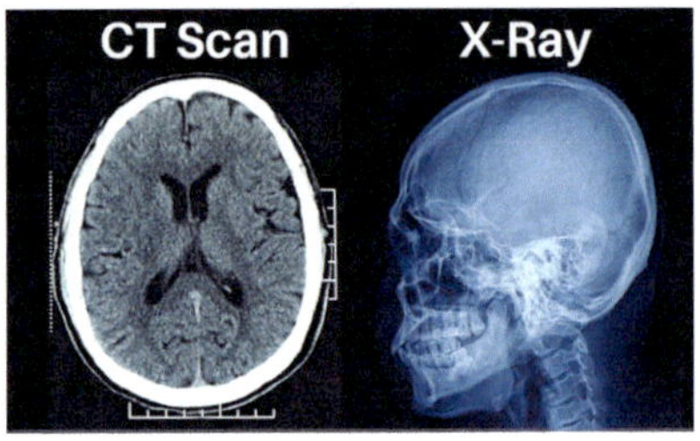

Figure 2.18. Magnetic resonance imaging (MRI) and computed tomography (CT) scans in bone analysis.

Source: https://external-content.duckduckgo.com/iu/?u=https%3A%2F%2Fkiranpetct.com%2Fwp-content%2Fuploads%2F2023%2F06%2FJobs-1200-x-720-SEO-1.jpg&f=1&nofb=1&ipt=63676487b834ba45373aaf53472a041ca0b79478892b14557a4b60ce47a1b8ea.

The high-resolution visualization capabilities of such imaging modalities enable detailed investigation of bone biomechanics and pathophysiology, which is crucial for formulating effective treatment plans. In addition, multimodal imaging approaches are now employed to leverage the strengths of both MRI and CT to offer comprehensive assessments of bone-related illnesses. With continued advances in research, understanding the implications of these imaging modalities will remain crucial for both clinical practitioners and research scientists, further illuminating the intricate interactions among factors that influence bone architecture and function (Abourachid et al., 2014) (Figure 2.18).

2.6.3. Bone Density Testing Methods

Bone mineral density tests are fundamental tools in the assessment of skeletal health, particularly the diagnosis and management of osteoporosis. The most common test is dual-energy X-ray absorptiometry (DXA), which is the precise measure of bone mineral density (BMD). The DXA technique employs two X-ray beams of different intensities to measure the bone density, especially in the femoral neck and lumbar spine, which are common sites for fractures. The method, which is painless, has revolutionized how practitioners assess fracture risk and manage osteoporosis. By providing a quantitative measure of BMD, DXA significantly enhances the ability to make an early diagnosis of osteoporosis and to initiate early treatment, with the potential to reduce fracture risk from the disease. In addition to DXA, quantitative computed tomography (QCT) has emerged as a valuable tool for bone density assessment. Unlike DXA, QCT can produce three-dimensional images of bone that enable more precise evaluation of bone architecture and differentiation between cortical and trabecular bone densities. Visualization of bone architecture offers advantages in identifying patient-specific fracture risk and in assessing bone mechanical properties. As described in the current work, the cancellous bone's architectural patterns can be used to make inferences about locomotor biomechanics, highlighting the significance of bone density assessment techniques not just in osteoporosis diagnosis but in inferential biomechanics in a broad variety of animals, including humans and theropod dinosaurs. The implementation of imaging technologies, such as QCT, in daily clinical practice may ultimately lead to more personalized treatment and the prevention of bone disease (Aamodt et al., 2018). Technologies such as high-resolution peripheral quantitative computed tomography (HR-pQCT) are the future of bone density measurement. HR-pQCT provides high-resolution images that enable detailed scanning of bone microarchitecture, allowing bone tissue quality and quantity to be analyzed in parallel. This is extremely useful when assessing treatments intended to strengthen bone structure and density, such as those for osteoporosis. Furthermore, studies have revealed that combining different imaging modalities can give an even more comprehensive view of the bone health of a person, in addition to traditional methods like DXA and QCT. The future of bone densitometry lies in the integration of multiple imaging technologies with robust biomechanical models, which will facilitate a deeper understanding of bone biology and structure. This incorporation not only supports the diagnostic capability but also therapeutic methodologies in the field of human osteology (Ahmed et al., 2017).

Test Your Knowledge

1. How are X-rays used in osteology, and why are they important for bone assessment?
2. How are MRI and CT scans employed to evaluate bone structure and pathology?

SUMMARY

In the investigation of bone structure and biology in human osteology, it is critical to appreciate the complex relationship between bone development and its biology. The evolution of ossified frameworks, such as the supraspinous ligaments found across species, indicates the flexibility of bone under mechanical stress. This is evident in the case of sauropod dinosaurs, where the supraspinous ossified rods have been highlighted by the evidence. The evolutionary importance of bone is noted to concern structural integrity and functional resilience. Further, examining the histological record of such structures reveals the intricate interactions among different bone tissue types in shaping total biomechanical performance. This data not only augments our understanding of the developmental processes underlying the evolution of bones but also aids modern studies of human osteology by providing comparative data on the evolution and adaptation of the human skeletal system. Furthermore, the recovery and analysis of disarticulated human remains call for a multidisciplinary approach in forensic practice. The complexity of handling such remains, particularly in biological profile identification, underscores the importance of bone architecture in forensic science. Bone structure poses problems for forensic professionals when skeletal remains are in fragments, like the recent instances involving legs and feet on beaches. The utility of accurate anatomical information may be appreciated, as each skeletal piece can convey individualized information about the biological identity of the individual. Increasing awareness of the skeletal features useful for human identification, as exemplified by the limited body of literature on the foot, underscores the need for more research and training in forensic osteology. This is consistent with the overall theme of bone in inferring human identity and biology. In general, bone biology and structure are a central subject in both biological and forensic studies. By integrating anthropological and forensic methods, the interaction between bone function and identification processes reveals the diversity of human skeletons and enables an inclusive understanding of human development and identity. With studies continuing daily, integrating viewpoints across departments will assuredly support practices used in the identification of remains and in understanding skeletal evolution. Last but not least, stimulating collaboration throughout the scientific community will pave the way for innovative research that honors both the complexity of bone biology and the practical necessities emerging in the science of human osteology, and for more effective identification and storage of human remains in forensic investigation.

The study of bone structure and biology in human osteology provides a basic foundation for interpreting the health and disease of the skeleton. Among the aspects of this study is the role of intervertebral cartilage, which plays a critical role in establishing the overall biomechanics of the vertebral column. Recent studies indicate that cartilage thickness and form vary widely across species, suggesting differences in mobility and posture. In the study of sauropods, for instance, intervertebral cartilage is stated to assist in maintaining an upright position of the neck that would not have been so valued without considering such anatomical considerations. Such an understanding relates to the function of cartilage in facilitating not only structural stability but also biomechanical function under load, as well as broadening our knowledge of vertebrate evolution and gait (Christian et al., 2013). The second essential factor integrates cancellous bone structure and its use to locomotor biomechanics. Cancellous or spongy bone is sensitive to mechanical stress, leading to dynamic responses that vary across species. This sensitivity allows one to infer locomotor patterns and indicates the variation in bone structure between extinct and extant taxa. For example, studies of theropod dinosaurs have revealed cancellous structures similar to those of humans, while avian birds exhibit adaptations related to their locomotor needs. Through the use of advanced imaging and analysis, these architectural patterns are offering significant knowledge of the trends in locomotion evolution, paving the way to more research into the factors of the musculoskeletal system that make up movement (Aamodt et al., 2018). Besides, bone structure knowledge also includes its application in clinical settings and the design of therapeutic interventions. Detection of variations in cancellous bone architecture can aid in forecasting fracture risk and the efficacy of certain medical interventions across populations. For instance, aging populations exhibit alterations in bone architecture and density, highlighting the need for a comprehensive view of bone biology in medicine. By putting together findings of work with both cancellous bone and cartilage with broader osteological systems, researchers can develop diagnostic and treatment techniques more proficiently and thus improve outcomes in the treatment of diseases of the skeleton. This connection between form and function underscores once more the fundamental role of bone biology in addressing both evolutionary questions and contemporary medical concerns.

KEY TERMS FROM THIS CHAPTER

- Bone Matrix
- Bone Remodeling
- Canaliculi
- Endochondral Ossification
- Haversian Canal
- Intramembranous Ossification
- Lamellar Bone
- Bone Mineral Density (BMD)
- Bone Resorption
- Collagen Fibers
- Epiphyseal Plate
- Hydroxyapatite
- Lacunae
- Osteoclasts

CRITICAL THINKING QUESTIONS

1. **What is the bone cell involved in resorption of bone?**
   a. Osteoblast
   b. Osteocyte
   c. Osteoclast
   d. Chondrocyte
2. **What is the principal organic component of the bone matrix?**
   a. Hydroxyapatite
   b. Collagen
   c. Calcium phosphate
   d. Magnesium
3. **What is the elementary building unit and functional unit of compact bone?**
   a. Trabecula
   b. Osteon
   c. Lacuna
   d. Canaliculus
4. **What is the primary work of the periosteum?**
   a. Mineral storage
   b. Repair of bone and growth
   c. Storage of fat
   d. Lubrication of joints
5. **Which mineral contributes most to bone mineralization?**
   a. Sodium
   b. Magnesium
   c. Calcium
   d. Iron

Short Answer Questions

1. What are the principal components of bone tissue, and how do they contribute to its strength and elasticity?
2. Describe how periosteum and endosteum contribute to health and healing of bones.
3. How is bone remodeling accomplished, and what regulates the process?
4. Describe the structural organization of an osteon in compact bone.
5. How is bone mineralization accomplished? What minerals are involved?
6. Describe the roles of hormones like parathyroid hormone (PTH), calcitonin, and vitamin D in regulating bone metabolism.

Answers to Critical Thinking Questions

1. (c); 2. (b); 3. (b) 4. (b); 5. (c)

REFERENCES

1. Bishop, P. J., Hocknull, S. A., Clemente, C. J., Hutchinson, J. R., Farke, A. A., Beck, B. R., Barrett, R. S., & Lloyd, D. G. (2018). Cancellous bone and theropod dinosaur locomotion. Part I—an examination of cancellous bone architecture in the hindlimb bones of theropods. *PeerJ*, *6*, e5778. https://doi.org/10.7717/peerj.5778Abdala, A., Abdala, A., Adams, A., Allin, E. F., Allin, C., Anthwal, N., Barghusen, H., et al. (2016). Morphological evolution of the mammalian jaw adductor complex. https://core.ac.uk/download/151161615.pdf (accessed on 18th July 2025).
2. Abdalla, O., Abdel Meguid, E. M., Barreto, C., Bonaparte, J. F., Bonaparte, J. F., Campos, D., Casal, G. A., et al. (2015). Histological evidence for a supraspinous ligament in sauropod dinosaurs. https://core.ac.uk/download/159287253.pdf (accessed on 18th July 2025).
3. Abourachid, A., Alexander, R. M., Allen, P. W., Allmendinger, C., Attene, F., Bakker, R. T., et al. (2018). Cancellous bone and theropod dinosaur locomotion. Part III—Inferring posture and locomotor biomechanics in extinct theropods, and its evolution on the line to birds. https://core.ac.uk/download/161818791.pdf (accessed on 18th July 2025).
4. Abourachid, A., Barnett, B., Bezuidenhout, C., Carter, C., Carter, R., et al. (2014). Three-dimensional anatomy of the ostrich (*Struthio camelus*) knee joint. https://core.ac.uk/download/36778017.pdf (accessed on 18th July 2025).
5. Abzhanov, A., Abzhanov, A., Abzhanov, A., Baggiolini, A., Baroffio, A., Beverdam, A., Chevallier, A., et al. (2019). Molecular and cellular mechanisms underlying the evolution of form and function in the amniote jaw. https://core.ac.uk/download/323079229.pdf (accessed on 18th July 2025).
6. Adams, C., Challands, T., Liston, J., et al. (2013). Growth, age, and size of the Jurassic pachycormid *Leedsichthys problematicus* (Osteichthyes: Actinopterygii). https://core.ac.uk/download/16460317.pdf (accessed on 18th July 2025).
7. Agnew, A. M., Al Qahtani, S. J., Anderson, T., Bennike, P., Ben-Amos, I., Britz, H. M., Burger, E. H., et al. (2019). Bone histomorphometry measures of physical activity in children from Medieval England. https://core.ac.uk/download/200153050.pdf (accessed on 18th July 2025).
8. Ahmed, F., & Maisano, J. (2017). ToScA North America (6–8 June 2017, The University of Texas, Austin, TX) Program. https://core.ac.uk/download/211334283.pdf (accessed on 18th July 2025).
9. Ahn, B., Bendele, B., Bialek, B., Bilezikian, J. P., Burnie, S., Candela, A., et al. (2014). Computed tomography analysis of guinea pig bone: Architecture, bone thickness, and dimensions throughout development. https://core.ac.uk/download/33574222.pdf (accessed on 18th July 2025).
10. Albert, C., Busse, B., Harris, G. F., Jameson, C., et al. (2013). 3D micron-scale imaging of the cortical bone canal network in human osteogenesis imperfecta (OI). https://core.ac.uk/download/213084385.pdf (accessed on 18th July 2025).
11. Alsaedi, A., Balasubramanian, M., Cabral, W. A., Cole, W. S., et al. (2017). Phenotypic spectrum in osteogenesis imperfecta due to mutations in TMEM38B: Unravelling a complex cellular defect. https://core.ac.uk/download/80840751.pdf (accessed on 18th July 2025).
12. Amling, M., Busse, B., Chushkin, Y., et al. (2019). Mechanical competence and bone quality develop during skeletal growth. https://core.ac.uk/download/286362743.pdf (accessed on 18th July 2025).

13. Arregui Dalmases, C., Galtés Vicente, I., Malgosa, A., Medallo-Muñiz, C., et al. (2017). New insights in the analysis of blunt force trauma in human bones. Preliminary results. https://core.ac.uk/download/132528495.pdf (accessed on 18th July 2025).

14. Barrett, B., Bidmos, M. A., Bidmos, F. A., Bidmos, R. A., Bilge, M., British Broadcasting Corporation, British Broadcasting Corporation, et al. (2014). The foot in forensic human identification–A review. https://core.ac.uk/download/30660095.pdf (accessed on 18th July 2025).

15. Benjamin, M., Camp, C. L., Castanet, J., Cope, E. D., Gauthier, J. A., Haines, R. W., Haines, R. W., et al. (2016). Anatomy, morphology, and evolution of the patella in squamate lizards and tuatara (*Sphenodon punctatus*). https://core.ac.uk/download/36779107.pdf (accessed on 18th July 2025).

16. Brouchoud, J. E. (2016). The effects of thermal alteration on saw mark characteristics. https://open.bu.edu/bitstream/2144/15348/1/Brouchoud_bu_0017N_10790.pdf (accessed on 18th July 2025).

17. Brun, K. (2016). The utility of histomorphometries in distinguishing between human and non-human rib bone: Osteon area, perimeter, and circularity. https://open.bu.edu/bitstream/2144/16028/1/Brun_bu_0017N_11052.pdf (accessed on 18th July 2025).

18. Buckberry, J. (2015). The (mis)use of adult age estimates in osteology. https://core.ac.uk/download/76945106.pdf (accessed on 18th July 2025).

19. Christian, A., Hultgren, B. D., Emerson, C. L., Holliday, C. M., Gilmore, C. W., Schwarz, D., Frey, E., et al. (2013). The effect of intervertebral cartilage on neutral posture and range of motion in the necks of sauropod dinosaurs. https://core.ac.uk/download/29026918.pdf (accessed on 18th July 2025).

20. Chyczewski, L., Kowalewska, J., Mackiewicz, Z., et al. (2012). Bone as a source of organism vitality and regeneration. https://core.ac.uk/download/268436446.pdf (accessed on 18th July 2025).

21. Curate, F. (2014). Osteoporosis and paleopathology: A review. https://core.ac.uk/download/pdf/151538188.pdf (accessed on 18th July 2025).

22. Gamble, J. A., & Gilmour, R. J. (2024). Bones at home supporting haptic learning and universal design beyond the biological anthropology laboratory. https://core.ac.uk/download/644028705.pdf (accessed on 18th July 2025).

23. Inchai, C., & Mahakkanukrauh, P. (2017). Biological markers associated with osteoarthritis. https://core.ac.uk/download/159613126.pdf (accessed on 18th July 2025).

24. Inthasan, C., & Mahakkanukrauh, P. (2017). Age estimation from clavicle by histomorphometry method: A review. https://core.ac.uk/download/159613125.pdf (accessed on 18th July 2025).

25. Lewis, M. (2017). Fetal paleopathology: An impossible discipline? https://core.ac.uk/download/42153730.pdf (accessed on 18th July 2025).

SKELETAL DEVELOPMENT AND ONTOGENY

3

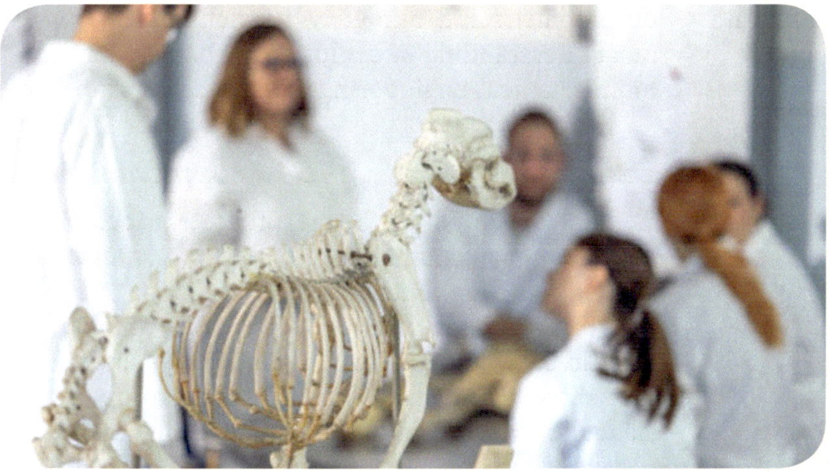

LEARNING OBJECTIVES

After studying this chapter, you will be able to:

1. Describe the basic anatomy of bonesDiscuss embryonic development of the skeleton
2. Highlight ossification processes
3. Understand bone maturation and growth
4. Highlight variations and abnormalities in the skeleton
5. Know physical activity and skeletal health

Introduction

The study of skeletal ontogeny and development is a multifaceted understanding of how skeletal structures emerge and develop throughout an organism's lifespan. Such medicine and veterinary science, where understanding of skeletal abnormalities can significantly impact therapy and care. Ontogeny is the developmental phase of an organism, through which the organism undergoes a series of developmental phases marked by specific morphological and physiological developments dictated by genetic determinants and environmental conditions. Hence, understanding skeletal development offers insight into the flexibility and robustness of different species, which are dictated by the complex interactions between genetic blueprints and developmental pathways. For example, the understanding of vertebral malformations offers a compelling case study in skeletal development. Recent studies have identified a number of anomalies, such as haemal vertebral compression and fusion (haemal VCF), which weaken the structural integrity of the vertebral column in certain aquatic animals. The term haemal

VCF indicates that developmental disruptions in early developmental phases result in profound morphological alterations that are typically not amenable to reversal upon reaching maturity. The results indicated that the frequency of such malformations reduces with age, and this could suggest a potential connection between early developmental challenges and subsequent levels of mortality. Such a note on the pathogenesis of skeletal malformations gives us better insight into evolutionary adaptation and indicates vulnerabilities in organismal development (Georgiou et al., 2013).

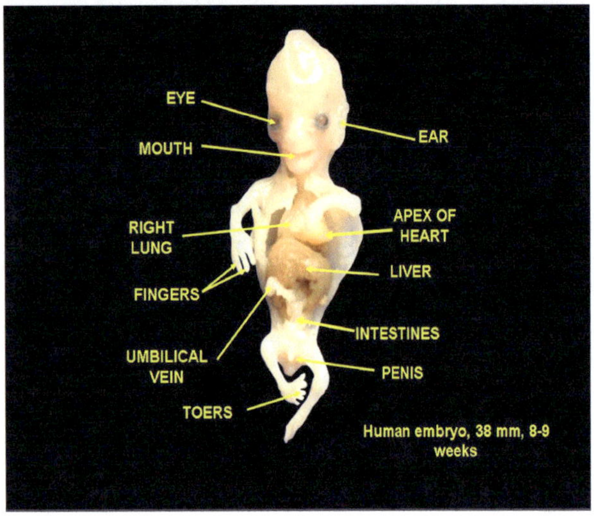

Figure 3.1. The study of skeletal development and ontogeny.

Source: https://upload.wikimedia.org/wikipedia/commons/thumb/c/c6/Human_embryo_8_weeks_2.JPG/960px-Human_embryo_8_weeks_2.JPG.

Similarly, avian groups, especially emus, exemplify the intricate dynamics between expansion and skeletal configuration. Emus possess remarkable growth rates, accumulating considerable mass from hatch to adulthood while still obtaining functional locomotion. Such growth is accompanied by changes in the physical properties of muscle and tendon that develop in accordance with allometric principles. The data indicate that in adult emus, muscle physiological cross-sectional area (PCSA) and tendon dimensions exhibit significant positive allometry, reflecting enhanced force production and capability. Understanding these ontogenetic trends not only informs us about the adaptations required for effective locomotion but also serves as a model for investigating rapid-growth biomechanics across other species (Abourachid et al., 2014). These investigations are particularly useful within the broader context of skeletal development and ontogeny, further informing our understanding of evolutionary biology and biomechanical engineering (Figure 3.1).

Definition of Skeletal Development

Skeletal development is the intricate process by which organisms develop their skeletal systems throughout various stages of life. The term implies constant interaction among genetic, environmental, and evolutionary factors that shape the formation and differentiation of skeletal tissues. Essentially, skeletal formation is regulated by a cascade of developmental events, beginning with embryonic development and continuing through to adult morphogenesis. During embryonic development, cells divide and differentiate along specific pathways to give rise to precursors of bone and cartilage, which will continue to form the adult skeleton. Understanding these processes is vital to understanding how the form of the skeleton relates to function and stability within the adult organism, particularly in the context of adaptations across various ecological niches. In echinoderms such as sea urchins, skeleton development exhibits an astonishing degree of sophistication, demonstrating the evolutionary significance of such processes. The micromere lineage of sea urchin embryos is predestined to provide the organism's skeleton before the onset of gastrulation. This early specification refers to the evolutionary innovation that led to the development of a biomineralized skeleton, essential for structural support in the organism.

The gene regulatory network (GRN) controlling this development has been established in detail and reveals that many differentiation genes in embryonic development are also important during adult skeletal development. As mentioned in recent reports, there is a clear difference in the regulatory pathways that govern these developmental phases, demonstrating that, whereas some genetic pathways have been conserved, others have diverged, and this is a manifestation of adaptation over evolutionary time (Arenas-Mena et al., 2008).

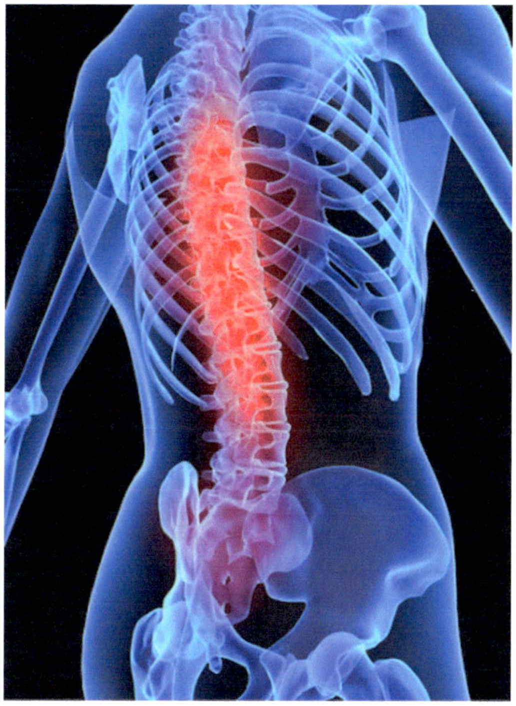

Figure 3.2. The term skeletal development encompasses the intricate process.

Source: https://lh4.googleusercontent.com/proxy/GffoCqYsupA4VgGaEU18gx5btWdJZPfQQqiJwDzcLsl-KAZLt6suWjFcKJmPLAZEKTTqlakU40GupmuGZ_0Us2KXwmXHtkH9pyzkbqzQ4GJFiznKRYXt.

In addition to the structural intricacies inherent in skeletal development, ontogenetic diversity in skeletal morphology also informs us about the evolutionary processes within species. For instance, research on the damselfish genus Dascyllus indicates major changes in morphology during ontogeny, especially in cranial and jaw structures across different body sizes. The chapter refutes the hypermorphosis hypothesis and speculates that giant species, rather than simply extending allometric trends in small species, exhibit unique allometric variations characterized by lateral transpositions. These facts are paradigms of how skeletal development and secondary adaptations are not caused solely by genetic forces but are also profoundly influenced by ecological pressures and functional demands (Frédérich et al., 2010). This holistic view of skeletal development as a developmental and evolutionary process is the door to understanding the complexity of vertebrate and invertebrate body forms (Figure 3.2).

Importance of Studying Ontogeny

The significance of ontogeny study is that it can uncover the dynamic mechanisms that control skeletal development. Understanding the stages of ontogeny provides insight into how organisms develop their adult form through intricate biological mechanisms. From embryonic development to adulthood, studying the formation of skeletal parts provides researchers with better insight into cell interactions and the impact of gene expression on anatomy. Moreover, ontogeny represents a system in which to study anomalies and developmental disease, possibly incurred by skeletal integrity. This analogy of normal to abnormal developmental events is particularly relevant to the areas of evolutionary biology and medicine, wherein this understanding may inform therapeutic modalities and interventions aimed toward restoring function or compensating for defects in skeletal form. Also, ontogeny provides an important system for studying the interplay between genetics and environment. Each developmental stage responds to both internal genetic pressures and external environmental signals in ways that illustrate how these components work together to adapt over time. As illustrated in the broiler chicken research, musculoskeletal health variability across developing stages can have important welfare and productivity consequences within farms. For instance, alterations in muscle structure and bone form, as reflected in the leg disorders noted, indicate the challenge posed by selection schemes. These regimens prioritize the growth rate at the expense of bone strength, putting emphasis on the necessity for ongoing inquiry into ontogeny in order to develop methods that weigh productivity against considerations of health. This type of research underscores the need for a comprehensive understanding of developmental processes to reduce issues in stock control and enhance animal welfare, in direct harmony with the principles of ontogeny.

Lastly, exploring ontogeny can also inform our understanding of evolutionary processes. By observing the development of skeletal systems across generations, scientists can identify selective forces that shape anatomical components with consequences for locomotion and agility. The effect of homeostasis across generations, as in developmental physiology, indicates that the organism's adaptive mechanisms become stabilized in its skeletal system (Torday et al., 2015). It is only by understanding these fundamental correlations that it is possible to decipher the evolutionary history of species, which reveals how specific traits have been sustained or modified in response to their environment. Repeated examination of ontogenetic changes, such as the growth of broiler chicken skeletons, shows the significance of timing and order in evolutionary modifications (Codd et al., 2014). This broad perspective reinstates the ontogeny-centered character of biological science as an integrating doctrine, uniting development, health, and evolutionary theory.

3.1. The Basics of Skeletal Anatomy

Learning Outcome

1. Structure of bones in the human skeleton
2. Principal functions of the skeletal system
3. Overview of bone make-up and anatomy

The human skeletal system is a fundamental body structure composed of 206 separate bones, grouped into two large categories: the appendicular skeleton and the axial skeleton. The axial skeleton, which makes up the skull, vertebral column, and rib cage, primarily provides support and protection for vital organs, except those of the cranial and thoracic cavities. On the other hand, the appendicular skeleton comprises the pelvic girdle and limbs, which are critical in supporting locomotion as well as body stabilization. It is worth comprehending this intricate arrangement because deviations from skeletal anatomy have a direct bearing on biomechanics, posture, and health. Interestingly, the structure of bones, e.g., their mineral composition and microstructure, directly correlates with their functional properties, underscoring the importance of additional research on the complexity of skeletal anatomy to elucidate its influence on development and throughout the human life course. Skeletal development, or ontogeny, is closely tied to the interaction of environmental, molecular, and genetic factors that shape bone formation and development. Mesenchymal stem cells are differentiated into osteoblasts and chondrocytes in embryonic development and form the foundation for cartilage and bone formation. Cartilaginous models formed early in development will subsequently ossify to form hard bone via processes such as endochondral ossification. Spatial and temporal skeletal patterns of development are also controlled by signaling molecules and transcription factors, dictating how skeletal elements form and adapt to functional demands. This complexity is all the more evident when considering cranial base synchondroses, whose functions as growth centers of the craniofacial skeleton underscore the possibility that abnormalities can cause a wide range of developmental conditions influencing overall skull morphology (Cendekiawan et al., 2010).

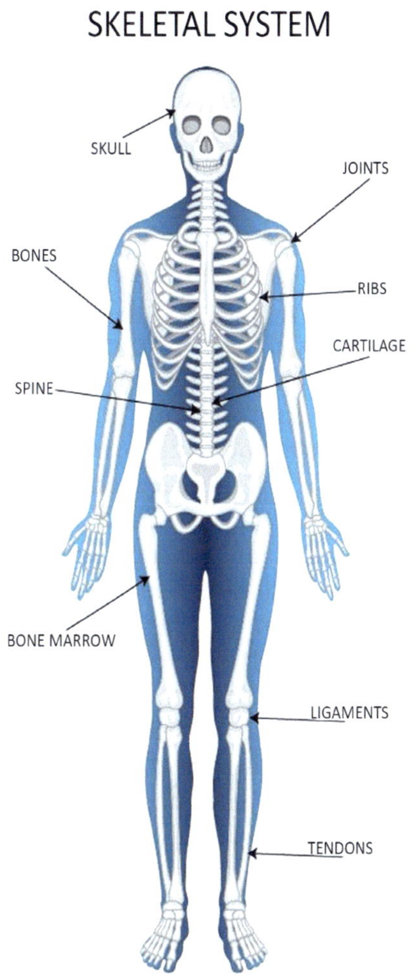

Figure 3.3. The human skeletal system serves as a fundamental framework for the body.

Source: https://ausoma.org/wp-content/uploads/2025/01/anatomy-and-physiology-skeletal-system.jpg.

In addition, skeletal system history reveals adaptive and functional diversity among species, particularly in the amniote jaw complex, a testament to the strong evolutionary forces that have shaped skeletal morphology. Jaw structure is a crucial evolutionary innovation that has enabled diverse feeding strategies to achieve survival and species diversification. Cranial neural crest mesenchyme plays a central role in jaw development with genetic and biomechanical regulation of craniofacial patterns (Abzhanov et al., 2019). These accounts of the adaptive basis of skeletal structure not only provide a framework for explaining species-specific variation but also emphasize the importance of recognizing how molecular and cellular mechanisms can lead to innovation in jaw architecture as well as to defects. Thus, research in skeletal anatomy is still in the process of exploring the complexities behind ontogeny and its applications in evolutionary biology and medicine (Figure 3.3).

3.1.1. Types of Bones in the Human Skeleton

The human skeleton is made up of different, distinct types of bones with specific structural and functional roles. Functionally classified, bones are categorized into four main categories: long bones, short bones, flat bones, and irregular bones. Long bones, such as the femur and humerus, are slender and elongated and are used for moving and supporting weight. They consist of a diaphysis, metaphysis, and epiphysis and are not only used for leverage during movement but also house bone marrow, where hematopoiesis occurs. Conversely, short bones, such as the carpals and tarsals, are typically cube-shaped and provide stability and support while allowing limited movement. Understanding these types is critical for examining how bone structure forms and alters during ontogeny, with implications for overall skeletal health and function. Flat bones, such as the sternum, ribs, and skull plates, are important defenders and muscle attachment points. Their flat, thin structure optimizes surface area, providing a robust but effective barrier against outside forces and supporting the muscles needed in respiratory and postural functions. Flat bones are developed through a process known as intramembranous ossification, in which mesenchymal cells transform directly into bone tissue, an important component of skull development in early periods in life. The irregular bones, e.g., the vertebrae and pelvic bones, possess complex shapes in agreement with the specific functions of support, protection of nerve function, and encasement of organs. Each is created by unique developmental processes, revealing the intricacy of skeletal ontogeny, answering to biological and biomechanical demands during the course of an individual's life.

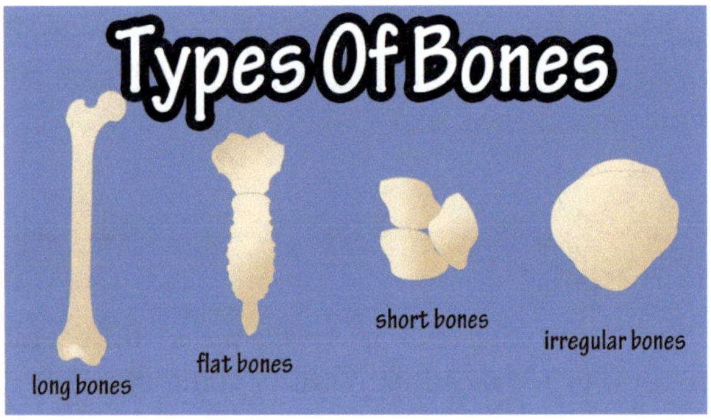

Figure 3.4. The human skeleton comprises several distinct types of bones.

Source: https://i.ytimg.com/vi/vDjW00S29l0/maxresdefault.jpg.

The structural diversity of the human skeleton demonstrates the evolutionary context of bone types, shaping their formation and adaptation. For example, cranial neural crest mesenchyme (NCM) is essential in the ontogeny of jaw bones and skull bones, controlling how these bones exhibit species-specific patterns (Abzhanov et al., 2019). Such a differentiation is a trade-off between adaptability and stability, significant for fitness during evolution. Further, adaptation of musculoskeletal systems can be seen in conditions involving genetic and environmental factors, as exemplified in cases such as broiler chickens, where anatomical adaptations influence function and movement patterns despite the absence of overt deficits (Codd et al., 2014). Incorporating bone type development with extrinsic pressures provides profound insights into the evolutionary foundation of skeletal morphology and function (Figure 3.4).

3.1.2. Major Functions of the Skeletal System

The skeletal system is the basic framework of the body, supporting and shaping the entire body structure. On a functional level, it supports the soft tissues and organs and maintains the body's shape. The body would lack the stability to stand upright or perform activities such as walking and running were it not for a rigid framework. Also, bones have attachment sites for muscles, facilitating movement through leverage. This is vital not only for basic locomotion but also for complex motor activities with coordination and force. Lastly, the skeletal system's ability to provide structural support has implications for mobility and physical functioning in individuals and therefore plays a significant role in general existence as well as in particular sporting activities. Apart from its structural function, the skeletal system plays a crucial role in protecting vital organs. The skull protects the brain from injuries, and the rib cage shields the lungs and heart from injuries from the outside. This protective role is critical, as damage to these organs can be lethal. In addition, the vertebral column shields the spinal cord, a main passageway for body neural impulses. Through further improvement in the skeleton, protective elements are enhanced in response to the needs of greater stability and defense against environmental stresses. Every anatomical adaptation is an evolutionary adaptation that enhances the survival potential of the organism by minimizing the risk of injury and thus demonstrates the dynamic role of the skeletal system to keep the individual healthy. Finally, the skeletal system contributes to hematopoiesis, the development of blood cells. Within the bone marrow present within certain bones, stem cells grow and form blood cells of all the various types, including red blood cells, white blood cells, and platelets. Not only does this keep the body's cellular products stable, but it also plays a central role in the immune system and overall health. Skeletal defects can predispose an individual to various hematologic disorders, underscoring the interrelationship between skeletal and overall well-being. The ontogeny of bone formation is the focus of the research into the development of skeletal systems, highlighting how bodily transformation affects such hemopoietic activities at various stages of life, as seen in cases like those presented in broiler chicken, whereby musculoskeletal well-being has a direct effect on locomotion as well as general biological function (Codd et al., 2014; Heers et al., 2018).

3.1.3. Overview of Bone Structure and Composition

Bone's intricate structure is a requirement for its purpose, offering tensile strength as well as elasticity. Bone is made up predominantly of a matrix of collagen fibers suspended in a mineralized environment, chiefly hydroxyapatite, a crystalline calcium phosphate. This composite structure allows the bones to withstand any forces while still being elastic. Osteocytes, osteoblasts, and osteoclasts are the primary cellular components responsible for bone construction, upkeep, and repair. Osteoblasts produce the bone matrix, while osteoclasts break down bone, so the bone material is in agreement with physiological needs and physical stress. It is critical to appreciate the microarchitecture of bone, both its trabecular (spongy) and cortical (compact) components, to grasp its response to mechanical loads during ontogeny, affecting growth and development from juvenile through adult. Continuing in the growth of the skeleton sees both the composition and the organizational structure of bone undergo radical alterations. This dynamism is particularly evident during phases of rapid growth, when the interaction between osteoblast activity and mineralization is the determining factor. That of growth factors and endocrine hormones, such as parathyroid hormone and calcitonin, becomes central in modulating these processes, directly affecting bone density and integrity. The differentiation of the bone structure also mirrors the plasticity of the skeleton, for instance, the transformation of cartilage to ossified bone is a critical phase in skeletal ontogeny.

A process like this relies on mechanical stress, as illustrated by changes in bone density under different loading conditions. The ability of bones to remodel to meet environmental demands is an evolutionary advantage that provides optimization of form and function throughout the life of an organism, for instance, the development that happens with the evolution of complicated facial and jaw structures in primates, which have evolutionary trends in skeletal development, particularly concerning expression and communication (Goswami et al., 2018).

In examining bone ontogeny, one must also deal with the applicability of anatomical development to locomotor function and overall functionality. For instance, in bird forms, the ontogeny of the pectoral limb demonstrates the convergence of skeletal form and locomotor activity. Experiments on developing birds have found that young organisms possess an excess of muscular potential, which is intricately involved in developing skeletal form. This interaction can take many forms, such as wing-assisted incline running (WAIR), which juveniles use long before they have fully attained flight. This kind of research informs us about how bone and musculature evolution are associated with movement adaptation, thereby placing a direct link between skeletal development and functional implications. The conclusions of these studies not only teach the biomechanics of living animals but also educate a paradigm of understanding the evolutionary pathways of extinct groups, such as theropod dinosaurs, and their locomotor adaptations (Heers et al., 2018) (Figure 3.5).

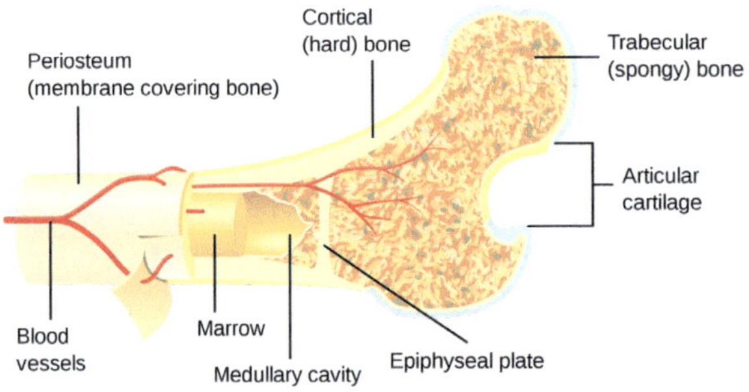

Figure 3.5. The intricate structure of bone is essential to its function.

Source: https://external-content.duckduckgo.com/iu/?u=https%3A%2F%2Fhumanbiology.pressbooks.tru.ca%2Fwp-content%2Fuploads%2Fsites%2F6%2F2019%2F06%2FBone_cross-section.svg_.png&f=1&nofb=1&ipt=050dec99f9a656fe7fdedb4a6ddc2df5d7dbd254ef0a8016dafd5b8089d13d63.

Test Your Knowledge

1. What is the basic structure of bones in the human skeletal system?
2. What are the principal functions of the skeletal system?

3.2. Embryonic Development of the Skeleton

Learning Outcome

1. Phases of embryonic development
2. Role of mesenchymal cells in bone formation
3. Genetic control over bone development

Formation of the embryonic skeleton is a complex process that occurs through several well-organized steps involving cellular differentiation, signal transduction, and structural formation. This formation begins with the production of mesodermal and neural crest cells, which are the progenitors of the skeletal framework. The progenitor cells undergo lineage differentiation to produce cartilage and bone. As embryonic development proceeds, cell-type-specific molecular signal-mediated interactions define the morphogenesis and growth of skeletal elements. Such early developmental phases provide insights into key windows when intervention could enhance skeletal integrity and health, especially in aquaculture, where high juvenile survival is essential to industry sustainability. Ideally, skeletal muscle ontogeny should be included because it is in a two-way relationship with the development of bony tissues, an aspect that largely determines aggregate juvenile quality and viability (Alami-Durante et al., 2013). During embryonic development, skeletal components undergo established phases of patterning and differentiation that ultimately give rise to the mature skeleton. It begins with the creation of the cartilaginous template, which serves as a scaffold for subsequent ossification. Throughout this phase, cranial neural crest mesenchyme is particularly important; its migration and incorporation into the template influence the production of craniofacial structures. Signaling pathways that regulate these events are most important in specifying proper anatomical identity and functional characteristics of bones. For instance, disruptions in molecular pathways can cause malformations, highlighting the fine balance that must be maintained during development. Understanding such mechanisms not only contributes to our fundamental vertebrate biology but also sheds light on potential evolutionary adaptations as variation arising in this intricate process might contribute to variability of body shapes within species, as elaborated upon through the study of jaw evolution in amniotes (Abzhanov et al., 2019). As embryonic skeletal development research continues to advance, increasingly it is apparent that environmental factors play a significant role in shaping developmental outcomes. For instance, nutritional issues and sensory stimulation may significantly impact the development and health of skeletal components during sensitive periods. In aquaculture, it is essential to determine the optimum nutritional regimes during larval stages to ensure maximum survival and growth potential. Moreover, taking an active account of the role biomechanical forces play can offer a clue to adaptive evolution between species. Such dynamics highlight the complexities of skeletal development and underscore the need to take a holistic view of both intrinsic cell mechanisms and extrinsic environmental influences. Thus, future research should continue to elucidate these interactions to identify gaps in knowledge of skeletal muscle and bone development, ultimately promoting enhanced outcomes in natural and cultivated environments (Alami-Durante et al., 2013) (Figure 3.6).

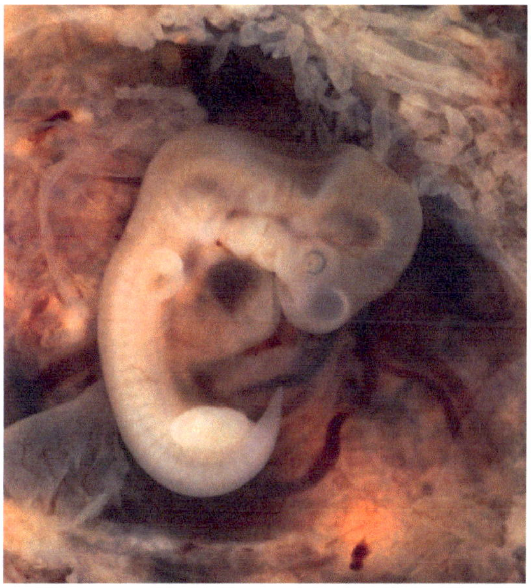

Figure 3.6. Embryonic development of the skeleton.

Source: https://files.mtstatic.com/site_7338/598/0?Expires=1750688501&S ignature =f6Utz A8jwBhlT8NyPwDPEVWhD725DPzce429VkJMq1dOtCfc1~QfFl3oH mQWo oWF OG710ejTEKlSRNbvaG5xOxeVVZ PI1Dsi2scQnlGBvcwWkOKa6ZKbveL2gXInELHQPqKAa9zmQ~Ve3WWZ5NAfumR-o1TR4N7hGlR7zNGITk_&Key -Pair-Id=APKAJ5Y6AV4GI7A555NA.

3.2.1. Stages of Embryonic Development

Embryo development is a complex process with different stages, beginning with fertilization and culminating in the formation of mature organs and systems. Each stage plays a significant role in establishing the foundation of the skeletal structure that will uphold the organism throughout its life. The zygote undergoes cleavage, resulting in a multicellular blastula that will give rise to the mesoderm, the tissue layer from which the skeletal tissues evolve. This transformation from one cell to a structured organism underlines the importance of cell division and differentiation, both of which have crucial roles in the formation of skeletal elements in vertebrates. As growth progresses towards gastrulation, the formation of germ layers establishes early cellular patterns that lay down the subsequent anatomical organization, such as the skeletal system, with systematic progress towards organogenesis. Entering the second phase of embryonic development, organogenesis is the intricate process through which tissues are differentiated and organs form.

In this process, mesodermal cells become cartilage and bone, demonstrating how embryonic development is a critical phase to the ontogeny of skeletal structures. The notochord, a basic feature at this point, plays a vital role not only in determining the dorsal-ventral axis but also in signaling pathways leading to vertebral element formation. A comparison of various species, including bats, as suggested by seminal work in evolutionary developmental biology, reveals how morphological changes arise through divergent developmental pathways such as acceleration and hypermorphosis. These adaptive differences may be the reason for the evolutionary diversity of skeletal forms, facilitating species with different ecological niches, showing the connection between developmental and evolutionary processes important in shaping skeletal form in the course of embryonic development. Development in the direction of subsequent stages involves utmost attention to the growth and elaboration of the skeleton. The fetal development stage is characterized by continuous development of bone elements, emphasizing the genetic and environmental factors on the integrity of the skeleton. Evidence indicates that these processes are crucial to consider when seeking to improve outcomes, e.g., in aquaculture, where the success of larvae hinges on growth conditions (Alami-Durante et al., 2013). These observations are not only critical for freshwater organisms that live in heterogeneous environments but also provide a general understanding of how skeletalogenesis is linked to overall organismal fitness. Beyond this, the identification of these stages of development is a context within which one can identify abnormalities in growth patterns or structural imperfections that could be established due to constraints in the availability of nutrients or environmental stresses. This comprehensive understanding of embryonic developmental stages underscores its significance in skeletal formation research and ontogeny (Figure 3.7).

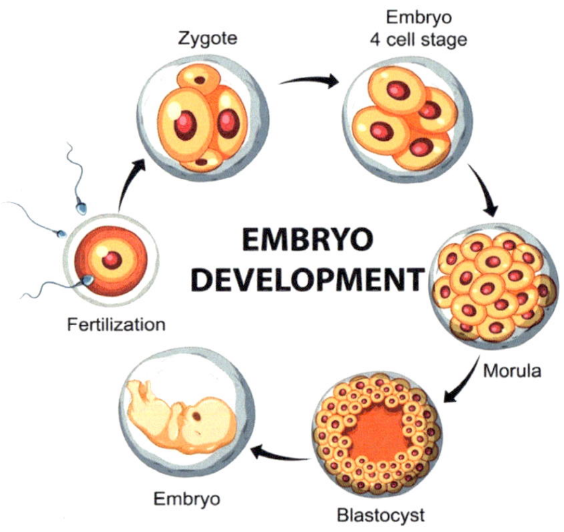

Figure 3.7. Stages of embryonic development.

Source: https://www.ferty9.com/wp-content/uploads/2025/04/Monsoon-Skin-Hair-Care-Tips-for-Kids-2023-03-28T192341.4121.png.

3.2.2. Role of Mesenchymal Cells in Bone Formation

Mesenchymal cells are essential for skeletal development and bone formation by producing numerous cell types that contribute to bone development. The multipotent stem cells reside in specific niches in the bone marrow, where they interact with other cells to maintain bone homeostasis and hematopoietic stem cell function. Both the vascular and endosteal niches are significant locations where mesenchymal stem/progenitor cells (MSCs) engage with osteoblasts, chondrocytes, and hematopoietic stem cells. Bidirectional communication between these cell types is critical for orchestrating bone remodeling, influencing osteogenesis and hematopoiesis. The sensitive equilibrium attained in such niches not only favors the differentiation of MSCs into osteoblasts, which build the bone matrix, but also highlights the necessity of their interaction to enhance skeletal function and integrity. Mesenchymal differentiation into osteoblasts is mainly governed by a multifaceted network of signaling pathways and transcription factors that direct gene expression relevant to bone growth. Important regulators such as bone morphogenetic proteins (BMPs) and Wnt signaling molecules regulate MSC differentiation into osteogenic cell lineages. Furthermore, these cell types can detect mechanical cues to a significant degree, integrating biomechanical information to enhance bone toughness and strength. The capacity of MSCs to communicate with the extracellular matrix also encourages their proliferation and differentiation into osteoblasts. Disruption of such developmental signaling pathways causes underdeveloped bone formation and many skeletal anomalies, underscoring the significance of mesenchymal cells in ensuring proper skeletal development and ontogeny. Mesenchymal cells play a significant role beyond differentiation; their interactions in the bone marrow microenvironment contribute to the complex network that ensures the structural and functional integrity of the skeleton. Experiments have revealed that these cells are not only involved in the formation of bone matrix but also regulate hematopoietic stem cells (HSCs) through niche-niche interactions. Recent findings indicate that a specific subset of osteoblasts maintains HSCs in the endosteal niche, thereby demonstrating the interdependence of hematopoiesis and bone formation. Besides, disruptions in vascular niche structure or function will compromise such crucial interactions necessary for hematopoiesis and lead to decreased bone formation. Such relationships clarify the complex regulatory interdependencies within the bone marrow microenvironment, as emphasized by studies of the homeostatic balance necessary for bone and immune cell function in this dynamic setting (Abzhanov et al., 2019; Agas et al., 2015).

3.2.3. Influence of Genetic Factors on Skeletal Development

Genetic factors and skeletal development are significant areas of research within the broader context of ontogeny. Genetic variation is primarily responsible for skeletal development and morphology, including size and form. Some genetic mutations lead to conditions such as non-syndromic orofacial clefts, demonstrating how genetic variation can alter craniofacial form. Research has shown that patients with such clefts exhibit complex morphological differences in their maxilla and mandible, suggesting that genes play a role not only in the development of the cleft but also in associated dentofacial deformities. These findings highlight the importance of understanding genetic effects as interdependent variables that shape skeletal development above the physical defect, as the produced dentoskeletal phenotype may be a product of an interaction between genetic tendencies and environmental interaction (Almpani et al., 2020). Additionally, modularity in skeletal development reaffirms the genetic nature of morphological diversity. Developmental modules constitute substructures of integrated characters that arise from special genetic instructions, facilitating different evolutionary adaptations in populations. Existing studies indicate that mutations may affect the covariance among characters without significantly altering overall craniofacial form. Modulation of skeletal characteristics illuminates the evolutionary potential of populations and suggests genetic causes create predisposed tracks for the development of the skeleton. In essence, the presence of cryptic patterns of modularity reveals that the craniofacial skeleton is not merely an outcome of random genetic variation but is underpinned by an orchestrated developmental program that can direct evolutionary outcomes (Albertson et al., 2018).

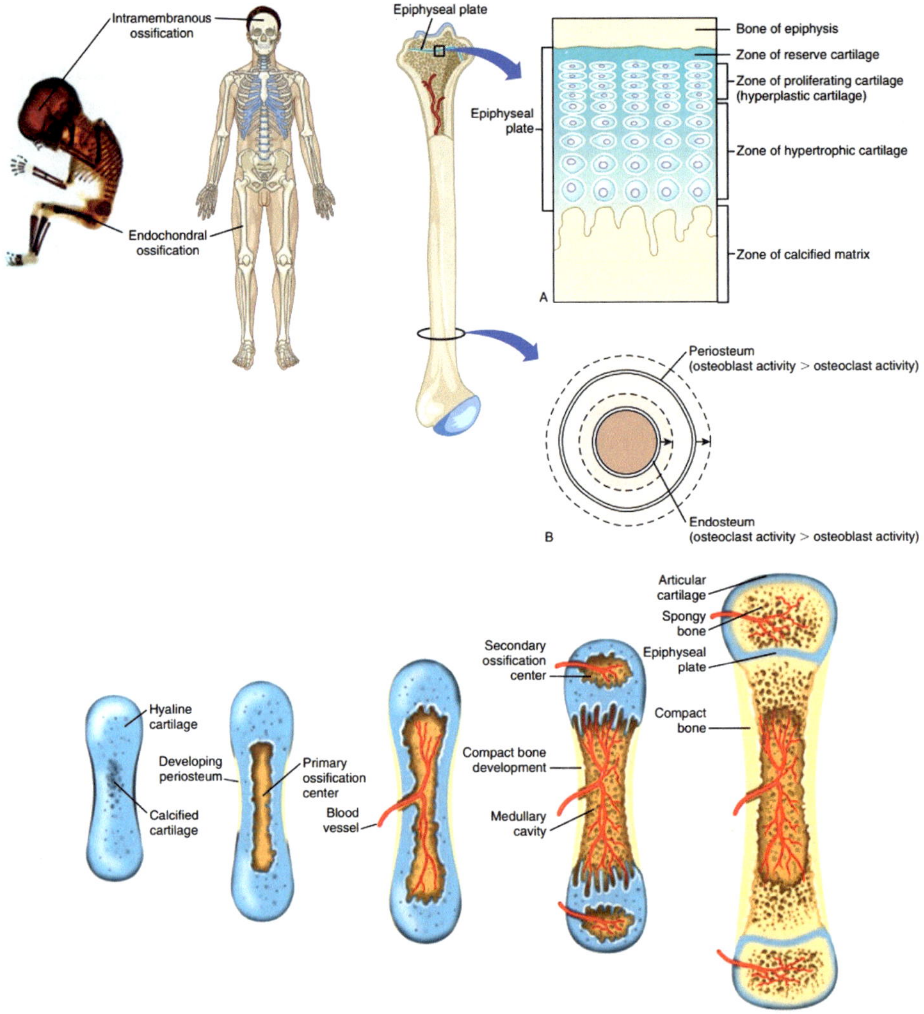

Figure 3.8. The interplay between genetic factors and skeletal development.

Source: https://www.pharmacy180.com/media/article/article-Growth-and-Developme-54R.jpg.

Secondly, awareness of the impact of genes on skeletal development is crucial for advancing therapeutic interventions for individuals with skeletal deformities. With the knowledge of the genetic causes of disorders such as craniofacial malformations, researchers can create therapies that will treat the structural deformities at their origin. This not only enhances the quality of life of those afflicted but also contributes to a deeper understanding of the processes involved in normal skeletal development. Recent research is actually tending towards the identification of gene interaction and their resulting influence on the phenotypic expression of the skeleton, which could unveil essential pathways for the therapeutic intervention. With additional advancements in genetic research, its significance for the ontogeny and development of the skeleton is sure to yield profound insights in both clinical and evolutionary biological contexts (Almpani et al., 2020) (Figure 3.8).

Test Your Knowledge

1. Explain the role of forensic pathologists.
2. Write a short note on post-mortem computed tomographic angiography (PMCTA).
3. What is exhumation?

3.3. Ossification Processes

Learning Outcome

1. Intramembranous ossification
2. Endochondral ossification
3. Factors influencing the rate of ossification

The mechanisms of ossification are crucial in developing skeletal structures, filling the gap between flexible cartilage templates and complex bone structures during ontogeny. The process is controlled primarily by two modes of ossification: intramembranous and endochondral. Intramembranous ossification occurs within mesenchymal tissue directly and is seen primarily in flat bones like the skull. Endochondral ossification, on the other hand, contains a precursor cartilage that exists when long bones like the femur develop. Ossification is highly regulated by numerous genetic and mechanical stimuli that vary significantly between species. As with seahorses, the timing and onset of ossification is important for growth and development, conferring evolutionary sensitivities that allow species like *Hippocampus subelongatus* to exhibit earlier than other relatives, and how this demonstrates the complexities and differences in skeletogenesis (Adriaens et al., 2014). In the examination of the processes of ossification, mechanical loading as a stimulus for bone formation must be taken into account. Experiments have shown the potential of mechanical forces to mold tissue differentiation in developing tissues, leading to specialized ossifications. Ostrich experiments had shown that some loading conditions in the patellar tendon could create multiple sesamoid bones. Since this observation shows the synergy between genetic programming and environmental forces in regulating skeletal development,. The evolutionary implications suggest that ossification is not merely a biological necessity but a process of adaptation that optimizes the morphology of the skeleton relative to various locomotory needs (Carter et al., 2017). The intersection of mechanical and biological signals is a multifaceted view of skeletal development and its evolutionary significance. Further examination of ossification processes reveals heterochronic shifts that can modify the timing of skeletal development. These shifts have the potential to cause variation with far-reaching implications for organisms' overall phenotype. For organisms like *Hippocampus reidi*, delayed ossification means slower development of the bony skeleton in comparison with its relatives. These differences in development form the basis of the evolution of these species, for example, in the case of the dwarf species *H. zosterae* whose small size is accompanied by a unique ossification schedule. These results not only provide insight into evolutionary biology but also emphasize the need for adaptive responses to environmental conditions. Thus, the deciphering of complex interactions between genetic and environmental components in ossification processes reveals an elaborate brocade of skeleton evolution worthy of exploration in evolutionary biology and comparative anatomy (Adriaens et al., 2014) (Figure 3.9).

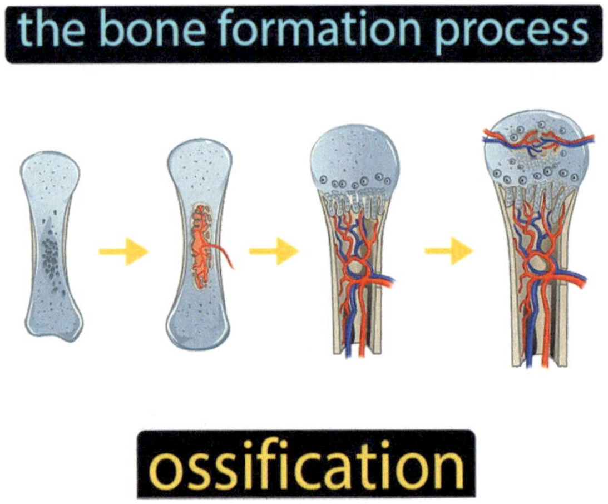

Figure 3.9. The ossification processes.

Source: https://i.pinimg.com/736x/6c/97/e1/6c97e1f84c7727539e63f23a1db6492e.jpg.

3.3.1. Intramembranous Ossification

Intramembranous ossification is one of the two central bone formation mechanisms, specifically making a distinct contribution to flat bone development, particularly that of the skull, face, and clavicles. Unlike endochondral ossification, where bone replaces hyaline cartilage, intramembranous ossification occurs within a fibrous connective tissue membrane directly. Intramembranous ossification begins when mesenchymal cells are transformed into osteoblasts, which then begin secreting the bone matrix. As matrix mineralization continues, osteoblasts become trapped and differentiate into osteocytes, forming the complex bone framework. Ossification is a significant process in fetal development, as it allows rapid growth of skeletal units required for protection and support, thereby contributing to structural integrity during initial growth. Intramembranous ossification is not only limited to bone formation in the simple sense but also plays roles in other aspects of skeletal development and ontogeny. It is the mechanism that enables the exquisite development of bones, demonstrating species-specific evolutionary adaptations. Comparative osteological research on different species, such as seahorses, illustrates how differences in ossification timing can yield spectacular functional consequences. For instance, certain seahorse species exhibit different patterns and rates of ossification, reflecting heterochronic changes that affect their evolutionary lineages. These differences highlight the complexity of intramembranous ossification and its role in facilitating environmental adaptations, which are responsible for a vast array of functional morphologies in vertebrates, including humans, where malformations in bone development can lead to developmental disorders. Since research continues to identify cellular and molecular mechanisms governing intramembranous ossification, how these results are integrated provides a better insight into bone development. The role of cranial neural crest mesenchyme

(NCM) in craniofacial structure development demonstrates how intramembranous ossification occurs together with other developmental processes. In addition, the interaction of biomechanical stress and genetic signaling mechanisms during ossification not only facilitates normal bone development but also supports the adaptive nature of skeletal morphology. Addressing both cellular dynamics and evolutionary significance, research on intramembranous ossification advances our understanding of skeletal ontogeny. This unification of biology and evolution provides windows into the appreciation of congenital defects and the adaptive utility of skeletal diversity within species, particularly as it pertains to human disease and health (Adriaens et al., 2014; Abzhanov et al., 2019) (Figure 3.10).

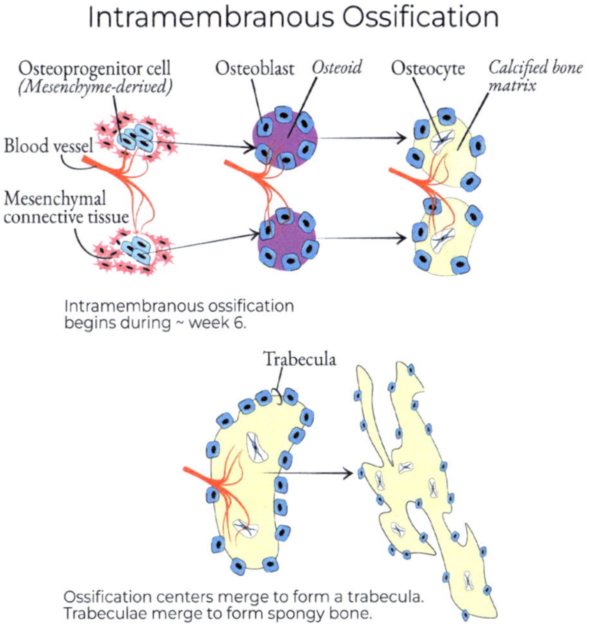

Figure 3.10. Intramembranous ossification represents one of the two primary processes of bone formation.

Source: https://d1j63owfs0b5j3.cloudfront.net/term/images/intramembranous-ossification-diagram-9535.jpg.

3.3.2. Endochondral Ossification

Endochondral ossification is a key mechanism in skeletal development and the primary process by which long bones and other skeletal tissues develop from hyaline cartilage. This intricate process involves of discrete steps, such as the proliferation, maturation, and hypertrophy of chondrocytes, and the synthesis and subsequent mineralization of cartilage matrix. It is against this background that angiogenesis, or the formation of new vessels, is significant, for it is the vascularization that is the basis of nutrient supply and cartilage-to-bone conversion. Apart from basic development, this process also occurs during fracture healing and in osteoarthritis-like conditions, indicating its fundamental clinical significance. By examining molecular and cellular mechanisms of endochondral ossification, researchers aim to uncover potential therapeutic strategies to enhance bone regeneration and treat degenerative joint diseases (Adams et al., 2018). Recent discoveries in endochondral ossification research have also challenged longstanding assumptions about the terminal differentiation of hypertrophic chondrocytes. Historically, these cells were thought to be destined to undergo apoptosis, but recent discoveries suggest they may have the capacity to transdifferentiate into osteoblasts. This information raises new questions regarding research avenues, suggesting that the fate of chondrocytes may be determined by their microenvironment, for example, the composition of the extracellular matrix (ECM) on which they grow. Of particular note, the epigenetic influences imparted by the ECM, unique to chondrocytes, would direct osteoblast behavior and bone quality. In view of this, understanding how these interactions influence the process of ossification not only will enhance our comprehension of the ontogeny of the skeleton but also inform new treatments for diseases like osteoarthritis and osteoporosis by targeted modulation of these pathways (Adams et al., 2018). In addition to the intrinsic regulation processes of endochondral ossification, mechanical forces outside also significantly impact the formation of the skeleton. For instance, sesamoid bone research, such as that of DeGAN, highlights the interaction between mechanical stress and gene effects involved in joint movement. The mechanical loading of tendons can induce differentiation of soft tissue into fibrocartilage, a key factor in the design of such augmentation structures as multiple patellae to enhance joint function. Finite-element simulations have demonstrated that the transition occurs preferentially in specific regions of the tendon under loading. This discovery of mechanical cues being the primary factors controlling the development of skeletal elements has served as the foundation for the extension of mechanobiological principles and their application to bone growth and health (Figure 3.11).

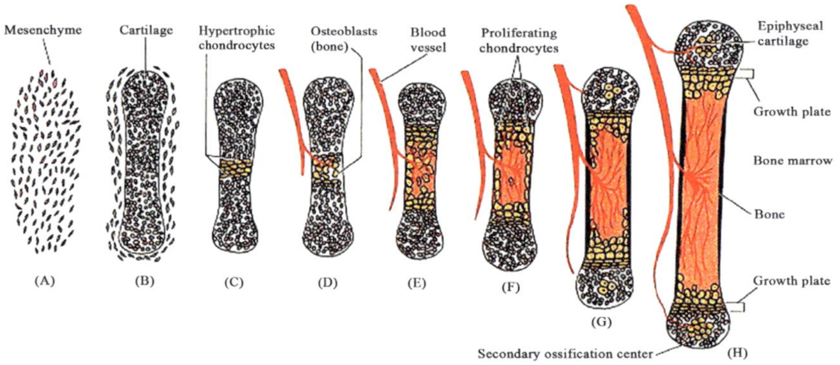

Figure 3.11. Endochondral ossification.

Source: https://www.researchgate.net/profile/Samir_Abdelmagid/publication/224929158/figure/fig11/AS:302569156038657@1449149516205/Endochondral-Ossification-A-B-Long-bones-such-as-humerus-femur-and-tibiae-develop.png.

3.3.3. Factors Influencing Ossification Rates

The process of ossification, which results in the formation of bone from cartilage, is extremely factor-sensitive during the growth of the skeleton. Genetic conditions are the most significant and earliest factors influencing ossification rates. Genes specifically governing the differentiation and expansion of chondrocytes, the cells responsible for producing cartilage, will dictate at what rate they will differentiate into bone. In addition, hormonal control limits the process; growth hormone and sex steroids, for instance, play a critical role in regulating osteoblast activity, the cells that form bone. Such hormone signals regulate the balance between bone formation and resorption, thereby determining the pace of ossification across the different components of the skeletal system. Further research into the interaction between genetics and hormones can shed insight into developmental abnormalities that manifest through abnormal ossification processes, as evidenced in the study of cranial base synchondroses and craniofacial growth (Cendekiawan et al., 2010). Environmental forces also play a strong role in influencing ossification rates, dictating the formation of the skeletal system in relation to what it senses from its external environment. Nutritional well-being, as reflected in the availability of calcium and vitamin D, is critical for bone development, as deficiencies can lead to faulty ossification and growth abnormalities such as rickets. Further, mechanical loading of the musculoskeletal system, through load-bearing exercise, promotes ossification by stimulating osteoblasts. This can be seen in the clinical area of dentofacial orthopedics, where mechanical stress is applied to cranial bones to induce growth changes during treatment for craniofacial deformities. Nutritional interactions with mechanical stress reveal the plasticity of the osteoskeleton and the ability of environmental cues to elicit the physiological adaptations necessary for normal ossification (Cendekiawan et al., 2010). Lastly, the contribution of growth rates to ossification should not be overemphasized, as they can also contribute to overall developmental stability. Variations in growth rates are revealed through studies to cause different levels of fluctuating asymmetry (FA), a measure of developmental instability. In non-human primates, studies have shown that species that grow more slowly exhibit greater developmental stability, as reflected in smaller FA values. For instance, craniofacial analysis in species such as Gorilla and Pan shows that details of growth rate are linked to developmental endpoints, demonstrating how environmental and biological stressors manifest in morphological characteristics. Understanding the relationship between ossification rates and these simple features of ontogeny yields basic knowledge of skeletal development and its evolutionary perspective, particularly in terms of adaptive responses to growth conditions.

Test Your Knowledge

1. What is endochondral ossification and how does it contribute to skeletal development?
2. What factors influence the rate of ossification in bones?

3.4. Growth and Maturation of Bones

Learning Outcome

1. Stages of bone growth
2. Hormonal control of growth of the skeleton
3. Impact of nutrition on bone health

Bone growth and development are complex phenomena reflecting the dynamic interaction between genetic, environmental, and mechanical factors influencing skeletal development. During fetal life, bone development begins with cartilage template ossification, a process that is critical for the organization of the skeleton. This initial phase lays the foundation for later bone growth, with endochondral ossification playing a central role in long-bone development. During growth, bones pass through stages marked by changes in density, form, and strength, all of which are required to support increasing body weight and activity. Knowledge of these phases of development helps account for how disruptions in normal developmental processes can lead to skeletal deficiencies or abnormalities, emphasizing the value of proper nutrient delivery and hormonal regulation during maturation. The influence of reduced blood supply on bone development is significant information regarding the physiological state in which skeletal maturation occurs. Experiments, even those conducted on the effects of reduced uterine circulation on postcranial bone development in animal models, illustrate how compromised circulation may lead to retarded bone development and alterations in morphological measurements. More specifically, findings indicate that certain bones are more susceptible to growth retardation due to vascular deficiency, reflecting sex-specific differences in growth development. It is essential here to consider what these findings mean for human development, particularly in cases of prenatal stress, which can have a widespread influence on skeletal quality throughout organism maturation. Appreciation for how blood flow intersects with bone formation deepens our understanding of the importance of vascular health during sensitive growth periods (Castro et al., 2010). Furthermore, the gross structure and properties of bone tissue are significant indicators of aging and growth, recording overall biological processes. As bones mature, they do not merely increase in size but also become denser and more mineralized, resulting in characteristic patterns that vary in species and gender. For instance, research has shown that cortical bone density increases significantly during early development but later diminishes after post-maturity in females, unlike in males. This indicates the impact of hormones, with estrogen being a central hormone that contributes to maintaining bone density across all stages of life. Recognition of these nuances underscores the complexity of bone maturation and the strategies involved in avoiding osteoporosis in adulthood (Hamada et al., 2012). Further, these observations provide a foundation for future research aimed at the development of preventive and therapeutic approaches to skeletal health (Figure 3.12).

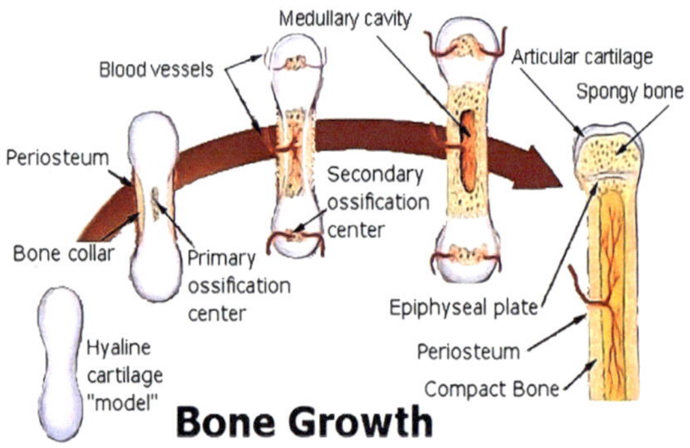

Figure 3.12. The growth and maturation of bones.

Source: https://cdn.storymd.com/optimized/VdKPRVswqK/original.jpg.

3.4.1. Phases of Bone Growth

The process of bone development is crucial for establishing the pattern of skeletal growth, as it defines the intricate mechanisms that direct the cartilaginous anlage toward an entirely ossified system. Primary bone growth occurs during embryogenesis, through endochondral ossification, where hyaline cartilage serves as a template for future bone growth. This phase is critical, as it sets the foundation for both the appendicular and axial skeleton and, indeed, for the whole body plan. This development is controlled in a multifactorial manner, involving cascading signals, mechanical tension, and hormonal control, which coordinately govern cellular differentiation and bone tissue replacement.

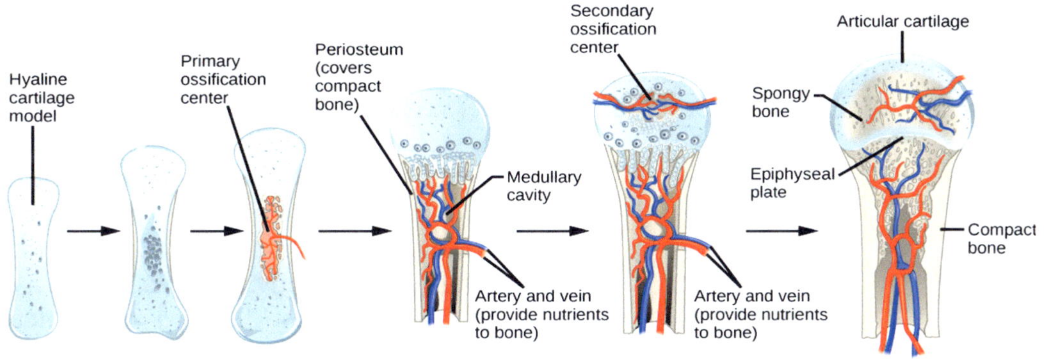

Figure 3.13. The phases of bone growth.

Source: https://s3-us-west-2.amazonaws.com/courses-images/wp-content/uploads/sites/1223/2017/02/08000442/Figure_38_02_06-1024x378.jpg.

Thus, the interaction of these factors underscores the importance of a dynamic homeostatic environment for balancing growth and adaptation throughout the life of the organism, in support of the argument that skeletal development is not merely a byproduct of geology but an adaptive biological function (Torday et al., 2015). Following the initial stages of ossification, bone growth proceeds through distinct remodeling and maturation phases. Bone growth is the activity of osteoblasts, whereas the function of osteoclasts is resorption of bone, both functioning in harmony to maintain a balance that is in favor of proper development. This interaction occurs when the long bones undergo extensive longitudinal growth in childhood and adolescence due to chondrocyte proliferation in the growth plates. Their closure indicates the beginning of a mature bony skeleton, completing longitudinal growth. But bone still needs to be modified throughout life due to ongoing remodeling processes, in which tissue is constantly replaced or renewed, responding to metabolic demands and mechanical loading. This modulation plays a vital role in bone resilience and strength, further illustrating the highly interdependent nature of bone growth with environmental and genetic variables (Adriaens et al., 2018). Moreover, the later phases of bone growth are especially important for assessing the evolutionary significance of vertebrate skeletal formation, particularly the refinement of form and function. Comparative studies across species provide insights into the isometric and allometric growth patterns of their skeletal systems. For instance, when paravian dinosaurs were examined, researchers observed diverse histological characteristics that paralleled osteohistological characteristics, indicating life-history variation associated with locomotion and flight proficiency. This indicates how evolutionary pressures affect bone growth, beneficial to survival and functionality in various ecological niches. Thus, the bone developmental stages not only describe the ontogeny of individual organisms but also point towards a broader understanding of evolutionary biology and the processes of skeletal adaptations over time. Understanding these stages can lead to an appreciation of the complexity involved in the development of the skeleton and the individual evolutionary routes taken within vertebrate lineages (Adriaens et al., 2018; Torday et al., 2015) (Figure 3.13).

3.4.2. Hormonal Regulation of Skeletal Growth

Skeletal growth is a multidimensional interaction of various hormones that affects the ontogenesis of the skeletal apparatus significantly. Growth hormone (GH) and insulin-like growth factors (IGFs), in particular, directly stimulate chondrocyte proliferation and osteoblast activity, thereby increasing bone size and weight. GH, released by the pituitary gland, stimulates the release of IGF-1 from the liver, which, in a local action in the growth plate, stimulates endochondral ossification. This is essential for optimal skeletal development, particularly in childhood and adolescence, when the growth plates are open. Dysregulation of GH signaling can lead to many growth disorders, again demonstrating the hormone's pivotal role in skeletal development and overall health. Understanding these hormonal mechanisms sheds light on those factors responsible for growth variation and the potential implications for the treatment of growth abnormalities. Furthermore, the estrogens and androgens also appear as essential growth regulators in the skeleton, particularly in the pubertal growth spurt. In addition to causing a sudden increase in height, these sex hormones also influence the maturation of the growth plates. In men, testosterone has been shown to enhance bone mineral density and stimulate longitudinal bone growth, whereas estrogens are responsible for the closure of growth plates, ultimately determining adult height. This hormonal regulation shows how complex bone growth is, as its effects vary by gender and developmental stage. Experiments have identified that a proportionate amount of these hormones is necessary; both excess or deficient levels of hormones have been linked to conditions such as hypogonadism or precocious puberty, leading to malformations of the skeleton. The interaction between estrogens and androgens is thus crucial for determining the skeletal template. The role of thyroid hormones in skeletal regulation cannot be excluded. T4 and T3 are also crucial for the healthy growth of cartilage and bone, influencing other cellular activities such as differentiation and metabolism. Thyroid hormones enable the formation of bone matrix and enhance osteoblast and osteoclast function, thereby controlling bone resorption and formation. Changes in thyroid hormone levels can lead to severe growth disturbances, including dwarfism or premature skeletal maturation. In aquatic animals, whose understanding of these hormonal impacts is in its infancy, studies suggest that alterations in thyroid hormone content are associated with growth rates and overall skeletal condition, and further studies are called for in this area. Understanding these hormonal pathways is critical to advancing aquaculture efforts to maximize skeletal growth and enhance juvenile quality, given the larger implications of hormonal regulation of skeletal development (Alami-Durante et al., 2013; Abzhanov et al., 2019).

3.4.3. Impact of Nutrition on Bone Health

Proper nutrition is required for optimal bone health, particularly during the periods of ontogeny and skeletal growth, as it directly influences bone strength and density growth and development. Components of the diet, such as calcium and vitamin D intake, play an important role in the bone mineralization process. Calcium is the primary mineral component of bone tissue, and vitamin D facilitates the intestinal absorption of calcium so it can be incorporated into the skeletal matrix. Deficiencies in nutrients during periods of peak development can result in lower bone density and possibly the onset of conditions such as osteoporosis in advanced age. Therefore, proper nutrition during childhood and adolescence, when bones are forming, is essential to the development of a good skeletal foundation for adulthood. Other micronutrients, including phosphorus, magnesium, and vitamins C and K, are also involved in bone health in addition to calcium and vitamin D. Phosphorus works together with calcium to form hydroxyapatite. This mineral complex makes bones hard. Magnesium regulates the activation of vitamin D to its biologically active metabolites and facilitates calcium absorption. At the same time, vitamins K and C play a vital role in the synthesis of bone-forming and remodeling proteins. A diet with these nutrients in balance has been shown in research to contribute not only to bone development but also to bone repair and maintenance at various life stages. Hence, an in-depth understanding of nutritional influence on bone health is critical in the development of efficient diet recommendations and interventions for lifelong skeletal integrity. Further, the intersection of nutrition and bone health highlights the importance of homeostasis in skeletal development. Homeostasis, commonly conceived in synchronic terms, also has diachronic analyses wherein it is perceived as functioning as physiological stability across generations. Nutritional status has been reported to influence the homeostatic regulation of bone remodeling, the continuous process of bone resorption and formation. As the body adapts to the alterations in nutritional inputs, such signals facilitate the optimization of bone tissue structure, survival, and adaptation to environmental requirements. This dynamic interplay between nutritional status and skeletal health signals developmental physiological pathways and a systems approach to the study of bone development, as emphasized in contemporary biology (Hooke et al., 2025; Torday et al., 2015). This systems approach can be used to shape public policy directed towards the promotion of nutrition and, with it, bone health in populations (Figure 3.14).

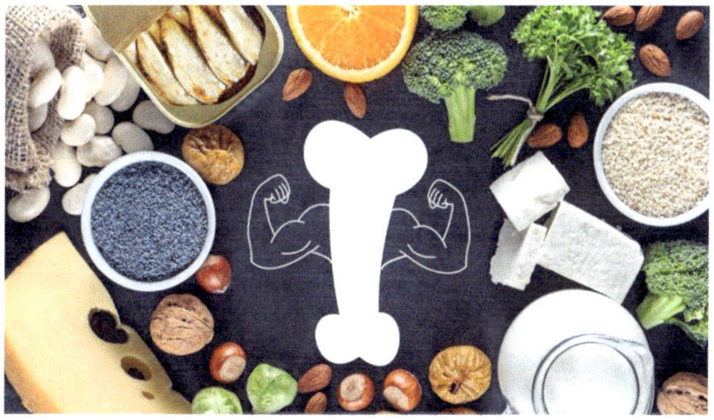

Figure 3.14. Proper nutrition is critical for optimal bone health.

Source: https://media.licdn.com/dms/image/v2/D5612AQE_6SknyIOESw/article-cover_image-shrink_720_1280/article-cover_image-shrink_720_1280/0/1724131132592?e=2147483647&v=beta&t=C6ECZvXnuKGBP9YQZ3WiQGka0WWIYxDs5YrgtBK2TZY.

Test Your Knowledge

1. What are the main stages of bone growth and maturation?
2. How do hormones regulate the growth and development of the skeletal system?

3.5. Skeletal Variations and Anomalies

Learning Outcome

1. Regular skeletal disorders
2. Genetic as opposed to environmental control of anomalies
3. Diagnostic methods of skeletal abnormality

Skeletal variations and anomalies form a significant aspect of skeletal development and ontogeny studies due to the range of morphological adaptability among populations. The variations may be caused by genetic, environmental, or a combination of causes, leading to typical shapes and structures in the skeletal system. Ailments such as non-syndromic clefts demonstrate how genetic susceptibilities interact with environmental factors to create specific skeletal defects. For instance, studies have shown that non-syndromic cleft lip and palate (nsCLP) patients often have complex dentofacial deformities that affect craniofacial morphology. These variations emphasize how identification of both ontogenetic growth trajectories and environmental factors that participate in skeletal variation in a species reinforces the reality that anomalies are not aberrations but also variations that reveal ontogenetic pathways that have evolved specifically to confront various environmental challenges (Almpani et al., 2020). The intricate interaction between skeletal anomalies and their genetic frameworks is also evident across diverse populations, revealing the nature of the relationship between development and evolution. For instance, specific skeletal malformations can be instructive in demonstrating past adaptations, suggesting how populations may have adapted to specific environmental pressures. Shape transformation analysis in animals, particularly at pivotal ontogenetic points, emphasizes examining broader aspects of development, such as ecomorphological controls. Using contemporary analytical methods, such as Self-Organizing Maps (SOMs) coupled with Elliptic Fourier Analysis, researchers can graphically represent the correspondence between morphological variation and ecological factors. This interfacing technique can unravel the adaptive significance of variations in bone, promoting more profound understanding of the evolutionary history of different species and mechanisms of resistance afforded by structural diversity (Cataudella et al., 2014).

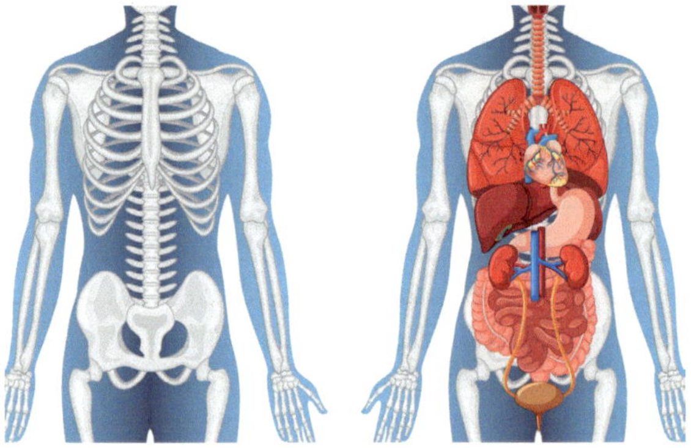

Figure 3.15. Skeletal variations and anomalies form a significant aspect of the study of skeletal development and ontogeny.

Source: https://udshealth.com/wp-content/uploads/2024/12/rib-cage-organs-scaled.webp.

Furthermore, beyond academic ends, the clinical application of information on skeletal variations and anomalies extends to shaping medical examination and management. Skeletal deviations or misalignments constitute serious issues in dental and orthopedic clinics, calling for well-thought-out intervention measures. For instance, understanding of the inherent skeletal variations among patients with conditions like nsCLP is crucial in formulating a feasible treatment plan. Such clinician awareness not only improves surgical outcomes but can be advantageous for the general health of afflicted subjects. By integrating comprehensive knowledge of skeletal development, variation, and anomalies, physicians can develop more effective treatment plans, underscoring the importance of skeletal studies in scientific inquiry and clinical therapy. Thus, the research into these topics increases our understanding of human development and the efficacy of intervention to promote skeletal health (Figure 3.15).

3.5.1. Common Skeletal Disorders

The cause of skeletal disorders is typically a complex interplay of genetic, environmental, and biomechanical factors. Acquiring an understanding of such musculoskeletal abnormalities requires a critical assessment of a number of disorders of skeletal integrity. For instance, in broilers, common leg disorders such as bacterial chondronecrosis with osteomyelitis and angular or rotational deformities have significant impacts on mobility and welfare. These are not only common across different developmental stages but also show how external and internal pressures influence skeletal growth. The morphological changes observed during periods of significant growth, especially at four to six weeks of age, emphasize the energetic cost of limb increase and heightened activity levels, demonstrating that the process of skeletal development must accommodate both genetic selection and environmental pressures (Codd et al., 2014). A core aspect of skeletal disorders concerns the molecular and cellular mechanisms underlying bone and cartilage formation. The intricacies of skeletal development, particularly in the craniofacial region, illustrate how disruptions at both embryonic and postnatal stages may result in various skeletal deformities. In the amniote mandibular jaw complex, for example, the role of cranial neural crest mesenchyme (NCM) is crucial for normal morphological development. Dysfunctions in its signaling pathways can lead to a range of defects in bone, muscle, and connective tissues. These disparities underscore the need to understand the ontogeny of the skeleton and how environmental and genetic influences may produce both evolutionary adaptations and disease. Thus, an appropriate analysis of these developmental pathways is essential for diagnosing common skeletal disorders and developing effective interventions (Abzhanov et al., 2019). The importance of skeletal disorders extends beyond acute physical well-being to shape overall welfare and quality of life. Mobility disorders can impair daily functioning, leading to secondary conditions such as obesity or chronic pain. In addition to direct physiological impact, the psychological impacts also cannot be overlooked; patients with skeletal disorders are stigmatized and also experience psychological distress due to their impaired mobility. This underscores the necessity of holistically oriented research approaches that include not only biological and biomechanical studies but also psychosocial evaluation. By gaining a thorough understanding of skeletal development and disorders, stakeholders can improve prevention, diagnosis, and treatment methods, ultimately enhancing the health of affected populations, whether livestock or human (Codd et al., 2014; Abzhanov et al., 2019).

3.5.2. Genetic vs. Environmental Influences on Anomalies

Research on anomalies in skeletal development calls for an advanced understanding of genetic-environmental interaction. Genetic factors play a central role in determining an organism's phenotypic traits, including skeletal anatomy. For instance, specific genes are implicated in craniofacial development, and mutations in these genes cause major skeletal abnormalities. The association of non-syndromic orofacial clefts with the dentofacial deformities that accompany them is proof of this fact, where structural alterations of the maxilla and mandible are present. Such circumstances imply that while genetic predispositions play a significant role, they do not act in concert. The actions of epigenetic determinants, such as environmental exposures during critical developmental periods, also become factors in accounting for these anomalies. Therefore, it is essential to define the actions of genetics relative to those of the environment in the broader context of skeletal development and ontogeny. Environmental factors play an important role in skeletal system development and can be held accountable for many anomalies that sometimes operate in intricate combination with genetic predispositions. Prenatal teratogenic exposures, maternal well-being, and nutrition are among the environmental factors that can have profound effects on skeletal morphology. It is conceivable, for instance, that deprivation of essential nutrients during critical developmental periods can lead to severe skeletal malformations, regardless of genetic background. Furthermore, research into pseudo-albinism in flatfish shows that environmental conditions can result in structural and functional tissue alterations rather than a defect in pigmentation. The evidence showed alterations in skin and intestine, showing interdependency between conditions within the environment and other biological systems, and exhibiting the complexity of anatomical development. Evidence such as this shows the need for an integrated approach to research, encompassing both genetic constitution and environmental conditions, when investigating skeletal anomalies. The combination of environmental and genetic factors is synergistic, making the analysis of anomalies more complex. For example, individuals with a genetic susceptibility to specific skeletal abnormalities can exhibit varying levels of expression depending on environmental factors. The interactions are usually noticeable in cases involving complex trait analysis. In syndromic orofacial clefts, environmental influences overlay genetic factors, thereby determining the appearance of the cleft itself. Furthermore, in studies of the pseudo-albino sole's gut microbiome, another microbial community was associated with pathological pigmentation, demonstrating the extent to which environmental conditions can influence genetic outcomes. This highlights the necessity of multilayered strategies that account for both genetic inheritance and environmental influences to further illuminate skeletal anomalies and their ontogeny, and to offer a holistic model for research and potential intervention strategies (Figure 3.16).

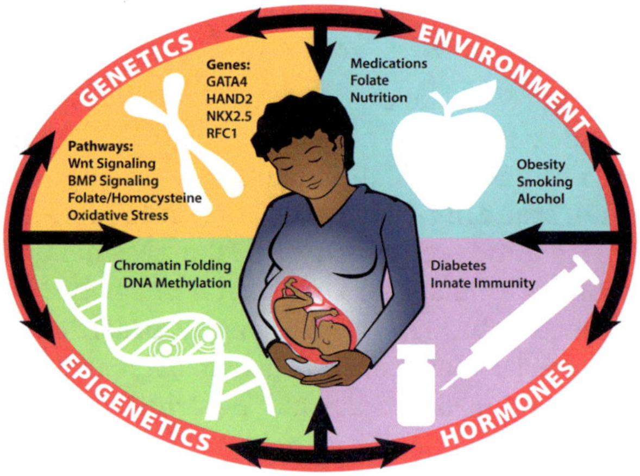

Figure 3.16. Genetic vs. environmental influences on anomalies.

Source: https://www.researchgate.net/profile/Daniel-Webber-6/publication/277331106/figure/fig2/AS:267901487808519@1440884100724/nteractions-between-genetics-epigenetics-maternal-hormonal-levels-and-environmental.png.

3.5.3. Diagnostic Methods for Skeletal Abnormalities

Precise diagnosis of skeletal abnormalities requires a multilayered approach that integrates traditional imaging techniques and advanced methodologies. Conventional radiographic imaging has long been the major skeletal assessment technique, allowing clinicians to visualize skeletal morphology in two dimensions. However, this method tends to be inadequate when defining complex anatomical relationships and subtle abnormalities. Therefore, three-dimensional imaging technologies such as CT and MRI have found increasing application for their ability to provide comprehensive images of skeletal morphology. These newer imaging techniques permit the more precise diagnosis of deformities by enabling three-dimensional reconstructions and volumetric measurements. Furthermore, these techniques can be complemented with geometric morphometric analysis, which provides greater insight into shape variation at a finer scale, thereby facilitating early diagnosis and intervention protocols. Alongside imaging, the integration of genetic and molecular diagnostic techniques has revolutionized the interpretation of skeletal abnormalities. Genetic screening and high-throughput sequencing can uncover dormant genetic predispositions, particularly in syndromic conditions. To illustrate, non-syndromic orofacial clefts are currently being studied intensively for their association with disruption of morphogenetic processes, which can manifest as skeletal deformities. By applying techniques such as full-skull cone beam computed tomography (CBCT), scientists can quantify differences in shape among affected individuals, as demonstrated in patient-based studies of non-syndromic cleft lip and palate. The studies determine significant correlations between genetic factors and the resulting skeletal forms, thereby informing therapeutic interventions and preventive care. As the field advances, integrating genetic data with imaging data will become necessary to continue refining diagnostic precision in skeletal malformations. Furthermore, quantification of bone mineral density (BMD) offers an attractive avenue for gaining additional insight into skeletal deformities, as in aquaculture studies on fish such as the gilthead sea bream. Techniques such as micro-computed tomography (micro-CT) enable three-dimensional, high-resolution assessment of BMD, correlating morphogenetic parameters directly with bone integrity. The finding that variations in BMD correspond to opercular deformations underscores the value of this quantitative technique in detecting skeletal abnormalities. However, one must recognize that mineralization patterns can vary across skeletal elements, underscoring the complexity of bone development. By combining state-of-the-art imaging technologies with quantitative assessments, researchers and physicians can develop integrated diagnostic approaches that can overcome the intricate challenges posed by skeletal defects, ultimately leading to enhanced patient outcomes in specific populations.

Test Your Knowledge

1. What are some common skeletal disorders and anomalies?
2. How do genetic factors differ from environmental factors in influencing skeletal anomalies?

3.6. The Role of Physical Activity in Skeletal Health

Learning Outcome

1. Effect of exercise on bone mass
2. The role of weight-bearing exercise.
3. Maintenance of skeletal health advice

The interconnection between bone health and physical activity is firmly rooted in the biological control of bone growth and maintenance. Repeated weight-bearing physical activity throughout life not only stimulates the formation of bone but also maintains structural characteristics and bone density with advancing age. If physical activity is sensibly integrated into the everyday routine, it is a potent stimulus for osteoblast activity, leading to high bone mass and improved mechanical toughness. This change is particularly crucial during periods of rapid growth, such as childhood and adolescence, when the skeleton is most susceptible to extrinsic physical stresses. Moreover, engaging in multiple physical activities, including resistance training and high-impact exercise, was discovered to have positive results in skeletal health, validating the hypothesis that active living encourages robust bone development and prevents diseases like osteoporosis in later years. In addition to immediate effects on bone density, physical activity influences the complex interaction between the hematopoietic and skeletal systems. The bone marrow niche, an environment critical for the maintenance of hematopoietic stem cells (HSC), and the bone scaffold surrounding it rely on physical exercise to ensure their functionality. Research has shown that mechanical loading during exercise enhances the osteogenic potential of osteoblasts, thereby maintaining HSC proliferation and activity. It is this interaction that underscores the importance of maintaining physical activity as much for bone health as for total immune system regulation. As interactions among the various cell populations within the marrow are closely linked to physical loading and bone strength, any disruption in these processes compromises bone formation and inhibits hematopoiesis, underscoring the importance of a clear understanding of these biological linkages (Agas et al., 2015). Moreover, the physical impacts of exercise on bone health extend beyond short-term benefits in bone strength and density; they also include a longer-term influence on preventing degenerative bone diseases. Longitudinal studies have established that individuals who exercise consistently throughout their lives have a significantly lower risk of osteoporotic fractures and other bone diseases. This protective effect arises from the cumulative benefit of ongoing physical training, which stimulates adaptive changes in the skeleton that last a lifetime. The bone plasticity theory, which emphasizes the skeleton's ability to remodel as a response to mechanical loading, supports the idea that lifelong activity is essential for ontogeny and skeletal development. Therefore, promoting exercise as an integral part of public health policy has widespread benefits for populations, ensuring healthier bones throughout life and minimizing the risks posed by age-related degenerative diseases (Hooke et al., 2025) (Figure 3.17).

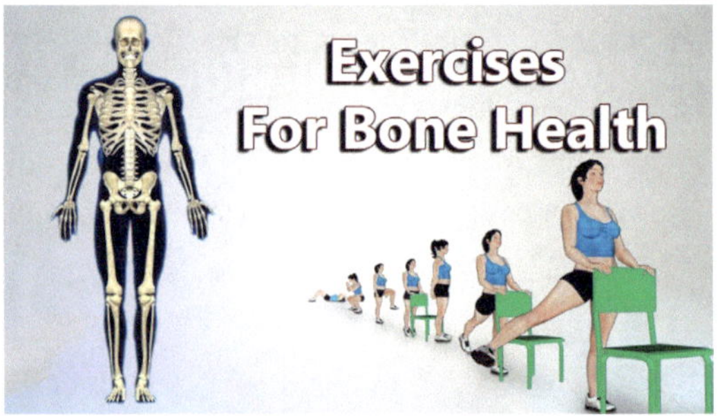

Figure 3.17. The role of physical activity in skeletal health.

Source: https://external-content.duckduckgo.com/iu/?u=https%3A%2F%2Fi.ytimg.com%2Fvi%2F9VF9TahVspg%2Fmaxresdefault.jpg&f=1&nofb=1&ipt=1904b56a63f967d033ddbecda549873e612dd7e83f8c4833b5bc5946a895ff9d.

3.6.1. Effects of Exercise on Bone Density

The interaction between exercise and bone density is a critical element of skeletal development and maintenance throughout ontogeny. Mechanical loading from exercise stimulates bone remodeling, the action of constantly reproducing bone tissue and strengthening it. Weight-bearing and resistance exercise trigger bone mass deposition through increased osteoblast activity, cells that build bones. In children and adolescents, regular physical activity may lead to greater peak bone mass, a significant determinant of adult skeletal health. The bone density acquired at these ages could delay or even obviate the onset of osteoporosis and fractures in old age. Thus, fostering an environment appreciative of exercise can pay substantial long-term dividends in skeletal toughness and durability. As people move through various stages of life, the impact of exercise on bone density can manifest differently. In young adults, regular participation in weight-bearing exercise has been found to preserve or even enhance bone density, reversing the natural losses that can occur with aging. The mechanotransduction process—by which cells detect and respond to mechanical stress—triggers signaling pathways that ultimately stimulate bone remodeling and increase bone density. Moreover, studies have shown that specific types of exercise, such as jumping or resistance training, are particularly useful for boosting bone mineral density and thus aiding skeletal health throughout an individual's lifetime. This is not only crucial for enhancing athletic function but also for avoiding injury and sustaining mobility later in life. Additionally, the role of exercise in strengthening bone density is magnified by its impact on hormonal and metabolic components. Exercise stimulates hormone release, such as growth hormone and insulin-like growth factor-1 (IGF-1), which play a central role in bone formation and remodeling. The increased muscle strength following exercise also enhances coordination and equilibrium, and therefore reduces risk of falls in the elderly—a significant problem with respect to bone integrity. The main effects of such physiological adaptations are a testament to the significance of exercise in promoting not only skeletal growth but also general health. Together, it is crucial to appreciate the intricate interplay among exercise, bone density, and underlying biological processes to design effective interventions that ensure lifelong bone health and avert degenerative bone disorders such as osteoporosis (Abourachid et al., 2014; Donaldson et al., 2025).

3.6.2. Importance of Weight-Bearing Activities

Weight-bearing exercise is an important determinant of mammalian ontogeny and skeletal growth. Mechanical loading from weight-bearing activity induces bone remodeling, leading to denser, stronger bones. This is particularly important during development when bones are more elastic and amenable to external influences. Repetitive exposure to weight-bearing exercise results in significant alterations in the trabecular and cortical bone structure, allowing for the skeleton to accommodate various mechanical stresses in which life is spent efficiently. These activities, executed by the developing organism, such as walking or climbing, progressive development of the bone material properties underlie its ability to withstand increased physical load with growth. This process shows that weight-bearing behaviors in early life are essential to creating a foundation for skeletal function and long-term skeletal health. The skeleton's structural responses to weight-bearing activity also highlight the influence of specific behaviors on bone and muscle development. Studies have shown that physical exercise, such as repetitive mechanical loading, alters the fiber type composition of muscle and its contractile properties, thereby affecting the structural maintenance of bones. For instance, coordination of myosin heavy chain (MHC) isoform expression and mechanical loading in the growth phases has been associated with muscle adaptations necessary to support weight-bearing activities. Particularly, MHC isoform ontogenetic transformation from fast-twitch to increased slow-twitch fiber content indicates a functional adaptation with increased utilization of the skeletal apparatus during activities such as nest construction in *Monodelphis domestica*, as observed in Budde et al. (2017).

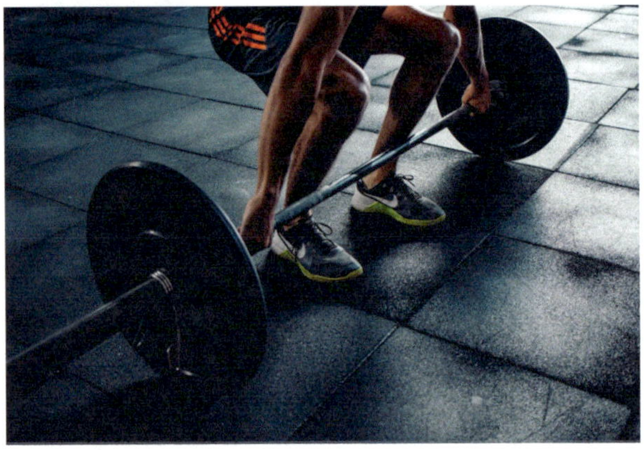

Figure 3.18. Weight-bearing activities play an essential role in the skeletal development and ontogeny of mammals.

Source: https://external-content.duckduckgo.com/iu/?u=https%3A%2F%2Fwww.rosycheeked.com%2Fassets%2Fmedia%2Ffile%2F22%2F43%2Fad3d6811c5073a4902a3fe9cd3b0c9d8.jpeg&f=1&nofb=1&ipt=ada8bb96bdbf82123335d81ced3e1f004fdfd7932c036518833f810c163d5440.

These findings indicate the intricate relationship between mechanical loading, muscle adaptation, and skeletal integrity throughout ontogeny. Furthermore, the role of weight-bearing activities is not merely physical growth; it is a vital aspect of healthy functional adaptation of joint structures. Research shows that trabecular bone's sensitivity to mechanical loading enables more accurate analysis of joint loading and use throughout an organism's life cycle. Maintaining healthy bone architecture through such activities helps prevent age-related illnesses such as osteoporosis. Moreover, understanding trabecular bone adaptations reveals how it can reconstruct behavioral patterns in living and extinct animals, as in Aerssens et al. (2016). By researching the adaptation of bones to the mechanical load of weight-bearing activities during growth, researchers can better comprehend evolutionary pressures that make skeletal morphology progress to its ultimate full understanding of skeletal development and ontogeny (Figure 3.18).

3.6.3. Recommendations for Maintaining Skeletal Health

Peak skeletal health relies on a complex process involving nutrition, exercise, and lifestyle. Nutrition is essential to skeletal development, with calcium and vitamin D being responsible for bone mineralization and maintenance. A balanced diet rich in these nutrients can significantly minimize the risk of osteoporosis and other bone disorders. For instance, calcium-rich milk products, spinach, and calcium-enriched foods provide the body with the calcium it needs, whereas vitamin D can be obtained through sunlight and some foods, such as fatty fish. Periodic assessment and adjustment of dietary habits are simple steps for anyone interested in maintaining skeletal health throughout life. Adding regular exercise is also vital in maintaining skeletal integrity. Weight-bearing exercises such as walking, running, and resistance training stimulate bone development and enhance bone density. An assortment of exercise programs not only develops muscle strength but also enhances coordination and balance, decreasing the risk of falls and ensuing injury. Furthermore, exercise stimulates the production of growth factors that promote bone formation, making it a critical component of skeletal development strategies. Exercise programs tailored to personal ability and choice can promote adherence and maximize bone health benefits with ongoing use. Besides dietary and exercise patterns, lifestyle influences contribute significantly to skeletal well-being. Prevention of smoking and heavy alcohol consumption may decrease the risk of acquiring bone density issues, while a normal body weight is also essential in ensuring skeletal integrity. Being aware of and controlling factors that may affect bone health, such as hormonal imbalances or chronic diseases, is equally important. Besides, individuals are supposed to be proactive when seeking a doctor's advice on their bones, especially those with a higher risk through genetics or age. With the introduction of these recommendations, individuals can significantly enhance bone growth and longevity, thereby ensuring a healthier future and reducing the complications of skeletal diseases (Bailey et al., 2018; Kenny et al., 2015).

Test Your Knowledge

1. How does regular physical activity affect bone mass and strength?
2. What strategies can help maintain skeletal health throughout life?

SUMMARY

In bringing together the complex findings on ontogeny and skeletal development, it is essential to understand the nuances of morphological adaptations in species. The evolutionary trajectories of the neotropical leaf-nosed bats illustrate that craniofacial developmental modifications entail acceleration and hypermorphosis as major processes shaping skull morphology. These developmental evolutionary patterns not only highlight the significance of ontogeny in revealing skeletal adaptations but also illustrate how environmental forces influence evolutionary strategy. Though adaptations lead to dietary diversification, peramorphosis as a process is a key element in the evolutionary history of bats, highlighting the interrelatedness of form, function, and evolutionary success during vertebrate development (Arthur et al., 2019). Similarly, research on seahorse skeletal development provides valuable insights into the divergence of ontogenetic processes in marine species. Comparative observations of ossification patterns among seahorse species illustrate not only the flexibility of skeletal structures within the family Syngnathidae but also the impact of heterochronic changes on evolutionary trails. The findings show that differences in the timing of skeletal maturation are not only side effects of the environment, but also key drivers of adaptive evolution, which allow species like *Hippocampus zosterae* to take up unique ecological niches. For this reason, the processes provide evidence for the thesis that ontogeny is a fundamental part of evolutionary biology, required for understanding how diversification occurs (Adriaens et al., 2014). Last but not least, the analysis of bone development across taxa highlights the paramount role of ontogeny in evolutionary biology. One begins to see that not only do developmental paths of single organisms establish physical characteristics of species, but developmental paths also reflect the evolutionary history and adaptive approaches governing survival. By integrating data across species like neotropical leaf-nosed bats and seahorses, we get a clearer picture of the intricate mechanisms of skeletal formation. The information is progressing toward enabling more knowledge of vertebrate evolutionary processes and the skeleton as an anatomical structure and as an evolutionary record of adaptation. Thus, future studies need to continue exploring these development processes to discover the complexities of evolution and their impacts on biodiversity (Adriaens et al., 2014; Arthur et al., 2019).

The exploration of skeletal development and ontogeny gives profound perspectives into the evolutionary processes of various species. Specifically, research on neotropical leaf-nosed bats has shown that differences in craniofacial growth significantly impact skull shape. The study applies three-dimensional geometric morphometrics that describe the complex interaction between evolutionary patterns and ontogenetic cranial structure modifications. Notably, the findings infer particular mechanisms, such as acceleration and hypermorphosis, that control skull morphogenesis in such bats. The investigation ultimately underscores the significant role of peramorphosis in dietary specialist evolution, a concept that describes the complex interaction between development and evolutionary biology (Arthur et al., 2019). Similarly, emu skeletogenesis provides a different angle from which to view ontogenetic changes in morphology. Emus experience significant increases in mass between hatching and adulthood while maintaining their bipedal mode of locomotion. Research on pelvic limb morphology in emus provides strong evidence on how various biomechanical parameters scale with increasing size. Muscles and tendons exhibit strong positive allometry, indicating greater force-generating capacity as these birds increase in size. Through the analysis of scaling patterns in muscle physiological cross-sectional area and tendon traits, we have a clearer understanding of how emus are morphologically prepared to cope with rapid growth and sustained locomotion, which are necessary for their survival and function in the wild (Abourachid et al., 2014). In concert, these studies illustrate the interaction between ontogeny and skeletal development across species and reveal that morphological adaptation reflects ecological niches and evolutionary pressures. The varied methods employed, from geometric morphometrics in bats to allometric scaling in emus, illustrate the variety of approaches employed to investigate development within a biological context. As scientists continue to investigate these intricate interactions, additional knowledge into the evolutionary developmental biology of different taxa is likely to ensue, allowing for an enhanced understanding of how skeletal morphology evolves and functions during ontogeny. These findings not only add to our understanding of species-specific adaptation, but they also illustrate the rule that development is both a byproduct of evolutionary history and an agent driving subsequent evolutionary directions (Abourachid et al., 2014; Arthur et al., 2019).

KEY TERMS FROM THIS CHAPTER

- Bone Modeling
- Bone Remodeling
- Cartilage
- Chondrocytes
- Endochondral Ossification
- Epiphyseal Plate
- Growth Plate
- Hypertrophy
- Intramembranous Ossification
- Mesenchymal Cells
- Mineralization
- Ossification
- Osteoprogenitor Cells
- Periosteal Apposition
- Pubertal Growth Spurt
- Skeletal Maturation

CRITICAL THINKING QUESTIONS

1. **What is bone development during embryonic stages called?**
   a. Mineralization
   b. Ossification
   c. Calcification
   d. Resorption
2. **What kind of ossification occurs inside the mesenchymal tissue directly?**
   a. Endochondral ossification
   b. Intramembranous ossification
   c. Secondary ossification
   d. Epiphyseal ossification
3. **What bones are formed by intramembranous ossification mainly?**
   a. Long bones
   b. Flat bones of the skull
   c. Vertebrae
   d. Carpals and tarsals
4. **In endochondral ossification, which structure serves as the template for bone formation?**
   a. Hyaline cartilage
   b. Fibrocartilage
   c. Elastic cartilage
   d. Mesenchymal cells
5. **What is the function of the epiphyseal plate in skeleton development?**
   a. Provides attachment for muscles
   b. Aids in bone resorption
   c. Facilitates longitudinal bone growth
   d. Prevents joint dislocation

Short Answer Questions

1. What is ossification, and why is it significant in the development of the skeleton?
2. Explain the role played by the epiphyseal plate in bone growth.
3. Why is hyaline cartilage significant in endochondral ossification?
4. Define endochondral ossification.
5. Define the role of growth hormone in bone development.
6. Define the role of nutrients like calcium and vitamin D in bone development.

Answers to Critical Thinking Questions

1. (b); 2. (b); 3. (b); 4. (a); 5. (c)

REFERENCES

1. Lamas, L. P., Main, R. P., & Hutchinson, J. R. (2014). Ontogenetic scaling patterns and functional anatomy of the pelvic limb musculature in emus (Dromaius novaehollandiae). *PeerJ*, *2*, e716. https://doi.org/10.7717/peerj.716Abzhanov, A., Abzhanov, A., Abzhanov, A., Baggiolini, A., Baroffio, A., Beverdam, A., Chevallier, A., et al. (2019). Molecular and cellular mechanisms underlying the evolution of form and function in the amniote jaw. https://core.ac.uk/download/323079229.pdf (accessed on 18th July 2025).
2. Adams, A., Aizawa, M., Akintoye, S., Amling, M., Bahney, C., Ballock, R., Behonick, D., et al. (2018). The chondro-osseous continuum: Is it possible to unlock the potential assigned within? https://core.ac.uk/download/155776524.pdf (accessed on 18th July 2025).
3. Adriaens, D., & Franz-Odendaal, T. A. (2014). Comparative developmental osteology of the seahorse skeleton reveals heterochrony amongst *Hippocampus* sp. and progressive caudal fin loss. https://core.ac.uk/download/55807543.pdf (accessed on 18th July 2025).
4. Adriaens, D., De Wolf, T., Dierick, M., et al. (2018). A 3D quantitative method for analyzing bone mineral densities: A case study on skeletal deformities in the gilthead sea bream, *Sparus aurata* (Linnaeus, 1758). https://core.ac.uk/download/188636251.pdf (accessed on 18th July 2025).
5. Adriaens, D., Godefroit, P., Hu, D. Y., Prondvai, E., et al. (2018). Intraskeletal histovariability, allometric growth patterns, and their functional implications in bird-like dinosaurs. https://core.ac.uk/download/153398302.pdf (accessed on 18th July 2025).
6. Aerssens, A., Alam, F., Almécija, S., Amling, M., Barak, M., Barak, G., Barak, M., et al. (2016). A review of trabecular bone functional adaptation: What have we learned from trabecular analyses in extant hominoids and what can we apply to fossils? https://core.ac.uk/download/46164630.pdf (accessed on 18th July 2025).
7. Agas, D., Douni, E., Marchetti, L., & Sabbieti, M. G. (2015). The unbearable lightness of bone marrow homeostasis. https://core.ac.uk/download/54653580.pdf (accessed on 18th July 2025).
8. Alami-Durante, A., Alami-Durante, A., Albalat, A., Albors, A., Almuly, A., Almuly, M., Almuly, O., et al. (2013). What determines growth potential and juvenile quality of farmed fish species? https://core.ac.uk/download/61514843.pdf (accessed on 18th July 2025).
9. Albertson, R. C., Crespel, A., Harris, M. P., Killen, S. S., et al. (2018). Conserved but flexible modularity in the zebrafish skull: Implications for craniofacial evolvability. https://core.ac.uk/download/157582972.pdf (accessed on 18th July 2025).
10. Almpani, K., Fung, P. W., Huang, J., et al. (2020). Craniofacial analysis may indicate co-occurrence of skeletal malocclusions and associated risks in development of cleft lip and palate. https://core.ac.uk/download/288166216.pdf (accessed on 18th July 2025).
11. Arenas-Mena, A., Armstrong, J. B., Benson, W. A., Bottjer, D. J., Cameron, R. A., Davidson, E. H., et al. (2008). Transfer of a large gene regulatory apparatus to a new developmental address in echinoid evolution. https://core.ac.uk/download/4878759.pdf (accessed on 18th July 2025).
12. Arthur, W., Baker, R. J., Darwin, C., Development Core Team, R., Dávalos, L. M., Ferrarezzi, H., Freeman, P. W., et al. (2019). Peramorphosis, an evolutionary developmental mechanism in neotropical bat skull diversity. https://core.ac.uk/download/286086786.pdf (accessed on 18th July 2025).

13. Bailey, R. A., Eckersall, P. D., & O'Reilly, E. L. (2018). A comparative study of acute phase protein concentrations in historical and modern broiler breeding lines. https://core.ac.uk/download/158368189.pdf (accessed on 18th July 2025).

14. Budde, J. E., Butcher, M. T., Chadwell, B. A., Thomas, D. P., et al. (2017). Ontogeny of myosin isoform expression and prehensile function in the tail of the gray short-tailed opossum (*Monodelphis domestica*). https://core.ac.uk/download/544278491.pdf (accessed on 18th July 2025).

15. Carballo, C., Codoñer, F. M., Costa, R. A., et al. (2019). Understanding pseudo-albinism in sole (*Solea senegalensis*): A transcriptomics and metagenomics approach. https://core.ac.uk/download/232150567.pdf (accessed on 18th July 2025).

16. Carter, D. R., Dye, S., Hogg, D. A., Lansdown, A. B., Macalister, A., Vickaryous, M. K., & Wren, T. A. (2017). Finite-element modelling of mechanobiological factors influencing sesamoid tissue morphology in the patellar tendon of an ostrich. https://core.ac.uk/download/82968870.pdf (accessed on 18th July 2025).

17. Castro, L. E., Cesani Rossi, M. F., Fucini, M. C., et al. (2010). Bone growth and sexual dimorphism at birth in intrauterine-growth-retarded rats. https://core.ac.uk/download/223030171.pdf (accessed on 18th July 2025).

18. Cataudella, S., Russo, T., & Scardi, M. (2014). Applications of Self-Organizing Maps for ecomorphological investigations through early ontogeny of fish. https://core.ac.uk/download/pdf/53860878.pdf (accessed on 18th July 2025).

19. Cendekiawan, T., Rabie, A. B. M., & Wong, R. W. K. (2010). Relationships between cranial base synchondroses and craniofacial development: A review. https://core.ac.uk/download/37901089.pdf (accessed on 18th July 2025).

20. Codd, J., Hutchinson, J. R., Manchester, P., Paxton, H. P., et al. (2014). Anatomical and biomechanical traits of broiler chickens across ontogeny. Part II. Body segment inertial properties and muscle architecture of the pelvic limb. https://core.ac.uk/download/36777728.pdf (accessed on 18th July 2025).

21. Donaldson, P. L., Garshnek, V., Hooke, L. R., et al. (2025). USSR Space Life Sciences Digest, issue 21. https://core.ac.uk/download/pdf/42828785.pdf (accessed on 18th July 2025).

22. Frédérich, B., & Sheets, H. D. (2010). Evolution of ontogenetic allometry shaping giant species: A case study from the damselfish genus *Dascyllus* (Pomacentridae). https://core.ac.uk/download/pdf/35112810.pdf (accessed on 18th July 2025).

23. Georgiou, A. N., Koumoundouros, G., Loizides, M., et al. (2013). A new type of lordosis and vertebral body compression in gilthead seabream, *Sparus aurata* Linnaeus, 1758: Etiology, anatomy and consequences for survival. https://core.ac.uk/download/55765477.pdf (accessed on 18th July 2025).

24. Goswami, A., Porto, A., Porto, A., Burrows, A. M., Esteve-Altava, B., Esteve-Altava, B., Esteve-Altava, B., et al. (2018). Primate modularity and evolution: First anatomical network analysis of primate head and neck musculoskeletal system. https://core.ac.uk/download/151211716.pdf (accessed on 18th July 2025).

25. Hamada, Y., Suryobroto, B., & Widiyani, T. (2012). Kepadatan tulang metacarpal simpanse usia 0 sampai 44 tahun. https://core.ac.uk/download/20334119.pdf (accessed on 18th July 2025).

26. Heers, A. M., Rankin, J. W., & Hutchinson, J. R. (2018). Building a bird: Musculoskeletal modeling and simulation of wing-assisted incline running during avian ontogeny. https://core.ac.uk/download/161515031.pdf (accessed on 18th July 2025).

27. Hooke, L. R., & Teeter, R. (2025). USSR Space Life Sciences Digest. Index to issues 1–4. https://core.ac.uk/download/pdf/42841024.pdf (accessed on 18th July 2025).

28. Kenny, T. S. (2015). Vitamin D status and bone mineral density in female collegiate dancers and cheerleaders. https://digitalscholarship.unlv.edu/thesesdissertations/2550 (accessed on 18th July 2025).

29. Romero, A. N. (2018). A comparison of craniofacial asymmetry in *Gorilla gorilla gorilla* and *Pan troglodytes troglodytes*. https://core.ac.uk/download/158200087.pdf (accessed on 18th July 2025).

30. Torday, J. S. (2015). Homeostasis as the mechanism of evolution. https://core.ac.uk/download/323075985.pdf (accessed on 18th July 2025).

CRANIUM – NEUROCRANIUM IN HUMAN OSTEOLOGY

4

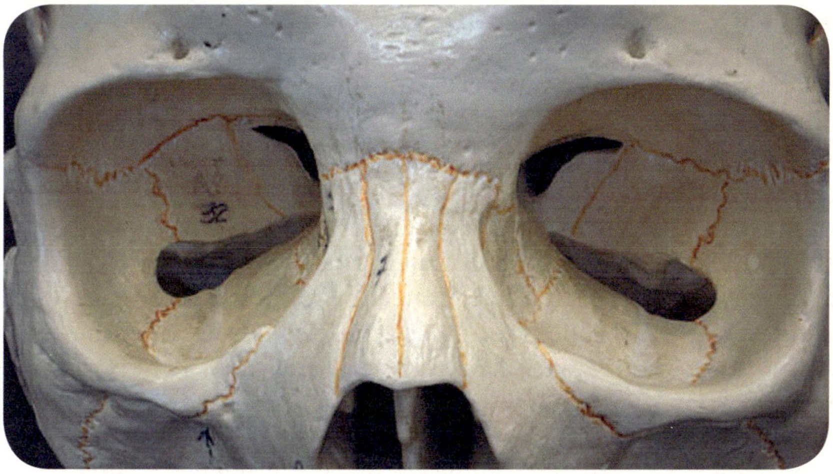

LEARNING OBJECTIVES

After studying this chapter, you will be able to:

1. Explain the anatomy of the neurocranium
2. Explain the development of the neurocranium
3. Emphasize neurocranium and brain protection
4. Explain the neurocranium in forensic anthropology
5. Identify the comparative anatomy of the neurocranium
6. Evaluate the clinical relevance of the neurocranium

Introduction

Human osteology is a highly inclusive branch of study that covers a wide range of skeletal morphology, particularly the cranium and its derivatives. Among them, the neurocranium is of great significance because it houses and protects the brain, the major organ of the nervous system. It is important to understand the neurocranium's structure to effectively review cranial anatomy, as it is the foundation for many neurological processes and overall human health. By examining its composition—eight cranial bones—scientists can discover how evolutionary pressures have shaped cranial morphology over time, impacting everything from the ability to think to the processing of sensory information. The combination of environmental and genetic factors has the most significant impact on the morphological variation between populations. In our case, research in some of these groups, such as the Sami, has shown specific variations between males and females in facial skeleton parameters, with implications suggesting adaptation to harsh living conditions (Borutskaya et al., 2017).

These findings reiterate the significance of the neurocranium as a structural component, but also due to evolutionary pressures that have determined its form. As researchers explore these differences in the skeleton, they expand knowledge of human resilience and adaptability, particularly in combating diverse environmental challenges. When studying the neurocranium, it is important to consider the roles that embryonic development and physiological factors play in increasing its complexity. The combination of several cellular and molecular processes in cranial development reflects the complex mechanisms behind craniofacial anatomy (Abzhanov et al., 2019). The interaction of different cell lineages affects not only the physical properties of the neurocranium but also its functional capabilities. By exploring these developmentally congruent processes, researchers can illuminate the relationship between structural variations and health conditions, thereby improving our understanding of cranial anatomy within an integrative model of human osteology. Such perspectives are central to advancing clinical practice and to better understanding cranial pathology and its effects on human health.

Definition of the Cranium

The cranium is an anatomical structure that plays a very significant role in the human skeletal system, serving as the shield for the brain. Composed of several bones that are fused, the cranium is also divided into two basic parts: the neurocranium and the viscerocranium. The neurocranium specifically houses and protects the brain, while the viscerocranium forms the skeletal structure of the face. This division emphasizes the cranium's multidirectional functions, conjoining protection and support. Its intricate shape not only supports the cerebral organs, but also closely relates to various anatomical systems, exhibiting required senses such as sight, hearing, and smell. It is crucial to have a clear understanding of the cranium's structure, particularly in fields such as anthropology and paleontology, where it provides significant insights into human evolution and anatomical population diversity. Of all the structures of the cranium, the neurocranium is of particular interest in the study of human osteology. constitute this part: the frontal, parietal, occipital, temporal, sphenoid, and ethmoid bones, which collectively contribute to overall protection and cranial vault structure. The neurocranium also significantly contributes to the support for of muscles and ligaments that aid in the movement and function of the head. Notably, studies reveal that sexual dimorphism occurs in the neurocranium, with males having larger and more voluminous cranial measurements than females, a pattern of growth with implications for sex estimation in forensic anthropology. Understanding the neurocranium's dimensions and morphological characteristics benefits not only biological anthropology but also the reconstruction of the appearance and way of life of ancient human populations, as shown by investigations of juvenile craniofacial development (Phillips et al., 2013). Exploring the evolutionary history of the cranium, particularly the neurocranium, offers useful insights into the development of early human species. The characteristic cranial morphology of fossil hominins, such as Homo neanderthalensis, reflects adaptations that are suggested to be responses to environmental pressures and phylogenetic legacy. The morphological changes over time, best reflected in the Middle and Upper Pleistocene periods, reflect fundamental changes in mode of life and habitat, influencing craniofacial structures. For instance, the Altamura Man, a Neanderthal human, is a fascinating glimpse into the past because its highly preserved cranial anatomy provides essential information for exploring the adaptive strategies of ancient populations. Such studies highlight the complex interplay between biology and environment in the formation of the human cranium, confirming its value as a subject of research in paleoanthropology and osteology (Buzi et al., 2020) (Figure 4.1).

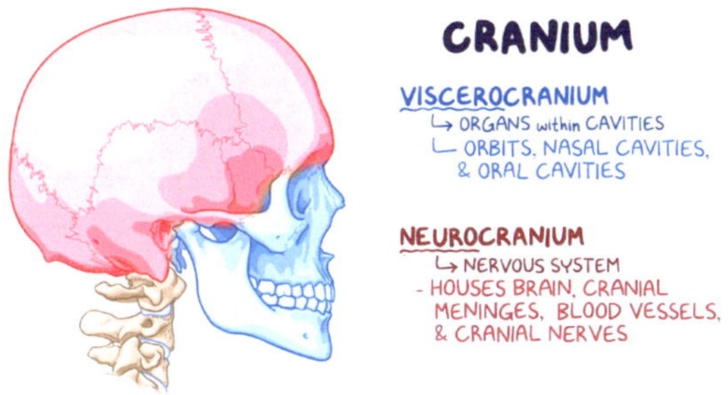

Figure 4.1. The cranium is an anatomical structure that serves a vital role in the human skeletal system.

Source: https://external-content.duckduckgo.com/iu/?u=https%3A%2F%2Fd16qt3wv6xm098.cloudfront.net%2FSrXGYa-0RXSwxrrl1s3t4hsYRp60Gmel%2F_.jpg&f=1&nofb=1&ipt=62a018cfb705c349dd1eaac413f03b134faf9e62ae4629eaa4b192dd495322c3.

Importance of the Neurocranium in Human Anatomy

The neurocranium is an essential protective structure in human anatomy that covers and protects vital neural structures, including the brain, cranial nerves, and associated vessels. Made up of eight individual bones, i.e., the frontal, parietal, and occipital bones, the neurocranium not only forms a hard protective covering from external trauma but also plays a decisive role in determining the overall shape and function of the skull. Its structural features enable integration with other musculoskeletal structures, such as the meninges and cranial ligaments, which provide additional protection for the neurocranium. This structural integrity is paramount as any alteration in the neurocranium would lead to neurological disturbances or disorders, underlining its central role in providing not only physical protection but also the functional equilibrium of the central nervous system. In addition to a protective role, the neurocranium is a key factor in craniofacial development and maturation. As the primary framework of the head, it sets facial symmetry, capacity, and disposition. Growth and morphogenesis of the neurocranium are subject to genetic and environmental factors that may also strongly impact other anatomical structures. Abnormal development patterns, for instance, such as craniosynostosis, can result from abnormal suture fusion in the neurocranium, and defective cranial form, alongside potential impairments to neurological function, ensues. Furthermore, neurocranial morphology has been correlated with general health and hereditary disorders in studies, which gives credence to the importance of neurocranial development studies in osteology and medical science (Carril et al., 2022). The neurocranium is thus an active structure rather than a passive one, playing a prominent role in the complexities of human anatomy. The neurocranium's functional interactions are also diverse in the scope of total cranial anatomy. For example, it is crucial to the skull's resonance, influencing speech and hearing capabilities. The intricate interdependence between the neurocranium and the surrounding structures provides balanced functionality for biological processes, from hearing and equilibrium to thinking function. The presence of frontal sinuses, for example, indicates how the neurocranium design is optimized according to some functional needs (Akbasak et al., 2013). The neurocranium's interconnectivity with the rest of the skull makes it significant for understanding human osteology. From the neurocranium's anatomical and functional features, students cannot only understand cranial integrity but also appreciate the broader evolutionary developments seen throughout human history. Thus, the neurocranium is a key subject to enjoy learning about when it comes to anatomical and pathological conditions that affect human health (Figure 4.2).

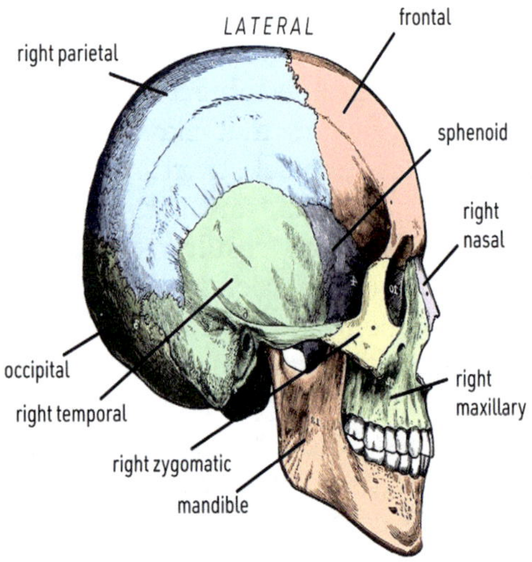

Figure 4.2. The neurocranium serves as a vital protective structure within human anatomy.

Source: https://external-content.duckduckgo.com/iu/?u=https%3A%2F%2Fanatomysystem.com%2Fdiagram%2FNeurocranium-Bones.jpg&f=1&nofb=1&ipt=1f7e7d3f18eb2a0e9cb222416a6a1c18fad1679a5ad16a591f31aef24b6846fb.

4.1. Anatomy of the Neurocranium

Learning Outcome

1. Description of the location of the neurocranium
2. Principal bones that constitute the neurocranium
3. Function of the neurocranium

The neurocranium is a vital architectural component of the skull, responsible for containing and protecting the brain. This bony structure develops from several embryonic tissues, primarily the neuroectoderm and mesoderm, which together contribute to its complex development. Central bones of the neurocranium include the frontal, parietal, temporal, occipital, and sphenoid bones. All of these parts are joined together by sutures, fibrous joints that provide flexibility during growth phases in development. The solidity of the neurocranium shields sensitive neural structures while allowing cranial nerve passage, thereby permitting important sensory and motor function. Knowledge of this anatomical organization is central to human osteology because differences in the pattern of neurocranium development will have profound effects on neurological health and craniofacial morphology throughout an individual's life. The discussion of developmental details of the neurocranium highlights the importance of cranial neural crest mesenchyme (NCM) in the formation of cranial structures. This single cellular component is of paramount importance for the development of bone and cartilage within the skull, providing both structural support and direction of growth patterns through evolutionary adaptations. The intricate interplay of signaling pathways directs proliferation and differentiation towards the diverse sizes and shapes of skulls that exist across species. Disruptions of these developmental processes can lead to congenital or other cranial defects, demonstrating the delicate balance maintained during cranial development. Such an understanding would suggest that a better insight into the neurocranium development will be helpful to detect pathological abnormalities and therefore contribute to the fields of clinical medicine and craniofacial rehabilitation. When comparative osteology is investigated, taxonomic variation of neurocranial shapes within and among species contains the most important evidence of adaptation to varied ecological niches during evolution. Examining basal cranial morphology, as with those in major clades such as catfishes, proves this principle of functional morphology. For instance, neurocranial specializations would allow taxa to inhabit specialized habitats, demonstrating spectacular evolutionary changes among teleosts. By studying the evolutionary significance of these developments in the cranial morphology, researchers can appreciate not only the mechanical functions of the neurocranium but also how these adaptations are extrapolated to the ecological forces that played on the species over geologic time. This multidisciplinary study of neurocranial anatomy increases our awareness of both human and non-human osteological morphology, enriching our appreciation of evolutionary biology and anthropological studies (Figure 4.3).

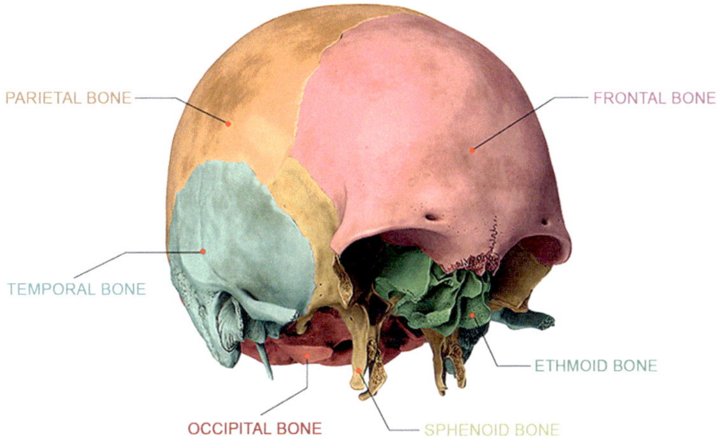

Figure 4.3. Anatomy of the neurocranium.

Source: https://external-content.duckduckgo.com/iu/?u=https%3A%2F%2Fanatomy.net%2Fuploads%2F03a137f5-7ca1-447d-bbe2-0cdbe55adaa4.png%3Fwidth%3D1200&f=1&nofb=1&ipt=d9260e701410fb71bc3dfb4675f3edc3fdca651dc9f648021bd7260428cdda69.

4.1.1. Description of the Neurocranium's Location

The neurocranium, an important component of the human cranium, is responsible for protecting the brain and maintaining cranial structures. It is located at the top of the skull, within the cranial cavity that houses the brain. This osseous component is composed of several bones that fuse as they develop to form a tough yet pliable structure, essential for protection and structural support. The neurocranium lies behind and above the face, whose border runs from the frontal bone in the forehead to the occipital bone in the back of the skull base. Paleontologists and medical professionals must understand the precise location of the neurocranium, as this involves cranial surgery, evolutionary biology, and anthropological studies of human skull morphological variation. Within the neurocranium, some bones demarcate specific regions that help in understanding cranial architecture. The frontal, parietal, temporal, sphenoid, and occipital bones are among the bones that demarcate different regions and help in understanding cranial morphology. Their orientation not only protects the central nervous system but also the areas of muscle and ligament attachment. Furthermore, the temporal fossa is a prominent feature of the neurocranium, providing space for the temporalis muscle, whose function is critical to the mechanism of mastication. Given that the neurocranium contains the brain, it assumes a morphology and structural features that accommodate the corresponding neural and vascular structures, testifying to the intricate interaction of cranial anatomy and neurological function, as demarcated by investigations into cranial development and adaptation (Abzhanov et al., 2019). The position of the neurocranium is particularly significant when considering the evolutionary adaptations that have led to its current state. Its strategic position allows for the accommodation of sensory organs and continuity from the brain to the spinal cord. Of note, the cranial base comprises numerous foramina that provide passage for cranial nerves and vessels, forming essential connections between the neurocranium and the rest of the body. This evolutionary perspective highlights the adaptive nature of the neurocranium among populations, as demonstrated in the comparative examination of the morphology of various human and hominin skulls. For instance, cranial remains from different localities, such as the Sami burials, reveal variations in cranial shape determined by environmental and biological factors (Borutskaya et al., 2017). Such findings bring to the fore the neurocranium's role not only as a covering but as an evolving structure under pressures of evolution (Figure 4.4).

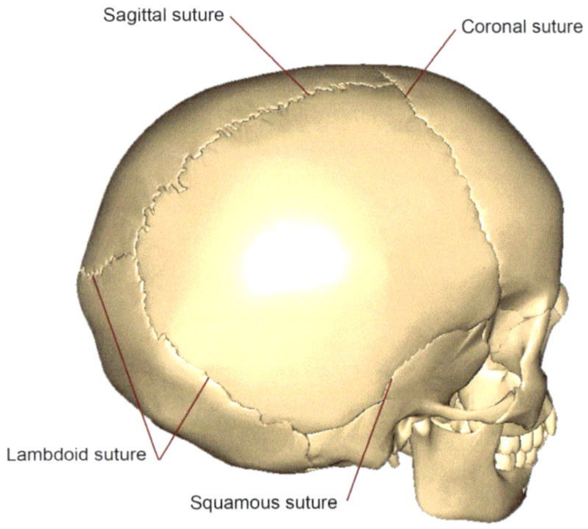

Figure 4.4. Description of the neurocranium's location.

Source: https://external-content.duckduckgo.com/iu/?u=https%3A%2F%2Fs3-us-west-2.amazonaws.com%2Fcourses-images%2Fwp-content%2Fuploads%2Fsites%2F102%2F2017%2F01%2F01213803%2FSutures.png&f=1&nofb=1&ipt=957a14400c90b3e1d958bcae5fb227e4f8c3022b154d210baa97e1bf29a59f5a.

4.1.2. Major Bones That Comprise the Neurocranium

The protective case of the human brain, the neurocranium, consists of eight principal bones: the frontal, parietal, occipital, temporal, sphenoid, and ethmoid bones. All these bones are important for the integrity of the cranium and the protection of the delicate structures contained within. The frontal bone forms the anterior portion of the cranium and is pivotal in bearing the forehead. The parietal bones shape the superior surfaces of the skull, which are sites for muscle attachment. The occipital bone at the rear of the skull gives passage to the spinal cord, demonstrating the neurocranium's important role in protection as well as provision of access between the brain and the body. The assembly of the bones produces a symphonic structure that shields the brain while leaving space for expansion in growth, demonstrating their significance in human osteology as they evolved. Moving closer to the center, the temporal bones that form the lateral walls of the skull hold essential components of the auditory apparatus, including middle and inner ear structures. Their fusion facilitates efficient sound transmission, underscoring the neurocranium's role in sensory reception. Lastly, the sphenoid bone, also known as the keystone of the skull, articulates with every cranial bone, further strengthening its role in providing cranial stability. This strategic location helps comprise a number of important structures, including the eye sockets and the base of the skull. The ethmoid bone, on the other hand, helps comprise the nasal cavity and plays a crucial role in olfactory functions. The relationship of these bones provides evidence not only of their roles in neural protection but also in sensation reception, underscoring the multifunctionality of the neurocranium within the human body. Understanding neurocranium development and structure provides significant insights into cranial variability and developmental craniopathies. The cells of the cranial neural crest mesenchyme (NCM) are particularly significant as they contribute to the formation of the majority of cranial structures during embryogenesis. Disruptions in these processes could lead to congenital anomalies, demonstrating that each bone's correct positioning and integration are crucial. Furthermore, biomechanical forces acting on the forming neurocranium significantly influence its geometry and structural properties. Exploration of these dynamics enhances our understanding of evolutionary adaptations in jaw morphology and cranial development, illustrating both the remarkable flexibility of the neurocranium and its disease susceptibility. Such knowledge is necessary to enhance medical understanding of cranial diseases and develop effective therapeutic treatments, paving the way for further studies in human osteology and cranial growth.

4.1.3. Functions of the Neurocranium

The neurocranium serves a variety of essential functions and is integral to both protection and structural integrity within the human cranium. It is the superior portion of the cranial space and houses the brain, shielding this essential organ from bodily injury. The neurocranium is more than protection, however, and is ideally suited to accommodate the complex anatomy of the brain itself, including its lobes and cranial nerves. This intricate structure is formed by the union of multiple cranial bones that contribute to the neurocranium's overall stability and resistance. The interaction of these bones provides some flexibility, which is very important during childbirth and in response to external pressure, helping reduce the risk of damage. Through this double layer of protection and flexibility, the neurocranium is not only a protective barrier but also an active structural component critical to the preservation of central nervous system function. In addition to protection, the neurocranium provides for variation in cranial shape, and such variation may be of evolutionary importance. During human evolution, selective forces selected cranial morphology for the evolution of sophisticated cognitive function and better sensory function. Genetic factors, as well as developmental environmental factors, affect neurocranium shape and size. For instance, deviations from typical neurocranial growth can result in congenital craniofacial deformities that affect neurodevelopment and overall health.

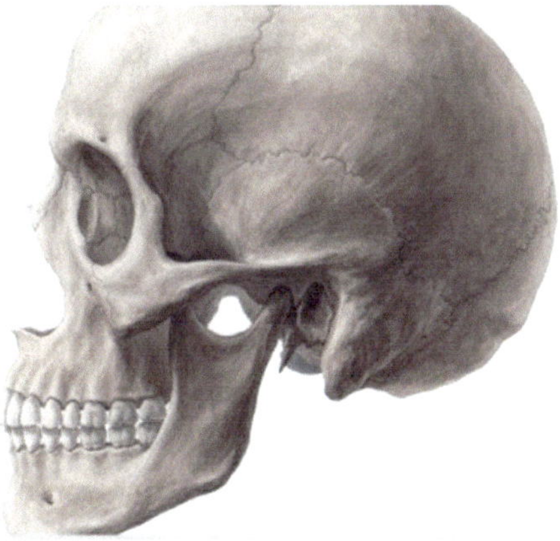

Figure 4.5. Functions of the neurocranium.

Source: https://i.ytimg.com/vi/c7_ZypQ94yQ/hq720.jpg?sqp=-oaymwEhCK4FEIIDSFryq4qpAxMIARUAAAAAGAElAADIQj0AgKJD&rs=AOn4CLArNRLRSwR9r2_HFMLVqountAtIGA.

This highlights the significance of studying the neurocranium, as understanding its morphogenic processes can address how cranial form affects neurological function. Variations in neurocranial form also serve to address human adaptation, biological variation, and the evolutionary course that has shaped our kind throughout history. The neurocranium is also crucial to the interface between the central nervous system and external sensory organs. Comprising the bony structure that supports important sensory modalities such as vision, hearing, and smell, the neurocranium is closely correlated with the functioning of these systems. The cranial base, for instance, houses inner ear and orbital structures and provides pathways through which cranial nerves connect to the brain via peripheral sensory organs. The neurocranium's anatomy is a model of evolutionary compromise that balances the need for protective encasement with the necessity of allowing sensory inputs critical to survival and interaction with the environment. An appreciation of these interrelationships is critical in the study of human osteology and in the exploration of how disruptions to cranial form can interfere with sensory perception and cognitive function, ultimately affecting quality of life (Figure 4.5).

Test Your Knowledge

1. Where is the neurocranium located in the human skull?
2. What is the primary function of the neurocranium?

4.2. Development of the Neurocranium

Learning Outcome

1. Embryological origins of the neurocranium
2. Childhood growth patterns
3. Aging changes in the neurocranium

Development of the neurocranium is a significant aspect of human osteology, intrinsically linking the evolution of cranial form with both form and function. This form is the bony casing that contains the brain, serving as a protective mechanism throughout life. The neurocranium forms mainly from the embryonal mesoderm and neural crest cells, which migrate early in development. The varying contributions of the cells are essential, as they define the fine details of bone formation that support the structural integrity of the neurocranium. As cells progress in differentiation, they undergo complex signaling interactions that ultimately result in the characteristic contours and spatial relationships of the neurocranium, thereby defining the upper boundaries of cranial architecture and protecting the neural tissue. When examining the neurocranium's development, both gene and environmental factors influencing its shape during development should be considered. Alterations in signaling pathways that control cranial neural crest mesenchyme can result in variations with a striking impact on jaw anatomy and the positioning of the entire craniofacial complex. Disruptions may lead to developmental anomalies or conditions that modify the functional properties of the jaw and surrounding structures. The built-in adaptive plasticity of these developmental stages is both fascinating and objectionable; while it permits considerable morphological diversity in response to environmental pressures, it also leaves the individual vulnerable to a range of craniofacial malformations. Thus, the investigation of neurocranium development extends beyond mere morphology to the long-term conditions it harbors for clinical pathology. Moreover, the evolutionary history of the neurocranium highlights its significance in human osteology. The neurocranial adaptations are not merely short-term, environment-responsive, but rather a manifestation of an evolutionary trend that has shaped cranial morphology across species. The evolutionary perspective sheds light on the interface of mechanical forces and molecular mechanisms governing the developmental process of the neurocranium. For instance, biomechanical forces' role in cranial development is critical because it influences both the physical growth and functional anatomy of the cranial framework. With increased scholarly research, it is increasingly evident that an understanding of the developmental intricacies of the neurocranium is central to understanding the intricacies of craniofacial morphology and its application to both evolutionary biology and human health (Adriaens et al., 2010; Abzhanov et al., 2019).

4.2.1. Embryological Origins of the Neurocranium

The embryological origin of the neurocranium begins early in development and is primarily contributed by the mesoderm and neural crest. The neurocranium, the cranial bony covering of the brain, originates from both paraxial mesoderm that goes into segmentation into somites and neural crest cells that migrate to the cranial region. During development, these cells undergo stereotypical movements and differences that give rise to the individual cranial bones. The fusion of several ossification centers, mostly derived from such lineage cells, is critical for the formation of the neurocranial structure. Understanding such origins not only indicates the complex processes that lead to cranial anatomy but also points to potential pathways for congenital abnormalities when embryological growth is compromised. Most crucial to the formation of the neurocranium is the role played by cranial neural crest mesenchyme (NCM) in patterning many of the cranial elements. NCM is also responsible for the patterning of bones, cartilages, and other supportive elements and therefore plays a fundamental role in form and function as well of the neurocranium. The relationship between NCM and surrounding tissues enables specialized patterning, allowing functional diversification and giving rise to various species. This molecular interaction sheds light on evolutionary processes that have led to cranial morphological adaptations in different amniotes. Analyzing how molecular processes regulate these variations will allow researchers to gain insight into the evolutionary significance of the neurocranium regarding jaw function and other craniofacial structures, thereby solidifying the relationship between embryology and osteology.

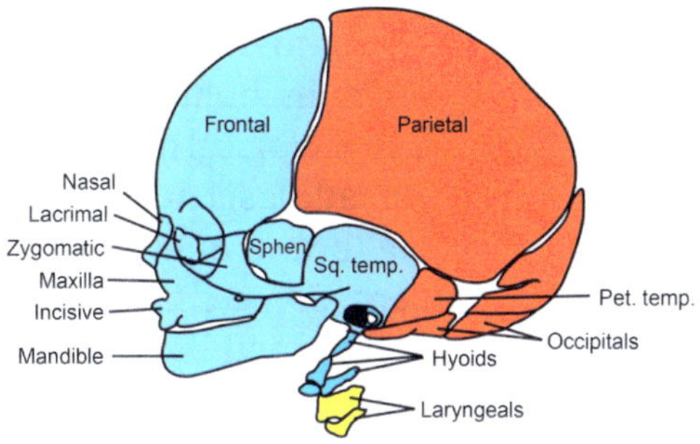

Figure 4.6. The embryological origins of the neurocranium begin during the early stages of development

Source: https://embryology.oit.duke.edu/craniofacial/headEmbryoImage11.jpg.

The newly updated anatomical terminology described in the 2019 version of Terminologia Anatomica, published by the Federative International Programme for Anatomical Terminology, is a necessary resource for students and professionals studying the human skull and neurocranium. Clarity and precision are the emphasis in this edition, which seeks to cover the often-complex head anatomy of the neurocranium and its structures. By democratizing this nomenclature, medical education students and educators are better equipped to address evolving terminology in anatomy. The changes are presented to make understanding and communication easier in both clinical and academic settings, particularly in light of challenges posed by traditional nomenclature. Expanding awareness of these nomenclature changes is important for advancing an inclusive approach to neurocranial anatomy and, thus, enhancing teaching and applied practice in the field of human osteology, as evidenced by controversies in cranial anatomy and human developmental diversity (Chmielewski et al., 2021) (Figure 4.6).

4.2.2. Growth Patterns During Childhood

Patterns of childhood growth, particularly in the neurocranium, are crucial to the understanding of overall development in human osteology. Development of the morphological neurocranium between infancy and adolescence , creating space for a growing brain and supporting functional development. Some changes involve coordination of resorption and bone formation across cranial sutures. The sutures maintain patency during this remodeling, allowing for growth and accommodation to environmental stresses. Trends in these processes are critical to understand, as they can inform broader developmental milestones and potential health relevance, such as the identification of growth abnormalities predictive of underlying pathologies or developmental disabilities (Das et al., 2022). In addition to general growth patterns, childhood craniofacial sex dimorphism also complicates the study of the neurocranium. Research has shown that male and female skulls become increasingly different as they grow. For instance, through the application of advanced imaging techniques, it has been confirmed that the male neurocranium grows lengthwise and widthwise more than that of a female, with greater anterior growth in the facial bones. Such differences have serious implications for anthropological analysis and forensic assessments. Awareness of such differences not only helps us understand human morphology but also enables the establishment of methodologies for sex estimation, which have achieved classification accuracy of 92% in populations of aged juveniles (Phillips et al., 2013). The results have implications for clinical practice and research protocols aimed at monitoring developmental norms and abnormalities. Also, the combination of environmental circumstances and hereditary tendencies determines the growth patterns in the neurocranium in infancy. While genetic factors lay the foundation for cranial development, environmental , such as nutrition, socio-economic status, and traditional practices, can alter the process. For instance, adequate nutrition during critical growth stages is essential to optimize craniofacial development, as malnutrition can lead to underdevelopment or deformities. The convergence of these factors is equally crucial in understanding the complexity of normal growth as opposed to pathologies. Clinicians and researchers must consider intrinsic and extrinsic factors when assessing cranial growth and potential growth disorders, as variations in growth patterns may indicate more extensive health issues that extend beyond skeletal maturation (Das et al., 2022) (Figure 4.7).

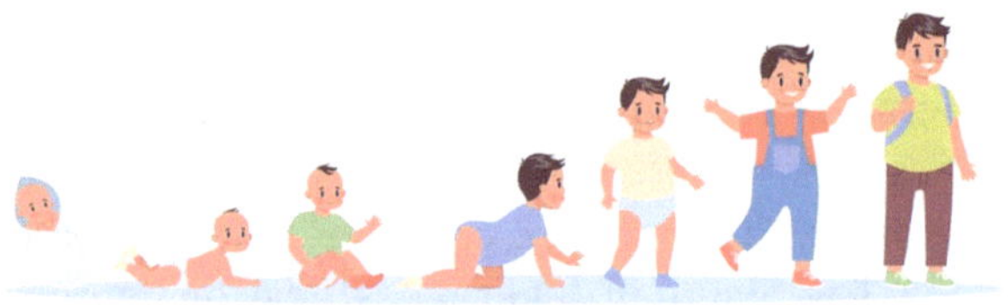

Figure 4.7. The growth patterns observed during childhood.

Source: https://www.shutterstock.com/image-vector/baby-growth-process-newborn-preschool-260nw-1680424801.jpg.

4.2.3. Changes in the Neurocranium with Aging

The neurocranium also undergoes significant morphological changes with aging, mirroring both environmental and physiological forces. Based on the literature, age-related changes in the skeleton can be diverse, so providing for specific time effects on the neurocranium must be acknowledged. The changes include cranial suture changes, where the complex interplay between bone resorption and bone deposition becomes evident. Patency, or openness, of the cranial sutures is preserved by a synchronized process of remodeling from infancy to adulthood. Remodeling is significant because it can affect cranial stability and overall head form with potential consequences for neurological function and health. Awareness of these alterations makes it easier to demarcate the line between normal aging processes and pathologic conditions, illuminating the template for future studies into the neurocranium's role in human osteology (Das et al., 2022). In addition, the morphological alterations in the neurocranium with increasing age also extend beyond the sutures, influencing the overall cranial shape and structural integrity. Research reveals that the internal architecture of the skull's trabecular and cortical bone changes in a way that may affect cranial capacity, as well as the brain's protective barriers. Such a change is a sign that there should be monitoring of craniofacial sexual dimorphism, which is sure to diminish with age. Specifically, reduced reductions in dimorphic areas have been documented, indicating the dynamic nature of the neurocranium as people progress through different stages of life. The ratio of unique morphological variation is central to forensic anthropology and biologic research because it explains demographic and evolutionary patterns in bones, which reveal something about the interrelations among aging, neurocranium shape, and individual identification (Suchá et al., 2024). In addition to these changes in form, the neurocranium's response to aging also has broader implications for disease and health. The heterogeneity of aging mechanisms necessitates a delicate assessment to distinguish normal from pathological states. Research indicates that aging-related progress is accompanied by changes in cranial sutures and cranial form, which are expressed through changes directly related to degenerative aging disorders, affecting cognitive and neurological well-being. This points to the significance of measuring cranial thickness and understanding its role as a marker of broader problems in the aging group. Thus, the investigation of neurocranial structures not only enriches human osteology but also serves important functional functions in medicine, anthropology, and archaeological analysis. By correlating patterns of aging changes with general wellness outcomes, researchers can enhance understanding of the complexities of skull morphology that emerge with aging and their implications (Das et al., 2022) (Figure 4.8).

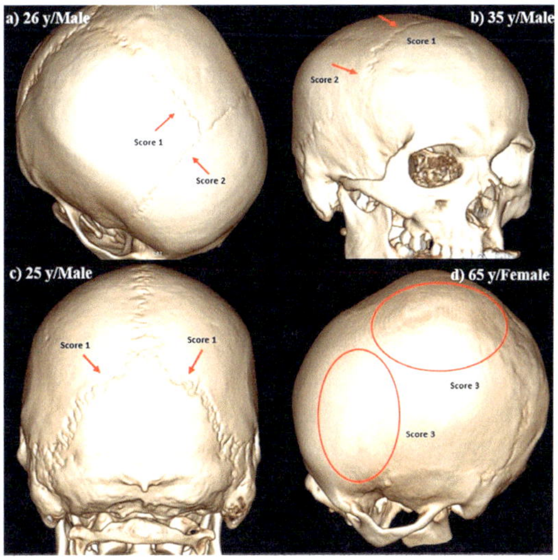

Figure 4.8. Changes in the neurocranium with aging.

Source: https://assets.cureus.com/uploads/figure/file/575906/article_river_f20a1080ba9611eda0a40d0d6dbdd3d0-thesis-image-final.png.

Test Your Knowledge

1. What are the embryological origins of the neurocranium?
2. How does the neurocranium change with aging?

4.3. Neurocranium and Brain Protection

Learning Outcome

1. Function of the neurocranium in protecting the brain
2. Effect of neurocranium structure on brain functioning
3. Typical injuries and their impact on the neurocranium

The neurocranium plays an important role in protecting the human brain, serving as a rugged encasement that is both physically protective and structurally supportive. Composed of several fused bones, such as the frontal, parietal, temporal, and occipital bones, this bony structure not only offers protection from external damage but also constitutes the overall anatomy of the skull. Developmental factors, such as sutural closure and sinus development, control the morphology of the neurocranium. Interestingly enough, the frontal bone, which consists of two halves that join after birth, can be affected by variations in the fusion of sutures, which can influence the development of the frontal sinus. These intricacies illustrate the interaction between brain protection and neurocranial morphology, such that an abnormality in bone formation will result in a series of complications that impact both structural integrity and intracranial pressure regulation (Georgiev et al., 2018). Apart from its structural role, the neurocranium also helps maintain the brain's homeostasis. The cranial vault contains cerebrospinal fluid (CSF), which cushions and protects neural tissues from mechanical stress. It also facilitates the transport of nutrients and elimination of waste products, thereby maintaining general brain health. Abnormalities in the craniofacial structures can compromise regular CSF flow and pressure, illustrating how neurocranium anatomy influences neurological function. Research shows that certain features of the orbit and the relationships among the cranial bones can indicate age, race, and gender, thereby enhancing forensic and clinical assessment. By studying the cranial vault's size and patterns, it is possible to uncover information about the defense mechanisms that prevent injury, highlighting the neurocranium's vital role in protecting the brain (Kong et al., 2015). Moreover, the awareness of the development and shape of the neurocranium is of significant value for clinical and surgical purposes. Variations or deformities, such as craniosynostosis, must be carefully considered since they impact brain development and protection.

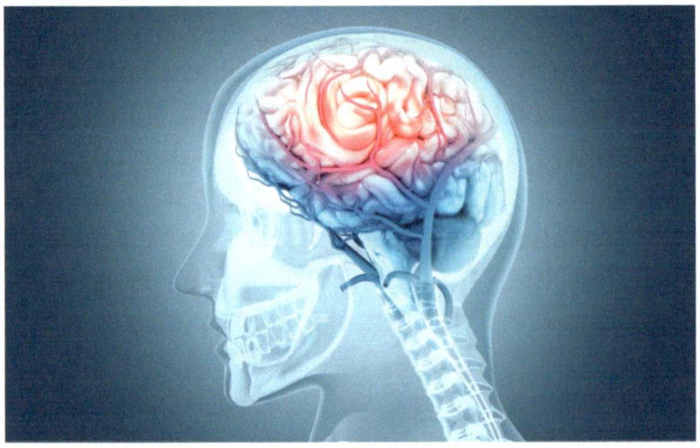

Figure 4.9. Neurocranium and brain protection.

Source: https://external-content.duckduckgo.com/iu/?u=https%3A%2F%2Fwww.grmedcenter.com%2Fwp-content%2Fuploads%2F2023%2F07%2FiStock-1421001995-scaled.jpg&f=1&nofb=1&ipt=6812225986f75aaef885de951191df7660e360727f95188b7e147a18b70284c8.

For instance, conditions like the failure to close the metopic suture are associated with alterations in the frontal bone as well as potentially influencing frontal sinus development. This association demonstrates how cranial abnormalities may manifest as structural and functional deficits, which are important to consider in medical interventions. As forensic anthropology and clinical radiology continue to evolve, a detailed understanding of neurocranial anatomy and its protective role will remain essential. Such information not only helps in diagnosing and treating cranial diseases but also contributes to the general understanding of human osteology and its influence on health outcomes (Georgiev et al., 2018) (Figure 4.9).

4.3.1. Role of the Neurocranium in Safeguarding the Brain

The neurocranium plays a crucial role in protecting the brain through its complex structure and composition. Composed of eight bones, including the frontal, parietal, and occipital bones, the neurocranium provides an immovable casing that protects the soft neural tissues from external physical damage. This protective bone structure not only shields but also facilitates essential functions, such as providing a house for the brain's support structures, like membranes and cerebrospinal fluid, that support the brain and serve to absorb impacts further. Moreover, the stability of the neurocranium is essential for optimal cranial pressure, which is essential for normal neurological function. Without such protective mechanisms, the brain would be vulnerable to injuries resulting from day-to-day activities, further stressing the evolutionary role of this skeletal element in human survival and physiology. Second, the neurocranium exhibits unique growth patterns that change throughout life, reflecting its dynamic protection of the brain. For instance, during infancy and early childhood, the sutures of the skull are open, allowing for cranial expansion due to growing brain size and accommodation to developmental changes. It is not a passive process; it is an active process that involves bone resorption and bone deposition, which adapts to genetic and environmental factors over time. With advancing age, cranial suture integrity and overall skull thickness can change, altering the protective function of the neurocranium. The changes hold the key to understanding how cranial structure evolves with age and influences neuroprotective functions, as identified in a study outlining age-associated skull alterations and their connection to cognitive health (Das et al., 2022). Eventually, the neurocranium's role is not merely physical protection but also its contribution to neuroanatomical mechanisms. The skull's construction allows for the incorporation of various brain regions while leaving essential vascular and neural tracts intact.

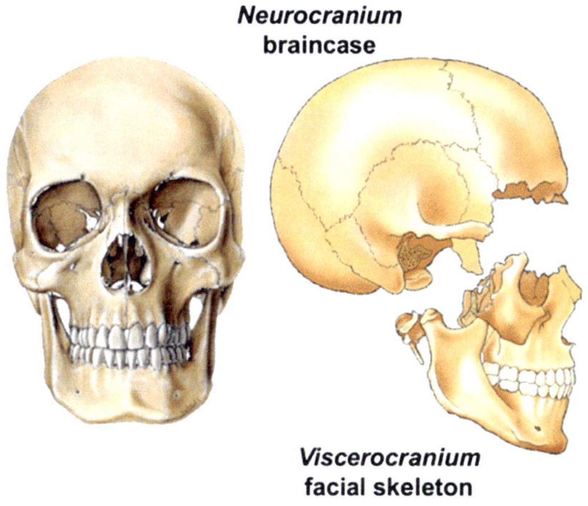

Figure 4.10. Role of the neurocranium in safeguarding the brain.

Source: https://external-content.duckduckgo.com/iu/?u=https%3A%2F%2Fo.quizlet.com%2FqJtUlsv8JB-Gb6A1KwaPAw.png&f=1&nofb=1&ipt=e802f680cdefcc9d32b691647ddf30c2a112407d5cad120930abe8ca29370679.

Such construction not only preserves cognitive functions but also guards against potential pathological abnormalities induced by structural flaws or age-related degeneration. Secondly, familiarity with the evolutionary accommodations of the neurocranium contributes to the interpretation of fossil evidence, offering insights into the morphological and behavioral evolution of early humans. As mentioned in the present study concerning cranial morphology, the neurocranium can symbolize both adaptation to environmental forces and evolutionary development of sophisticated cognitive abilities in hominins (N/A, 2017). Thus, the neurocranium is not only essential for safeguarding the brain but also for understanding human evolution and osteological development (Figure 4.10).

4.3.2. Impact of Neurocranium Structure on Brain Function

The structure of the neurocranium plays a crucial role in defining the brain's various functions, especially in how it is supported and safeguarded. Composed of numerous bones that enclose the cranial cavity, the structure of the neurocranium facilitates the normal development and functioning of the brain. For instance, the cranial vault not only provides physical protection to the brain but also serves a vital role in accommodating cerebrospinal fluid, essential for cushioning the brain against external mechanical forces. Such cushioning is particularly necessary given that the brain requires an unchanging state of existence for its functionality. Furthermore, the thickness and solidity of the neurocranium can influence intracranial pressure, impairing neuronal communication and overall brain well-being, thereby highlighting the critical interdependence of cranial form and brain function. Structurally supportive as it is, the neurocranium is also intimately connected to the brains functional systems by means of development and morphology. The correspondence between cerebral development and cranial growth patterns illustrates the accommodative nature of such structures. Morphological variation of the neurocranium may affect brain growth by increasing brain expansion during development and producing distinct functional effects. For example, studies show that morphological abnormalities of the neurocranium can induce developmental disorders and cognitive dysfunction, underscoring the importance of regular morphological patterns in maintaining unimpaired brain function. Knowledge of how variation in neurocranial shape is connected to neurological function has the ability to inform the evolutionary development of humankind and the specialization of particular brain regions, ultimately influencing cognitive function and processing ability. The significance of neurocranium shape transfers to functional purposes in areas such as forensic science and medicine. For example, anthropometric research on cranial dimensions has been critical in historical and demographic research, accounting for racial and gender differences in neurocranial anatomy.

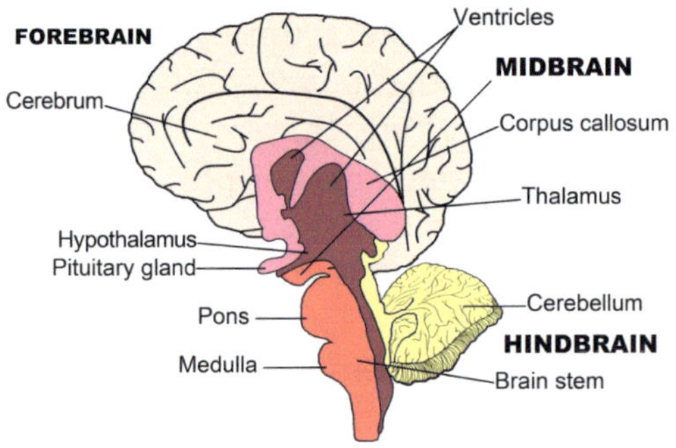

Figure 4.11. The structure of the neurocranium plays a pivotal role in determining various functions of the brain.

Source: https://external-content.duckduckgo.com/iu/?u=https%3A%2F%2Fwww.nbia.ca%2Fwp-content%2Fuploads%2F2014%2F03%2Fbrain-structure1.jpg&f=1&nofb=1&ipt=2c81d557465c87d40265de506364444fed0311022ae498abbfeecbb8d8712611.

Evidence indicates measurable differences in dimensions such as the width and height of the orbit, which can be important to account for in explaining the cranium's development and its impact on brain function across different populations (Kong et al., 2015). These findings underscore the importance of exploring neurocranium variations, not only for anthropological inquiry but also for clinical applications such as neurosurgical interventions and orthodontic treatments. Ongoing research on neurocranial morphology and its relationship to brain function can yield further insights into human evolution, health disparities, and novel therapeutic approaches to craniofacial abnormalities, thereby improving our general understanding of the intricacies of human osteology (Figure 4.11).

4.3.3. Common Injuries and Their Effects on the Neurocranium

The neurocranium, which houses the brain, is most vulnerable to various types of injury, mainly blunt trauma-induced injuries. Blunt trauma-induced injuries, commonly a result of accidents or brawls, tend to result in severe structural damage to the cranial bones. Not only do these traumas increase the chances of fractures, but they also contribute to secondary injuries like concussions, contusions, and intracranial hemorrhages. An extensive review of traumatic trauma emphasizes the importance of understanding the mechanisms of forces to the skull. Biomechanical examinations of blunt force trauma emphasize how the impact site, severity of force, and surface geometry cooperate to produce specific patterns of injury. Human skeletal analysis expertise, as documented in more recent studies, facilitates the reconstruction of the environment in which injuries occurred (Marinho et al., 2013). This assists in guiding forensic trauma analysis in court. The implications of neurocranium injuries extend beyond physical impacts. They often have wide-ranging cognitive and psychological impacts that manifest over the long term. Patients may acquire perceptual shifts, memory processing problems, and emotional lability following severe cranial injury. The relationship between structural harm, such as fractures or contusions, and neurologic outcomes is complex, relying on the person's age, overall physical health, and the existence of comorbidities. It is also critical to consider the impact of repeated head trauma, which is common in contact sports, as accumulative trauma can lead to chronic traumatic encephalopathy (CTE). This makes it imperative to ensure proper medical evaluation and treatment following occurrences of neurocranium injuries, considering a larger public health concern surrounding head trauma and its consequences (Das et al., 2022). In addition to the psychological and cognitive effects, the physical alterations resulting from the injury to the neurocranium can be problematic when they heal. The neurocranium has a complex structure that may require extensive medical intervention to facilitate full recovery. Fractures not only distort the cranial structure but also the peripheral soft tissues, producing complications such as infection or elevated intracranial pressure. Since cranial sutures follow age-related patterns that change over time through bone remodeling, this information is fundamental for the assessment and management of injuries and trauma (Marinho et al., 2013). The constant research regarding the interaction between cranial sutures, aging, and trauma serves to reinforce the essence of making informed judgments regarding the handling of head injuries (Marinho et al., 2013). Lastly, the effects of trauma to the neurocranium extend far past immediate harm to the body, and there is a host of potential effects determined by biology and situation.

Test Your Knowledge

1. How does the neurocranium protect the brain?
2. What are common injuries to the neurocranium, and how do they affect its function?

4.4. Neurocranium in Forensic Anthropology

Learning Outcome

1. Identification of people by cranial details
2. Study of trauma and pathology in the neurocranium
3. Application of neurocranium to ancestry determination

The neurocranium is crucial in forensic anthropology because it provides a solid basis for estimating demographic features, such as age, sex, and ancestry, from bone remnants. The unique morphology of cranial sutures, which have growth and closure phases during development, allows forensic anthropologists to assess age accurately. Research highlights the importance of understanding the synchronized remodeling of cranial sutures, with these advancements maintaining patency because of bone deposition and resorption from childhood to young adulthood. The relationship between cranial sutures and aging underscores how morphological characteristics can yield insights into individuals' biological profiles. Therefore, using the neurocranium as a point of reference in forensic analysis not only enables the creation of a biological profile but also enhances the precision of age estimates in human skeletons, which are critical for efficient identification procedures in the forensic environment (Das et al., 2022). Determination of ancestry in juvenile skeletons remains a challenging field for forensic anthropologists. Despite the existence of standard protocols for obtaining biological profiles from adults, subadult remains are limited for estimating ancestry because few studies have examined nonmetric traits across ages. Studies on prominent collections of skeletons like the Hamann-Todd and Terry Osteological Collections reveal that even in younger humans, variation existed among the ancestral groups, although scoring the nonmetric traits was difficult. These findings point to the neurocranium as a major source of subadult ancestry determination in remains, providing evidence that juvenile cranial characteristics warrant further examination to enhance forensic methods. As a result, addressing the complexities of subadult ancestry determination could help more fully interpret forensic demographic patterns (Reinman et al., 2019). The application of neurocranium analysis extends beyond mere identification; it provides evidence of the biological and environmental forces that shape human skeletal development. Morphological alterations in the neurocranium can provide insights into genetics, diet, and health throughout an individual's life course.

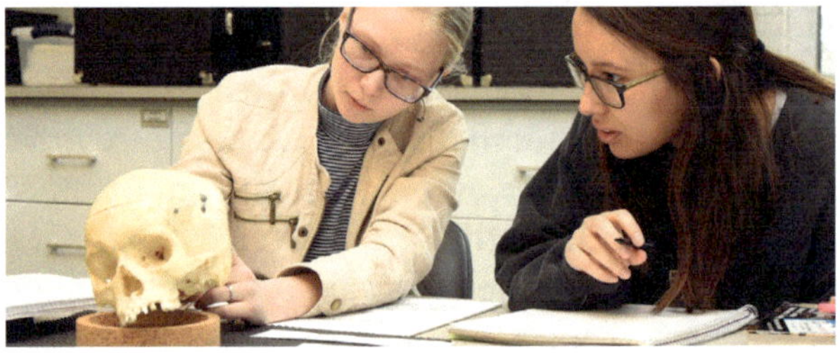

Figure 4.12. The neurocranium serves a vital function in forensic anthropology.

Source: https://external-content.duckduckgo.com/iu/?u=https%3A%2F%2Fwww.washburn.edu%2F_redesign2018%2F_files%2Fimages%2Finterior%2Fforensics%2FRS2014_DSC_8596.jpg&f=1&nofb=1&ipt=12277f04979848d6662496f3a157935981e507e2df3c01bac7ef90174d897aa4.

The intersection of developmental pathways and forensic anthropology is particularly valuable when considering age variation and biological profiles. The ability to separate normal variation from pathological conditions via cranial morphology is a valuable forensic anthropologist's skill. Second, recognizing the trajectory effect, or the splitting of the biological and chronological age, and further acceleration with aging, enhances human skeletal aging knowledge in forensic practice. The neurocranium is thus a vital part not only to recognize an individual but also to put their life story into perspective regarding demographic factors and health conditions (Das et al., 2022) (Figure 4.12).

4.4.1. Identification of Individuals Through Cranial Features

An individual's identification based on cranial features has become a prime area of study in human osteology, making it feasible for forensic experts and anthropologists to determine sex, age, and even ancestry from bones. The neurocranium, which houses the brain, is the most significant one because it has comparatively consistent morphology along with characteristic features that can be different between an individuals and. For instance, the systematic comparison of cranial dimensions can reveal phenotypic differences connected with biological sex. Studies have determined that males' crania exhibit higher dimensions and strength compared to women, with classification accuracy ranging from 66%–92% based on age group and method used, as indicated in current research that builds on previous success in such research (Phillips et al., 2013). Aside from sex determination, the neurocranium also has an important role in age estimation, particularly in juvenile remains. The patterns of growth in the craniofacial anatomy are manifestations of biological processes associated with maturation. As children mature, certain indicators within the neurocranium—such as suture closure and cranial vault proportions—can indicate an individual's stage of development. Investigation with sophisticated imaging techniques, such as CT scans, can capture fine cranial details that might otherwise be missed during routine examinations. These techniques are vital for formulating classification models that leverage visually derived data, which aid in building detailed profiles of skeletal remains (Phillips et al., 2013). This focus on cranial morphology not only enriches forensic applications but is also pertinent to the broader anthropological study of population variation over time. Cranial morphology is not solely the result of biological processes; it is also influenced by environmental and genetic processes operating in individual identification. The intricate interplay between cranial morphology and ancestry has been elucidated in studies of the impact of evolutionary pathways on craniofacial morphology. For example, specific neurocranial characteristics can be shown to represent previous adaptations influenced by climate and geography. These variations are important data for forensic identification, where determining a person's geographic and ethnic origin could assist in unidentified-remains cases. With phylogenetic research still underway to shed light on the evolutionary background of cranial morphology, they reinforce the need to rely on neurocranial features as reliable indicators for establishing identity and making sense of human diversity. Finally, the multi-dimensionality of cranial identification through neurocranial features promises fertile grounds for exploration in human osteology (Figure 4.13).

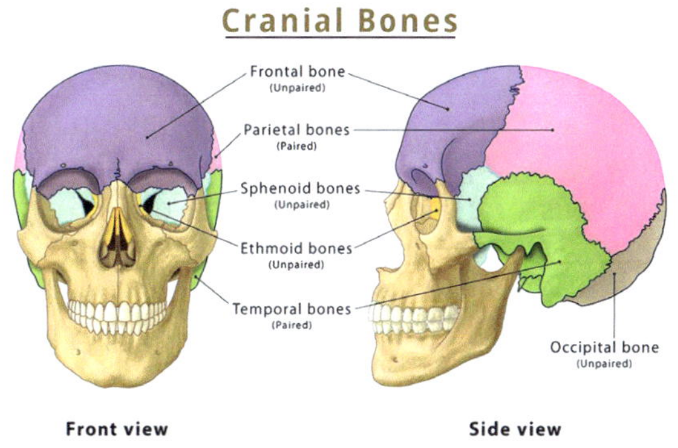

Figure 4.13. Identification of individuals through cranial features.

Source: https://external-content.duckduckgo.com/iu/?u=https%3A%2F%2Fwww.theskeletalsystem.net%2Fwp-content%2Fuploads%2F2022%2F03%2FCranial-Bones-Labeled.jpg&f=1&nofb=1&ipt=e3d544c8a62494979f3010fa6be8c9eae6cf1a5764291ae6f00dcc3806b7fbd7.

4.4.2. Analysis of Trauma and Pathology in the Neurocranium

Analysis of trauma and pathology within the neurocranium provides important insights into human osteology and structural integrity in response to external energy. Protective architecture for the brain, the neurocranium consists of primary elements such as the frontal, parietal, temporal, and occipital bones. It may be influenced by different forms of trauma, either caused by blunt trauma, penetrating trauma, or illness. These traumas can alter its form and function. Determining alterations to these necessitates understanding a combination of biomechanical stresses and adaptive body mechanisms. For instance, the assessment of cranial trauma caused by traumatic injury typically employs imaging modalities in order to determine fractures or distortions, which may have particular significance to neurological health and cognitive functions. Results of such analyses are invaluable in uses like forensic science, where etiology of cranial injury aids in determining the cause of death and circumstances of traumatic injury. Deviations in states of the neurocranium often arise from a multitude of intrinsic and extrinsic stimuli that compromise bone strength. Osteoporosis, for instance, significantly alters the mechanical properties of cranial bones such that they are susceptible to fracture and deformation. This condition could be particularly heightened in the instance of castration history, with studies showing that anthropological analysis was employed to highlight cervical vertebrae alterations associated with prolonged singing practice in castrati. Here, castration hormonal effects led to higher occurrences of osteoporosis, and this furthered the risk for cranial trauma (Bonati et al., 2016). These observations emphasize the importance of identifying discrete pathological markers in the neurocranium, which are particularly important for determining the effects of genetic and environmental interactions on normal and abnormal cranial growth. Advances in imaging and anthropometric analysis have also enhanced our knowledge of trauma and pathology within the neurocranium, enabling better clinical management. Computed tomography (CT) scan-based studies quantifying orbital measurements reveal age, race, and gender correlations that affect cranial shape (Kong et al., 2015). By highlighting correlations in measurements like orbital height and width, variability in such measurements can provide critical information for clinical application in all aspects, from maxillofacial surgery to forensic identification. Besides, generating baseline anthropometric data not only enables surgical precision but also helps us understand normal cranial variations, thereby improving trauma assessment and aftercare. Understanding these relationships is essential in the development of population-specific interventions, including the mechanical trauma effects and occult pathologies that predispose individuals to neurocranial trauma.

4.4.3. Use of Neurocranium in Determining Ancestry

The neurocranium is responsible for contributing immensely to defining human ancestry, as the morphological variations usually match the genetic population adaptations over time. Several environmental factors, such as climate and lifestyle, have influenced cranial feature development and can be traced to an ancestral origin. Researchers study characteristics such as the shape and size of the neurocranium to demarcate boundaries among groups based on the evolutionary mechanisms that lead to differences manifesting in physical traits. Because these characteristics are passed down through generations, the neurocranium serves as an entry point into an individual's genetic inheritance, yielding information about their lineage. This influential association illustrates not only the function of cranial morphology but also its role in mapping human evolutionary history. Identification of ancestry using neurocranial morphology is also complemented by technological advances such as discriminant function analysis. This method allows precise discrimination of skull features and has been used successfully in research to distinguish between various population groups. For example, research has shown strong sexual dimorphism in craniofacial growth, implying that skulls of males and females possess different characteristics that can be employed to deduce ancestry. Research carried out on juveniles has implied that neurocrania morphologies are involved in the determination of ancestry, as some forms of growth occur, which concern sex and age. This systematic analysis emphasizes the importance of neurocranial measurements in anthropology so that scientists are able to make more accurate classifications and interpretations of human populations' migratory and evolutionary histories, corroborating the importance of the neurocranium in estimating ancestry. Furthermore, neurocranium form and age have important roles in establishing ancestry. During growth, the human skeleton undergoes many changes, particularly in cranial sutures and overall cranial architecture. Knowledge of such changes is fundamental for assessing biological ancestry and chronological age, indicating the correlation between skeletal changes and age and genetic background. Researchers note that age markers should exhibit uniform characteristics that change in a single direction, thereby making ancestry estimation more precise over time. For instance, variations in cranial suture morphology provide clues to the identification of the biological and environmental determinants of skull shape among populations. Therefore, the inclusion of age-related changes in neurocranium analysis enables a more advanced understanding of human ancestry, thereby justifying the application of cranial studies in anthropological research (Phillips et al., 2013; Das et al., 2022).

Test Your Knowledge

1. How is the neurocranium studied to identify trauma and pathology in forensic anthropology?
2. How can neurocranial features be used to determine ancestry in forensic investigations?

4.5. Comparative Anatomy of the Neurocranium

Learning Outcome

1. Differences between human and non-human organisms' neurocranium
2. Evolutionary significance of neurocranium differences
3. Lessons from comparative anatomy in anthropology

The comparative anatomy of the neurocranium provides valuable insights into the evolutionary adaptations of various species, particularly those of the amniotic lineage. The architecture of the neurocranium is necessary not only for its protective function over the brain but also because it covers sensory organs and enables the various modes of life to perceive their surroundings. When two neurocrania from different species are compared, one finds vast variability across environmental and developmental contexts. For instance, variation in the shape and size of the neurocranial elements may reflect different functional demands, such as sensory information and feeding modes. These changes are backed by sophisticated molecular and cellular mechanisms underlying cranial character evolution, pointing to the role of cranial neural crest mesenchyme in shaping cranial form and function throughout evolution (Abzhanov et al., 2019). The evolutionary significance of the neurocranium can also be illustrated through research in particular groups. An examination of the Sami populations inhabiting Kolsky Bay illustrates how cranial elements develop to accommodate unfavorable environmental conditions. The comparative study observed that there was a range of variations between male and female skulls regarding their facial skeletons, highlighting how genes and environment interact during cranial development. Such flexibility implies neurocranial traits are dynamic but instead vary based on social, ecological, and biomechanical stresses. Understanding these differences enriches our understanding of human osteology by situating cranial development within a broader evolutionary context and demonstrating the intricate interaction between form and function across different human populations (Borutskaya et al., 2017). Lastly, comparative neurocranial anatomy extends beyond the field of plain morphology, allowing us to extrapolate deeper insights into the progression of vertebrate evolution, including that of human beings.

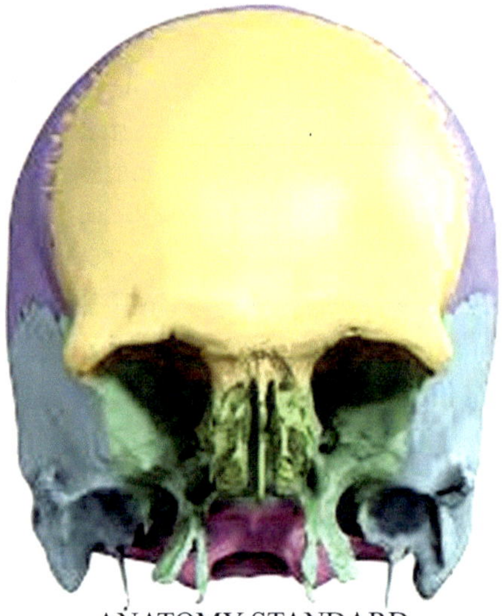

Figure 4.14. The comparative anatomy of the neurocranium.

Source: https://encrypted-tbn0.gstatic.com/images?q=tbn:ANd9GcSX6ROMhabdZftzsN4nVskNKSEgO_aDPDQYTg&s.

By comparing neurocranial morphology across a series of animals, scientists trace out the significant evolutionary lines that have led to the highly developed shapes we observe. Neurocranium evolution is inextricably bound to adaptive modes, as observed in the amniote jaw complex, revealing the subtle interplay of genetic, environmental, and developmental processes that shape cranial form. By further exploring variations within and between species, we can better understand how neurocranial structure not only helps to ensure the survival of the individual but also contributes to the diversity of life forms that have evolved over the course of evolutionary history (Abzhanov et al., 2019) (Figure 4.14).

4.5.1. Differences Between Human and Non-Human Neurocranium

Comparing the human and non-human neurocranium, one finds that each has been significantly shaped by evolution, with the necessary effects on their anatomical structures. Human beings possess a relatively larger neurocranium than facial structures compared to non-human primates, and this is strongly linked to cognitive development and the capacity to execute higher-order functions. This proportional enlargement mirrors the development of higher brain systems responsible for advanced reasoning, language acquisition, and social interaction. On this basis, the vertical height of the human neurocranium is most pronounced, with an increasingly rounded cranium that differs markedly from the elongate or flattened crania of the majority of non-human species. These morphological differences are also reflective not only of the evolutionary record but also of the differing functional stresses on the neurocranium across species, implying a complex interrelationship between morphology and intellectual capacity. Moreover, the integration of the cranial elements presents an attractive perspective on the evolutionary divergence of humans from non-human neurocrania. It has been evidenced that morphological integration is somewhat dissimilar, with human humans tending to have low integration than other primates, such as baboons, with high levels of skeletal integration between cranial components (Hemingway et al., 2017). Differences in integration could be attributed to different genetic and developmental mechanisms as well as functional adaptations. For example, the vault, facial skeleton, and cranial base of humans exhibit unique covariation patterns compared to those of non-human primates. Modularity of this kind is important for maintaining organismal viability, facilitating solitary adaptations while preserving general cranial function. This differentiation highlights how evolutionary forces have shaped the neurocranium to meet the particular requirements of humanity, supporting the contention that cranial shape is inextricably tied to biological fitness and interactions with the external world. The consequences of these structural variations extend beyond simple morphology to shape the functional potential of the neurocranium for communicative and sensory functions. The human neurocranium has space for evolved auditory and vocal capabilities, an evolutionary adaptation favorable to the emergence of language. Non-human primates, with evolved communication systems, exhibit variable neurocranial structure in line with their specific social and environmental demands, which lean towards visual or olfactory aspects rather than vocal expression. The distinctive pattern of neurocranial elements is also the basis for sensory information processing, thereby differentiating humans from non-humans in their cognitive and communication practices. Hence, the study of differences in neurocrania not only advances knowledge of human osteology but also identifies the evolutionary processes that have shaped the distinctive cognitive and communicative arenas we observe between species today (Abzhanov et al., 2019).

4.5.2. Evolutionary Significance of Neurocranium Variations

The neurocranium, or braincase, is one of the most significant evolutionary adaptations that has diversified across vertebrate species in response to varied ecological and biological stresses. Neurocranium variations are of extreme significance in interpreting functional anatomy, particularly neuroanatomy and sensory function. Neurocranium differences are of utmost significance in human evolution. For instance, the size and shape of this structure evolved over time in response to changes in brain size and intellectual capacity, pointing to a connection between cranial shape and neurological development. The correlation suggests that the evolution of the neurocranium provides testimony regarding alterations in social behavior and environmental adaptation, emphasizing its pivotal position within the hominin phylogenetic landscape. Furthermore, the ontogeny of neurocranial features demonstrates how such differences can confer evolutionary advantages in response to environmental niches. Cranial morphologies across species, including the damselfish, are explored through research demonstrating that various skeletal units have evolved to support specific environmental demands. As evidenced, the more varied the neurocranial form, the more environmentally flexible, suggesting that differences in shape can determine survival and reproductive success under changing environments. For instance, the evolution of damselfish from larvae to adults illustrates significant changes in neurocranial morphology that are correlated with shifts in diet and habitat use, supporting the contention that cranial specializations are often an immediate reflection of selection pressures in specific environmental contexts (Cardini et al., 2011). Moreover, the recognition of neurocranium variations is not merely about anatomical comparison; it also informs discussions of ancestry and demographic profiling in forensic anthropology. As has been proposed by recent studies, the neurocranial characteristics can provide significant information for the reconstruction of identities from skeletal remains. This is particularly crucial in subadult individuals, where neurocranium variations can serve as excellent markers for determining ancestry. By examining nonmetric characteristics of the neurocranium, researchers can uncover patterns that can be observed to have evolutionary significance for population migrations and interbreeding events in ancient human populations. These findings are significant for the neurocranium not only from a biological perspective but also in terms of its role in anthropological studies of human variation and the evolutionary process that characterizes our kind (Reinman et al., 2019) (Figure 4.15).

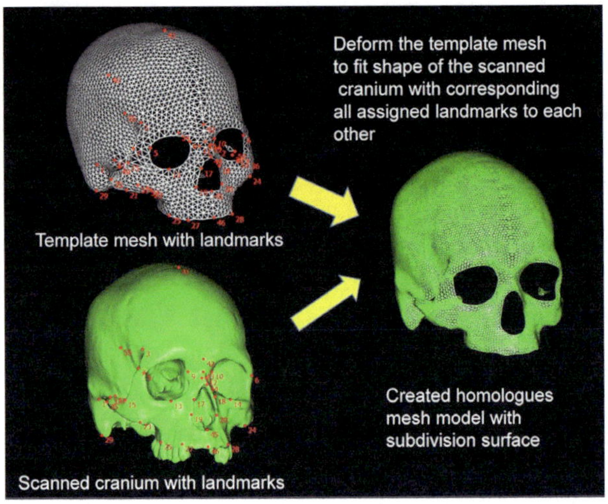

Figure 4.15. Evolutionary significance of neurocranium variations.

Source: https://media.springernature.com/lw1200/springer-static/image/art%3A10.1038%2Fs41598-022-15883-3/MediaObjects/41598_2022_15883_Fig1_HTML.jpg.

4.5.3. Insights From Comparative Studies in Anthropology

Comparative anthropology gives profound insight into human cranial evolution, particularly the role of the neurocranium in informing cognitive ability. Osteological analysis is used by anthropologists to uncover differences in cranial anatomy across populations, providing a window into evolutionary changes over millennia. For instance, by examining the neurocranium's structure, researchers can see how cranial shape and neurological development influence one another. Such research is relevant because it shows how the forces of the environment have influenced cranial morphology and sheds useful light on human adaptation and survival in various environmental settings. Besides, the comparative findings assist in disentangling the complexities of human phylogeny by mapping the lineage and adaptation trajectories that have marked Homo sapiens and their ancestors over time. Additionally, some case studies corroborate the role of comparative anthropological research in explaining geographic differences between human populations. For example, the investigation of hominid skulls from Sarstedt provided significant data on the anatomical characteristics associated with the Arteria meningea media and their significance within the hominidae group (Czarnetzki et al., 2012). Such targeted research contributes to a rich background for the investigation of cranial morphology, shedding light on the potential means by which different anatomical features might be linked to broader behavioral and cognitive adaptations. By placing these anatomical variations within the context of environmental factors, anthropologists can paint a more complete picture of human development. Such an understanding not only enlightens us as to human biology but also addresses the controversy surrounding the interaction of environment and inborn abilities. The study of specific groups, such as the Sami of the Kolsky Bay region, also illustrates the utility of the anthropological comparative method in explaining the variability of human cranial traits. Specifically, the study of Sami graves involved collecting and examining skeletal material and demonstrated significant differences in facial skeleton parameters between men and women (Borutskaya et al., 2017). Such comparative anthropology helps to clarify how genetic factors and adaptive strategies are manifested in cranial morphology. Distinguishing characteristics revealed through skeletal analyses can be applied to broader discussions of human adaptation to harsh environments, highlighting the interplay between genetic variation and environmental adaptation. Consequently, such findings not only enhance our understanding of human osteology but also deepen our appreciation for the subtle interplay among anatomy, nature, and culture in anthropology.

Test Your Knowledge

1. What are the key differences between the human neurocranium and that of non-human organisms?
2. How is comparative neurocranial anatomy applied in anthropological studies?

4.6. Clinical Relevance of the Neurocranium

Learning Outcome

1. Medical conditions related to neurocranium
2. Surgeries involving the neurocranium
3. Advances in imaging technologies used for neurocranium assessment

The neurocranium, with its brain and protective cover against extrinsic pressure, is of utmost clinical significance in neurology and craniofacial surgery. Its structural deformities lead to many neurological abnormalities in cognitive function and overall health. For instance, structural abnormalities like craniosynostosis, with its early suture closure of cranial bones, can restrict brain expansion, leading to increased intracranial pressure and developmental issues. Recognition of the usual variations and potential abnormalities of the neurocranium is critical to ensuring timely intervention and diagnosis and to influencing long-term patient outcomes. Nikolova et al. (2015) highlight the importance of identifying such anatomical variations since significant alterations can provide significant information on underlying pathology and hence affect therapy planning. It is against this kind of variation that anatomical data is translated from a theoretical foundation into an accessible tool in the clinic. The application of variations of the neurocranium extends beyond the initial medical examinations; it is also important in the formulation of surgical approaches in cranial reconstructive surgery. For surgeons, recognition of the variations aids in planning how best to carry out effective and safe interventions, particularly in children, where the neurocranium is developing. Abnormalities such as atlas occipitalization, documented by Nikolova et al. (2015), require specialized operative techniques to account for altered anatomical structures and thereby prevent procedural complications. In addition, the operative techniques used in procedures should consider the specific regions of the neurocranium to prevent damage to adjacent neurological structures. The combination of unique anatomical features and the surgical techniques employed underscores the clinical relevance of the neurocranium, highlighting the crucial role of in-depth anatomical knowledge in the successful execution of lucrative surgical operations with reduced patient risk. Besides, molecular mechanisms of neurocranial formation and osteogenesis are added to the clinical importance in studies.

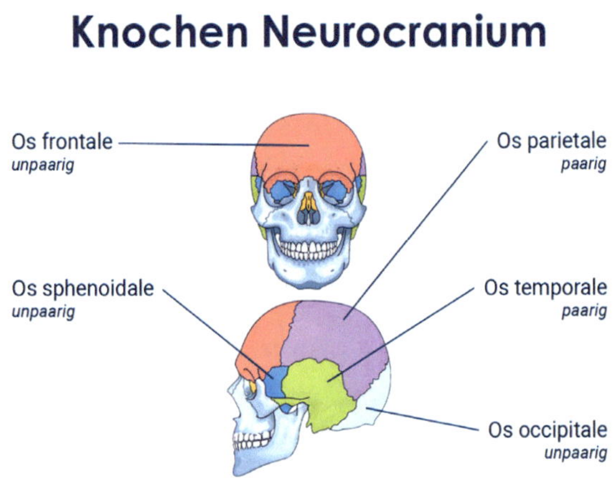

Figure 4.16. Clinical relevance of the neurocranium.

Source: https://external-content.duckduckgo.com/iu/?u=https%3A%2F%2Fwww.medi-karriere.de%2Fwp-content%2Fuploads%2F2024%2F03%2FGrafik-Neurocranium-e1709815539460.jpg&f=1&nofb=1&ipt=fc337e429576fdb9eedf635de99a316adcd153b5cae2354c2555fa1d2f821887.

Research such as this demonstrates that environmental factors, i.e., temperature, influence bone development, which can manifest in neurocranial changes. Understanding the inherent biological mechanisms of osteogenesis guides clinical use in cases of growth disorders or neurocranium deformities. It reveals the extent to which external conditions shape cranial morphology, traditionally linking environmental conditions with cranial health and development. This comprehension is part of advancing preventive interventions and treatment strategies that are appropriate to specific patient needs, hence emphasizing the neurocranium's clinical relevance in contemporary osteological practice and studies. As more studies are conducted, it becomes evident that a deep knowledge of neurocranial anatomy provides important insights into broader health perspectives in pediatric and adult populations (Figure 4.16).

4.6.1. Neurocranium-Related Medical Conditions

The neurocranium, which consists of the cranial vault and base, contains and safeguards the brain, and as such, is central to general health and function. Some clinical conditions directly affect the neurocranium and have tremendous implications for clinical practice. Conditions such as craniosynostosis, or premature closure of one or more sutures on the cranium, stop the growth of the skull and can result in increased intracranial pressure, retardation of development, and a host of cognitive defects. The necessity for prompt surgical treatment to reopen the closed sutures and permit normal brain development underscores the necessity of understanding neurocranial disorders in pediatric populations. These conditions also mirror the relationship between cranial anatomy and neurological health and indicate the greater implications for surgical procedures and rehabilitation, which can impact patient outcomes for individuals with neurocranium-related medical conditions. In addition, the neurocranium can also show sexual dimorphism in its anatomy, which is clinically important. Research has shown that males tend to have a broader and larger neurocranium compared to their females, with remarkable development in the anterior facial region (Phillips et al., 2013). These variations in form may influence diagnostic activities, particularly in forensic anthropology and orthodontics. For instance, understanding these variations is crucial when developing methods for age and sex estimation based on cranial measurements. Such knowledge enhances the accuracy of clinical decision-making, particularly for treatments that can alter cranial form, such as orthodontic treatment or reconstructive surgery. Furthermore, the distinct growth patterns observed in juveniles underscore the need for a refined approach to neurocranium-associated conditions, particularly when weighing treatment options for both genders. Another key component of neurocranium-associated medical illnesses is the enormous array of genetic and environmental determinants of cranial development. The intricate embryological processes that regulate neurocranial development are responsible for a host of disorders, ranging from congenital malformations to acquired conditions resulting from trauma or infection. Abzhanov et al. (2019) emphasize the role of cranial neural crest mesenchyme in the developmental processes that shape the jaw and surrounding tissues, which become aberrant when disrupted. For instance, diseases such as cleft palate exhibit complex interactions between genetic predisposition and environmental triggers, with significant implications for craniofacial growth. These insights contribute not only to pathophysiology knowledge of neurocranium-related conditions but also require interdisciplinary input from genetics, developmental biology, and clinical practice to ensure improved management and treatment paradigms.

4.6.2. Surgical Interventions Involving the Neurocranium

Surgical procedures on the neurocranium are essential techniques in modern medicine, used to manage many neurological disorders and cranial defects. Surgical operations conducted on the neurocranium, which include the brain's covering, involve surgical interventions such as craniotomies in which part of the skull is cut away to access the underlying tissue. The technique is mainly applied in managing traumatic brain injury, brain tumors, and hydrocephalus. For instance, in traumatic brain injury, craniotomy removes pressure from cerebral edema and thereby reduces the risk of brain herniation. Furthermore, technological developments in imaging enhance the precision of these interventions, enabling neurosurgeons to refine their skills for specific pathologies of the neurocranium. The variability of skull development and abnormalities further complicates the interaction between neurocranial anatomy and surgical intervention. Surgical planning must account for the neurocranium's specific anatomical features, including conditions such as a persistent metopic suture or a frontal sinus malformation. Research indicates that these variations can influence not only surgical planning but also the risk of complications, such as sinus atrophy, during surgery. Specifically, the correlation between persistent metopic sutures and abnormal frontal sinus development has been identified as important, underscoring the significance of preoperative imaging (Akbasak et al., 2013; Georgiev et al., 2018). Specifically, pneumatization of the frontal sinus is not excluded by the presence of a metopic suture; however, its significance for surgical outcomes requires strict evaluation. Lastly, ongoing studies and strict evaluation of surgical outcomes further reinforce the clinical context for neurocranial operations. An understanding of the nuances of neurocranial anatomy, particularly in relation to developmental anomalies, is paramount to optimizing surgical techniques. Studies on the relationship between anomalies, such as persistent metopic sutures, and frontal sinus morphology illustrate the complexities surgeons must contend with. Furthermore, the addition of preoperative assessment, such as high-end imaging modalities, can significantly enhance the effectiveness and safety of neurocranial surgery. With the evolution of neurosurgical expertise driven by technology, a deep appreciation of the variability in human osteology will remain crucial to advancing patient care and surgical creativity in the context of neurocranium procedures (Figure 4.17).

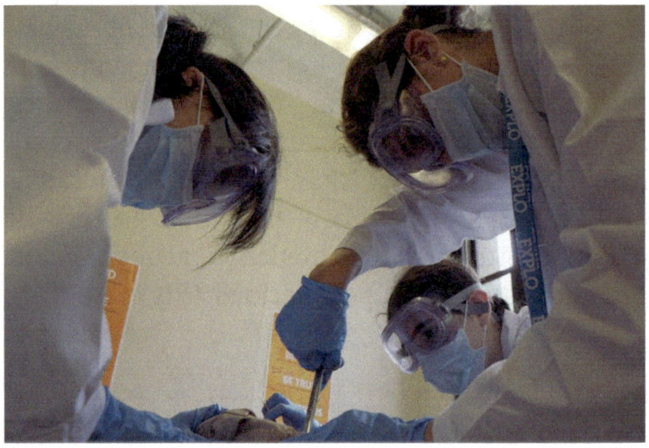

Figure 4.17. Surgical interventions involving the neurocranium.

Source: https://external-content.duckduckgo.com/iu/?u=http%3A%2F%2Fblog.explo.org%2Fhubfs%2Fyale%2Facademics%2Fslideshows%2F20170629_103615%2F6-29_Surgical_Interventions_-_13_of_20.jpg&f=1&nofb=1&ipt=af024266c9391c4e6a6c0b5349c5f4e3eab5baa2de28af822dfe396f16ba22fb.

4.6.3. Advances in Imaging Techniques for Neurocranium Assessment

Technological advancements in imaging techniques have greatly improved the assessment of the neurocranium in recent years, enabling greater visualization and analysis of cranial structures. Among these technological improvements, computed tomography (CT) and magnetic resonance imaging (MRI) stand out for their ability to generate high-resolution, three-dimensional images of the neurocranium. These modalities enable accurate examination of cranial anatomy, which is essential in both clinical and forensic contexts. With high-tech reconstruction software, radiologists can now examine cranial features with unprecedented accuracy, providing vital information for anthropological research. Furthermore, the technologies permit the examination of pathological alterations in the neurocranium and, hence, a better understanding of various cranial abnormalities, along with their epidemiology, as seen in the HUSM population study, to establish anthropometric information correlating orbital dimensions with gender and age (Kong et al., 2015). In forensic imaging, the synergy between novel imaging techniques contributes to the reconstruction of cranial profiles and assists in identification procedures. Recent studies have shown the effectiveness of multi-modal imaging approaches integrating CT and MRI findings for the overall description of the neurocranium. Double imaging not only enhances the imaging of small cranial details but also the validity of forensic conclusions based on imaging findings. Superimposition ability of various imaging datasets is helpful in distinguishing between various demographic parameters, such as age and gender, which are critical in forensic anthropology. Additionally, as seen in recent geoscience imaging literature, multi-modal concepts can be transferable to other scientific domains, thus facilitating interdisciplinary research (Ahmed et al., 2017). The future neurocranium assessment is set to be even more innovative, particularly as technological advancements continue in the development of imaging modalities and their applications. The potential of high-resolution X-ray computed tomography (HRXCT) is intriguing, especially for evaluating fine cranial details beyond the capabilities of routine imaging. By heightened image resolution and contrast, HRXCT can provide improved delineation of cranial sutures, fontanelles, and other structures critical to clinical diagnostics and anthropological research. As imaging technologies become increasingly advanced, there is a critical need for researchers and practitioners alike to develop standardized methods for applying these advances so that new anthropometric information is correctly assimilated into clinical use and forensic methodologies. The integration of imaging technology and the evaluation of the neurocranium ultimately expand our understanding of human osteology and its application across various fields of study.

Test Your Knowledge

1. What are some medical conditions associated with the neurocranium?
2. What types of surgical procedures involve the neurocranium?

SUMMARY

A summary of current research on the neurocranium in the field of human osteology identifies the intricate interrelationships between cranial anatomy and various demographic factors, such as sex, age, and geographical variation. As demonstrated by comparative observations of bone remains, distinct patterns in craniofacial morphology mimic the adaptability and evolutionary nature of human populations. For instance, homogeneity-group analysis of Sami graves demonstrates that variation in facial skeleton parameters is consistent with environmental adaptation in the Arctic, highlighting the impact of long-term survival mechanisms on body features (Borutskaya et al., 2017). This demands that one be aware of neurocranial structures not only from a clinical or anatomical perspective but also within the context of their sociocultural relevance. Moreover, evidence of sexual dimorphism in craniofacial growth carries far-reaching consequences for anthropological research and forensic applications. The results of greater male neurocranial size than females, along with accurate classification rates across age categories, indicate the potential for even more specialized uses of cranial size in age and sex estimation (Phillips et al., 2013). These results add weight to the argument for holistic approaches that can enhance the precision of sex estimation. Interestingly, such morphological variations are relevant to numerous fields, ranging from biological anthropology to archaeology, broadening the area of inquiry into human skeletal remains. In summary, the intricate aspects of the neurocranium are critical points of entry to the appreciation of general themes in human osteology. These results not only demonstrate variation in cranial morphology but also suggest the need for further studies that integrate multidisciplinary research encompassing genetics, anthropology, and environmental science. The future studies should be aimed at expanding the cranial measurement database for various populations and using the latest imaging technologies to refine our understanding of neurocranial development further. Finally, a closer examination of these associations will result in a more complete explanation of human evolution and adaptation across various ecological environments, with significant information regarding our species' history and relevance for current and future research.

Understanding the neurocranium in the analysis of human osteology provides significant insights into cranial bone growth and sexual dimorphism. Research shows that male and female subjects exhibit distinct craniofacial growth patterns, with males possessing a larger, longer neurocranium than females. This was supported by computed tomography imaging of juvenile subjects, which showed that male skulls exhibit greater anterior development in the facial region. The findings show that accurate sex estimation using cranial measurements can be achieved, with classification accuracies of 66%–85% across age group. The neurocranium's correlation with growth patterns implies its significance not only in understanding the development of the skeleton but also in forensic examination and anthropology, providing crucial information for discriminating between male and female skeletal elements (Phillips et al., 2013). Ageing changes have profound consequences for the neurocranium, underscoring the complexity of skeletal modification throughout human life. Determining age from cranial shape relies on understanding the multifaceted relationships between cranial sutures and remodeling forces during development. With increasing age, the sutures remain patent through a coordinated process of bone formation and resorption, illustrating their capacity to respond to various biological stresses. Normal and pathological ageing differ, especially in forensic contexts where skeletal remains analysis is conducted. Understanding these markers of age and their unidirectional changes enables attempts to exhaustively explore the timing and order of skeletal change, so that chronological ages may be determined accurately (Das et al.,

2022). In: Furthermore, the inclusion of several specimens in craniofacial morphology and ageing offers a broad view of the human neurocranium. Comparison of epiphyseal growth patterns with cranial suture remodeling highlights the dynamism of the skeletal structure. . Researchers have highlighted epiphyseal appearance and union to provide important information on growth pathways, particularly in immature subjects. As studies continue to explore the relationships between genetics, environmental factors, and morphological changes, the nuances of both biological and chronological ageing become clearer. These insights contribute significantly to the overall understanding of human osteology, laying the groundwork for further studies that could improve methods of age estimation and sex determination in various scientific fields (Das et al., 2022).

KEY TERMS FROM THIS CHAPTER

- Bregma
- Cranial Vault
- Ethmoid Bone
- Frontal Bone
- Parietal Bones
- Sphenoid Bone
- Cranial Base
- Crista Galli
- Foramen Magnum
- Occipital Bone
- Sella Turcica
- Temporal Bones

CRITICAL THINKING QUESTIONS

1. **Which of the following bones is NOT a component of the neurocranium?**
   a. Frontal bone
   b. Temporal bone
   c. Maxilla
   d. Parietal bone
2. **How many bones constitute the neurocranium?**
   a. 6
   b. 8
   c. 10
   d. 12
3. **Where is the foramen magnum located in the neurocranium?**
   a. Frontal bone
   b. Occipital bone
   c. Temporal bone
   d. Parietal bone
4. **What is the function of the ethmoid bone in the neurocranium?**
   a. Forms the forehead
   b. Contains the auditory canal
   c. Contributes to the floor of the anterior cranial fossa
   d. Provides articulation for the mandible
5. **Which two bones form the sides and top of the cranium?**
   a. Parietal bones
   b. Temporal bones
   c. Sphenoid bones
   d. Occipital bones

Short Answer Questions

1. Define the neurocranium and its primary function.
2. What is the role played by the frontal bone in the neurocranium?
3. Explain the role played by the occipital bone in the cranium.
4. Identify the paired bones of the neurocranium.
5. Explain the role played by the parietal bones in the cranium.
6. Explain how the external and internal surfaces of the neurocranium differ.

Answers to Critical Thinking Questions

1. (c); 2. (b); 3. (b); 4. (c); 5. (a)

1.

REFERENCES

2. Woronowicz, K.C., Schneider, R.A. Molecular and cellular mechanisms underlying the evolution of form and function in the amniote jaw. *EvoDevo* **10**, 17 (2019). https://doi.org/10.1186/s13227-019-0131-8Adriaens, D., Baskin, J. N., & Coppens, H. (2010). Evolutionary morphology of trichomycterid catfishes: About hanging on and digging in. https://core.ac.uk/download/55867718.pdf (accessed on 18th July 2025).
3. Ahmed, F., & Maisano, J. (2017). ToScA North America (6–8 June 2017, The University of Texas, Austin, TX) Program. https://core.ac.uk/download/211334283.pdf (accessed on 18th July 2025).
4. Akbasak, A., Bilgin, S., Duymus, M., et al. (2013). Association between frontal sinus development and persistent metopic suture. https://core.ac.uk/download/268451143.pdf (accessed on 18th July 2025).
5. Bisconti, M., Bosselaers, M., & Lambert, O. (2017). Revision of *"Balaena" belgica* reveals a new right whale species, the possible ancestry of the northern right whale, *Eubalaena glacialis*, and the ages of divergence for the living right whale species. https://core.ac.uk/download/pdf/154802660.pdf (accessed on 18th July 2025).
6. Borutskaya, S., & Vasilyev, S. (2017). Anthropological study of Sami from the Kola Peninsula (Russia). https://core.ac.uk/download/93130857.pdf (accessed on 18th July 2025).
7. Buzi, C. (2020). Morphology of the inner structures of the facial skeleton in *Homo neanderthalensis* and the case-study of the Neanderthal from Altamura (Bari, Italy). https://core.ac.uk/download/288656530.pdf (accessed on 18th July 2025).
8. Capilla, E., Costa, R., Gisbert, E., et al. (2018). Temperature responsiveness of gilthead sea bream bone; an *in vitro* and *in vivo* approach. https://core.ac.uk/download/225163048.pdf (accessed on 18th July 2025).
9. Cardini, A., Cardini, A., Ivanovic, A., Lo-Yat, A., Loy, A., Sampey, A. R., et al. (2011). Bipartite life cycle of coral reef fishes promotes increasing shape disparity of the head skeleton during ontogeny: An example from damselfishes (Pomacentridae). https://core.ac.uk/download/pdf/8554410.pdf (accessed on 18th July 2025).
10. Carril, J., de Mendoza, R. S., Degrange, F. J., et al. (2022). Redefining the simplicity of the craniomandibular complex of nightjars: The case of *Systellura longirostris* (Aves: Caprimulgidae) by means of anatomical network analysis. https://core.ac.uk/download/603308720.pdf (accessed on 18th July 2025).
11. Chmielewski, P. P. (2021). New Terminologia Anatomica: Cranium and extracranial bones of the head. https://core.ac.uk/download/268450419.pdf (accessed on 18th July 2025).
12. Czarnetzki, A., von Rautenfeld, D., & Samii, M. (2012). The phylogenetic principles of MMA: A hypothetical biostratigraphy model. https://core.ac.uk/download/pdf/1569968.pdf (accessed on 18th July 2025).
13. Das, A., & Mohanty, S. (2022). Closure of cranial sutures and expansion of epiphysis of bones as indicators of ageing in forensic sciences: A review. https://core.ac.uk/download/622609390.pdf (accessed on 18th July 2025).
14. Georgiev, I., Lazarov, N., Nikolova, S., et al. (2018). Relation between metopic suture persistence and frontal sinus development. https://core.ac.uk/download/322438178.pdf (accessed on 18th July 2025).

15. Hemingway, J. (2017). Exploring patterns of morphological integration in the crania of *Papio hamadryas ursinus* and *Homo sapiens*. https://core.ac.uk/download/188775577.pdf (accessed on 18th July 2025).

16. Lee, C. K. (2015). CT-based three-dimensional measurement of adult orbit in Hospital Universiti Sains Malaysia. https://core.ac.uk/download/158571016.pdf (accessed on 18th July 2025).

17. Marinho, L. M. O. (2013). Perimortem blunt force trauma analysis: On the reconstruction of the circumstances of death of human skeletal remains. https://core.ac.uk/download/43586847.pdf (accessed on 18th July 2025).

18. Nikolova, S. Y., & Toneva, D. H. (2015). Metopic skull with occipitalization of the atlas. https://core.ac.uk/download/542906545.pdf (accessed on 18th July 2025).

19. Phillips, C. E. B. (2013). The use of craniometrics in the estimation of juvenile sex by means of discriminant function analysis: A revised method. https://open.bu.edu/bitstream/2144/12187/6/Phillips_Chase_2013_nosig_nocv.pdf (accessed on 18th July 2025).

20. Reinman, A. (2019). Ancestry assessment in subadult skeletons. https://core.ac.uk/download/223096314.pdf (accessed on 18th July 2025).

21. Rippa Bonati, M., Scattolin, G., Zampieri, F., et al. (2016). Occupational markers and pathology of the castrato singer Gaspare Pacchierotti (1740–1821). https://core.ac.uk/download/53529342.pdf (accessed on 18th July 2025).

22. Suchá, B. (2024). Klasifikace pohlaví na základě 3D modelování lebky v multipopulačním souboru. https://core.ac.uk/download/624142384.pdf (accessed on 18th July 2025).

CRANIUM – VISCEROCRANIUM (FACE) IN HUMAN OSTEOLOGY

5

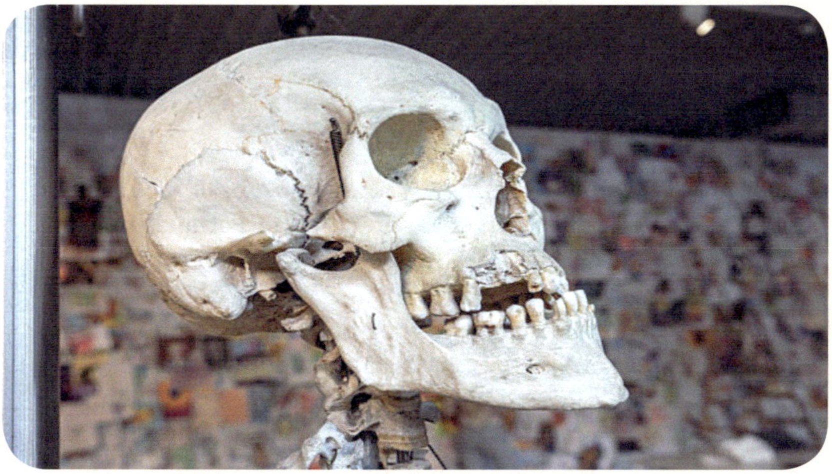

LEARNING OBJECTIVES

After studying this chapter, you will be able to:

1. Discuss the anatomy of the cranium
2. Give a general overview of the viscerocranium
3. Describe viscerocranium development
4. Understand the functional anatomy of viscerocranium
5. Know viscerocranium pathology
6. Focus on comparative osteology

Introduction

The facial skeleton or viscerocranium is a vital component of the science of human osteology because it is at the heart of both functional anatomy and identification of individual variation. It is composed of various bones, including the maxilla, mandible, and nasal bones, which enable functions such as respiration, mastication, and articulation. Its complex constitution is an expression of evolutionary innovations that have enabled human beings to exist in diverse environments. The viscerocranium is the product of intricate genetic and molecular mechanisms by which the cranial neural crest mesenchyme contributes to the shaping of facial bones. Having insight into the mechanisms is important as their interference can lead to congenital malformations, underscoring the relevance of studying the viscerocranium for osteological research (Abzhanov et al., 2019). Sexual dimorphism is another prominent characteristic of the viscerocranium that provides excellent information on human osteology. Research confirms extensive differences in craniofacial development between males and females, which affect the viscerocranical morphology. A computed tomography scan revealed that male juveniles had a longer, wider neurocranium than females, whose more precise classification rates notwithstanding, their sample was smaller (Phillips et al., 2013). These findings underscore the importance of accounting for sex differences in anatomical science and forensic practice, as facial differences can influence both anthropometric measurements and skeletal identification.

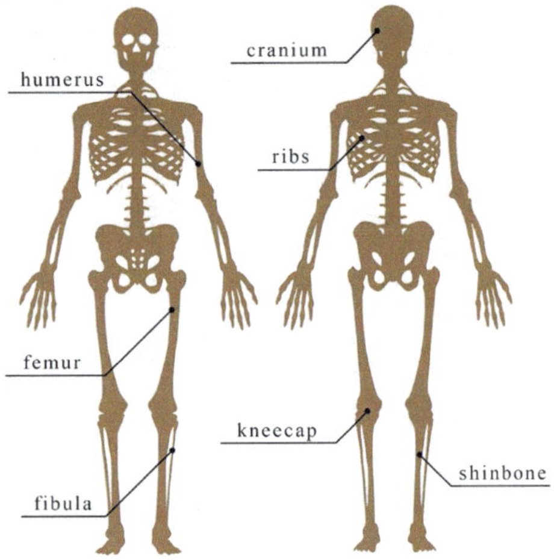

Figure 5.1. Cranium – Viscerocranium.

Source: https://img.freepik.com/free-vector/parts-skeleton_23-2147537320.jpg?semt=ais_hybrid&w=740.

This knowledge also adds to understanding human variation and fosters an integrated perspective within osteology. Besides, viscerocranium is not only utilized for functional purposes but is also an incredibly significant factor in anthropological studies as well as evolutionary biology. By analyzing morphological adaptations in the viscerocranium, scientists can determine the evolutionary history of modern humans and their ancestors. The dynamic among environment, biomechanics, and developmental processes has generated a heterogeneous array of facial morphologies that reflect adaptive strategies across diverse environments. As highlighted by studies of jaw morphology and its associated structures, an understanding of the viscerocranium provides a framework for examining human development and evolutionary processes. Such an examination draws us closer to understanding anatomical variation, completes the dialogue between osteology and anthropology, and establishes the viscerocranium's role in the broader scheme of human osteology (Abzhanov et al., 2019) (Figure 5.1).

Definition and Significance of Human Osteology

Human osteology, the science of bones and skeletal structures, is a foundational field of study within anthropology for understanding the human cranium and viscerocranium, or face skeleton. Human osteology studies the morphology, growth, and other processes of bones in order to enable researchers to define individual and population characteristics through the examination of the skeleton. The applicability of osteology extends beyond raw anatomical interest; it plays a central role in forensic anthropology, archaeology, and bioarchaeology, where analysis of skeletal remains can yield information on demographic attributes such as age, sex, health, and even behavioral trends of prehistoric cultures. A proper understanding of osteological foundations is thus crucial for both applied work and theoretical research in anthropology. The viscerocranium, which comprises the facial bones, is of particular interest in human osteology because it is implicated in many biological and social processes. Structurally, these bones protect vital sensory organs and support essential functions such as respiration and mastication. Moreover, viscerocranium is highly sexually dimorphic, and studies have shown that male craniofacial structures not only become larger but are also more powerful relative to female structures. These differences impact forensic anthropological practice, and accurate measurement of these differences determines the sexual identification of unknown skeletons. Studies have shown that craniofacial development follows different patterns in the two sexes, indicating the need to use advanced methodologies to enhance classification reliability, especially in juveniles, as suggested by ongoing research (Phillips et al., 2013).

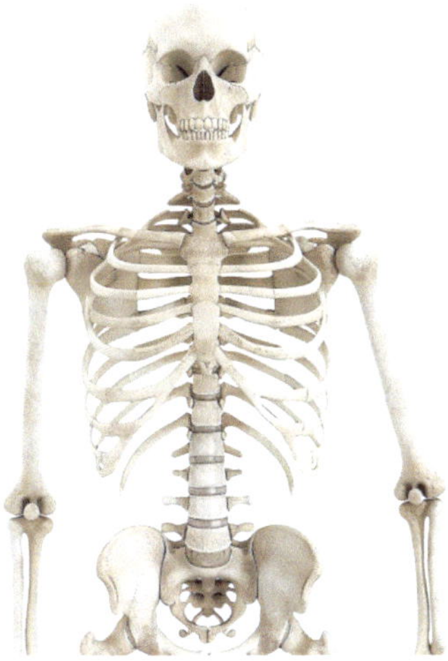

Figure 5.2. The significance of human osteology.

Source: https://external-content.duckduckgo.com/iu/?u=https%3A%2F%2Fstatic.vecteezy.com%2Fsystem%2Fresources%2Fpreviews%2F044%2F183%2F312%2Foriginal%2Fa-clear-look-at-human-osteology-bones-unveiled-free-png.png&f=1&nofb=1&ipt=e957e2da329049cdfd1de4c8b58483ae13527501d59f2ba7586835747eeb983d.

Furthermore, continuous advances in osteological research methodologies continue to expand our knowledge of craniofacial morphology. New techniques, such as analysis of the exocranial surface of skulls to estimate sex, have been highly accurate, with up to 91% success in some populations (Suchá et al., 2024). Such methodological sophistication reflects the deeper integration of technology and anthropology, enabling more refined deciphering of craniofacial elements in the context of biodiversity and evolutionary biology. In addition, the age-related changes in craniofacial morphology are an aspect of understanding the social and biological nature of human development. Hence, the significance of human osteology, particularly its relevance to the viscerocranium, extends beyond the interpretation of past human populations to its application in present forensic techniques and anthropological research (Figure 5.2).

Overview of the Cranium and Its Components

The cranium, a vital part of the human skeleton, serves to contain and shield the brain and provide structural support to the face. It is composed of two major components: the neurocranium and the viscerocranium or facial skeleton. The neurocranium is formed by a series of flat and irregular bones fused to create a protective vault around the brain's delicate tissue. In contrast, viscerocranium comprises bones that form the facial structure, hosting sensory organs and the oral cavity. This intricate design not only protects critical neural structures but also supports diverse functions, including respiration, mastication, and communication. Recognition of these components is core to disciplines such as anthropology, forensic science, and medicine, in which the skull's morphological attributes can yield information on evolutionary patterns and personal identity. Within the viscerocranium are numerous discrete bones that contribute to functional and aesthetic facial attributes. Foremost among these are the maxilla, mandible, nasal bones, and zygomatic arches, each playing a significant role in facial morphology and function. The maxilla forms the upper jaw and the position of the upper teeth, whereas the mandible comprises the lower jaw that facilitates the movement required for chewing and speech. The nasal bones contribute to the bridge of the nose, whereas the zygomatic bones facilitate the prominence of the cheek. These bones are very interdependent and undergo complex developmental patterns, which continue to develop further at different stages of life, as indicated by the extensive alterations in cranial sutures, which are present in a dynamic state for development and adaptation. Such integration makes one think it is significant to study cranial morphology according to physiological function as well as evolutionary development (Das et al., 2022). Morphological integration of the cranium's components illustrates its structural complexity. Research shows that growth patterns within the cranial vault, the cranial base, and the facial skeleton are regulated by genes and environment (Hemingway et al., 2017).

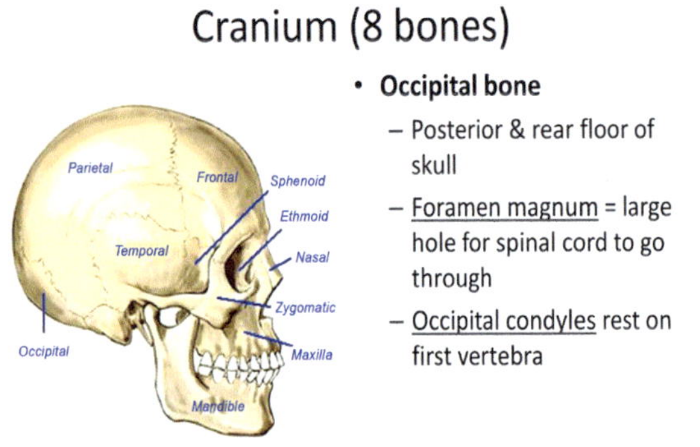

Figure 5.3. The cranium, a vital feature of the human skeletal system.

Source: https://external-content.duckduckgo.com/iu/?u=https%3A%2F%2Fimage1.slideserve.com%2F2065371%2Fcranium-8-bones2-l.jpg&f=1&nofb=1&ipt=5933accc2394031ed8153bf9e33e6fcfc627e65738a481da75b766124b79d77a.

The degree of integration among these areas varies, with modules forming independently yet cooperatively within the overall cranial structure. This modularity enhances the cranium's flexibility, enabling organisms to accommodate diverse functional needs, including the coordination of senses and the spatial arrangement of facial structures. The study of such integration patterns is therefore of great value in the study of cranial structure evolution, as it concerns the adaptation of the cranium to both functional needs and environmental forces. Understanding the dynamics is essential in comprehending human osteology as a whole in a modern and evolutionary context (Figure 5.3).

Importance of Studying the Viscerocranium

The viscerocranium, the facial skeleton, is a crucial part of human osteology, particularly in light of its functional and evolutionary significance. Understanding viscerocranial morphology and structure is central to a full appreciation of growth in the face, with top-down influences on varied biological functions such as respiration, mastication, and communication. The viscerocranium houses critical structures such as the orbits, nasal airway, and teeth, making it at the focal point of disciplines ranging from anthropology to forensic odontology. By analyzing this part of the skull, researchers can disentangle the developmental processes that underlie facial shape and explore the significance of these variations for environmental adaptation and evolutionary history, thereby providing valuable insights into past populations' biological profiles and their environmental contexts. Apart from its biological significance, the viscerocranium is an important forensic anthropological parameter, particularly for identifying human remains. The facial skeleton carries significant information in constructing a biological profile since it provides clues regarding an individual's age, sex, and ancestry, and more significantly, such details are important in subadult remains cases. Subadult skeletal analysis remains a challenging area; nonetheless, new evidence is emerging indicating that nonmetric characteristics of the viscerocranium are helpful in differentiating ancestral populations, even within juvenile samples. This draws considerable emphasis to the viscerocranium not just in anatomical investigation but also in the practical application of forensic investigation, where accurate identification can be heavily reliant on the proper investigation of this intricate structure (Reinman et al., 2019). Moreover, the evolutionary perspective on viscerocranium emphasizes its adaptive function and intraspecific complexity of cranial growth. Comparative analysis of significant morphological features among primates, particularly African apes, can shed light on human cranial evolution, revealing patterns of growth underlying sexual dimorphism and intraspecific diversity. By leveraging contemporary analytical methodologies and age-specific sample populations, science provides greater understanding of the viscerocranium's ontogeny and insight into how evolutionary pressures affect cranial form. Information yielded as a consequence not only adds greater depth to human origin but also informs ongoing anthropological debate regarding variation, adaptation, and functional morphology. With further advances in research in this field, the use of data on the viscerocranium is becoming increasingly important for both theoretical and practical applications in anthropology and related sciences (Massey et al., 2018).

5.1. Anatomy of the Cranium

Learning Outcome

1. Definition and terminology of the cranium.
2. Major bones of the cranium;
3. Functions of the cranial bones;

The anatomy of the cranium consists of a highly developed series of bones that are vital to structure and function. Comprising two major divisions—the neurocranium and the viscerocranium—the cranium houses the brain and forms the base of the face. The neurocranium is made up of eight bones, including the frontal, parietal, and occipital bones, while the viscerocranium consists of 14 bones that contribute to facial forms and support. Understanding the intricate interrelations among the bones is essential to enjoy various clinical significances, like craniofacial deformities and their evolutionary significance. The functions of cranial neural crest mesenchyme in molding these bones highlight the intricate developmental processes underlying the unique morphology of each human cranium, thereby pointing to functional and adaptive elements in human osteology (Abzhanov et al., 2019). The viscerocranium also facilitates important functions such as mastication, respiration, and phonation. The viscerocranium's bone structure not only provides the structural support but also creates cavities that influence sound resonance and airflow. Surprisingly, changes in the shapes and dimensions of these bones can be induced by both genetic and environmental factors. For instance, repeated metopic sutures, located on the frontal bone, highlight the dynamic interaction between bone development and structural form. Research has shown that variations in frontal sinus development are associated with these sutures (Akbasak et al., 2013), although a causal relationship has yet to be established. Such a discovery underscores the importance of continued investigation into cranial anatomy to unravel the interaction between genetic predisposition and the environment in human osteology. Furthermore, the significance of the cranium extends far beyond its anatomical structure to encompass far-reaching implications in disease and health. Perturbations in cranial development have the potential to create defects that are detrimental to an individual's overall health, function, and well-being. Anomalies of the frontal sinus, for instance, which can result from conditions like metopism, are a reminder of how the cranium's anatomy is connected to physiologic processes. The interplay highlights the need for multidisciplinary methods to explore cranial anatomy, including contributions from genetics, evolutionary biology, and clinical medicine. By studying cranial disparities and their functional implications, researchers can extend their understanding of craniofacial anomalies and, quite possibly, inform surgical practices aimed at remedying these conditions. The study of the cranium remains, therefore, at the forefront of osteological inquiry as well as clinical application, illustrating the manner in which its anatomy nicely scales form with function (Figure 5.4).

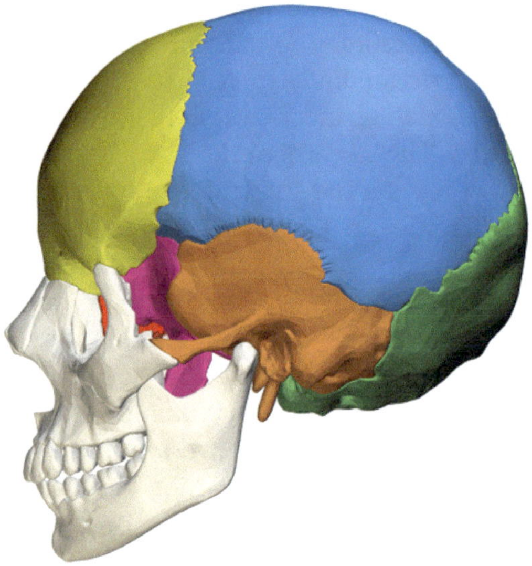

Figure 5.4. The anatomy of the cranium.

Source: https://external-content.duckduckgo.com/iu/?u=https%3A%2F%2Fo.quizlet.com%2Fptxo8FUVaYP218mw14O0HA_b.png&f=1&nofb=1&ipt=c1de4a25f56a8d25ba83c1e187e98bcea7ff10863c94785d4fd9369f1da521df.

5.1.1. Definition and Classification of the Cranium

The cranium is a critical component of the human skeleton that serves as a protective case for the brain but also supports facial structures. Its definition goes beyond protection and encompasses the intricate interactions of bone morphology necessary for functions such as mastication, respiration, and sensory perception. The cranium is generally separated into two primary components: the neurocranium and the viscerocranium. There are eight bones in the neurocranium, the frontal, parietal, and occipital bones, which make up the cranial vault that houses the brain. The viscerocranium, also referred to as the facial skeleton, consists of 14 bones, such as the maxilla, mandible, and zygomatic bones, which comprise the face structure. This distinction is essential to understanding the anatomical and functional variation of cranial morphology in human osteology. Within the classification of the cranium, sexual dimorphism describes differences in morphological features between male and female skulls. Observations reveal that males have more extensive and heavier cranial features than females, primarily in the neurocranium and some facial structures. For example, Gonzalezs study noted that male heads are generally taller and longer, and there was a clear distinction in craniofacial developmental patterns between the sexes (Phillips et al., 2013). Not only does this dimorphism influence physical anthropology and forensic anthropology, but clinical practice as well, where identifying the differences among the sexes is useful in sex estimation from cranial remains correctly. Surprisingly, the accuracy of such estimations has been reported to range from 66% to 92%, depending on age group and the methodologies employed. The classificatory nature of viscerocrania also revolves around their dynamic interrelation with dental condition and anatomical variations resulting from tooth loss. Structural changes resulting from edentulous conditions complicate the identification of sex and ancestry from cranial remains, particularly when working with underrepresented groups. As illustrated in the white South African crania study, tooth loss completely alters the maxillary alveolar ridges and may lead to misestimates of cranial morphology (Small et al., 2016). The use of advanced methods, such as geometric morphometrics, provides greater insight into the effects of tooth loss on cranial classification. This information is important to forensic anthropologists, as it enhances the validity of biological profiles constructed from fragmented or absent cranial remains, ultimately strengthening the integrity of anthropological analysis and advancing the science of human osteology (Figure 5.5).

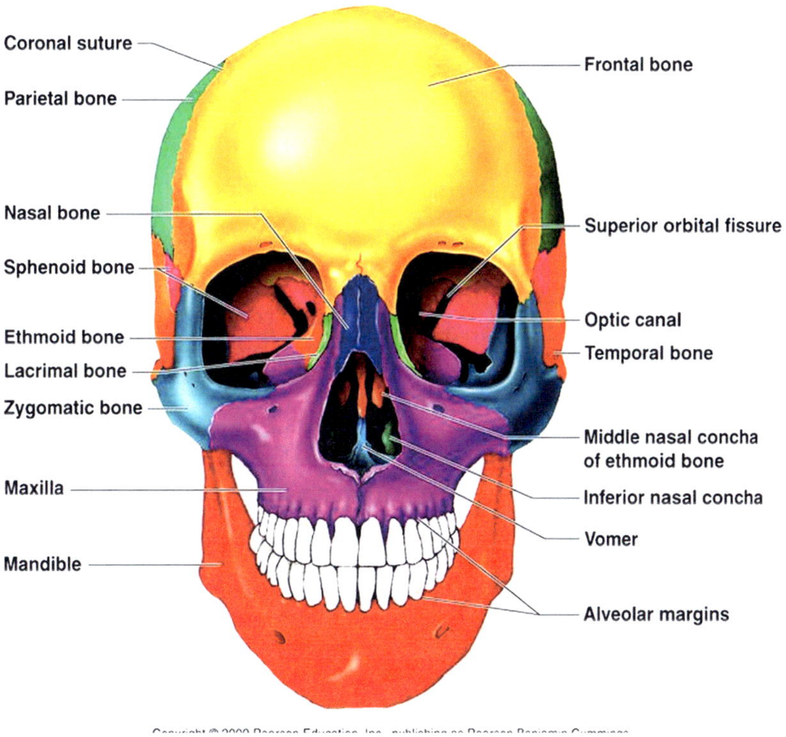

Figure 5.5. Classification of the cranium.

Source: https://external-content.duckduckgo.com/iu/?u=https%3A%2F%2Fi.pinimg.com%2F736x%2Fc2%2Fd5%2F52%2Fc2d552de912cac7a169fd75f15477ce6--skull-anatomy-long-dresses.jpg&f=1&nofb=1&ipt=ce43bfdcdb6f50a3598008c114925b7c20a9d7442310b90366ffbbdb7ea396ac.

5.1.2. Major Bones of the Cranium

The cranium, which encloses the brain and supports the facial framework, is composed of numerous bones divided into two large categories: the neurocranium and the viscerocranium. The neurocranium, composed of the frontal, parietal, occipital, temporal, sphenoid, and ethmoid bones, is most important for accommodating the brain. The frontal bone at the forehead is significant in both the development of the anterior cranial fossa and in contributing an area for muscular attachment, hence influencing facial beauty. Besides this, parietal bones that are placed bilaterally along the skull constitute the upper structure and cover of the brain as well as formation of the sagittal suture. All these bone elements play a paramount role in protecting vulnerable neural tissues and facilitating complex interactions with neighboring bones. The viscerocranium, or facial skeleton, is made up of those bones that act to support and structure the face. They include the maxilla, mandible, and nasal bones, among others including zygomatic bones, each contributing distinctive features required for breathing, mastication, and facial expression. The maxilla, for instance, forms the upper jaw and holds the upper teeth, whereas the mandible forms the lower jaw and is the sole movable skull bone. This mobility is vital for several functions, including articulation and mastication. Also, the unique geometry of the nasal bones to produce the bridge of the nose indicates the viscerocranium's function not just in use but in the general facial appearance of humans as well. It is essential to know about the interaction between the neurocranium and the viscerocranium to proceed to study human osteology thoroughly. The ontogenetic patterns of these bone structures provide evidence on evolutionary adaptation, as testified by variations resulting due to biomechanic loads and functional requirements. Research shows that interference with cranial bone development can lead to evident deformities affecting overall craniofacial morphology. Most interesting are results indicating the metopic suture persistence to be associated with abnormal frontal sinus development as outlined in recent literature; while the character of these associations requires more research for a better comprehension of their impact on skull development and underlying pathological conditions (Akbasak et al., 2013; Abzhanov et al., 2019). This intricate web of relationships between cranial bones, functional as well as aesthetic, demonstrates the cranium's pivotal role in the anatomy and evolution of humans (Figure 5.6).

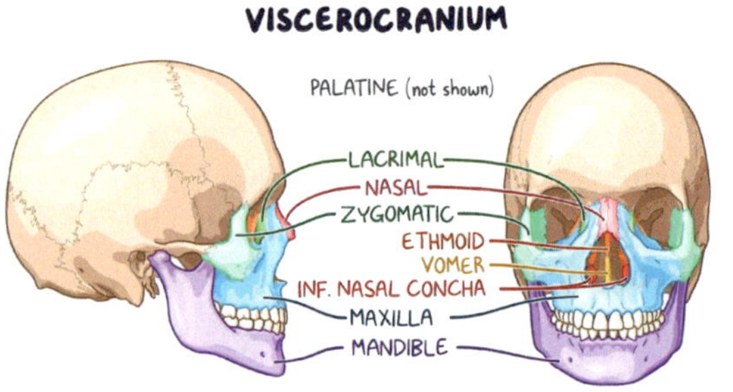

Figure 5.6. Major bones of the cranium.

Source: https://www.osmosis.org/_next/image?url=https%3A%2F%2Fd16qt3wv6xm098.cloudfront.net%2FzCPy5ljxRf_TRbEpWpGVi98mQnGq_tCt%2F_.jpg&w=3840&q=75.

5.1.3. Functions of the Cranial Bones

The cranial bones perform several major functions essential to human physiology and anatomy. Most centrally, they have a protective function, containing the brain and shielding it from external trauma. This encasement is critical, given that the brain is one of the most delicate organs and susceptible to injury. The irregular shapes of cranial bones, combined with the composition of the bones, allow them to absorb and dissipate forces that would otherwise cause catastrophic harm. In addition, particular areas within the cranial bones grow into sinuses and cavities and are involved in important physiological activities, such as reducing skull weight and improving the resonance of the voice. These processes are fundamental to maintaining intellectual function and overall cranial stability within the viscerocranium complex of human osteology. Furthermore, cranial bones also contribute to the formation of facial features and human expression, with specific functions that play a role in human identity. The facial bones, or viscerocranium, form features that make up individual appearances, including the mouth, eyes, and nose. Not only do these bones add structure, but also the positioning needed for significant functions like eating, speaking, and breathing. The dynamic relationship between the cranial bones and other soft tissues, like muscles and nerves, creates expressions that are intrinsic to human social interaction and communication. Such types of interactions also play an essential role in non-verbal communication, reinforcing social relationships and aiding survival through the expression of emotions and intentions. The roles of the cranial bones thus extend beyond structural functions to encompass broader social and evolutionary roles in human interaction. In addition to protection and cranial form, cranial bones have developed the ability to respond to some physiological demands that vary with age. With increasing age, morphological alterations in cranial sutures occur, which not only influence the overall shape of the skull but also the inner architecture. Notably, observations are illustrated graphically to demonstrate how the changes relate to age, reflecting a synaptic link between bone alterations and chronological estimates of aging (Das et al., 2022). Cranial bone and suture remodeling is a complex process controlled by environmental and genetic factors that underlie human variation in bone structure. Understanding these changes enhances understanding of cranial bone function throughout the human life span, providing information on craniofacial development and health. This dynamic view locates cranial bones not simply as stationary structures, but rather as active participants in a continuous process of adaptation and evolution as individuals grow up and interact with their environments (Abzhanov et al., 2019) (Figure 5.7).

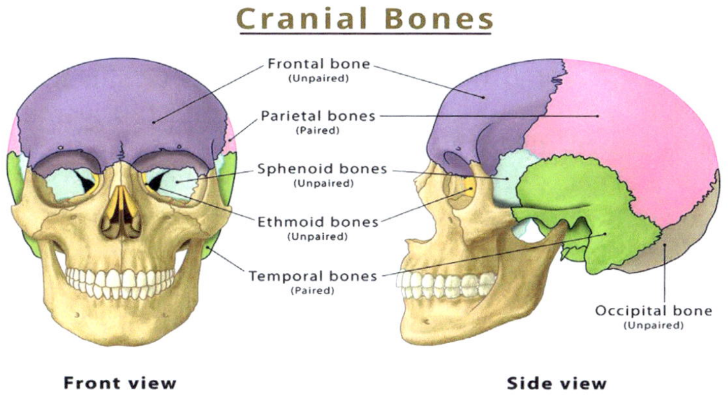

Figure 5.7. The cranial bones serve multiple essential functions.

Source: https://www.theskeletalsystem.net/wp-content/uploads/2022/03/Cranial-Bones-Labeled.jpg.

Test Your Knowledge

1. What are the major bones that make up the human cranium?
2. How is the cranium divided into the neurocranium and viscerocranium, and what are their functions?

5.2. Overview of the Viscerocranium

Learning Outcome

1. Definition and distinction from the neurocranium
2. List of bones forming the viscerocranium
3. Role of the viscerocranium in face structure

The viscerocranium, or face skeleton, is made up of a series of bones that underpin the structure and function of the face. There are 13 different bones, including the nasal bones, maxillae, zygomatic bones, and mandible, among others, that work together to generate the face structure. The bones do not just provide shape and support to the face, but also take part in some of the most important activities like breathing, chewing, and speaking.

The viscerocranium interacts with the cranial component to establish an anatomical equilibrium that supports aesthetic and physiological integrity. Besides its structural function, the viscerocranium plays a leading role in sensory processes such as vision, olfaction, and taste, highlighting the complex interplay between anatomy and sensation. Considering the viscerocranium in analysis, the dynamic aspects of its development and aging processes need to be kept in mind. Viscerocranium is influenced by environmental and genetic variables which confer variation in bone morphology and structure. Research shows that as age progresses, signs of skeletal change become evident, particularly in cranial suture development and closure. The constant remodeling and integrity of the facial bones, the viscerocranium, suggest not only chronological time but also unique biological aging processes. As has been explored in previous studies, awareness of how age changes are represented in the viscerocranium is imperative for correctly interpreting skeletal remains, determining biological age, and distinguishing between normal aging and pathological processes that can debilitate individuals over time (Das et al., 2022). Furthermore, the viscerocranium is an essential element of sexual dimorphism, which is crucial for anthropological inquiry and forensic assessment. Characteristics of the viscerocranium are highly variable in both males and females, making identification possible in poorly preserved fossil remains. Studies on some markers, i.e., the maximal size of the palatinal foramen and the size of the maxillary torus, reveal that such morphological traits are good sex determinants regardless of age and environment (Suriyanto et al., 2006).

This sexual differentiation is not only advantageous to archaeology and paleoanthropology but also enhances understanding of human population variation and evolutionary adaptations. By synthesizing information on the viscerocranium with methods for skeletal analysis, scientists can gain crucial insights into the biological and cultural history of ancient human populations (Figure 5.8).

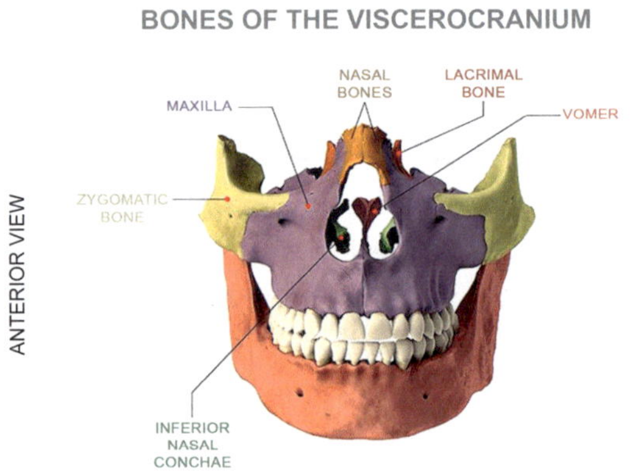

Figure 5.8. The viscerocranium, also known as the facial skeleton.

Source: https://admin.anatomy.app/Media/images/6d665c97-d5ed-4952-b83e-96c2536fb7e2_large.jpg.

5.2.1. Definition and Distinction From the Neurocranium

Anatomically, the cranium is divided into two regions: the neurocranium and the viscerocranium, each serving distinct functions of encasing and supporting different biological structures. The neurocranium includes the superior cranial vault, which encloses and protects the brain and, therefore, is a critical part of neurological function. There are eight bones in this section, including the frontal, parietal, and occipital bones, that form a protective covering over the brain. The viscerocranium, or facial skeleton, is composed of 15 bones that play a crucial role in supporting the facial structures, such as the maxilla and mandible, and that harbor sensory organs. An appreciation of such distinctions is important in fields such as anthropology and forensic science, where accurate recognition of cranial components can reveal information about biological profiles and evolutionary streams. To proceed further, morphologically, the neurocranium and viscerocranium exhibit specific developmental and integration characteristics that bear on both evolutionary biology and forensic anthropology. As explained by Hemingway et al. (2017), the unification of cranial areas is under the control of numerous genetic and functional factors that lead to disparity in morphological patterns. For instance, although the neurocranium is usually relatively constant across species in its rudimentary structure, the viscerocranium is flexible in response to dietary and environmental requirements. This diversity is particularly relevant when used to consider sexual dimorphism, which Small et al. (2016) explain has been shown to influence cranial morphology in different populations significantly. Hence, the difference between such areas is not merely based on anatomical variation, but has significant impacts on functional adaptations and evolutionary mechanisms. The interaction between the viscerocranium and neurocranium also underscores the need for coordinated function of both to preserve primary functions such as respiration, mastication, and sensory integration. The viscerocranium not only gives support to the face but also has a direct effect on the functional efficiency of the neurocranium via its interaction with the cervical spine and associated musculature. The intricate interactions between these regions, as revealed by studies of morphological integration, show how their evolutionary paths are intertwined (Hemingway et al., 2017). Furthermore, the development of morphological assessment techniques, as explained in Small et al. (2016), has better informed us about how sexual dimorphism, among other factors, affects an individual's cranial anatomy. This emergent knowledge of cranial function and structure serves to pinpoint the significance of distinguishing between the viscerocranium and neurocranium within the broader contexts of human osteology and evolutionary biology.

5.2.2. List of Bones Comprising the Viscerocranium

In human osteology, the viscerocranium, or facial skeleton, consists of some exceedingly significant bones that all work to contribute to the entire structure and function of the face. This section of the cranium includes the nasal bones, maxillae, zygomatic bones, palatine bones, lacrimal bones, inferior nasal conchae, and mandible. They all play a crucial role in the formation of the orbital, nasal, and oral cavities, thus facilitating essential functions such as respiration, mastication, and articulation. The intricate relationships among these bones also shape facial beauty and symmetry, underscoring the viscerocranium's significance in both biological and social realms. Viscerocranium development is affected by multiple biological processes, most notably the function of cranial neural crest mesenchyme (NCM) during embryogenesis. Elucidating how such derived tissues communicate through molecular and cellular processes helps reveal the evolutionary adaptations witnessed in jaw morphology throughout species. For instance, disturbances of these cellular pathways could lead to diverse anatomical variations or abnormalities, affecting ratios and ultimately function in the jaw complex. In terms of their anthropological and clinical significance, studies of such morphogenetic determinants have helped raise interest in understanding how these factors transfer to normal and pathological states in human individuals (Abzhanov et al., 2019). Additionally, viscerocranium bone abnormalities can have significant clinical relevance, particularly in dental and orthodontic applications. For example, persistence of metopic sutures—a developmental anomaly—can be related to abnormal development of the frontal sinus, illustrating the connection between cranial structures and their health implications (Akbasak et al., 2013). Apart from this, an understanding of the intricate relationships between these bones and various soft tissue structures can enhance practice in reconstructive and orthognathic surgery, as practitioners must consider not only the bony structure but also how it will affect surrounding structures. Hence, having a total perception of the viscerocranium can offer medical practitioners the knowledge required to overcome clinical difficulties.

5.2.3. Role of the Viscerocranium in Facial Structure

The viscerocranium, or facial bones, is an important part of deciding the human face's architecture and aesthetics. Composed of several bones, including the maxilla, mandible, zygomatic, and nasal bones, the viscerocranium provides the underlying structure of the face. This bone network protects not only the face's soft tissues but also houses important structures, including the oral and nasal cavities. The morphological patterns of such bones are of evolutionary significance; variations in viscerocranium structure embody adaptations to diet, environmental changes, and social behavior over time. The mutual interaction between genetic and environmental pressures shapes the viscerocranium, marking its significance as a field of research in human osteology and evolution. In embryonic development, the viscerocranium is greatly influenced by cranial neural crest mesenchyme, which, through intricate signaling pathways and mechanical forces, creates the facial bones. This mesenchyme is itself derived from embryonic neural crest cells, which migrate and differentiate into many of the tissues that compose the viscerocranium. This period of development can be disrupted by congenital abnormalities, underscoring the importance of facial skeleton development in clinical and evolutionary contexts. In addition, the viscerocranium's connection with the craniofacial morphology highlights the manner in which cranial neural crest-derived tissue is involved in the functional diversification of the jaw complex.

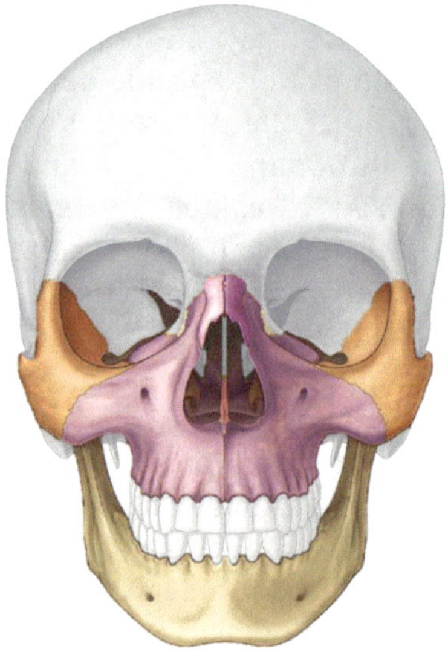

Figure 5.9. Role of the viscerocranium in facial structure.

Source: https://external-content.duckduckgo.com/iu/?u=https%3A%2F%2Fo.quizlet.com%2FIMKM3f8uGFn6GPDekwsmnA_b.png&f=1&nofb=1&ipt=ad715671c18e5353834c0ce7d24cb2f5c050d8caf844e7df655963b56c17c1e2.

The evolutionary significance of such modifications is evident in the diversification of facial structures across species, which has led to the viscerocranium being described as a paramount field of investigation for human ontogeny and phylogeny (Abzhanov et al., 2019). Aging affects the viscerocranium's structure extremely profoundly, with other morphological and physiological modifications being observed throughout the life of a subject. Research indicates that remodeling of cranial sutures and the consequent alterations in facial bones are complexly correlated with aging, which is typically controlled by environmental and genetic factors. For instance, patency in cranial sutures is maintained through coordinated remodeling processes involving resorption and bone deposition. The transformation emphasizes the importance of the viscerocranium for facial attractiveness and functional needs, as facial appearance typically changes with progressive aging. Understanding age-related changes in the viscerocranium can yield insights into broader anatomical and biological processes, which can translate into more efficient methods of age estimation and highlight the interconnection between skeletal aging and overall health (Das et al., 2022) (Figure 5.9).

Test Your Knowledge

1. What is the viscerocranium, and what are its primary functions in the human skull?
2. Which bones constitute the viscerocranium, and how do they support facial structures?

5.3. Development of the Viscerocranium

Learning Outcome

1. Embryological origins of the viscerocranium
2. Growth patterns and changes during development
3. Common developmental disorders of the viscerocranium

Viscerocranium formation is a complex process that depends on subtle interactions among various embryonic tissues, particularly the input of cranial neural crest cells (NCCs). They form early during embryogenesis and travel enormous distances to form the foundation of the jaw and face. The viscerocranium is composed of several bones, including the maxilla, mandible, and nasal bones, all of which derive from NCCs that give rise to mesenchyme. Communication between these cells and their surrounding tissues is essential, as it dictates each component's anatomical identity and the morphology of the viscerocranium. Disruptions in this development can lead to structural malformations, highlighting the finely tuned processes of cells that allow for evolution and adaptation of the amniote jaw complex (Abzhanov et al., 2019). In addition to cell migration forming the viscerocranium, biomechanical forces are a critical consideration during development. These forces are produced by functional processes such as respiration and mastication, which alter bone growth and form. Throughout craniofacial development, mechanical stresses continuously interact with developing tissues, eliciting adaptive responses that enhance the structural integrity of the viscerocranium. This adaptive plasticity is essential to the functional and evolutionary differentiation of facial structures across species. Furthermore, the ability to accommodate adaptations driven by external forces underscores the importance of a coordinated developmental program that also accounts for genetic and environmental influences (Abzhanov et al., 2019). As development proceeds, aging is also a critical consideration in the interaction between cranial sutures.

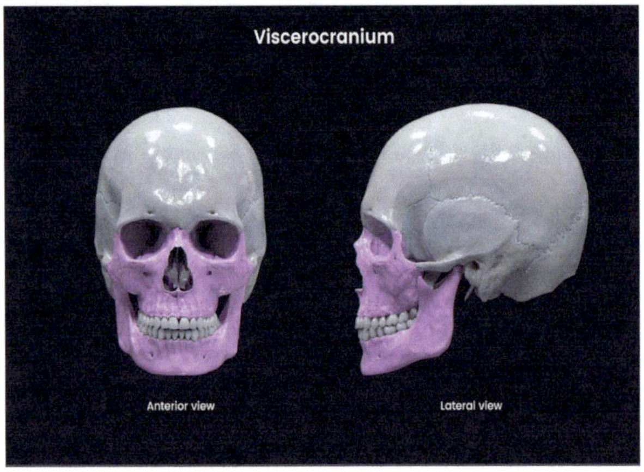

Figure 5.10. The development of the viscerocranium.

Source: https://admin.anatomy.app/Media/images/skull-head-neck-skeleton-parts-viscerocranium-anterior-lateral-view_20240906053640_large.jpg.

The study of cranial sutures yields details on the manner in which viscerocranium can evolve over the course of an individual's life. The sutures are maintained patent through coordinated bone remodeling, an activity that advances from infancy to young adulthood. This dynamic phenomenon, responsible for providing growth space, is similarly associated with the aging process, during which sutural morphological differences can serve as indicators of chronological age. Such changes are informative both in paleontological studies of human ancestors as well as clinical evaluation of craniofacial growth in the living population. The interconnectedness of these developmental and aging processes further underscores the significance of cranial measurements in anthropological research and clinical practice (Figure 5.10).

5.3.1. Embryological Origins of the Viscerocranium

The facial skeleton, or viscerocranium, develops during embryogenesis through intricate processes involving differential cellular origins and interactions. The viscerocranium is mainly developed from the mesoderm and the neural crest cells. Neural crest cells arise from the neural tube edges and play a fundamental role in the development of facial structures. Cells that migrate develop cartilage and bone in the maxillary and mandible regions. By allowing multiple facial components to amalgamate, they develop into an integrated skeletal structure for facial functional adjustments. Thus, a familiarity with embryological origin of the viscerocranium explains significant pathways of facial growth and associated malformations based on disruptions of these pathways. Cell-to-cell interactions between the neural crest mesenchyme (NCM) and other embryonic structures form the basis of viscerocranium formation. The complex dynamic interactions among signaling pathways during embryogenesis dictate the formation of specific anatomical features, so that the viscerocranium becomes an entity not only in terms of individual bones but also as an integrated whole, with functionality in mind. Interfering with these molecular signals results in a spectrum of congenital malformations of facial morphology. For instance, signaling pathway aberrations that regulate NCM migration result in defects such as cleft lip and palate, demonstrating how the proper coordination of development is responsible for correct facial architecture. Furthermore, this cell integration is accompanied by an evolutionary aspect, in which variation is shown to induce adaptive changes in facial shape across species. With ongoing embryological research, it becomes increasingly clear why existing anatomical nomenclature should take precedence.

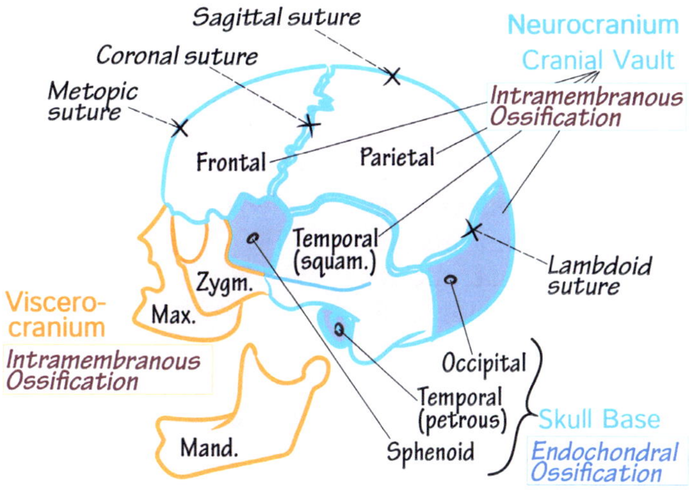

Figure 5.11. Embryological origins of the viscerocranium.

Source: https://d1j63owfs0b5j3.cloudfront.net/term/images/skull-development-skull-fetus-neurocranium-viscerocranium-1378.png.

The 2019 revisions published by the Federative International Programme for Anatomical Terminology (FIPAT) aim to refine the terminology used to define cranial structures, including the viscerocranium. This type of revision offers a clearer understanding of anatomical relationships and developmental mechanisms, which is critical to medical research and study. By exposing clinicians and students to current terminology, the complexities of the viscerocranium become easier to understand. This book also offers greater insight into the intricate development of facial structures and their functional significance, underscoring the need for a solid foundation of knowledge when studying human osteology and its relevance to the clinic. This emerging vocabulary will be an invaluable tool to appreciate the significant detail of cranial structure and development within the broader context of medical education (Figure 5.11).

5.3.2. Growth Patterns and Changes During Development

Growth patterns and developmental changes are important concepts in human osteology, especially as they relate to the viscerocranium. Primary growth begins early in embryonic development, when the cranial neural crest mesenchyme (NCM) shapes facial structures. Through the intricate interplay of cellular signaling, these mesenchymal cells give rise to various tissues that constitute the viscerocranium, including bone, cartilage, and muscle. These processes are strictly regulated, where any perturbation can lead to congenital anomalies or variations in jaw morphology. Abzhanov et al. (2019) illustrate this intricate relationship by outlining how variations in molecular and cellular responses can lead to the promotion of normal variation as well as pathological deviation in jaw development and function, reflective of the significance of being aware of these growth patterns not just for their normative importance but also for their evolutionary and clinical importance. During continuous development, cranial dynamics of growth change. Post-embryonic changes, for example, those documented from infancy to adulthood, illustrate continuous remodeling of cranial sutures and their interactions with bordering osseous elements. Patency of cranial sutures is maintained by the combined effect of bone resorption and deposition, a phenomenon heavily influenced by the biomechanical environment of the organisms. The remodeling is what allows the skull to adapt to functional loads and regular age-related changes. As noted in Das et al. (2022), the line of demarcation between normative development and pathological processes may be thin; hence, the need for a robust understanding of how these sutural changes, in addition to reflecting age, reflect various health states. Therefore, cranial growth needs to be researched with consideration of both biological and chronological age to accurately measure developmental pathways. Also, aging involves profound morphological transformations of the viscerocranium, further complicating our understanding of craniofacial development. During aging, several markers are used to quantify physiological changes in cranial structures. For example, the epiphyseal closure of long bones gives information about overall skeletal maturity and any potential growth patterns, which can have a significant impact on determinations related to the viscerocranium. The trajectory effect theory, as outlined in Das et al. (2022), emphasizes the distinction between biological and chronological age and demonstrates how these factors are responsible for misinterpreting developmental status. Proper cognition of these processes of aging is important for professionals in the field of osteology and medicine as it not only enhances diagnostic accuracy but also directs intervention against craniofacial developmental abnormalities throughout the lifespan.

5.3.3. Common Developmental Disorders Affecting the Viscerocranium

Developmental disorders of the viscerocranium encompass a range of congenital anomalies with the potential to have a significant impact on facial function and morphology. Among the most widely known conditions is cleft lip and palate, which occurs due to the inadequacy of the normal union of embryonic tissues forming the upper lip and the palate. This malformation not only affects the aesthetic look but also can lead to functional issues such as feeding disorders, speech disorders, and ear infections. The prevalence of clefts varies across populations, highlighting the contributions of genetic and environmental factors during development. Other conditions, such as craniosynostosis, involve premature closure of cranial sutures, which can lead to abnormal skull shape and aberrations in brain development, further underscoring the complexities of viscerocranium formation and its implications for overall health and wellness. Another significant category of developmental disorders of the viscerocranium is represented by skeletal developmental abnormalities, particularly those involving the cranial neural crest mesenchyme. The cranial neural crest plays a pivotal role in facial bone formation and development, and disruptions in its migration or signal can result in a variety of dysmorphic features. Syndromes like Treacher Collins syndrome, characterized by hypoplastic facial bones and soft tissues, result from mutations in genes that affect neural crest function. These syndromes underscore how intricate cellular and molecular processes define craniofacial integrity. As highlighted in relevant studies, an understanding of these mechanisms is at once a promise of advancement in treatment strategy and a paradigm for understanding the plasticity and flexibility of craniofacial form, and how these anomalies play their part in evolutionary discussion of human anatomy (Abzhanov et al., 2019). Apart from that, the complexities of sexual dimorphism in craniofacial form can impact the incidence and expression of developmental disorders specific to the viscerocranium. Experiments have shown that there are cranial measurements that are extremely variable across males and females, with statistical considerations for disorder diagnosis, like maxillary hypoplasia or zygomatic irregularities. Among populations characterized by extreme edentulism, as is indicated by research on the morphology of the cranium, the association between edentulous statuses and morphological differences can equally make sexual dimorphism analyses complicated (Small et al., 2016). Proper assessment of such disorders is crucial for clinicians and forensic anthropologists alike, as it will ascertain biological profiles and develop individualized treatment strategies. Understanding how genetics, the environment, and anatomy interact in craniofacial disorders can have direct benefits for patients and may advance the study of human osteology.

Test Your Knowledge

1. What are the main stages of viscerocranium development during embryogenesis?
2. How do genetic and environmental factors influence the growth of the viscerocranium?

5.4. Functional Anatomy of the Viscerocranium

Learning Outcome

1. Role in mastication and speech
2. Contribution to sensory functions
3. Function in facial aesthetics and identity

The viscerocranium, or the facial skeleton, plays a vital role in respiration, mastication, and articulation. This complex framework is composed of various bones that not only provide the face with its shape and protect it, but also serve as attachment sites for muscles. The bones of the viscerocranium, such as the maxilla, mandible, zygomatic, and nasal bones, possess a complex embryological origin, predominantly from the cranial neural crest mesenchyme. This cell divergence enables morphological plasticity, allowing adaptive mechanisms to respond to environmental stress over evolutionary time. The functional significance of the viscerocranium centers on its structural strength and elasticity, underscoring its role in understanding human osteology and the phylogenetic history of craniofacial morphology, as examined through analyses of amniote jaw evolution and the molecular mechanisms underlying it (Abzhanov et al., 2019). Furthermore, viscerocranium is sexually dimorphic, making it an essential focus of anthropological and forensic studies. Size, shape, and epigenetic characteristics of certain features may play a role in sex determination based on the skeleton. For instance, in skull samples, it has been demonstrated that measurements of the palatinal foramen and the expression level of torus features can be used to easily differentiate between male and female sex in viscerocrania. Such a capability is particularly relevant to paleoanthropological and archaeological work, which usually entails working with fragmentary and poorly preserved human skeletons. Being able to ascertain sex from skeletal traits, independent of age and race, is a vital tool for scholars. This rich appreciation makes rich contributions to our knowledge of human variation and evolution, with the viscerocranium's place in the broader landscape of human osteology (Suriyanto et al., 2006). In addition to utilitarian functions, the viscerocranium is also richly involved in sensory and communicative processes.

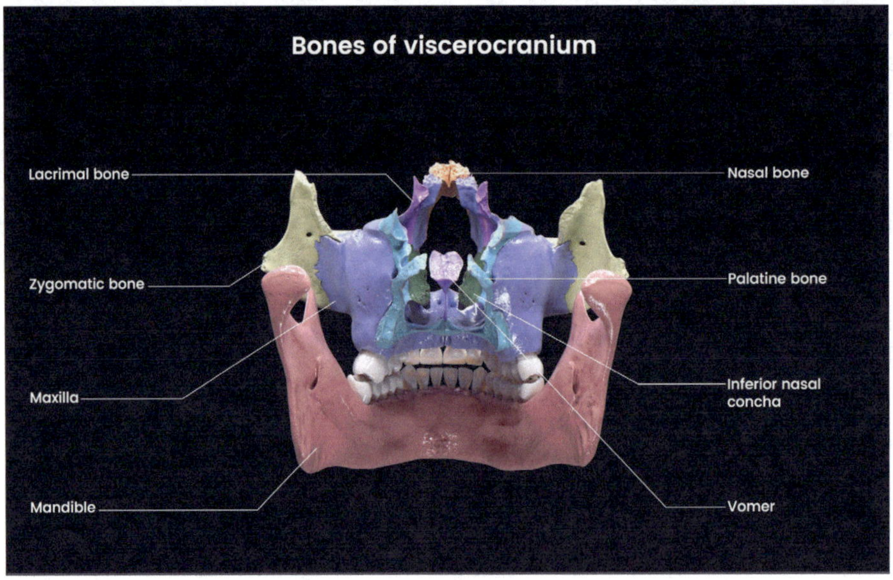

Figure 5.12. Functional anatomy of the viscerocranium.

Source: https://external-content.duckduckgo.com/iu/?u=https%3A%2F%2Fadmin.anatomy.app%2FMedia%2Fimages%2Fskull-cranium-head-neck-parts-viscerocranium-bones-posterior-view_20240912033703_large.jpg&f=1&nofb=1&ipt=4e94522b84fbb146fe87504bc5b0647951f0568acc24d1d8354399580c2ab6e3.

The bones of the face house organs of sight, taste, and smell, thereby facilitating rich engagement with the environment. The articulation of the mandible with the temporal bone forms a specialized joint structure that can accommodate the broad movement necessary for mastication and pronunciation. In addition, the facial skeleton offers a functional platform for a number of musculature of facial expressions, which play a vital role in non-verbal communication. The viscerocranium's multidirectional nature is indicative of its fundamental role in physiology and social interaction. A recognition of these correlations increases our sensitivity to the viscerocranium's role in evolution, showing how specializations of anatomy in turn mirror survival requirements and social behavioral complexity in human groups (Abzhanov et al., 2019) (Figure 5.12).

5.4.1. Role in Mastication and Speech

The viscerocranium, or facial skeleton, is also a highly significant component of both speech and mastication, serving as the structural framework supporting the soft tissues of these functions. The maxilla and mandible are particularly significant structures in this role because they house the dental arches, where the chewing teeth are located. Correct stability and alignment of these bones enable the temporalis and masseter muscles to act, which are critical to the development of the force level required for adequate mastication. Moreover, during chewing, these bones must work together with joints and ligaments so that motion is smooth and coordinated, suggesting harmony in the anatomy of the viscerocranium. This structural-functional coordination also points to the way craniofacial structure directly impacts nutritional lifestyle and overall health, thereby tracing an archaic correlation between food intake and skeletal morphology. The complexity of the viscerocranium does not begin or end with mastication, since speech production is also required. The coordination of the mandible, maxilla, and other bones of the face allows for variations in tongue movement and position, which are necessary for the articulation of different phonemes. In addition, the nasal cavity size and position, which are defined by the skull structure, have an effect on resonance and voice quality. Specific structures of the viscerocranium, like the pterion region where various cranial bones converge, also play a role in speech production. This area of overlap represents a convergence of evolutionary specializations based on both phylogenetic context and biomechanical requirements for the production of complex sounds. Such anatomical configurations can thus be considered evolutionarily preserved traits, substantiating the double functions of mastication and speech as bases for human adaptation and social behavior (Gamet et al., 2017). Research on the viscerocranium has provided invaluable insights into how it functions, compared with similar activities from an evolutionary perspective. The biomechanics of mastication can influence craniofacial structures in subtle ways over time, leading to variations that affect speech functions and dietary adaptation. Particularly, different species informs about the adaptive significance of the viscerocranium in food processing and speech sound production, and, therefore, places it in a broader functional context. Functional consequences have been linked to extreme sexual dimorphism in craniofacial bones, with differences among populations based on specific diet and communicative habits. Thus, the viscerocranium's role in mastication and speech transcends immediate bodily needs, highlighting deeper evolutionary processes that characterize human anatomy and behavior (Suchá et al., 2024).

5.4.2. Contribution to Sensory Functions

The facial skeleton, or the viscerocranium, plays a fundamental role in offering varied sensory functions required for human interaction with the environment. This is where the buildings that harbor the sensory organs of the senses of sight, taste, smell, and even hearing are. The orbital cavities, for instance, provide protection and housing for various eyes, while the nasal cavity is crucial for olfactory purposes as it facilitates the sense of smell. Again, the maxilla and mandible are involved in tasting through the connection of the taste buds with the ingested material. Collectively, these structures emphasize the coordinated nature of sensory inputs, enabling effective interpretation and response to stimuli in humans. Such an appreciation of the contribution of human osteology provides better insight into anatomical configurations that influence sensory ability and, hence, behavioral adaptations. In addition to housing the sensory organs, the viscerocranium also has a significant supportive role in the sensory processing hierarchy. The craniofacial configuration provides stability, essential for sensory integration, when information from several modes is combined and used to make decisions. Chewing, for example, with its delicate mechanisms facilitated by the mandible and its articulation with the temporal bone, is inherently linked with gustation and flavor sense in general. This anatomical reliance underscores a typical evolutionary pattern: the evolution of viscerocraniums has been driven by the demands of functional morphology in an environment of rich sensory input. The interaction between cranial form and sensory function reflects a complex relationship that has evolved, augmented by specific concessions in the face and jaw that accommodate both the demand for sensory processing and the mechanical demands of so doing. Morphological integration of the viscerocranium's elements also elucidates its function in sensory processes.

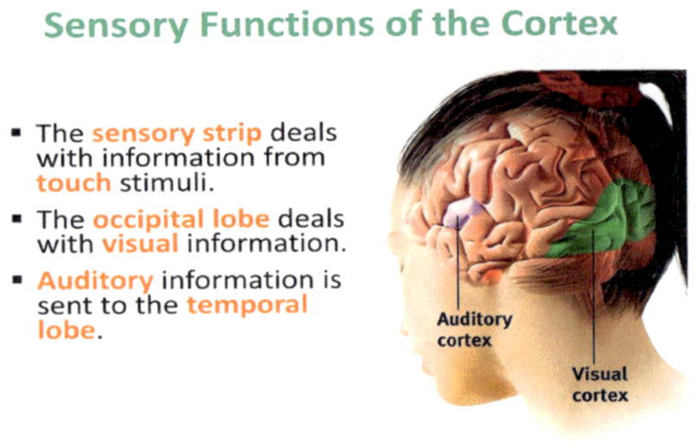

Figure 5.13. Contribution to sensory functions.

Source: https://external-content.duckduckgo.com/iu/?u=https%3A%2F%2Fimage3.slideserve.com%2F5624366%2Fsensory-functions-of-the-cortex-l.jpg&f=1&nofb=1&ipt=172af3995b2d59fda8d2dd363990c18670be234c086760c16b72edcfaf39dd64.

The structural similarity among the different elements of the face, sculpted by genetic, developmental, and functional forces, enables communication among the nasal, oral, and ocular regions. As recent studies have demonstrated, allometric development might mask weak patterns of integration, especially regarding how the sensory systems may be developing relative to one another. For instance, human beings exhibit lower levels of morphological integration than other primates, which necessarily suggests that craniofacial structural associations are subject to different evolutionary forces. These differences introduce new facets into the understanding of sensory functionality in the viscerocranium by claiming that the structure of the cranium is not a series of distinct elements but a single entity that serves to enhance sensory capabilities and thus different interactions with the environment as well as social behavior (Hemingway et al., 2017; Abzhanov et al., 2019) (Figure 5.13).

5.4.3. Importance in Facial Aesthetics and Identity

The connection between facial aesthetics and identity is deeply embedded in human biology and culture. In the world of human osteology, the viscerocranium has a central role to play in creating an individual's overall looks and, consequently, their identity. The arrangement of facial elements—such as the nasal area, orbital cavities, and dental structure—adds to the basic components of aesthetics. For instance, craniofacial measurements show that slight variations can make a big difference in beauty and attractiveness judgments across cultures. Being familiar with the anatomical foundation of facial beauty, scientists can better understand how facial features can serve as identifiers and expressions of social and cultural identity. Such findings are priceless in forensic anthropology and anthropometry, where facial feature reconstruction can help identify individual identities, especially when primary identifiers like DNA are not possible. Facial beauty is beyond outward appearances; it plays an integral role in the social and psychological processes of identity construction. The characteristics of the viscerocranium may influence an individual's self-perception, social relationships, and even opportunities in other aspects of life, such as work. Recent craniofacial studies, particularly those involving some individuals, suggest an interaction between genetically determined facial traits and environmental influences on facial growth. Research such as the evaluation of facial approximations in purpose samples of populations supports that it is crucial to understand craniofacial structure in order to understand identity, since culturally derived perceptions about beauty shape personal self-esteem and social status. The viscerocranium, therefore, ought to be viewed not only as a biological template but also as a significant component of identity formation. Interestingly, the record of artificial cranial modification (ACM) is a paradigm case of how facial aesthetics may represent social identity and culture. Historical ACM practices that altered cranial shapes for various cultural reasons demonstrate a complex intertwinement of biology and sociocultural explanations. Studies indicate that styles of modification can affect not only epigenetic traits but also specific facial dimensions, making it challenging to apply linear notions of beauty and identity (Boston et al., 2012). By studying such modifications, anthropologists can glean rich insights into past social hierarchies and ethnic identities. Furthermore, the recognition of the effects of ACM on morbidity and mortality demonstrates how deeply physical appearance is intertwined with cultural practice. In examining the viscerocranium, one can easily see that facial attractiveness exceeds biological definition, as it is closely linked to the intricate matrix of human identity and social interaction.

Test Your Knowledge

1. How does the viscerocranium support the functions of mastication, respiration, and sensory perception?
2. What role do the bones of the viscerocranium play in facial expression and muscle attachment?

5.5. Pathology of the Viscerocranium

Learning Outcome

1. Common diseases and disorders of the viscerocranium;
2. Trauma and impact on facial bones;
3. Surgical alternatives and implications.

Viscerocranium, a component of the human skeleton, encompasses the facial bones, which play critical structural and functional roles in preserving the integrity and function of the face. Illnesses in this region can seriously debilitate several physiological processes such as breathing, chewing, and speech. Cleft palates, caused by defective fusion of palatine processes, are a good example of the impact of developmental disorders on the viscerocranium. Furthermore, persistent metopic sutures have been associated with distorted development of the frontal sinus, thereby further complicating craniofacial morphology and likely leading to functional impairment. Studies indicate that approximately 9.7% of individuals exhibit persistent metopic sutures, which may be associated with other pathological manifestations of the frontal region, suggesting that these structural abnormalities warrant further study in osteological research on craniofacial anomalies (Akbasak et al., 2013). Trauma to the viscerocranium generally leads to a range of pathologies, including fractures that can have long-term implications for form and function. Blunt trauma, for example, is often associated with mid-facial fractures, which can interfere with the continuity and alignment of facial structures. The biomechanical analysis of such injuries has a significant role to play in determining the circumstances of the death of an individual, insofar as it discusses potential mechanisms of trauma. Forensic examination has shown that nearly 59.1% of reconstructed death scenarios are consistent with observable traumatic events in cranial remains (Marinho et al., 2013).

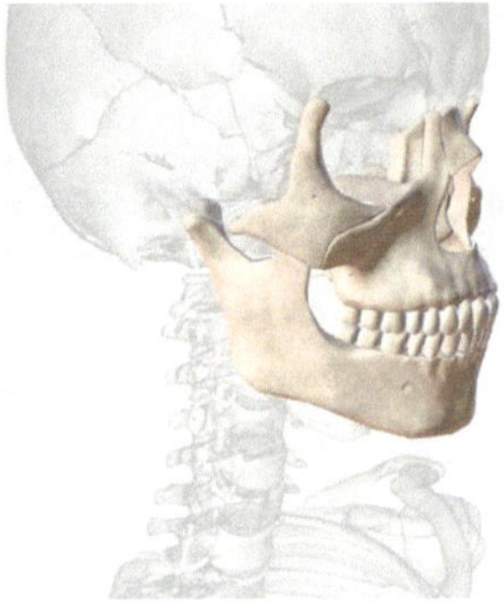

Figure 5.14. The viscerocranium, an integral part of the human skeleton.

Source: https://external-content.duckduckgo.com/iu/?u=https%3A%2F%2Ft4.ftcdn.net%2Fjpg%2F07%2F17%2F07%2F19%2F360_F_717071985_2qswCg8snTMGbJNFazYt4zi10SvrXpit.jpg&f=1&nofb=1&ipt=1c81a1fe77c585682abb2178709640016bc044acf5e4d47d0b507257297d177c.

The results highlight the importance of examining viscerocranial integrity following trauma and further advancing techniques to elucidate the relationship between trauma and the intrinsic factors of death in forensic science. Pathological status and the viscerocranium have a significant impact on one another, well into the field of genetics and congenital disease. Genetic mutations can result in craniofacial syndromes that express in extremely varied forms, impacting the morphology and function of the viscerocranium. Syndromes such as Treacher Collins syndrome are a classic example of the wide-ranging impact of genetic abnormalities on facial growth and development, leading to dramatic variations in bone structure and soft-tissue positioning. These congenital disorders overlap with environmental factors to produce complex clinical presentations that pose diagnostic challenges. Explaining viscerocranial pathology of genetic predispositions not only enhances knowledge of craniofacial anomalies but also directs future research towards more targeted therapeutic strategies, bringing into the limelight the need for multidisciplinary research in the field of human osteology (Akbasak et al., 2013) (Figure 5.14).

5.5.1. Common Diseases and Conditions Affecting the Viscerocranium

The viscerocranium, or facial bones, is prone to some diseases and conditions that can affect both structural integrity and function profoundly. Osteomyelitis, a bone infection, is a particular hazard to the viscerocranium. This is usually a complication of an infection in the oral cavity, especially in the maxilla or mandible, and can lead to serious complications such as bone necrosis and systemic disease unless treated.

The unique anatomical characteristics of the facial bones, which differ from those of other cranial bones in their vascular supply and density, influence the evolution and management of osteomyelitis. Hence, knowledge of the processes beneath this illness is fundamental for forensic anthropologists analyzing skeletal remains, as a diagnosis of osteomyelitis can provide significant data on the health of the individuals at the moment of death, revealing potential causes of death or the aftermath of trauma (Marinho et al., 2013). Facial trauma, whatever its cause (accidents, violence, or pathologic processes), is also a fundamental point to alter the viscerocranium. Blunt trauma injuries, in particular, often lead to fracture of facial bones and thus complicate facial reconstruction of facial contours in forensic and clinical contexts. The biomechanics of such injuries can also be employed to prove the cause resulting in trauma, and forensic examiners would gain valuable information regarding the circumstances of a person's death. However, as research indicates, arriving at a direct causal connection between perceived skeletal trauma and death circumstances is still challenging. A deep exploration of traumatic patterns will assist in uncovering legal investigations and medical interventions that warrant a keen osteological examination to ascertain possible underlying causes of such injuries (Reinman et al., 2019). Another significant condition that arises in the viscerocranium is the development of congenital abnormalities, such as cleft lip and palate. These abnormalities not only have environmental and genetic implications but also entail a wide array of functional limitations, including difficulties with eating, speaking, and hearing. Investigation of these abnormalities in the viscerocranium is imperative since they must be treated and repaired through multidisciplinary approaches. Surgical interventions are typically necessary, and craniofacial surgeons play a paramount role in correcting structural deficits to improve patient outcomes. Besides, new imaging techniques can provide detailed information on the gravity and implications of these conditions, enabling personalized treatment plans. By analyzing bone remains with congenital malformations, forensic anthropologists may also provide insights into past prevalence and consequent health implications (Marinho et al., 2013).

5.5.2. Impact of Trauma on Facial Bones

The viscerocranium of man, which consists of many facial bones, is particularly vulnerable to trauma and can drastically alter its function and structure. Facial bones, unlike the more rigid cranial vault, possess a multifunctional architecture that is highly developed for supporting soft tissues and sensory organs. Trauma to such bones can result from various causes, such as blunt trauma, falls, or road traffic accidents, causing fractures, dislocation of the jaw joints, and soft tissue injuries. The ensuing trauma not only impairs the cosmetic presentation but can even hamper life-sustaining functions like mastication and respiration. Since the majority of the facial skeleton injuries occur in violent or sports-related scenarios, an awareness of the biomechanical outcome and possibility of long-term complications becomes crucial in clinical and forensic practice (Marinho et al., 2013). Facial bone injury usually affects the treatment approach to the injury and recovery from it. Fractures can be straightforward and undisplaced or complex, comminuted fractures, requiring meticulous reconstruction. Facial anatomy restoration is essential to preserve both form and function, and it is of paramount importance in social behavior and mental well-being. The intricate relationship between facial bones, soft tissues, and sensory organs presents a challenge for surgeons, as they must contend not only with skeletal damage but also with the surrounding musculature and nerves (Abzhanov et al., 2019). Also, complications from post-trauma, such as infection, improper healing, or malunion, may further complicate recovery, and thus it becomes important to have adequate treatment protocols to enhance the healing and minimize long-term aesthetic and functional deformity. In understanding the impact of trauma on the viscerocranium, one needs to appreciate the broader implications on the patient who suffered facial trauma. The psychological effect of facial injury may be extreme; disfiguring injury causes anxiety, depression, or reduced self-esteem among many patients. The social emphasis on facial attractiveness, allied with the impact of trauma on a patient's sense of identity, can provoke such psychological disturbances (Marinho et al., 2013). Outreaches on health education for traumatic injury impact and the necessity of early treatment will render healthcare-seeking behavior more acceptable. Furthermore, ongoing research on the trauma and recovery pathway will aid in improving clinical practice in the treatment of facial injuries, ensuring that individuals receive comprehensive care that heals both physical and psychological wounds (Abzhanov et al., 2019) (Figure 5.15).

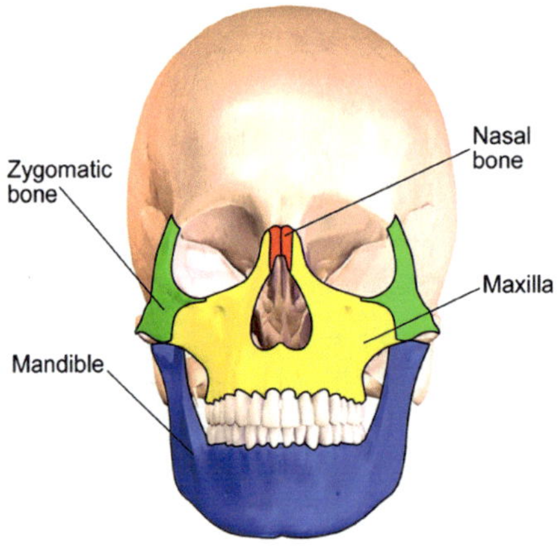

Figure 5.15. Impact of trauma on facial bones.

Source: https://external-content.duckduckgo.com/iu/?u=https%3A%2F%2Fwww.physio-pedia.com%2Fimages%2Fthumb%2F5%2F54%2FBlausen_0393_FacialBones_01.png%2F600px-Blausen_0393_FacialBones_01.png&f=1&nofb=1&ipt=c1596ec11394003bdb99703ded534d9fb90448e4c679b45320923939b22716c5.

5.5.3. Surgical Interventions and Their Implications

The investigation of operations on the viscerocranium and cranium is of significant importance for the acquisition of cranial anatomy and the diagnosis of cranial pathological conditions. Surgical interventions such as craniotomies and reconstructive facial surgery are significant in treating trauma or birth deformities. Surgical interventions alter the integrity of cranial structures and alter bone morphology. To illustrate, craniotomies can disrupt the association between the calvaria and the brain structures beneath it, potentially making it difficult for future imaging interpretation. Beyond that, with evolving innovations in contemporary surgery, the application of devices and implants can also affect osteological analyses more. This dynamic intricacy necessitates a solid foundation of insight into the normal and pathological conditions of cranial bones, which is imperative for sound assessment in forensic anthropology and bioarchaeology. As such, incorporating surgical procedures into cranial anatomy learning broadens the range of techniques available to correct craniofacial malformations. The impacts of surgical procedures are not only limited to bone structures but also extend to personal identification in forensic investigations. Surgical or traumatic abnormalities provide helpful information for personal identification when compared with ante-mortem clinical records and post-mortem skeletal remains. Previous research has established that healed fractures and surgical devices are significant markers that can help forensic scientists link unidentified remains to individuals with known identities. However, how reliable such markers are remains debatable. For example, while some conditions, such as the presence of surgical implants, can be highly individualizing, others, such as healed rib fractures, might be underreported and thus pose a challenge for identification. The recurring threat of non-alignment between recorded medical procedures and actual skeletal evidence underscores the importance of attention to detail in forensic analysis, as suggested by studies of skeletal collections (Maijanen et al., 2014). Moreover, the transformation of cranial sexual dimorphism with age in relation to surgical procedures illustrates the active interaction between osteological features and surgical history. Research indicates that the degree of sexual dimorphism is reduced significantly with age, along with any treatment that may alter craniofacial shape. These findings are highly relevant in cases where surgical interventions are capable of modifying the visibility of sexual dimorphism. Knowledge of these associations is most valuable not only for surgical planning but also for understanding the broader implications of anthropological studies of the human cranium. For instance, advances in surgery can affect later interpretations of sexual dimorphism both in recent and archaeological populations. Therefore, including surgical intervention data in osteology makes sex estimation methods more accurate and enables a more sophisticated understanding of cranial morphology, as seen in recent research (Suchá et al., 2024).

Test Your Knowledge

1. What are common pathological conditions that affect the viscerocranium, such as fractures or congenital deformities?
2. How can diseases or trauma of the viscerocranium impact facial function and aesthetics?

5.6. Comparative Osteology

Learning Outcome

1. Differences in human and non-human viscerocranium
2. Evolutionary significance of viscerocranium
3. Companions to comparative studies in anthropology

The facial skeleton or viscerocranium is significant in comparative osteology as it highlights evolutionary divergences among species. As a complex structure, the viscerocranium is made up of a few large bones that form the facial portion's framework, and they significantly contribute to operations like respiration, mastication, and social signaling. Comparative research indicates that variation in external morphology, bone structure, and size among species can help us understand functional adaptation to different ecological niches. For example, specific adaptations observed in primate species, such as variation in maxillary and mandibular morphology, can indicate particular food habits and sociality. Identification of such adaptations not only enlightens facial evolutionary processes but also enables reconstruction of ancestral morphology and relationships among mammals, a goal at the very center of comparative osteology. The contribution of cranial neural crest mesenchyme (NCM) to viscerocranial architecture cannot be overstated. It is directly responsible for embryonic development of the facial skeleton, bone and cartilage formation, and the delicate interactions among signaling pathways that define the shape of the face. The evolution of the jaw and associated structures appears to be heavily influenced by the plasticity in NCM, which enables it to accommodate differential functional pressures across species. Experiments show that perturbations during the migratory and signaling phases of NCM yield distinct morphological consequences, accounting for the vast variability in amniote jaw forms. These results are critical for appreciating the evolutionary mechanisms governing the viscerocranium and its morphological variation across taxa, and for emphasizing the need for a fine-grained analysis of cranial development processes in comparative osteology (Abzhanov et al., 2019).

Besides providing insights into evolution, the utilitarian application of research into the viscerocranium includes forensic and archaeological contexts. Knowledge of sexual dimorphism in facial morphologies enhances the competence of sex determination of bones, which plays a vital role in anthropology and archaeology. Research on specimens such as the Gilimanuk skull has shown that some epigenetic characteristics, including the size and expression of the palatine foramen and the torus structures, are effective in discriminating between male and female viscerocrania. This utility is particularly increased with fractured or degraded remains, where traditional morphological methods will be insufficient. Ongoing analysis of such sexually dimorphic characters in the viscerocranium not only enriches anthropological research but also world debates on human variation and health, and therefore underscores the significance of comparative osteology in informing the interpretation of our species record (Suriyanto et al., 2006) (Figure 5.16).

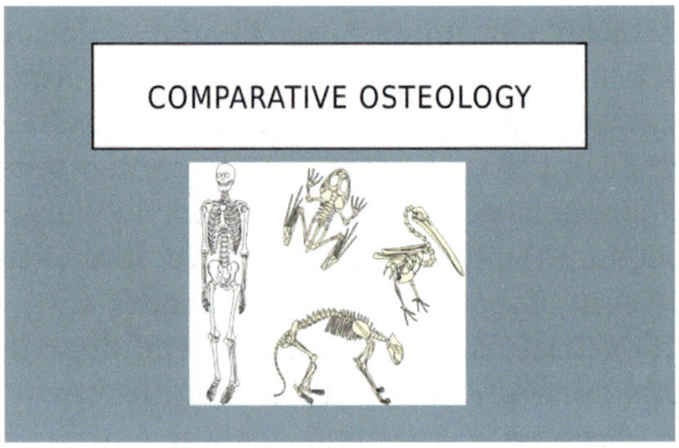

Figure 5.16. Comparative osteology.

Source: https://external-content.duckduckgo.com/iu/?u=https%3A%2F%2Fs2.studylib.net%2Fstore%2Fdata%2F027010541_1-1786726f86b1d702fe521ef96d502907-768x994.png&f=1&nofb=1&ipt=9c866e9b8c1011f3753624087ca7fc5c7712f6329c04380d940112c2d9677f09.

5.6.1. Differences Between Human and Non-Human Viscerocranium

The viscerocranium, or facial skeleton, is multipurpose in human and non-human animals but has remarkable differences in morphology and structure. In humans, the viscerocranium is not large and is flat in facial profile, enabling speech and the creation of complex facial expressions. This development is closely related to the evolution of human-specific social and cognitive behavior. By contrast, the majority of non-human animals possess clearly defined facial morphologies that are adapted to their environments. The canine long snouts and the clearly defined mandibles in carnivores, for instance, correspond to their nutritional needs. In contrast, herbivorous species possess wider, less curved facial bones that enable efficient grinding of plant matter. Such morphological changes are indicative of differences between viscerocranian morphology and the functional demands imposed by contact with the environment. The developmental biology of the viscerocranium also varies significantly between human and non-human organisms. The amniote jaw complex in non-human animals displays a remarkable diversity of morphology, shaped by diverse embryonic sources and cellular signals. The complexity of the viscerocranium in such creatures is driven by molecular and cellular regulatory variation, as witnessed in studies on the role of cranial neural crest mesenchyme (NCM) in jaw development (Abzhanov et al., 2019). The result in non-human creatures generates a higher number of jaw adaptations (such as broader feeding behavior varieties) that also influence dental functions such as vocalization and defense mechanisms. This biological plasticity underlies the species-specific morphological specializations of the viscerocranium during vertebrate evolution.

The impact of evolutionary forces on the viscerocranium tells us about the adaptive tactics of various species. Human viscerocranium adaptations are preeminent for social cognition and communication, reflective of our complex social existence. In comparison, non-human species present with adaptations that enhance survival, such as powerful jaw structures for predator capabilities and specialized cranial structures to enhance sensory functions. Comparing the upper viscerocranium across populations provides insight into how environmental stresses maintained populations apart and influenced their morphological evolution over time. For instance, epigenetic variation in the viscerocranium observed in Bali and East Nusa Tenggara illustrates how geography and environmental settings shape human facial morphology, with a complex interplay among environment, genes, and bone (Suriyanto et al., 2007). In conclusion, the study of variations between human and non-human viscerocranium tells us much about the evolutionary processes of the vertebrate lineage.

5.6.2. Evolutionary Significance of the Viscerocranium

The viscerocranium, or facial skeleton, plays a significant role in the evolution of mammals, including humans. This structural innovation has resulted from complex interactions of environmental, embryological, and genetic forces that together determine craniofacial morphology. Jaw evolution in amniotes is a prime example, in which viscerocranial modifications enabled diverse feeding modes and social behaviors. The incorporation of embryonic cell lineages, especially cranial neural crest mesenchyme, is pivotal in viscerocranium development. These cellular mechanisms allow for accurate anatomical orientation and structure, facilitating the viscerocranium's functional adaptability over time. The ability to analyze the developmental pathways can tell us not only about evolutionary adaptation but also about potential variation that leads to the emergence of jaw shapes, and it highlights the viscerocranium's role in allowing survival and species diversity across evolutionary timescales (Abzhanov et al., 2019). The adaptive role of the viscerocranium is also evident through its role in social signaling and communication between species. Facial bones' distinctive shape and the structural pattern in some way contribute to non-verbal communication, both at the social and the individual hierarchical level. As hominins developed toward a more advanced social existence, the viscerocranium evolved both to support the functional requirements of feeding and to express the nuances of social conduct through facial expression. This dual responsibility illustrates how evolutionary forces have shaped the viscerocranium to serve two capacities, thereby optimizing survival. In addition, differences in viscerocranial structure across populations can be explained by environmental factors, demonstrating the dynamic interrelationship between ecological settings and evolutionary processes. Understanding these lines of evolutionary action provides a broader perspective on the viscerocranium's requirements beyond bodily subsistence (Suriyanto et al., 2006). In addition, the study of the viscerocranium has significant implications for anthropology and paleontology, particularly for sex determination and population analysis. For instance, examining distinctive epigenetic features in cranial morphology can provide valuable insights into the demography of ancient human populations. Research indicates that the size of the palatine foramen and the presence of several bone structures are features responsible for the division of male and female viscerocrania, which is helpful for analyzing fractured or fragmented archaeological materials. This discrimination of individuals based on craniofacial remains can enhance understanding of social organization, variability of the gene pool, and adaptability in past human populations. Thus, the viscerocranium is not only a component of anatomical study but also a vital element in reconstructing the evolutionary history of humans and society (Suriyanto et al., 2006) (Figure 5.17).

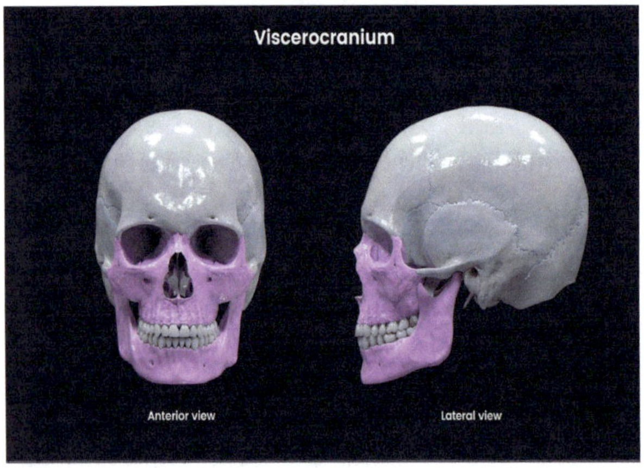

Figure 5.17. The viscerocranium, often referred to as the facial skeleton.

Source: https://admin.anatomy.app/Media/images/skull-head-neck-skeleton-parts-viscerocranium-anterior-lateral-view_20240906053640_large.jpg.

5.6.3. Insights from Comparative Studies in Anthropology

Comparative anthropology studies are a fundamental model for understanding human osteology, particularly when working with the viscerocranium. The viscerocranium that contains the facial bones is a window into the adaptive and evolutionary strategies of anthropological populations. Differences in craniofacial structure between populations can lead anthropologists to infer the effects of environmental, genetic, and social factors on skeletal form. The zygomatic arch shape and nasal passage, for instance, can be shaped by diet or climatic adaptation, thereby conveying the interaction between environment and biology. These analyses not only deepen our insight into hominin evolution but also enable applications in forensic anthropology, where skull differences can be used to identify sex and estimate ancestry. Comparative anthropology's ability to utilize quantitative methods in the analysis of the skull is one of the significant developments of this discipline, as it adds more precision in the determination of sexual dimorphism in remains. The analysis of the Gilimanuk skull sample demonstrates that some morphological traits can effectively distinguish between male and female crania, even when confronted with challenging, fragmented archaeological materials. Traits such as palatinal foramen depth and the formation of toroidal traits are particularly relevant here, as they are stable indicators regardless of race, age, or environmental influences. Such a methodological approach not only makes identification processes easier in paleoanthropological investigations but also raises the scholarly level of human osteology, allowing more systematic and scientifically validated conclusions about ancient populations. Furthermore, comparative geometric morphometry-based studies have provided a robust technique for analyzing cranial shape variation, broadening our understanding of functional and evolutionary processes. For instance, studying skull morphology in Wistar albino rats accounts for gender dimorphism and its effects on the structural integrity of the neurocranium. Through principal components analysis to track shape differences across different areas of the skull, researchers can highlight anatomical differences that may be present across taxa. These cranial morphological findings not only add to the fundamental knowledge base of anthropology but also make possible cross-disciplinary applications in biology and archaeology. Integrative studies of this nature again underscore the central position of comparative methods in expanding our understanding of human anatomical variation and its chronological context in the investigation of the viscerocranium.

Test Your Knowledge

1. What is the purpose of comparative osteology in studying skeletal remains?
2. What techniques are used to compare human and non-human skeletal structures in osteology?

SUMMARY

In condensing the complex relationship of the cranium to the viscerocranium in the framework of human osteology, it is clear that the structural make-up and evolution of the facial skeleton are crucial for both functional morphology and clinical value. The viscerocranium, which consists of many bones that create the face, has a complex interplay of environmental and genetic forces during development. This fusion of anatomical components not only gives the facial architecture its distinctive features but also shows evolutionary concessions for optimal biomechanical function. An understanding of these features not only offers insights into normal craniofacial development but also explains the complexities associated with many types of congenital anomalies and pathologies likely to result from changes in these developmental processes, warranting multi-disciplinary treatment of such conditions. The significance of sex dimorphism in craniofacial growth, particularly among juveniles, also underscores the relevance of anatomical diversity to the viscerocranium. Based on studies, neurocrania and facial forms tend to be larger in males than in females, a trend supported by quantitative comparisons such as those reported in allied research. These results emphasize the variability in cranial morphology, which can impact everything from anthropology to forensic science. Knowledge of these sex-differentiated distinctions increases the effectiveness of classifying and interpreting craniofacial data, enriching our understanding of human biological diversity and its evolutionary history. The identification of these traits not only guides clinical practice but also shapes broader discourse on human adaptation and evolutionary biology. The convergence of molecular and cellular mechanisms governing jaw development is at the forefront of our understanding of craniofacial anatomy. Awareness of the roles of cranial neural crest mesenchyme and biomechanical forces in embryogenesis illuminates the dynamic process by which the viscerocranium develops. As seen in previous studies, variation among these lines of development can have implications that extend across a broad spectrum, affecting jaw morphology, evolutionary processes, and the well-being of individuals. Future studies will have to push forward in exploring the implications of these findings within clinical settings, particularly in terms of jaw defects and disease that have a material impact on quality of life. By combining clinical osteology and developmental biology, we better understand craniofacial complexities and gain insight into future therapeutic approaches, ultimately advancing our understanding of human skeletal evolution.

The viscerocranium or facial skeleton is crucial for the structural stabilization of the human skull as well as for the functional abilities of the oral and nasal cavities. This part of the cranium consists of several significant bones that contribute to facial beauty and the protection of sensitive organs. These are the maxilla, mandible, zygomatic, and nasal bones, each with its own distinct function while simultaneously working together with the rest to provide integrity for the facial structure. Knowledge of the anatomical relationships and developmental patterns of the viscerocranium contributes to the assessment of variations and abnormalities that may develop throughout life, particularly in the context of growth and sexual dimorphism, as highlighted in current studies (Phillips et al., 2013). Such knowledge of craniofacial anatomy is the foundation of advances in fields ranging from forensic science to orthodontics. A closer look at the viscerocranium reveals the importance of identifying sex dimorphism in craniofacial morphology, particularly during developmental stages. Recent literature identifies quantifiable differences in craniofacial morphology between males and females as indicating that males tend to develop more anteriorly and possess larger cranial size (Marinho et al., 2013). This study, conducted on juvenile specimens using advanced imaging techniques, revealed the most salient differences between the neurocranium and the face areas influenced by nasopharyngeal growth. Identification of these patterns is not only of interest to anthropological classification but also of relevance to clinical application in reconstructive surgery and individualized orthodontics. With the help of accurate CT imaging analysis, researchers have measured these disparities to further our understanding of human craniofacial variation. The peak of studies on the viscerocranium and its associated growth patterns underscores the value of a multidisciplinary approach in human osteology. By integrating data from biomechanical analysis of perimortem trauma and anatomical studies of the facial skeleton, researchers are better able to reconstruct individuals' life histories from their bones. Understanding the perimortem trauma implications, for instance, enhances forensic assessment by linking skeletal findings to specific events in the time before death (Marinho et al., 2013). The interaction between anatomical information and trauma analysis underscores the foundational importance of the viscerocranium across fields such as anthropology, medicine, and forensic science. Through further enhancing methodology and fostering interdisciplinary approaches, future research can address the intricacies of human craniofacial variation while strengthening investigative techniques in osteological research.

KEY TERMS FROM THIS CHAPTER

Alveolar Process	Inferior Nasal Concha
Infraorbital Foramen	Lacrimal Bone
Mandible	Maxilla
Mental Foramen	Nasal Bone
Nasal Septum	Orbit
Palatine Bone	Ramus of Mandible
Vomer	Zygomatic Arch

CRITICAL THINKING QUESTIONS

1. **Which of the following bones is NOT part of the viscerocranium?**
   a. Maxilla
   b. Zygomatic bone
   c. Temporal bone
   d. Mandible
2. **How many bones make up the viscerocranium?**
   a. 12
   b. 14
   c. 16
   d. 18
3. **Which bone makes up the lower jaw in the viscerocranium?**
   a. Maxilla
   b. Mandible
   c. Zygomatic
   d. Nasal
4. **What bone forms the front portion of the nasal septum?**
   a. Vomer
   b. Ethmoid
   c. Palatine
   d. Nasal
5. **Which bone is involved in the formation of the cheekbones?**
   a. Maxilla
   b. Zygomatic bone
   c. Nasal bone
   d. Lacrimal bone

Short Answer Questions

1. Define the viscerocranium and its primary function.
2. How many bones make up the viscerocranium, and how are they divided?
3. Describe the role of the maxilla in the facial structure.
4. Explain why the lacrimal bone is important in the viscerocranium.
5. Describe how the zygomatic bone and temporal bone are connected.

Answers to Critical Thinking Questions

1. (c); 2. (b); 3. (b); 4. (a); 5. (b)

REFERENCES

1. Woronowicz, K.C., Schneider, R.A. Molecular and cellular mechanisms underlying the evolution of form and function in the amniote jaw. *EvoDevo* **10**, 17 (2019). https://doi.org/10.1186/s13227-019-0131-8Akbasak, A., Bilgin, S., Duymus, M., et al. (2013). Association between frontal sinus development and persistent metopic suture. https://core.ac.uk/download/268451143.pdf (accessed on 18th July 2025).
2. Boston, C. E. (2012). Investigations of the biological consequences and cultural motivations of artificial cranial modification among northern Chilean populations. https://core.ac.uk/download/61633397.pdf (accessed on 18th July 2025).
3. Chmielewski, P. P. (2021). New Terminologia Anatomica: Cranium and extracranial bones of the head. https://core.ac.uk/download/268450419.pdf (accessed on 18th July 2025).
4. Das, A., & Mohanty, S. (2022). Closure of cranial sutures and expansion of epiphysis of bones as indicators of ageing in forensic sciences: A review. https://core.ac.uk/download/622609390.pdf (accessed on 18th July 2025).
5. Demiraslan, Y., & Gürbüz, İ. (2025). Wistar albino ratların kafatası şekil analizi: Bir geometrik morfometrik çalışma. https://core.ac.uk/download/643189032.pdf (accessed on 18th July 2025).
6. Dorfling, H. F. (2017). Aspects of facial features in a South African sample as applicable for facial approximations. https://core.ac.uk/download/528265907.pdf (accessed on 18th July 2025).
7. Gamet, N. (2017). Investigating pterion from two perspectives: Phylogenetics and biomechanics. https://core.ac.uk/download/232704524.pdf (accessed on 18th July 2025).
8. Hemingway, J. (2017). Exploring patterns of morphological integration in the crania of *Papio hamadryas ursinus* and *Homo sapiens*. https://core.ac.uk/download/188775577.pdf (accessed on 18th July 2025).
9. Maijanen, H. M. K. (2014). The prevalence of pathological conditions in a modern skeletal collection–Implications for forensic anthropology. https://core.ac.uk/download/268768805.pdf (accessed on 18th July 2025).
10. Marinho, L. M. O. (2013). Perimortem blunt force trauma analysis: On the reconstruction of the circumstances of death of human skeletal remains. https://core.ac.uk/download/43586847.pdf (accessed on 18th July 2025).
11. Massey, J. (2018). Pattern of cranial ontogeny in populations of *Gorilla* and *Pan*. https://core.ac.uk/download/211367170.pdf (accessed on 18th July 2025).
12. Phillips, C. E. B. (2013). The use of craniometrics in the estimation of juvenile sex by means of discriminant function analysis: A revised method. https://open.bu.edu/bitstream/2144/12187/6/Phillips_Chase_2013_nosig_nocv.pdf (accessed on 18th July 2025).
13. Reinman, A. (2019). Ancestry assessment in subadult skeletons. https://core.ac.uk/download/223096314.pdf (accessed on 18th July 2025).
14. Small, C. (2016). Sexual dimorphism in white South African crania. https://core.ac.uk/download/188770744.pdf (accessed on 18th July 2025).

15. Suchá, B. (2024). Klasifikace pohlaví na základě 3D modelování lebky v multipopulačním souboru. https://core.ac.uk/download/624142384.pdf (accessed on 18th July 2025).

16. Suriyanto, R. A. (2006). Dimorfisme seksualitas dalam karakteristik epigenetis upper viscerocranium dari sampel tengkorak manusia Gilimanuk (Bali). https://core.ac.uk/download/539561277.pdf (accessed on 18th July 2025).

THE VERTEBRAL COLUMN IN HUMAN OSTEOLOGY

6

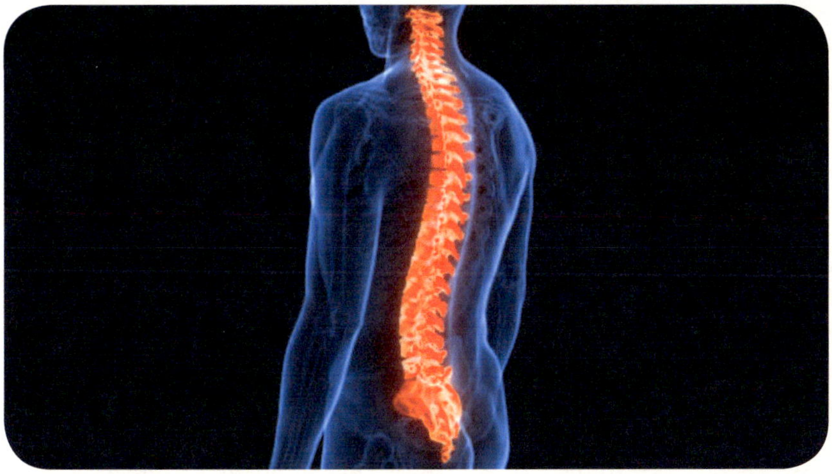

Introduction

The vertebral column, or spine, is one of the fundamental structural components of human osteology and plays a central role in posture support, spinal cord protection, and motion. The intricate structure consists of individual vertebrae, further subdivided into the cervical, thoracic, lumbar, sacral, and coccygeal regions. Each of these regions possesses specific characteristics that mold it to perform specific biomechanical functions. The vertebral column not only supports the weight of the upper body but also allows movement in different directions, providing flexibility during activities that require twisting and bending. Understanding the intricate anatomy of the vertebral column is important across disciplines such as medicine, anthropology, and forensic science, as variations in its structure can provide clues to human evolution and aid in diagnosing injuries. Vertebral column analysis increasingly emphasizes the importance of identifying anatomical variation, which can play a significant role in clinical and forensic outcomes. For instance, some morphoscopic characteristics,

LEARNING OBJECTIVES

After studying this chapter, you will be able to:

1. Discuss the anatomy of the vertebral column
2. Explain the development of the vertebral column
3. Understand the function of the vertebral column
4. Focus on pathologies of the vertebral column
5. Know diagnostic techniques
6. Learn about treatment options

such as differences in the number of thoracic and lumbar vertebrae, are of decisive importance in the process of remains identification. One study analyzing the John A. Williams Documented Human Skeletal Collection identified numerical variations in vertebral structures and concluded that not all such variations are anomalies but may actually reflect significant biological trends within populations (George et al., 2022). Forensic experts would need to recognize such variations, as they can facilitate identification of skeletal remains and yield more accurate results in forensic cases. Also, variations in the vertebral column observed go beyond mere identification; they can even illuminate broader anatomical and evolutionary trends within human populations. Findings suggest that the patterns of variation observed within the vertebral column could account for evolutionary distances and adaptive adaptation among populations (George et al., 2022). Furthermore, research has also emphasized the extent to which similar patterns of variation across other species, for example, in sauropods, expose evolutionary specializations to certain ecological niches (Taylor et al., 2013). Such comparative analysis emphasizes the importance of the vertebral column as part of human anatomy and as a window into our evolutionary history. Accordingly, continuous study of this crucial structure clarifies theoretical and applied branches of osteology, thereby increasing our understanding of human physical diversity.

Definition of the Vertebral Column

The vertebral column, or spine, is an essential structural component of the human skeleton. Composed of an aggregate of individual vertebrae piled one upon another, the column is a strong yet elastic central axis on which the head and trunk are supported and by which a limited freedom of movement is facilitated. Composed typically of 33 vertebrae, the column is also divided further into five distinct regions: cervical, thoracic, lumbar, sacral, and coccygeal. All such areas play specific functions; for instance, cervical vertebrae facilitate head movement, whereas lumbar vertebrae maintain upper body weight support. The vertebral column also supports the spinal canal, which contains and protects the spinal cord, an extension of the central nervous system for the transmission of nerve impulses throughout the whole body. Thus, anatomical knowledge of the vertebral column is crucial in osteology. Apart from the protective and structural role, the vertebral column also plays a significant role in posture and balance. Alignment of vertebrae, along with intervertebral discs interspersed between them, ensures shock absorption as well as mobility during locomotion. These discs, composed of a gel-like inner nucleus pulposus and a more fibrous outer annulus fibrosus, act as shock absorbers that prevent vertebrae from rubbing against each other. Proper alignment of the vertebral column is essential for optimal function, as excessive or improper alignment can lead to many musculoskeletal disorders, including pain and restricted movement. Similarly, this importance also exists across different physiological conditions; e.g., traumas such as those documented at historical sites—witnessed by fractures and degenerative diseases found in archaeological specimens—demonstrate the impact of structural faults on overall wellbeing, as reported in research from the Akhetaten cemetery (Hodgin et al., 2012). Additionally, the vertebral column is essential to our understanding of evolutionary biomechanics and suggests adaptation over time in bipedalism in humans. The human spine's unique curvature characteristics, lordosis and kyphosis, reflect evolutionary adaptations that enable bipedalism and optimal load distribution within the body. Such innovations are contrasted with findings in other vertebrates, revealing how vertebral morphology has been adapted to meet functional demands in diverse environments. Studies of fossilized vertebrae, such as those of sauropod dinosaurs, having similar structural characteristics, contribute to our knowledge of vertebral evolution. Additionally, histological analysis of the structures can reveal the functional relevance of vertebral differences, as evidenced by ossified ligaments in extinct animals (Abdalla et al., 2015). Appreciation of the complexity of the vertebral column, therefore, helps to bring out its fundamental importance to both the human skeleton and, more widely, vertebrate history, in **Figure 6.1.**

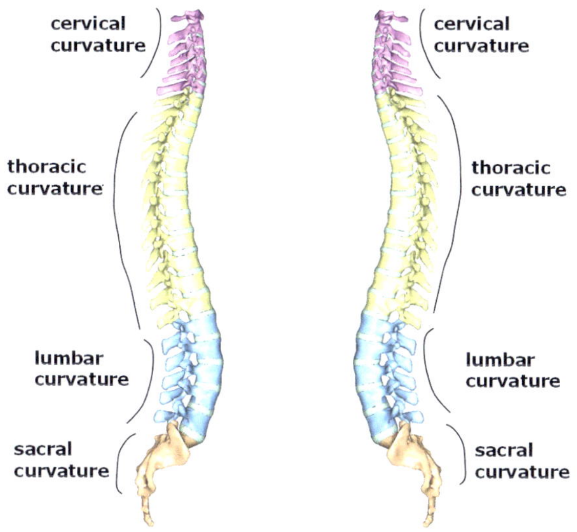

Figure 6.1. The vertebral column.

Source: https://external-content.duckduckgo.com/iu/?u=https%3A%2F%2Fbio.libretexts.org%2F%40api%2Fdeki%2Ffiles%2F39573%2Fclipboard_e0fe9872a9ee3e941d8271a88d6d7fad8.png%3Frevision%3D1&f=1&nofb=1&ipt=81f001be4f0abb5d34dd7477240e67c54267fea504bf144b2995dfa1877bc27e.

Importance in Human Anatomy

The vertebral column, or spine, is a vital part of human anatomy that plays a central role in maintaining posture, facilitating movement, and protecting the spinal cord. Composed of 33 individual vertebrae that are organized into cervical, thoracic, lumbar, sacral, and coccygeal segments, the vertebral column provides structural support as well as a conduit for the nervous system. Alignment and health of the vertebrae are integral to the overall function of the musculoskeletal system. Diseases such as scoliosis or bulging discs can lead to severe impairments, affecting their role in daily life, and their ability to adapt across different periods of life, particularly during growth spurts and senility, underscores their dynamic nature and utility in the human body. The anatomy of the vertebral column is specifically designed to facilitate a range of movements while ensuring stability and protection. Every vertebra has unique features, such as intervertebral discs that provide shock absorption and flexibility, and zygapophyseal joints that can permit controlled movement. The seven vertebrae of the cervical spine are especially significant in supporting the head and providing rotational movement, which is of crucial significance for functions such as visual orientation and balance. Also, the lumbar region, which has wider vertebrae, is essential for bearing much of the body's weight when performing tasks like lifting and bending. Of particular value in human osteology, an awareness of the specific adaptation of the vertebrae to their particular functions highlights the vertebral column's intrinsic function not only as a body support but also as facilitating complex movement. The evolutionary origin of the vertebral column underscores its fundamental role in human physiology and anatomy. As a primary structural component, the vertebral column has undergone impressive adaptations across species, attesting to its critical importance for movement and general function. Long-necked sauropod dinosaur vertebral morphology, for instance, demonstrates diverse adaptations that enabled the animals to survive and thrive in their environments, such as changes in vertebral size and structure that optimized neck length for feeding (Taylor et al., 2012). The present human vertebral column demonstrates similar adaptations, including the configuration of points of muscle attachment and intervertebral cartilage that assist in strength and flexural capability. Interestingly, the functional significance of these anatomical features comes to light in evolutionary contexts where the spine's efficiency has been handy for bipedal locomotion, thus vindicating its role in the interpretation of human osteological complexities (Christian et al., 2013) (Figure 6.2).

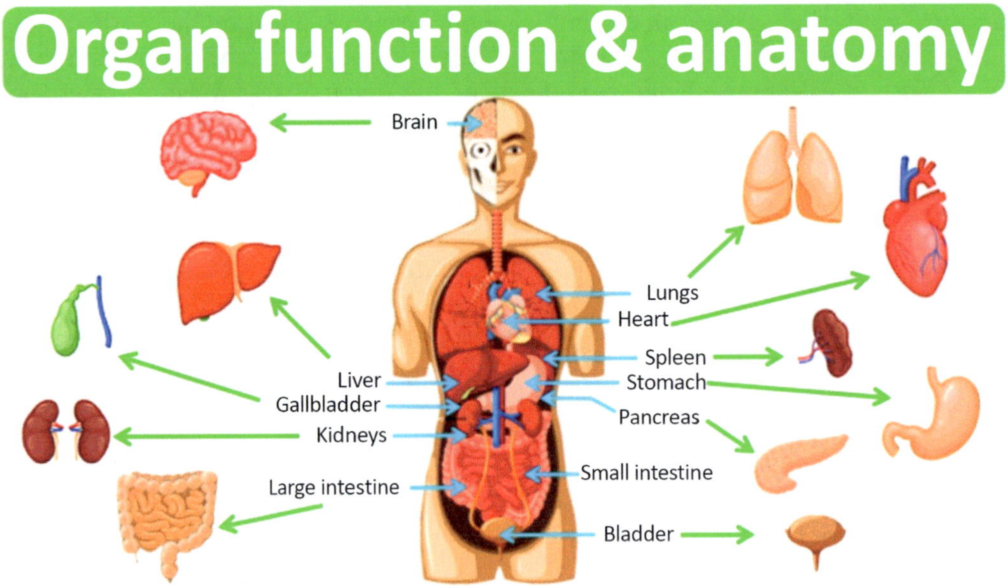

Figure 6.2. The vertebral column.

Source: https://external-content.duckduckgo.com/iu/?u=https%3A%2F%2Fi.ytimg.com%2Fvi%2Fk_F1oZKVPMw%2Fmaxresdefault.jpg&f=1&nofb=1&ipt=6da3f711f492bd645a1c6c9183006b9eb957c9c1c86347158807cbdd0deea091.

6.1. Anatomy of the Vertebral Column

Learning Outcome

1. Number of vertebrae and their classification;
2. Parts of the vertebral column;
3. Intervertebral discs and their role.

The spine, or vertebral column, is a dynamic and complex structure of significance to human anatomy and overall function. It contains 33 individual vertebrae, grouped into cervical, thoracic, lumbar, sacral, and coccygeal regions. The vertebral column plays an essential role in supporting posture and protecting the spinal cord. Every vertebra possesses its own specific anatomical features that enhance its specific function, such as the distinctive lordosis and kyphosis curves that enhance the columns strength and flexibility. Also, intervertebral discs act as shock absorbers between adjacent vertebrae, providing a degree of motion and helping prevent damage during physical stress. The intricate arrangement of ligaments and muscles covering the vertebral column also increases its stability and mobility, underscoring its dual functional role in human osteology and physiology. In order to assess the functional meaning of the vertebral column's structure, it is necessary to examine the inter-relationships between its different parts. For instance, the cervical vertebrae are specifically designed to facilitate greater movement of the head and neck, supporting critical functions such as vision and balance. In contrast, the thoracic vertebrae, which are part of the rib cage, provide protection and stability for critical organs in the thorax while facilitating respiratory mechanics.

The lumbar region bears much of the body's weight and is anatomically so constructed for strength and bearing, and therefore susceptible to trauma. The sacral and coccygeal regions, while traditionally considered vestigial, are significant structures that provide pelvic mobility and stability. A realization of these anatomical differences is key to realizing the vertebral column's general functional significance in human osteology. Recent advances in imaging technology have enabled more detailed probing of the anatomy and biomechanics of the vertebral spine. Studies involving computer-assisted instruction (CAI) and technology-enhanced learning (TEL) have indicated that incorporation of these technologies in osteology coursework may significantly affect understanding of the anatomy of the spine and its clinical significance. Improved access to quality pictures and interactive learning modules allows students to explore the three-dimensional anatomy of the vertebral columns and their dynamic intervertebral joints. This shift in practice mirrors the focus on pedagogical innovation, a movement exemplified by modules such as the one treating the vertebral column, which combine anatomical data with application and clinical insights (Eckel et al., 2021). As the profession develops, a profound appreciation of such anatomical subtleties will be necessary for future healthcare professionals to accurately diagnose and treat spinal pathologies (Figure 6.3).

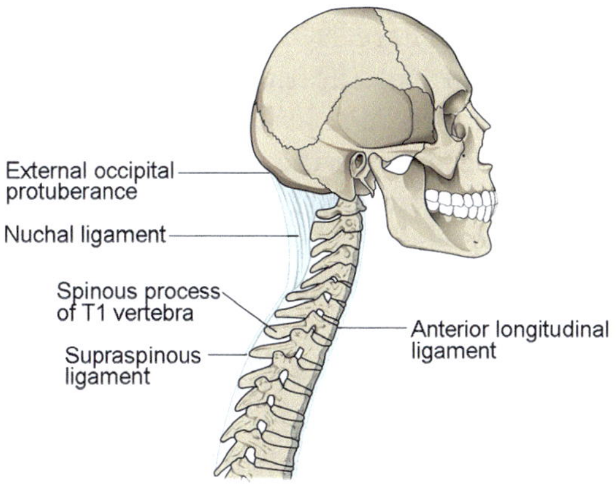

Figure 6.3. The vertebral column, also known as the spine.

Source: https://external-content.duckduckgo.com/iu/?u=https%3A%2F%2Fs3-us-west-2.amazonaws.com%2Fcourses-images%2Fwp-content%2Fuploads%2Fsites%2F1512%2F2017%2F04%2F04232006%2F729_Ligaments_of_Vertebral_Column.jpg&f=1&nofb=1&ipt=428b54e5903e85a254c4ce100550e709cb6a22eea08b360a1c020315c8da593b.

6.1.1. Number of Vertebrae and Their Classification

The vertebral column is one of the most fundamental parts of human osteology, and its classification is based on the number of vertebrae in different regions. The vertebral column in the human body typically consists of 33 vertebrae, all of which are classified into five discrete regions: cervical, thoracic, lumbar, sacral, and coccygeal. There are seven cervical vertebrae that support the neck and allow diverse movement. This is followed by the 12 thoracic vertebrae, which each join up with a pair of ribs, providing stability to the ribcage. The lumbar region, made up of five vertebrae, is designed to bear heavy weight. Then there are the sacral and coccygeal regions, made up of five fused sacral vertebrae and three to five coccygeal vertebrae, respectively, and designed to bear the pelvis as well as act as an anchor for ligaments and muscles. There is excellent variation of this structural classification, primarily among the thoracic and lumbar vertebrae. Research indicates differences in the number of vertebrae, with some individuals having 11 or even 13 thoracic vertebrae and four or six lumbar vertebrae. These morphological characteristics, or morphoscopic characteristics, are essential to enable practitioners to distinguish individual anatomical variations in skeletal remains, which can be pretty significant in forensic identification processes.

These variations can inform practitioners about the anatomical norm and deviation, thereby making them more effective at making accurate judgments in clinical and forensic contexts. Besides, understanding the prevalence of these variations helps formulate effective methods for identifying the skeleton, ultimately contributing to improved results in both medical and forensic sciences. The classification of vertebrae into categories based on their number and morphology also provides future practitioners with knowledge of human anatomy. With access to resources such as the John A. Williams Documented Human Skeletal Collection, students are taught directly how to examine and recognize naturally occurring differences in the vertebral column. Learning from these experiences sheds light on how anatomical differences can affect clinical practice, particularly in fields like orthopedics and forensic anthropology. Handling such skeletal structures allows students to appreciate the complexity of human variation with a focus on the significance of proper documentation in anatomical studies. Such a significant understanding of anatomical variation allows healthcare practitioners and scientists to better appreciate unique characteristics that can contribute to forensic identification, ultimately bridging the gap between theoretical knowledge and practical application in human osteology.

6.1.2. Regions of the Vertebral Column

The vertebral column or spine consists of particular parts that are both structural and functional of the human skeleton. It is divided into five major regions, namely cervical, thoracic, lumbar, sacral, and coccygeal. The cervical part consists of seven vertebrae (C1–C7) and is designed to support the skull while offering much freedom of the head's movement. The cervical vertebrae are characterized by their relatively lighter and particular features, such as the transverse foramen, which accommodates the vertebral arteries. This region plays a critical role in protecting the spinal cord and allowing movement, forming the foundation of the head's rotational and flexural capacity. Thus, information regarding the cervical region is important in studies of human anatomy and in its clinical application to neck pain and trauma, indicating its significance in the field of human osteology. Progressing to the thoracic region, the 12 thoracic vertebrae (T1–T12) are also important as they house and protect the thoracic organs such as the heart and lungs. Unlike the cervical vertebrae, the thoracic vertebrae are greater in size and have articular facets that connect them to the ribs to form the rib cage. The structure is central to respiratory mechanics in that it allows the rib cage to contract and expand during respiration. The thoracic spine also contributes to postural stability by balancing mobility and support. Their attachment to ribs forms a movable yet stable column that underscores the region's biomechanical importance for both movement and protection. Moreover, thoracic vertebral pathologies, such as scoliosis, can have widespread effects on not only spinal health but also respiratory function, linking anatomical studies with potential clinical impact. The lumbar spine, consisting of five vertebrae (L1–L5), is significant due to its load-bearing function and support for the upper half of the body. This segment of the spine consists of larger, stronger vertebrae designed to withstand the stresses of day-to-day activities such as bending and lifting. The anatomy of the lumbar vertebrae is unique, with features such as larger vertebral bodies and extensive flexion and extension, providing greater mobility in the lower back than in the remaining spine. This mobility comes at a price, since the lumbar region is highly susceptible to injuries, such as herniated discs and strain. An understanding of the anatomical and functional complexities of the lumbar region is crucial to medical professionals when treating back pain and related disorders. By studying the regions of the vertebral column, we can understand both the normal function of the spine and the effects of pathological conditions, ultimately enhancing our knowledge of human osteology (Figure 6.4).

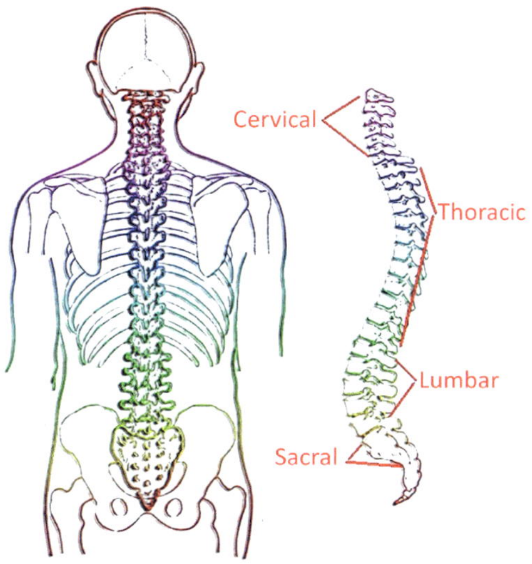

Figure 6.4. Regions of the vertebral column.

Source: https://external-content.duckduckgo.com/iu/?u=https%3A%2F%2Fthisdancinglife.com%2Fwp-content%2Fuploads%2F2019%2F07%2FVertebral_column_regions.jpg&f=1&nofb=1&ipt=7dc1eaa09c9b6f45ac5d2b4e7294bb3bc53aff7c1aa4c08067a562a1269e4750.

6.1.3. Intervertebral Discs and Their Function

The intervertebral discs are the key anatomical structures of the spinal column, which are situated between the vertebrae with mechanical and physiological roles important to human movement and stability. They both have an outer fibrous covering, the annulus fibrosus, and an inner gel-like material, the nucleus pulposus. This unique structure allows the discs to withstand compressive loads effectively while simultaneously providing flexibility to the spine, permitting a full range of motion in acts such as twisting and bending. The annulus fibrosus's superior tensile strength, coupled with the elastohydraulic constitution of the nucleus pulposus, allows the discs to bear heavy mechanical loads, absorbing shock among the vertebrae during the performance of daily activities and movements. Further, intervertebral discs help maintain healthy spinal alignment by ensuring that the spacing and positioning of the vertebrae are appropriate. Proper weight distribution along the spinal column occurs with healthy discs, which also relieve excessive stress on the muscles and ligaments surrounding the spinal column. This dynamic balance permits a successful mechanical function of the vertebral column, reducing the risk of injury and pain, which may happen in conditions such as a herniated disc or degenerative disc disease. An understanding of the function of intervertebral discs in general spinal mechanics is critical to the development of rehabilitation methods and prevention programs aimed at maximizing the duration of spinal health within diverse populations, especially as they mature and undergo lifestyle alterations that threaten spinal integrity. Research on interspecies variability of intervertebral disc composition is critical to understanding its evolutionary significance. Studies of the intervertebral cartilage have shown great diversity in mammals and other animals, such as birds, which employ synovial joints in the neck but not intervertebral discs. This suggests that intervertebral discs have evolved in some lineages. The structural differences between the discs lead to distinct biomechanics of range of motion and posture in mammals, as evidenced by differences in cartilage thickness ratios across species, with mammals generally having thicker cartilage than birds, potentially indicating locomotion and lifestyle adaptations (Christian et al., 2013). As we proceed to discover these anatomical adaptations, we appreciate that understanding intervertebral discs and their functions provides critical information not only about human osteology but also about the extensive evolutionary history of vertebrates (Synstelien et al., 2001).

Test Your Knowledge

1. What are the major regions and types of vertebrae in the human vertebral column, and how are they structurally distinct?
2. How do intervertebral discs, ligaments, and spinal curves contribute to the overall stability and flexibility of the vertebral column?

6.2. Development of the Vertebral Column

Learning Outcome

1. Embryological origins
2. Growth and maturation processes
3. Common developmental disorders

The vertebral column, a critical part of the human skeleton's overall structure, is formed significantly during embryonic and postnatal development. The vertebral column arises initially in the somites, the segmented structures that form along the neural tube early in embryogenesis. All somites mature into individual components that provide sclerotome cells, which eventually form the vertebrae. This is a tightly regulated morphogenetic process, since several signaling pathways and regulatory genes control it. In the course of embryonic development, the sclerotomal cells proliferate, migrate, and form intervertebral discs and articulating surfaces that are required for spinal mobility and stability. Mechanical forces also play a critical role in morphological adaptation during this stage of development, as vertebral bodies adapt to increased load and motion stresses. With maturity occurring within the vertebral column, regional specialization is observed in its most solid manifestation, consistent with the demands placed upon it. In humans, the vertebral column is divided into cervical, thoracic, lumbar, sacral, and coccygeal regions, each containing structures suited to their respective functions in movement and load transmission. The cervical region, for instance, bears the load of the skull but has a significant amount of motion, facilitated by the presence of intervertebral foramina and the unique cervical vertebra shape. In contrast, the thoracic spine originates anchorage for the ribs. It is comparatively fixed to accommodate the thoracic organs, whereas the lumbar spine can bear a significant amount of weight and stabilize the body during bipedal gait. Such regional adaptation indicates how developmental forces have shaped the vertebral column not only to bear bipedalism but also to optimize respiratory and circulatory functions within the thoracic cavity. The subsequent stages of vertebral column development also involve the incorporation of soft tissue, such as ligaments and intervertebral discs, which play crucial roles in spine health and function. The development of these structures is regulated by mechanical stress and the biochemical environment, demonstrating the synergistic interplay between genetics and environmental factors during maturation. Studies on the vertebral morphology of other vertebrate classes, i.e., dinosaurs, provide insight into the variety of vertebral modifications. The existence, for example, of supraspinous ossified rods in some sauropods suggests a similar process of metaplastic ossification due to mechanical demands, as seen in humans, with evidence of evolutionary convergence in the development of the vertebrae between species (Abdalla et al., 2015). Furthermore, the pneumatic patterns found in sauropod vertebrae indicate secondary and advanced adaptations not commonly met in human osteology (Taylor et al., 2013). This comparative approach enhances our understanding of vertebral column development and the evolutionary context's role in creating skeletal forms within various taxa (Figure 6.5).

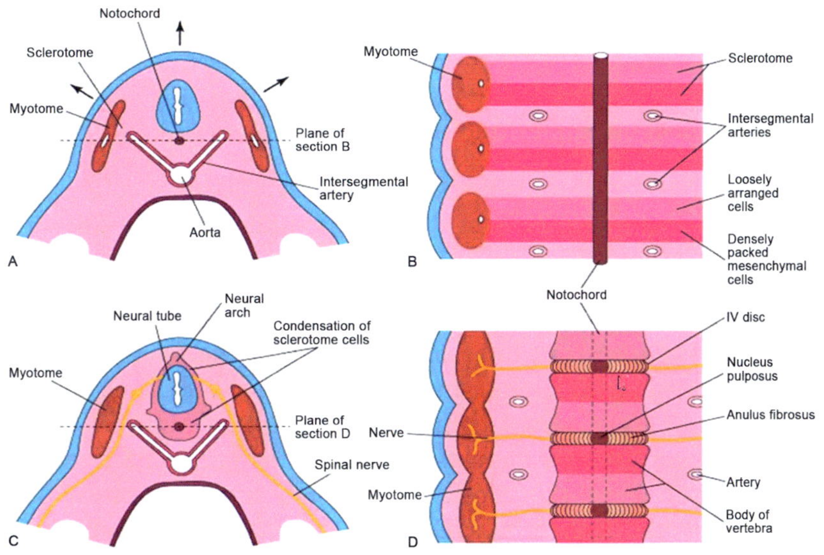

Figure 6.5. Development of the vertebral column.

Source: https://external-content.duckduckgo.com/iu/?u=https%3A%2F%2Fi.ytimg.com%2Fvi%2FR9Q2ThMbHU8%2Fmaxresdefault.jpg&f=1&nofb=1&ipt=7b60e389eee164ed064b240156d09240ee904e23d1d99404fe54c952555cd754.

6.2.1. Embryological Origins

The embryological development of the vertebral column is fundamental to understanding its structural and functional evolution in human beings. During early embryogenesis, the notochord serves as the original axis upon which the vertebral column forms, dictating the formation of vertebrae by a process termed endochondral ossification. Somites, in turn, derive from paraxial mesoderm and give rise to sclerotomes that ultimately form cartilaginous precursors of the vertebrae. The precise regulation of gene expression during this differentiation is critical since abnormalities can result in congenital spinal malformations. Moreover, the differentiating vertebral column must undergo a series of morphogenetic alterations, including segmentation and fusion of vertebral units, to establish the correct anatomical organization. Understanding these embryonic mechanisms provides excellent insight into how vertebral malformations arise and serves as a paradigm for studying spinal structure evolution in health and disease.

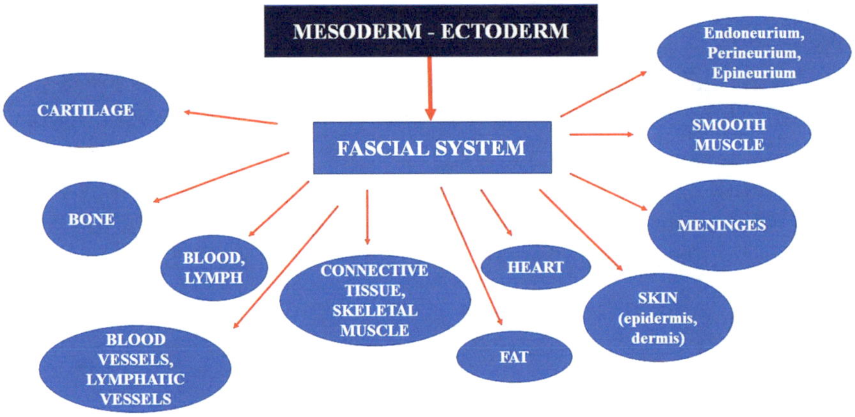

Figure 6.6. The embryological origins of the vertebral column.

Source: https://www.researchgate.net/profile/Matthew-Varacallo/publication/335969177/figure/fig3/AS:805733608202240@1569113270420/The-figure-illustrates-the-different-embryological-origins-of-the-system-or-fascial.png.

Profound genetic impacts on embryonic development also emphasize the stepwise evolution of vertebral morphology. Recent studies of homeotic genes show their role in establishing vertebral identity and segmental arrangement. Evolutionary developmental changes along the body axis are typically controlled by gradients of homeotic genes and account for the morphological diversity observed in mammalian lineages. An analysis of homeotic gradients across 250 mammalian species found that changes in vertebral identity can lead to new body plans and thus convergent features among different species. Therefore, while human beings have a specific vertebral structure, the underlying genetic processes are shared with most other mammals, which show a complex interaction of evolutionary pressures over millions of years. This information, obtained from such studies, enhances our knowledge of vertebral evolution and is extremely vital for deciphering common anatomical details among species (Keith et al., 2007). Moreover, embryological origins are also explored in understanding the epigenetic features of the vertebral column because these are key indicators of ancient genetic links between populations. Vertebral epigenetic features have been found relevant in clarifying genetic patterns and social organization in ancient populations through studies of skeletal remains in archaeological sites. For example, vertebral features from the Kellis 2 cemetery in Egypt have provided evidence of patrilocal and patrilineal organization within the group, suggesting that vertebral features can reflect broader social patterns. The existence of an intrinsic link between embryological features and sociocultural evolution also underscores the importance of the vertebral column in human osteology. Thus, the inclusion of such embryological perspectives not only adds to our knowledge of vertebral development but also underscores the significance of vertebral growth in historical population genetics and evolutionary biology (Sarfo et al., 2014) (Figure 6.6).

6.2.2. Growth and Maturation Processes

The vertebral column maturation and growth process is part of human osteology that encompasses the delicate interactions between genetic, hormonal, and environmental forces that mold the developmental pattern of bone. There are substantial changes in the shape and size of vertebrae during early life, as they evolve from cartilaginous to ossified vertebrae. This is crucial for maintaining structural integrity and mobility. As growth continues, vertebral growth is not uniform, and there are phases, particularly adolescence, during which growth is rapid owing to hormonal activity. Clinicians and researchers must understand the processes of maturation because it accounts for normal bone development and identifies deviations which can predispose to scoliosis or kyphosis with long-term effects on health and function. In vertebrate maturation, cervical vertebral maturation (CVM) is a reliable method for estimating skeletal age and can be used to predict growth spurts and the timing of peak growth velocity. The CVM method categorizes the stages of vertebral development and has been extensively studied for reproducibility and clinical use. Research indicates that the accuracy of skeletal age assessment is significantly enhanced by operator calibration and accuracy methods, as evidenced by a study of 104 female subjects aged 8–14. Improved definitions and new phases in the CVM system make it more reliable, making it a valuable tool for orthodontic assessment and treatment planning. Such measurements align with the general aims of osteology, facilitating understanding of developmental milestones and their health consequences. Further exploration of the interplay between vertebral development and overall patterns of growth provides substantial implications for tailored treatment strategies within clinical practice. Inquiries into growth patterns and variations call for the necessity of tailoring interventions based on the individual patient's unique development curve. For example, determining the phases of CVM can guide orthodontists in selecting the optimal timing of intervention, thereby ensuring the best possible outcome. Additionally, understanding the complexity of vertebral column maturation enables practitioners to better anticipate potential complications arising from atypical developmental patterns. An intimate understanding of these growth and maturation processes advances the science of human osteology and enables more nuanced methods for addressing musculoskeletal wellness throughout life, as encouraged by recent advances in clinical methods focused on patient-centered medicine (Jamal et al., 2008).

6.2.3. Common Developmental Disorders

The vertebral column plays a central role in the investigation of common developmental disorders that impact the skeleton's integrity in human osteology practice. The most prevalent condition is scoliosis, which is an abnormal lateral curvature of the spine. Scoliosis may result from genetic, environmental, or muscular factors, ultimately leading to complications that may affect not only posture but also organ function. Individuals with scoliosis have structurally abnormal vertebrae, which makes treatment and management even more challenging. The consequences extend beyond mere appearance, e.g., severe cases that necessitate surgery to prevent respiratory complications and chronic pain. Awareness of these developmental disorders enhances our understanding of the vertebral column's functional adaptations and the nuances of skeletal well-being throughout life. Spina bifida is another developmental disorder related to the vertebral column, a congenital anomaly resulting from a failure of the neural tube to properly close during embryonic development. This condition may lead to any level of neurological impairment and physical disability, depending on the extent and location of the defect. The most common anatomical defects in the vertebrae occur in spina bifida and affect not only the spinal cord but also the musculature and the adjacent soft tissues. The resultant sensory and motor deficits are typically best managed with an interdisciplinary regimen that includes physical therapy, surgical intervention, and long-term follow-up. From an osteological perspective, research on spina bifida offers a glimpse into the mechanisms regulating vertebral formation during development and is also important to individual outcomes and quality of life. Other conditions, including congenital vertebral malformations, further demonstrate the complexity of human vertebral development and the myriad of disorders. Such malformations may appear as hemivertebrae or block vertebrae, which can have a tremendous impact on spinal alignment and movement. Appreciating these phenomena, it is critical to understand the mechanisms of vertebral formation, as disruptions during crucial developmental stages can cause a range of deformities. This knowledge is essential in deploying proper diagnostic and therapeutic management in clinical practice. As demonstrated in fetal paleopathology research, our comprehension of these developmental pathologies further illuminates the life experiences of those with such afflictions, both in the past and present, by way of informed ideologies of vertebral column disease and health (Abramoff et al., 2012; Lewis et al., 2017) (Figure 6.7).

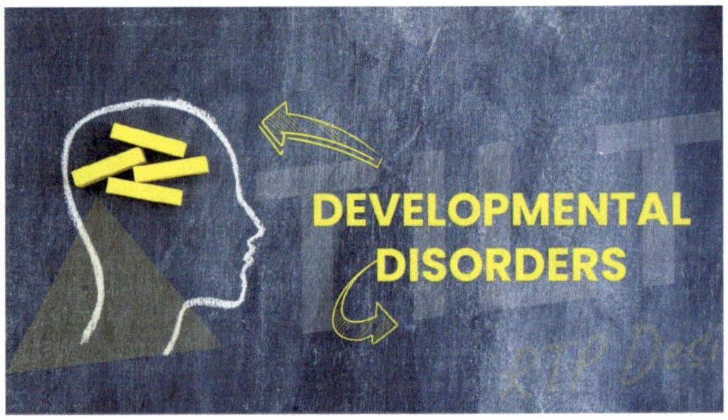

Figure 6.7. The vertebral column plays a crucial role in understanding common developmental disorders that can affect skeletal integrity.

Source: https://external-content.duckduckgo.com/iu/?u=https%3A%2F%2Fsp-ao.shortpixel.ai%2Fclient%2Fto_auto%2Cq_lossless%2Cret_img%2Cw_1263%2Ch_700%2Fhttps%3A%2F%2Ftriangletiltrtp.com%2Fwp-content%2Fuploads%2F2023%2F03%2FWhat-are-Developmental-Disorders-1.jpg&f=1&nofb=1&ipt=504d2afdef5235fa90509ccbcd005f259d4a42d77fda95444fae9fc59173682a.

Test Your Knowledge

1. How does the vertebral column develop during embryonic and postnatal stages, including the formation of primary and secondary curvatures?
2. What genetic and environmental factors influence the normal growth and alignment of the vertebral column?

6.3. Function of the Vertebral Column

Learning Outcome

1. Body support and stability
2. Protection of the spinal cord
3. Role in movement and flexibility

The vertebral column, or spine, performs a variety of essential functions that support the structural integrity and overall functioning of the body. One of its roles is to support the upper body weight, providing a rigid axis for the ribs and pelvic girdle to articulate. This support allows an upright posture, so that humans can perform several activities of daily life with stability. The vertebral column protects the spinal cord, a significant component of the central nervous system, by encasing it in the bony vertebrae. This protective function is required to safeguard nerve routes through which communication between the brain and the remainder of the body can coordinate movement and reflexes. The second prominent function undertaken by the vertebral column is facilitating mobility and flexibility. There are 33 vertebrae in the spine, divided into various regions: cervical, thoracic, lumbar, sacral, and coccygeal. Each region allows different movements; e.g., the cervical region allows rotation and lateral flexion of the neck, while the lumbar region allows bending and lifting. Intervertebral discs, which are between vertebras, are shock absorbers when in movement and are cushions to reduce impact forces. The intricate composition of the vertebral column, its curves, and mobile joints provides stability and mobility during any physical exercise, adding to the overall functional capacity of an individual. Moreover, the vertebral column is also involved in hematopoiesis and calcium storage and influences broader physiological functions. Vertebral bodies house bone marrow where the red and white blood cells are produced that contribute to the body's immune surveillance system and oxygen supply system. Additionally, vertebral bones serve as reservoirs of phosphorus and calcium, which are essential for biochemical reactions and bone strength. This multifunctional feature emphasizes the importance of the vertebral column within the human body because not only does it provide structural integrity and motion, but it also actively participates in essential metabolic processes. This understanding strengthens learning in human osteology because it stresses the vertebral column's direct role in sustaining life and physical activity in a number of different forms.

6.3.1. Support and Stability of the Body

The vertebral column has a critical role to play in the stability and support of the human body, the major skeletal framework that protects the spinal cord but allows some movement. With 33 vertebrae, this intricate system of bones consists of identifiable sections: cervical, thoracic, lumbar, sacral, and coccygeal. All vertebrae are specifically designed to perform their particular functions, supported by intervertebral discs for cushioning and flexibility. Vertebrae shapes and orientations also play an important role in maintaining the posture and alignment of the body as they allow upright locomotion and balance the pelvis, head, and spine. Also, the vertebral column provides attachment for various muscles and ligaments to aid movement without compromising stability, illustrating the critical balance of support and movement inherent in human osteology. Understanding the structure of the vertebral column reveals the evolutionary adaptations that support stability and load-bearing. For instance, the sacrum, formed by the fusion of five vertebrae, is a powerful base for the spine, transferring weight from the upper body to the pelvis and lower limbs. Such support is particularly vital for walking on two legs, allowing human beings to walk efficiently on two legs. Furthermore, the lumbar region is designed to resist mechanical strains with larger and stronger vertebrae compared to the cervical and thoracic regions. Such anatomical specialization emphasizes the vertebral column's functional importance in providing not only structural support but also flexibility for normal movement. Vertebral variations also accentuate these adaptations, allowing diverse physical abilities while maintaining overall body stability, providing evidence of the delicate balance required in human biomechanics. Apart from structural stability, the vertebral column is also a key component of the protection of the central nervous system, particularly the spinal cord traversing the vertebral foramen. This stabilization role is most critical, as damage to the spinal cord can lead to severe neurological compromise or paralysis. The vertebrae must also work together to maintain proper posture and prevent injury. Scoliosis or bulging discs can compromise this alignment, leading to instability and pain. Based on comparative vertebrate anatomy observations, unique human vertebral column features, like its curvatures, provide an evolutionary advantage compared to other animals in terms of both support and mobility. The relationship between mechanical stability, anatomical structure, and protective functions demonstrates the complexity of human osteology and vertebral columns' critical role in maintaining body support and stability under different circumstances, supporting its critical significance in human movement and health (Mallison et al., 2015; Taylor et al., 2012).

6.3.2. Protection of the Spinal Cord

Spinal cord protection is critical for maintaining neurological integrity and body function. The vertebral column, consisting of independent vertebrae, is a rigid bony column containing the spinal cord and providing static as well as dynamic support. Each of these vertebrae is designed with some curvature so that the columns are shock-absorbing with movement but resist mechanical stress to a very great extent. Further, intervertebral discs between the vertebrae act as shock absorbers, supporting axial load transmission and minimizing the risk of spine damage. Such an anatomical configuration not only guards the spinal cord against external damage but also facilitates ease and mobility, allowing individuals to perform various motions without compromising nerve protection, forming a critical balance of rigidity and beauty inherent in human movement. In addition, the significance of protecting the spinal cord is emphasized by the need for other stabilizing components such as muscles and ligaments. The anterior and posterior longitudinal ligaments run parallel to the vertebral bodies and help maintain spinal stability. The ligaments, together with the musculature surrounding them, protect the spinal cord from abnormal motion that could lead to severe damage or neurological impairment. Moreover, the complex anatomy of the cervical spine highlights the protective features that preserve cord function while permitting a tremendous range of motion. Because cervical structures innervated by spinal nerves (C1 - C3) are a source of neurological disorders, it is important to understand their biomechanics to evaluate spinal health. Efficient treatment interventions, such as mobilization procedures, may alleviate tension-induced pain due to malfunction of these structures and thus emphasize the importance of both protective and therapeutic care in spinal health (Pharris et al., 2000). The relationship between the protective systems of the vertebral column and associated conditions further emphasizes the importance of comprehensive spinal health. Understanding the complexities of the spinal anatomy and the role of protective mechanisms will help toward better diagnostic and therapeutic intervention of this region's conditions. Cervicogenic headaches, for instance, resulting from dysfunction of cervical vertebrae, can indicate how misalignment and other issues can impact not only the vertebral column but also the integrity of the spinal cord and overall neurobiology. Hence, the role of the vertebral column is more than mere structural support; it is a crucial framework that combines physical protection with potential neurological function. The more research that is conducted to determine the complex interactions in the spine, the clearer it becomes that protecting the spinal cord is imperative for maintaining structural integrity alongside neural functioning in the human body (Bailey et al., 1984) (Figure 6.8).

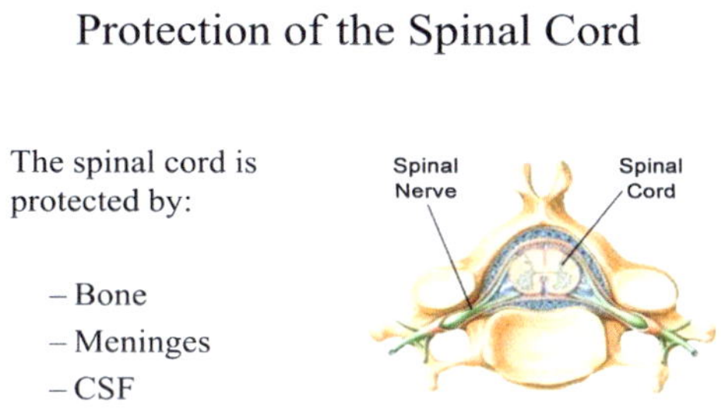

Figure 6.8. The protection of the spinal cord.

Source: https://external-content.duckduckgo.com/iu/?u=https%3A%2F%2Fimage5.slideserve.com%2F9393935%2Fprotection-of-the-spinal-cord-l.jpg&f=1&nofb=1&ipt=2360d5614b5af1dd4ceba5d2c8b32cf6b865b59da8a1b6a373b182c56b1197eb.

6.3.3. Role in Movement and Flexibility

The vertebral column is a key organ of movement and flexibility of the human skeletal system and serves as the base of most of the body's movements. Composed of a series of individual vertebrae coupled by intervertebral discs, this anatomical structure provides a substantial range of motion while maintaining structural stability. The intervertebral discs, which consist of a jelly-like nucleus pulposus contained within an annulus fibrosus, have a key role in enabling flexibility. The shock-absorbing cushions allow the spine to twist and bend, thereby facilitating a wide range of activities, including bending, twisting, and lateral flexion. Without the dynamic function provided by the vertebral column's flexible shape, the human body would be severely limited in mobility, hindering athletic performance and routine activities. Second, the specialized anatomical configuration of the vertebrae, including differences in form and size, contributes to the diverse range of motion present in the human spine. Each portion of the vertebral column—cervical, thoracic, and lumbar—contains adaptations that maximize motion in various ways. For example, the neck region is composed of more freely movable, smaller vertebrae, allowing extensive rotation and flexion to facilitate head movement. In contrast, the lumbar region is designed for support and stability with limited but strong capacity for flexion and extension. The zygapophyses also form intervertebral joints that facilitate gliding motion, contributing to the spine's flexibility. An understanding of how these body structures function to allow the spines to move underscores the importance of the vertebral column's position in the overall functionality of the human body. Comparing the vertebral column with that of other animals, such as sauropod dinosaurs, underscores the evolutionary importance of vertebral structure in providing space for movement and flexibility. Sauropods, owing to their long necks and certain anatomical structures, are a perfect example of how vertebral structures can be utilized to improve motion (Taylor et al., 2012). Sauropods provide the best example of vertebral flexibility, with features such as pneumatic chambers and long cervical vertebrae allowing them to have a wider range of motion than most of their modern counterparts. This evolutionary viewpoint explains the human vertebral column's flexibility, which has evolved to reconcile flexibility and stability in a range of locomotor functions. Through the comparison of human and non-human vertebrates, it can be seen that the vertebral columns function in enabling movement and flexibility, which is a complex but essential part of osteological function across different organisms (Christian et al., 2013) (Figure 6.9).

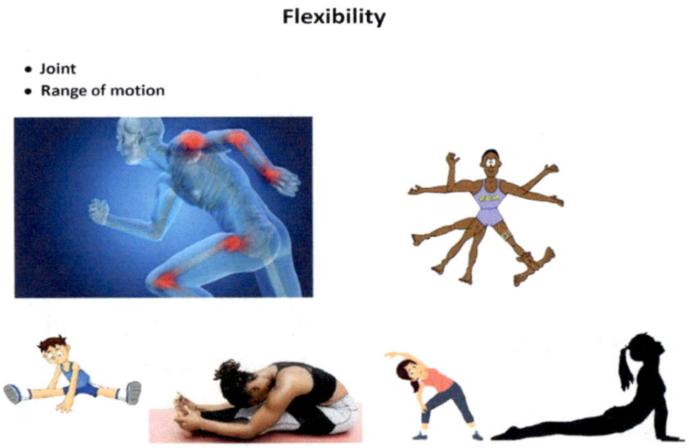

Figure 6.9. Role in movement and flexibility.

Source: https://external-content.duckduckgo.com/iu/?u=https%3A%2F%2Fimgv2-1-f.scribdassets.com%2Fimg%2Fdocument%2F598322750%2Foriginal%2F8c27c76b79%2F1674049094%3 Fv%3 D1&f=1&nofb=1&ipt=f2b057296cbb171e66c6a03bcdf82ce832b92508fa1e0ed79d3932862a081fc8.

Test Your Knowledge

1. How does the vertebral column support the body's weight, protect the spinal cord, and allow movement?
2. What role do the vertebral curves and intervertebral discs play in shock absorption and balance?

6.4. Pathologies of the Vertebral Column

Learning Outcome

1. Prevalent spinal disorders (e.g., scoliosis, herniated discs)
2. Effects of changes with age
3. Trauma and its effects

The vertebral column is an important structural element of the human skeleton, and its pathologies have a notable effect on general health and mobility. Several conditions may affect the vertebral column, including scoliosis, kyphosis, and disc herniation, which all present different diagnostic and treatment complexities. Scoliosis, characterized by an abnormal lateral curvature of the spine, can lead to trunk asymmetry and pain or discomfort over time. Kyphosis, typically characterized by overcurvature of the thorax, may result from degenerative disease or developmental disorders. It is worthwhile to understand morphoscopic variation within the vertebral column because it enables medical practitioners to identify and document these conditions more effectively, ultimately leading to the establishment of treatment tailored to a person's particular skeletal composition. Understanding pathologies of the vertebral column also largely aids forensic anthropology, particularly skeletal identification. When handling differences like the presence of extra thoracic or lumbar vertebrae, forensic anthropologists have to be very good at recognizing such pathologies in a way that can differentiate human bones from animal bones. The complexity of vertebral pathologies makes them difficult to recognize, particularly when variations such as an odd number of lumbar vertebrae are present. It requires good understanding of normal anatomical variations in order not to misidentify. Research in this field, for example, George et al. in the Williams Collection, is concerned with the dominance of morphoscopic characters and how such variations can be applied in the forensic identification process, ultimately enhancing the efficacy of recovery and identification methods (Sanford et al., 2024). Outside the forensic community, the implications of vertebral pathology identification are also immense, as these conditions carry significant medical significance. Accurate recording of common vertebral column-related diseases can help inform prevention and treatment strategies in the clinical setting. As patients present with vertebral disease, clinicians are encouraged to consider the prevalence of specific diseases in specific populations. For instance, thoracic and lumbar vertebral numbers may be associated with ethnic or demographic factors as indicated by skeletal collections. Such demographic data can influence how diagnosis and treatment are managed in the clinical setting, to the advantage of both health providers and patients. In addition, the integration of research findings into training practices can render medical and forensic experts well-equipped to handle the intricacies and variations encountered in vertebral column pathologies (Fourshee et al., 2022) (Figure 6.10).

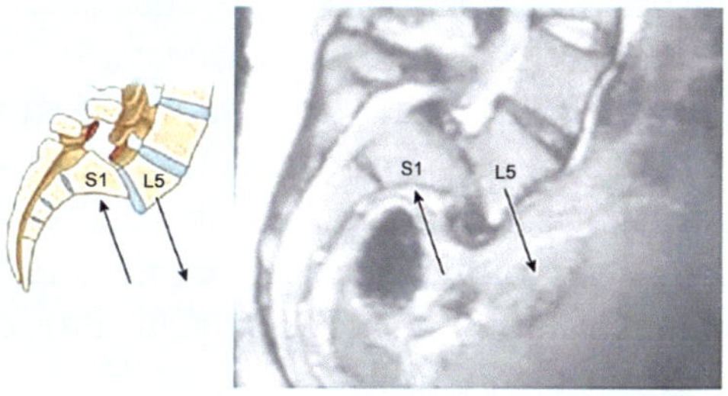

Figure 6.10. Pathologies of the vertebral column.

Source: https://external-content.duckduckgo.com/iu/?u=https%3A%2F%2Fo.quizlet.com%2FJrO4ZV68lWKvBVH5YDUQ0Q.png&f=1&nofb=1&ipt=d55d05f7fe664f8324af58c5c11a7b373ec4133ec4b90cd797edb9b4dd24779c.

6.4.1. Common Spinal Disorders (e.g., Scoliosis and Herniated Discs)

Knowledge of normal spinal disorders is essential to understanding the complexity of the vertebral column. Among these disorders, herniated discs and scoliosis are common and can significantly impact a person's quality of life. Scoliosis, or a structural lateral curvature of the spine, usually develops in adolescence and can be caused by genetic or idiopathic factors. This curvature can lead to imbalance and discomfort, warranting observation and, in severe cases, surgery. As the spine is a central body structure, learning about the effects of its abnormality, such as those of scoliosis, places the vertebral column at center stage in human osteology and overall body function. Disc hernias are another common spinal condition resulting from damaged intervertebral discs, which are shock-absorbing pads between the vertebrae. The condition occurs when the softer inner material of the disc bulges out through a tear in the tougher outer layer, typically compressing the nerves. Shooting pain down the limbs, numbness, and muscle weakness are typically the symptoms. Incidence of herniated discs serves to underscore the fundamental pairing of spinal health and mobility. Above all, surgical intervention is sometimes necessary, particularly for nonresponsive individuals receiving traditional treatment regimens. Present research indicates early surgical intervention can markedly improve outcomes, particularly in individuals with chronic sciatica, as demonstrated through recent clinical research (Puneeth et al., 2016).

Consequently, the prevalence and impact of herniated discs are of utmost importance in vertebral column studies. The role of newer diagnostic modalities, particularly magnetic resonance imaging (MRI), has revolutionized spinal disorder diagnosis and treatment, such as scoliosis and herniated discs. MRI provides high-resolution imaging of spinal anatomy, detecting disc degeneration, bulging, and other nonspecific abnormalities that may not be visible on standard imaging. For instance, diffusion-weighted MRI has been effective in quantifying the changes of intervertebral discs following trauma and determining the relationship between structural features and patient symptoms (Kerttula et al., 2001). Through the clinical application of MRI, medical professionals gain valuable information about the anatomical and functional status of the spine, thereby enabling individualized treatment regimens. The inclusion of these advanced imaging modalities in osteological research significantly expands our understanding of spinal disorders, leading to improved patient outcomes and innovative surgical techniques.

6.4.2. Impact of Age-Related Changes

The vertebral column, a significant aspect of human osteology, undergoes significant age-related changes that affect its function and structural integrity. With aging, the structure and morphology of the vertebrae change, and bone density and intervertebral disc condition deteriorate, leading to progressive osteoporotic bone loss and increased susceptibility to stress fractures and possible spinal deformity. Disruption of disc elasticity and hydration results in decreased shock absorption and mobility, which may contribute to the development of conditions such as degenerative disc disease. Determining the mechanism of such alterations is critical; it yields information regarding preventive strategies or interventions that may reduce the pace of age-related degeneration. Additionally, the functional implications of age-related changes extend far beyond physiological effects to encompass the general quality of life. Total loss of spinal stability may lead to chronic pain, reduced mobility, and increased susceptibility to injury. Segmental instability caused by compromised vertebrae and injured discs is generally a serious threat. Elderly individuals are often found with decreased range of motion, which contributes to more sedentary behavior and, as a result, worsens musculoskeletal disorders.

By understanding these effects, healthcare professionals are better able to address the needs of older adult populations, providing therapeutic interventions to address improvements in spinal well-being and functional capabilities. Examination of intervertebral cartilage is also crucial in understanding the impact of aging changes on the vertebral column. As noted in studies of modern vertebrates, diversity in intervertebral cartilage morphology influences joint function and overall biomechanics. Research has shown that cartilage-to-bone ratios are significant parameters for evaluating spinal joints, and age-related changes are likely to influence cartilage thickness and composition. This becomes essential when considering the adaptability and response of human vertebrae to mechanisms of aging. For instance, it is of essence that healthy cartilage is maintained because its loss has a profound impact on the lifespan of the joints and on movement. Broadly, studies of vertebral change throughout life illuminate not only the osteology of human beings but also the importance of guiding interventions to preserve spinal health over a lifetime because it reflects broader implications regarding mobility and independence in later life (Figure 6.11).

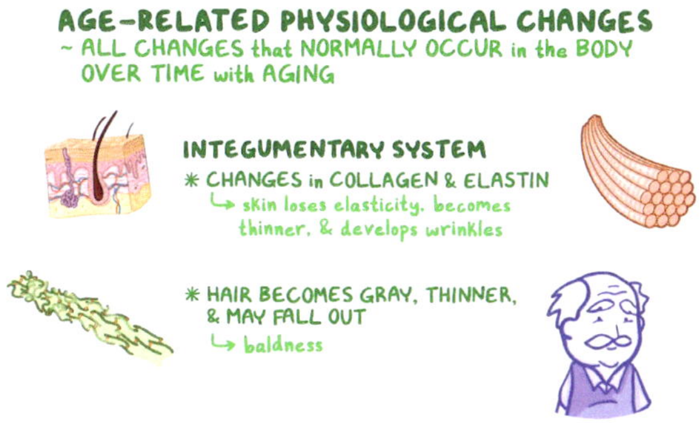

Figure 6.11. Impact of age-related changes.

Source: https://www.osmosis.org/_next/image?url=https%3A%2F%2Fd16qt3wv6xm098.cloudfront.net%2F5_CioGyNRrOhN10wLNoZTG1fR5KkgPlz%2F_.jpg&w=3840&q=75.

6.4.3. Injuries and Their Implications

When considering the importance of injuries in the vertebral column, consideration should be given as to how these physical injuries might affect overall skeletal function and health. The vertebral column is more than a structural component of the skeleton; it also plays a critical role in housing the spinal cord and supporting the body's posture. Trauma to this area can lead to a range of complications, including chronic pain, neurological deficit, and alteration of mobility. These conditions not only diminish the patient's quality of life but also have broader implications for social organisation, particularly among populations that are physically based. Appreciation of the nature and frequency of injuries like these is essential to making sense of their importance for the past, as they tend to reflect the stresses and strains placed on people in their worlds.

The archaeological record at sites such as Akhetaten informs us about the types of injuries people suffered in ancient societies and what those injuries reveal about previous lifestyles. The traumatic injuries present among the individuals excavated, particularly those linked to the building activities in the region, give insight into the physical demands imposed on workers. Among the interesting discoveries is the trace of chronic ulnae stress fractures and other spinal issues like Schmorl's nodes and spondylolysis, which shows a trend of repetitive physical exertion significantly linked with hard work (Hodgin et al., 2012). In addition, the correlation between trauma to the skeleton and activity attests to the close integration of work and health in these groups and offers an engaging analysis of people's ordinary experience in ancient Egypt. Also, integrating fetal paleopathology into the analysis accentuates the multiscalar importance of skeletal health over generations. The research emphasizes the types of information to be obtained from the examination of fetal remains, such as the relationship between maternal health and fetal development under conditions of bodily injury (Lewis et al., 2017). This branch of osteology shows how conditions and injuries experienced by the mother can affect fetal outcomes, extending the discourse to also cover the broader implications of injury within family and societal groups. The exploration of these intergenerational relations not only advances our understanding of osteological evidence but also fosters a multidisciplinary approach to the examination of historical patterns of health, ultimately for its potential contribution to a fuller portrait of human life over the centuries.

Test Your Knowledge

1. What are the common vertebral column disorders, such as scoliosis, kyphosis, and herniated discs, and how do they affect function?
2. How can degenerative changes like osteoarthritis impact the mobility and structural integrity of the vertebral column?

6.5. Diagnostic Techniques

Learning Outcome

1. Imaging methods (X-rays, MRI, CT scans)
2. Techniques for physical examination
3. Early diagnosis and its significance

Diagnostic techniques in the study of human osteology are particularly significant, especially in the vertebral column. The ability to accurately distinguish human remains from nonhuman remains is paramount for forensic anthropologists. Forensic contexts generally require a close inspection of skeletal features, especially when dealing with fragmented or decomposed remains. Morphological examination, comparative osteology, and advanced imaging techniques are vital to determining skeletal origins. The data acquired from these approaches enhance understanding not only of the vertebral column but also of the broader scope of human skeletal variation, thereby supporting more accurate identification in both forensic and clinical settings. Further, the increasing complexity of skeletal analysis necessitates further research into the most common species involved in forensic cases. For instance, studies indicate that the mammalian remains most frequently encountered in forensic investigations can complicate identification, as their shape and size closely approximate those of human bones. Hence, forensic anthropologist training programs should place even more emphasis on differentiating human from nonhuman skeletal elements. The analysis of bones of nonhuman animals, such as white-tailed deer or domestic cattle, can play a determinant role in field and case analysis improvements. Extensive training in diagnostic practices ensures that forensic analysts can minimize misidentifications, thereby enhancing the quality of forensic inquiry (Fourshee et al., 2022). Apart from morphological techniques, resource compilation remains very important for better diagnostic practice in osteology. Investigational studies aiming at creating comparisons of the fauna of an area provide a valuable source of materials for forensic anthropologists. A comprehensive manual covering the cranial and postcranial segments of the skeletons of local species, for example, enables anthropologists to quickly identify and distinguish skeletal remains in a medicolegal case.

Not only does this ease identification, but it also advances forensic anthropology by providing graphical documentation of the most diagnostic features within species. The development of these guides allows for the systematic determination of species-specific descriptions during enquiries, thereby maximizing overall accuracy and efficiency in forensic analysis and significantly adding to knowledge regarding the vertebral column in human osteology (Dewey et al., 2013) (Figure 6.12).

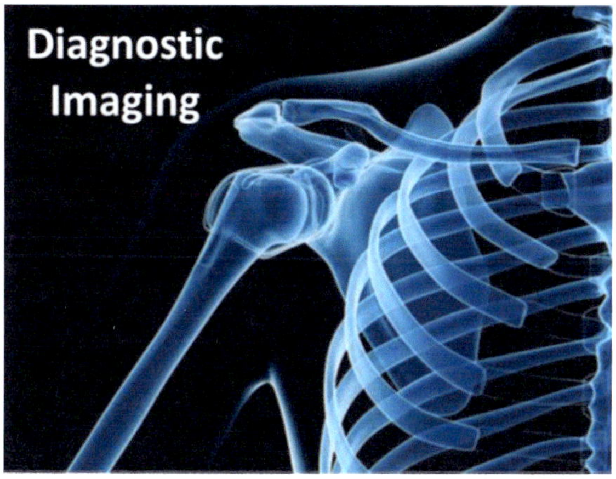

Figure 6.12. The diagnostic techniques play a crucial role.

Source: https://external-content.duckduckgo.com/iu/?u=https%3A%2F%2Fdryuc24b85zbr.cloudfront.net%2Ftes%2Fresources%2F6410646%2Fimage%3Fwidth%3D500% 26height%3D500%26version%3D1394553856000&f=1&nofb=1&ipt=14653b646e0e1b541934ebc46133d7f7135ce7e7f3c5c3e78d4c1e83911f8912.

6.5.1. Imaging Methods (X-rays, Magnetic Resonance Imaging (MRI), Computed Tomography (CT) Scans)

The application of advanced imaging methods, such as X-rays, MRI, and CT scans, has revolutionized the examination of the vertebral column in human osteology by providing precise visualization of bone architecture and surrounding tissues. X-rays provide the foundation, enabling quick, low-cost images that facilitate the diagnosis of fractures, degenerative disorders, and overall skeletal alignment. Their ability to detect bone pathology or deformity makes them a valuable tool in assessing conditions such as disc herniations or scoliosis. The limitations of X-rays, such as decreased soft-tissue contrast, also necessitate the use of supplemental imaging modalities to evaluate the vertebral column better. On the other hand, MRI offers greater contrast between soft tissues and is very valuable for detection of spinal cord injury, intervertebral disc disease, and associated nerve root disease. The capacity is particularly relevant in evaluating complicating factors from the vertebral column, such as tumors or inflammatory processes. The validity of osteometric data acquired from MRIs has been established by studies comparing MRI and cadaver measurements, concluding that MRI can accurately capture osteological data, including vertebral measurements. Such methods enhance the information on vertebral morphology and aid in the development of accurate biological profiles, further establishing the usefulness of MRI in osteology (Brits et al., 2016). CT scans are another radiological innovation, with high-resolution cross-sectional images that allow good visualization of the spine's anatomy. The technique is better in the evaluation of complex fractures or congenital malformations often missed by plain X-rays. As observed in studies of vertebral pathology, CT scans are highly significant for preoperative planning and for guiding surgical procedures. Besides, CT capacity for 3D reconstructions adds to our understanding of the vertebral columns' anatomical relationship and population differences. In reference to biomechanical research, an integrated approach using these imaging modalities illustrates a comprehensive view of vertebral morphology and functioning, and ultimately contributes to improved clinical practice and optimal patient outcomes (Mallison et al., 2015) (Figure 6.13).

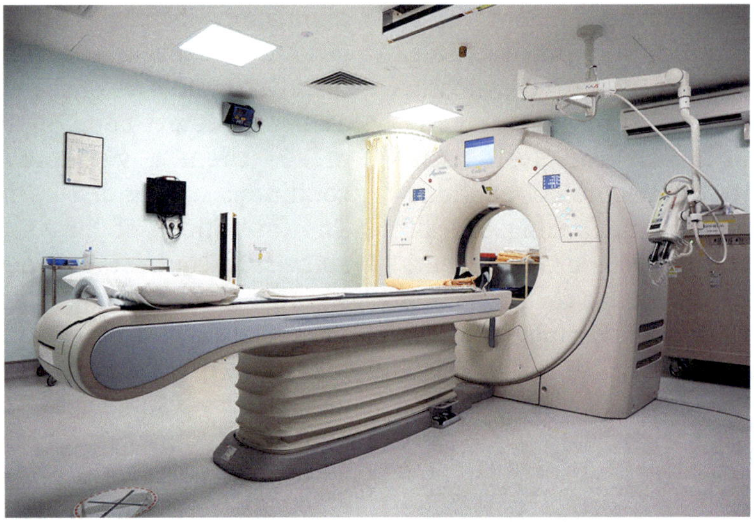

Figure 6.13. The utilization of advanced imaging methods such as X-rays.

Source: https://external-content.duckduckgo.com/iu/?u=https%3A%2F%2Fwww.srikotamedical.com%2Fwp-content%2Fuploads%2F2021%2F02%2FCt-Scan-2.jpg&f=1&nofb=1&ipt=acf10772b6d8ec3a8335153500a203542e79b87ec0abcdc28b956eda080db0c1.

6.5.2. Physical Examination Procedures

The institution of physical examination procedures is an essential necessity when assessing the vertebral column in human osteology. These tests typically begin with a proper visual checkup, where the clinician examines for any abnormality of postural, alignment, and symmetry of the spinal column. Initial palpation of the vertebrae allows assessment of tenderness, misalignments, or deformities such as scoliosis or kyphosis. Moreover, the evaluation of the range of motion by specific tests helps differentiate the functional impairments capable of affecting the spine's overall well-being. Deliberate investigation is important in such tests because the vertebral column is not only essential for structural integrity but also for the protection of the spinal cord. Therefore, judiciously applied physical examination can facilitate early detection of conditions that, if left untreated, would result in severe morbidity. After initial assessment, specialty-based physical examination methods may further refine insight into the specific pathologies affecting the spinal column. Clinical tests such as the straight leg raise or Spurling's test help to identify nerve root irritations or herniated discs, which are key locations in anatomical and forensic studies. Anthropologists and forensic specialists who analyze skeletal specimens need to be well-versed in these functions, particularly when distinguishing human from nonhuman bones. For instance, pathological alterations in vertebral structure are employed to provide bioarchaeological inferences about past populations' age, sex, and health. This translates into a broader understanding of the socio-medical context in ancient societies and can shape the approach to examination techniques for assessing cremated remains and skeletal anatomy in modern times, as illustrated by biases in cremation studies (Kurila et al., 2015). In addition, meticulous physical exam protocols are also essential in cases involving trauma or post-mortem. The role of forensic anthropologists is to differentiate between ante-mortem and post-mortem modifications of the skeleton, which often have a significant influence on case determination. The work is likely to consist of evaluating fracture mechanics of the vertebral column, ultimately resulting in conclusive findings regarding cause and mode of death. The distinction between human and nonhuman skeletal remains is also emphasized in forensic environments, where species identification can be outcome-determining in an inquiry (Fourshee et al., 2022). Analysis in such environments emphasizes the interconnectedness of anatomy, function, and pathology, enabling anthropologists to demand large-scale training in the identification of various aspects of vertebral column pathologies. Lastly, well-established physical examination methods enhance our understanding of the vertebral column, advancing both osteology and forensic science.

6.5.3. Importance of Early Diagnosis

There can be no overemphasis on the importance of early diagnosis of the vertebral column in human osteology. Early diagnosis of spinal diseases such as scoliosis, disc hernia, and vertebral fractures is paramount in preventing further complications and providing improved management results. Early diagnostic technology, including cutting-edge imaging techniques such as MRI and CT scans, enables a better understanding of conditions that may not present symptoms right away. By diagnosing these issues early on, doctors can tailor interventions that not only relieve pain but also enhance the quality of life. Further, early diagnosis helps document changes in spinal conditions over time, thereby contributing to the overall field of osteological research and to the success of rehabilitation. Beyond individual health outcomes, in human osteology studies, the effects of early diagnosis extend to population health trends. Early identification of abnormal vertebral features in skeletal material gives valuable insight into previous health trends, population growth, and nutrition. For instance, skeletal analysis will verify the prevalence of specific musculoskeletal disorders, which either environmental or genetic factors can cause.

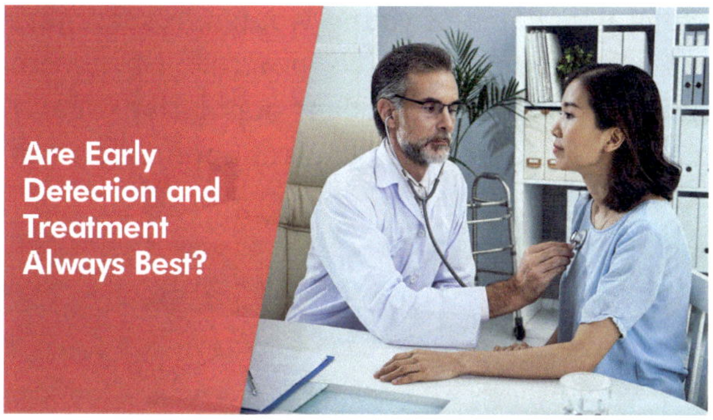

Figure 6.14. The importance of early diagnosis.

Source: https://external-content.duckduckgo.com/iu/?u=https%3A%2F%2Fgerman-heart-centre.com%2Fwp-content%2Fuploads%2F2023%2F03%2F980398a66baf8e801a3c9124bb9bcd5c.jpg&f=1&nofb=1&ipt=7a7aee77940b07637cdacd3d9757fe85c00f08e64477cc9e154248c188bbd4e6.

The analyses highlight the importance of early detection in the archaeological record, where skeletal data show the stewardship of collective health over various periods of time. These findings further build on an understanding of how early intervention techniques, suggested by osteological investigation, can significantly improve health and diminish the long-term burden of diseases associated with the vertebral column across generations. Additionally, early diagnosis exemplifies the intersection of current medical practices with paleoarchaeological research.

As stated, increased emphasis is currently placed on understanding the health of mothers and babies through fetal paleopathology, placing early critical stages of life on the agenda for influencing long-term health outcomes. Such multi-disciplinary approaches contrast with conventional thinking focused on adult skeletons, such as in the research paper that addresses medieval society, where artifacts primarily portray adults' existence (Lewis et al., 2017). By applying more recent techniques and a wider, more diverse sample, such as the skeletal remains of young women, researchers can chart an inclusive portrait of health stratification within ancient populations. Early diagnosis not only has clinical application but also dramatically increases our understanding of how health was described in the past and how societies were organized (Lewis et al., 2015) (Figure 6.14).

Test Your Knowledge

1. What imaging methods are commonly used to diagnose vertebral column pathologies, and what information does each provide?
2. How do physical examinations and neurological assessments complement imaging in evaluating spinal disorders?

6.6. Treatment Options

Learning Outcome

1. Non-surgical treatment (exercise, medication)
2. Surgical treatment (spinal fusion, laminectomy)
3. Rehabilitation and healing measures

Ablation options for vertebral column disorders and injuries are significant for continued patient outcomes and the restoration of functional mobility. Conservative treatments generally include physical therapy, pain relief by medication, and lifestyle changes to reduce stress on the spine. Those approaches aim to alleviate symptoms and improve strength without invasive techniques. Where conservative techniques fail or structural instability is identified, surgery may be required. Interventions via surgery are likely to stabilize the spine, decompress neural structures, or remediate deformity consistent with evidence-based orthopedic medicine. For example, advances in surgical techniques have enabled more minimally invasive procedures, resulting in reduced recovery time and fewer complications. Hence, it is essential for health practitioners treating conditions of the vertebral column to be aware of these treatment modalities. Surgical techniques employed in the treatment of vertebral column conditions range from decompression operations to spinal fusions. For example, anterior cervical discectomy and fusion with plating (ACDFP) is a common procedure used in treating cervical disc degeneration or herniation. Recent biomechanical studies have shown that certain fixation techniques, e.g., posterior lateral mass screw fixation, may provide greater stability than ACDFP in specific injury situations. The importance of choosing surgical methods based on individual patient anatomy and injury patterns cannot be overemphasized. Cutting-edge biomechanical research, as outlined in new studies, recognises the complex interplay between injury type and treatment effectiveness, thereby informing the development of more standardised surgical procedure protocols to achieve optimal outcomes for patients with cervical spine injuries (McLachlin et al., 2013). Reactive arthropathy treatment as part of vertebral column disease is another aspect of treatment. Reactive arthropathy may be caused by infections, with resulting inflammation and complications in spinal tissues. Military personnel have been historically exposed to infections that might lead to such a condition, and knowledge of the processes at play is essential to allow therapeutic strategies to be designed. Management is frequently successful through a multidisciplinary approach, with pharmacologic interventions to suppress inflammation and physical rehabilitation to restore function. The recognition of such an association supports not only the need for comprehensive investigations but also highlights the importance of infection prevention and control interventions that can exacerbate vertebral column diseases, as noted in previous military environments (Banton et al., 2014). Thus, a coherent understanding of treatment is essential to improving patient outcomes and care in vertebral column pathologies.

6.6.1. Non-Surgical Interventions (Physical Therapy and Medication)

Non-invasive therapies are critical in the treatment of vertebral column disorders, particularly in osteological conditions such as scoliosis and other spinal curvatures. Physical therapy has become an essential form of treatment, focusing on improving strength and mobility. Depending on individual assessments, therapists may devise customized regimens involving exercises to improve core stability and spinal alignment. The following targeted therapeutic methods are instrumental in children, in which treatment before the scoliosis progresses is possible. The effectiveness of physical therapy not only in curing current symptoms but also in ensuring long-term spine health aligns with the principle of maintaining a functional, well-aligned vertebral column in human osteology. Out of many non-surgical treatments, medication is another simple method used in pain alleviation and inflammation minimization. Nonsteroidal anti-inflammatory drugs (NSAIDs) are commonly employed to alleviate pain secondary to a large number of spinal pathologies, which translates into improved quality of life in patients with back pain or degenerative disease.

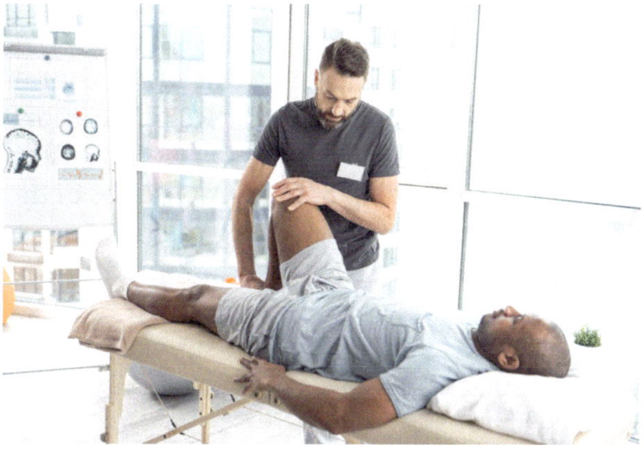

Figure 6.15. Non-surgical interventions.

Source: https://external-content.duckduckgo.com/iu/?u=https%3A%2F%2Fnyboneandjoint.com%2Fwp-content%2Fuploads%2F2021%2F07%2FHow-Physical-Therapy-Can-Help-Replace-Pain-Medication.jpg&f=1&nofb=1&ipt=af18e356e1bdd9e87b67c862c6d3588554895eb298e33ddf01de5b48599222bb.

On occasion, muscle relaxants can be used to reduce muscle spasm associated with spinal pain. Pharmacologic management of this type is a vitally important adjunctive therapeutic modality when combined with physical therapy, since it can enable patients to engage in rehabilitative maneuvers. Consequently, successful medication protocols significantly enhance compliance with physical therapy protocols, enabling optimal recovery channels for spinal patients. The use of innovative practices, such as Magnetically Controlled Growing Rod (MCGR) systems, reflects advancements in non-surgical treatments, particularly for children with Early-Onset Scoliosis (EOS). The MCGR technique appears to have shown encouraging results at an early stage, as it achieves spinal lengthening through office-based techniques and thus reduces the need for frequent surgeries associated with traditional methods. The technology is a significant milestone in treatment modalities, as it significantly reduces adverse effects associated with surgical interventions. Interestingly, studies indicate that these techniques offer equal spine correction to conventional processes, with better overall outcomes and fewer unnecessary complications from surgery (Akbarnia et al., 2012). With greater understanding of the complexities of the vertebral column, such non-surgical innovations are embraced, along with a greater appreciation of the importance of fine-tuning treatment modalities to enhance prognosis and patient care (Cheung et al., 2012) (Figure 6.15).

6.6.2. Surgical Procedures (Spinal Fusion and Laminectomy)

Spinal surgery, particularly surgery such as spinal fusion and laminectomy, has transformed the management of many vertebral column diseases. Spinal fusion aims to stabilize segments of the spine by permanently locking two or more vertebrae together to reduce pain and promote function. It is often employed in cases of degenerative disc disease, scoliosis, and spinal stenosis, ailments that can significantly sap mobility and quality of life. Surgeons enhance fusion and spinal structural stability through the use of bone grafts and instrumentation, such as rods and screws. Not only does the surgery alleviate pain, but it is also important in order to prevent future deformity and complications of spinal diseases. Laminectomy, a critical surgical intervention, involves the removal of a segment of the vertebral arch to relieve compression of the spinal cord or nerve roots. This is primarily performed to alleviate conditions such as herniated discs, spinal stenosis, and tumors. By removing the lamina, the operating physician creates additional space in the spinal canal, which can significantly relieve leg pain, numbness, and weakness.

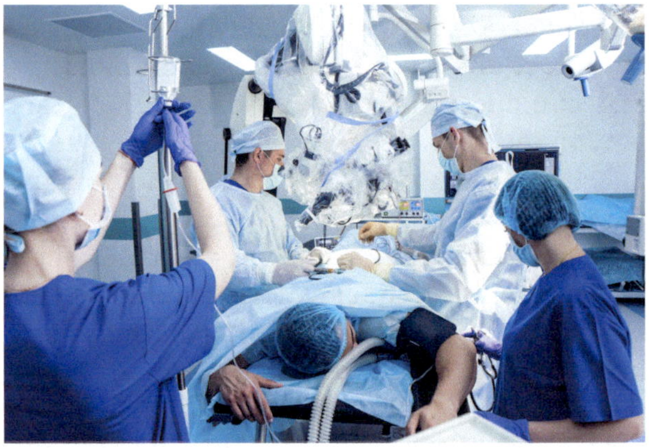

Figure 6.16. Surgical procedures.

Source: https://external-content.duckduckgo.com/iu/?u=https%3A%2F%2Fpremiaspine.com%2Fwp-content%2Fuploads%2F2023%2F02%2Flumbar-laminectomy-with-fusion.jpg&f=1&nofb=1&ipt=c9de936c40a665dcfa67f86fd2fd4d98b00f69616378c4021d4f99c62c8a53c6.

Peculiarly, the laminectomy may be performed as a stand-alone procedure or together with spinal fusion when stability is needed. Whether it is performed singly or in tandem typically hinges on the patient's true diagnosis and condition, which underscores the meticulous attention required in spinal surgical interventions. Surgical and technological advancements have significantly improved outcomes in spinal surgery, as evidenced by recent research and clinical data. Innovations such as pedicle screw fixation have been practical regarding enhancing deformity correction in adolescent idiopathic scoliosis (AIS) with the preservation of spinal balance and fusion of levels. Techniques like the alternate level screw technique (ALSS) are included in these advancements, implying more customized surgical methods. The identification of congenital conditions such as Klippel-Feil Syndrome (KFS) also underscores the variability of spinal conditions and the need for specialized surgical approaches to improve quality of life for people with such conditions (Cheung et al., 2012; Herman et al., 2012). Such continuous development in surgical procedures validates the irreplaceable role of these interventions in human osteology and the treatment of spinal disorders (Figure 6.16).

6.6.3. Rehabilitation and Recovery Strategies

The vertebral column is an indispensable part of the structural mobility and stability of the human skeleton, so rehabilitation and recovery strategies are of key importance after spinal disorders or injury. practical recovery plans also integrate occupational and physical therapies focused on the individual's needs and designed to restore mobility and function. Specific exercises, for instance, can strengthen the stabilizing musculature, improve posture, and enhance flexibility, ultimately improving spinal health. Pain management techniques also form part of rehabilitation, using modalities of heat, cold, or electrical stimulation to reduce pain. Through an integrated rehabilitation system, patients can achieve a recovery track that not only meets immediate needs but also fosters long-term wellness and prevents future damage. Integrating multidisciplinary practice is vital when developing high-quality rehabilitation procedures for spinal injury. Such a process involves teamwork among healthcare professionals, including physiotherapists, occupational therapists, and pain management experts, who can mutually facilitate healing processes. There is data to support that tailored therapeutic intervention is much more effective than generalist programs, as they consider the diversity of types of injuries, personal history of diseases, and life problems. By conducting intensive evaluations, clinicians can create personalized rehabilitation plans that may include exercise regimens, ergonomic assessments, and even dietary guidance to support overall healing. Understanding the bioarchaeological context, such as previous injury patterns and recovery methods at sites like Turkey Creek Pueblo, can be beneficial for understanding current practices and signaling the importance of individualized strategies in achieving the best recovery outcomes (Ralston et al., 2023). Furthermore, ongoing evaluation of recovery is necessary to dynamically adjust rehabilitation strategies. Continued assessments allow medical experts to assess improvements or reversals in recovery, enabling appropriate adjustments to the rehabilitation program. This continuous feedback process keeps the patient engaged in their recovery process and provides them with a sense of control over their recovery. In addition, new technologies such as virtual reality and biofeedback have been found effective in enhancing spinal injury rehabilitation outcomes. By providing innovative ways to engage patients in rehabilitation activities, these technologies have the potential to advance adherence to rehabilitation regimes and reduce recovery times. Such insight into the historic management of trauma, as witnessed in decapitated burials in Romano-British periods, also underlines the significance of integrated strategies towards rehabilitation since there is the ability to reap from experience under conditions of trauma (Tucker et al., 2012).

Test Your Knowledge

1. What non-surgical treatments, including physiotherapy and pharmacological interventions, are used for vertebral column disorders?
2. When are surgical interventions necessary, and what types of spinal surgeries are commonly performed to correct vertebral pathologies?

SUMMARY

Together, the vertebral column forms a keystone of structural reinforcement and functional movement in the human skeleton. Bridging otherwise unconnected anatomical structures, it facilitates movement while protecting the spinal cord, a significant component of the central nervous system. The vertebral column's structure, with articulated vertebrae, intervertebral discs, and ligaments, promotes not only flexibility but also resistance to mechanical stress. Developments in the understanding of spine mechanics highlight its evolutionary significance, particularly with respect to human adaptations—such as terrestrial bipedal locomotion—that place greater stress on spinal shape and function. These adaptations equate to both health and locomotion consequence, rendering the vertebral column of prime concern in human anatomical research. Moreover, the vertebral column's evolutionary history also shows compelling similarities with other archosaurs, including anatomical adaptations that have optimized locomotion across multiple environments. The evolution from sprawling to erect locomotion, as observed between reptilian and avian lineages, underscores the confluence of skeletal shape and functional need adapting to meet new environments better. The vertebral column's role in stabilizing various modes of locomotion in dinosaurs, as argued in discussions regarding the biomechanical specificity between *Mussaurus patagonicus* and *Crocodylus johnstoni*, illustrates the evolutionary versatility so important to vertebrate survival. A study of the vertebral column, therefore, does not simply shed light upon human anatomy but also upon its broader vertebrate context, revealing interspecies connections. Lastly, the implications of our knowledge on the vertebral column are not limited to anatomical studies; they guide clinical practice in spinal health and musculoskeletal disorders. With changing patterns of human activity, the possibility of spinal complications is of growing concern. Studies on the evolution of vertebral structures can guide therapeutic interventions and rehabilitation of spinal deformities or injuries. The vertebral column as a whole is not just an underlying system of support; it is a sophisticated tale of evolution and adaptation that mirrors broader biological phenomena in the vertebrate lineage. By synthesizing data from both osteological research and evolutionary biology, we can gain a deeper understanding of the human spine as a multifaceted subject of study, thereby reflecting on its significance in the discipline of human osteology.

The vertebral column is a complex structure that not only supports the human body but also plays a key role in biomechanics and locomotion. The column consists of 33 vertebrae segmented into cervical, thoracic, lumbar, sacral, and coccygeal areas that are all uniquely formed with varied functions, which all contribute to achieving physical stability. The cervical vertebrae, for instance, are smaller and more mobile, allowing head movement, while the lumbar region is best suited for heavy weight-bearing, showing vertebral morphological versatility. This evolutionary vertebral specialization meets the demands of human bipedal locomotion by balancing stability and flexibility to suit various activities (Christian et al., 2013). Additionally, human vertebrae and other animals' vertebral columns' comparative analysis accounts for the human spine's unique adaptations. For example, vertebral adaptations that allow vertebrae to undergo significant elongation and serve this function are documented in research on sauropod dinosaurs. These adaptations range from pneumatic cavities that reduce the weight of vertebrae while maintaining structural support to a feature that affects the understanding of vertebral evolution (Taylor et al., 2012). These findings suggest that while human vertebrae are uniquely suited for bipedal walking, comparative studies of the evolutionary histories of other animals provide valuable lessons about more general vertebral morphology and adaptation to specific ways of life and environments. In summary, the vertebral column is a demonstration of evolutionary ingenuity, as tension between form and function is offset by a dynamic exchange. Special points of focus are the structural differentiation between vertebral regions, the biomechanical performance implications of the differences, and comparative anatomy, which informs our knowledge of human osteology. This study not only highlights the intricate architecture of the spine in human physiology but also extends the concept by examining how vertebral components have evolved across various species over millions of years, thereby stimulating further research into their evolutionary background and biomechanics (Taylor et al., 2012; Christian et al., 2013).

KEY TERMS FROM THIS CHAPTER

- Cervical Vertebrae
- Thoracic Vertebrae
- Lumbar Vertebrae
- Sacrum
- Vertebral Foramen
- Transverse Process
- Lamina
- Pedicle
- Intervertebral Disc
- Facet Joint
- Transverse Foramen
- Annulus Fibrosus
- Nucleus Pulposus

CRITICAL THINKING QUESTIONS

1. **How many adult human vertebrae are in the vertebral column?**
   a. 24
   b. 26
   c. 33
   d. 30
2. **Which region of the vertebral column has the most vertebrae?**
   a. Cervical
   b. Thoracic
   c. Lumbar
   d. Sacral
3. **Which vertebra is also called the "atlas"?**
   a. C1
   b. C2
   c. T1
   d. L1
4. **What is the primary function of the intervertebral discs?**
   a. To protect the spinal cord
   b. To give flexibility and shock absorption
   c. To attach muscles to vertebrae
   d. Supply blood to the spine
5. **Where are transverse foramina located in the vertebral region?**
   a. Thoracic
   b. Lumbar
   c. Cervical
   d. Sacral

Short Answer Questions

1. Define the vertebral column and its primary functions.
2. How many vertebrae make up the adult human vertebral column?
3. Explain the structure and function of intervertebral discs.
4. Explain primary and secondary curvatures of the spine and how they differ from each other.
5. Explain the function of the spinous and transverse processes of a vertebra.
6. Explain the clinical significance of the intervertebral foramina.
7. How is the vertebral column protective of the spinal cord?
8. Explain the occipital bone to the atlas articulation.

Answers to Critical Thinking Questions

1. (b); 2. (b); 3. (a); 4. (b); 5. (c)

REFERENCES

1. Cerda, I. A., Casal, G. A., Martinez, R. D., & Ibiricu, L. M. (2015). Histological evidence for a supraspinous ligament in sauropod dinosaurs. *Royal Society Open Science*, *2*(10), 150369. https://doi.org/10.1098/rsos.150369Abramoff, B., Bick, B., Brochu, B., Byron, C., Carpenter, C., et al. (2012). Histology-based morphology of the neurocentral synchondrosis in *Alligator mississippiensis* (Archosauria, Crocodylia). https://deepblue.lib.umich.edu/bitstream/2027.42/89542/1/21495_ftp.pdf (accessed on 18th July 2025).
2. Akbarnia, B. A., Cheung, K. M. C., Dannawi, Z., et al. (2012). Next generation of growth-sparing techniques: Preliminary clinical results of a magnetically controlled growing rod in 14 patients. https://core.ac.uk/download/38035632.pdf (accessed on 18th July 2025).
3. Allen, V., Hutchinson, J. R., Otero, A., et al. (2017). Forelimb muscle and joint actions in Archosauria: Insights from *Crocodylus johnstoni* (Pseudosuchia) and *Mussaurus patagonicus* (Sauropodomorpha). https://core.ac.uk/download/141887609.pdf (accessed on 18th July 2025).
4. Bailey, J. W., & Heidt, G. A. (1984). Postnatal osteology of the northern grasshopper mouse, *Onychomys leucogaster*. https://core.ac.uk/download/84121570.pdf (accessed on 18th July 2025).
5. Banton, M. E. (2014). Examining reactive arthropathy in military skeletal assemblages: A pilot study using the mass grave assemblage from the Battle of Towton (1461). https://core.ac.uk/download/79496181.pdf (accessed on 18th July 2025).
6. Brits, D. M. (2016). Stature estimation in South African juveniles and adult females. https://core.ac.uk/download/188773243.pdf (accessed on 18th July 2025).
7. Cheung, K. M. C., Cheung, W. Y., Leung, Y., et al. (2012). Selection of fusion levels in adolescent idiopathic scoliosis (AIS) using the fulcrum bending radiograph prediction: Verification based on pedicle screw strategy. https://core.ac.uk/download/37987465.pdf (accessed on 18th July 2025).
8. Christian, A., Hultgren, B. D., Emerson, C. L., Holliday, C. M., Gilmore, C. W., Schwarz, D., Frey, E., et al. (2013). The effect of intervertebral cartilage on neutral posture and range of motion in the necks of sauropod dinosaurs. https://core.ac.uk/download/29026918.pdf (accessed on 18th July 2025).
9. Dewey, J. (2013). Survey of comparative human and non-human osteology: Common Florida species. https://core.ac.uk/download/236292661.pdf (accessed on 18th July 2025).
10. Eckel, C., Fiallo, M., Mas, J., et al. (2021). Osteology modules for the human structure course. https://core.ac.uk/download/657567126.pdf (accessed on 18th July 2025).
11. Fourshee, J. L. (2022). Differentiating human from nonhuman bone: Insights from a medical examiner's collection, Kenosha, Wisconsin. https://core.ac.uk/download/554010999.pdf (accessed on 18th July 2025).
12. Herman, J., Khalluri, P., Lubicky, J. P., et al. (2012). 'Clinical triad' findings in Klippel-Feil patients. https://core.ac.uk/download/37987463.pdf (accessed on 18th July 2025).
13. Hodgin, R. M. (2012). Trauma at Akhetaten (Tell el-Amarna): Interpersonal violence or occupational hazard. https://core.ac.uk/download/84118993.pdf (accessed on 18th July 2025).

14. Jamal, B. (2008). Cervical vertebral maturation stage as a growth predictor. https://core.ac.uk/download/571283978.pdf (accessed on 18th July 2025).
15. Keith, A., Keith, A., Minelli, A., Minelli, A., Rokas, A., Stollewerk, A., Stoltzfus, A., et al. (2007). Homeotic evolution in the Mammalia: Diversification of therian axial seriation and the morphogenetic basis of human origins. https://core.ac.uk/download/pdf/7715930.pdf (accessed on 18th July 2025).
16. Kerttula, L. (2001). Magnetic resonance imaging of the intervertebral disc: Post-traumatic findings and the value of diffusion-weighted MR imaging. https://core.ac.uk/download/628862336.pdf (accessed on 18th July 2025).
17. Kurila, L. (2015). Cremation as limitation? A paleo demographic inquiry into the accuracy of macroscopic analysis of cremated human remains based on an East Lithuanian sample. https://core.ac.uk/download/43658404.pdf (accessed on 18th July 2025).
18. Lewis, M. (2017). Fetal paleopathology: An impossible discipline? https://core.ac.uk/download/42153730.pdf (accessed on 18th July 2025).
19. Lewis, M., Shapland, F., & Watts, R. (2015). The lives and deaths of young medieval women: The osteological evidence. https://core.ac.uk/download/42153597.pdf (accessed on 18th July 2025).
20. Mallison, H., Pittman, M. D., & Schwarz, D. (2015). Using crocodilian tails as models for dinosaur tails. https://core.ac.uk/download/38080310.pdf (accessed on 18th July 2025).
21. McLachlin, S. D. (2013). An investigation of subaxial cervical spine trauma and surgical treatment through biomechanical simulation and kinematic analysis. https://core.ac.uk/download/61638378.pdf (accessed on 18th July 2025).
22. N/A. (2017). III. Observation of internal morphology. https://core.ac.uk/download/94868602.pdf (accessed on 18th July 2025).
23. Pharris, M. (2000). Cervicogenic headache: A manual therapy approach. https://core.ac.uk/download/235074309.pdf (accessed on 18th July 2025).
24. Puneeth, K. (2016). Study of outcome of early versus delayed surgery in lumbar disc prolapse: A prospective study. https://core.ac.uk/download/235658308.pdf (accessed on 18th July 2025).
25. Ralston, C. E. (2023). Gendered bodies, engendered lives: Bioarcheological exploration of the intersectionality of gender, health, and trauma at Turkey Creek Pueblo, Arizona (AD 1225–1286). https://digitalscholarship.unlv.edu/cgi/viewcontent.cgi?article=5768&context=thesesdissertations (accessed on 18th July 2025).
26. Sanford, L. A. (2024). Numerical variations in the thoracic and lumbar vertebrae within the John A. Williams skeletal collection, Western Carolina University, Cullowhee, NC (USA). https://core.ac.uk/download/610528747.pdf (accessed on 18th July 2025).
27. Sarfo, T. A. (2014). A statistical investigation of nonmetric vertebral traits with a skeletal population sample from the Dakhleh Oasis, Egypt. https://core.ac.uk/download/61655207.pdf (accessed on 18th July 2025).
28. Synstelien, J. A. (2001). Differences in the os coxae between blacks and whites: A musculoskeletal approach to human variation. https://core.ac.uk/download/588287985.pdf (accessed on 18th July 2025).

29. Taylor, M. P., & Wedel, M. J. (2012). Why sauropods had long necks; and why giraffes have short necks. https://core.ac.uk/download/29026739.pdf (accessed on 18th July 2025).
30. Taylor, M. P., & Wedel, M. J. (2013). Caudal pneumaticity and pneumatic hiatuses in the sauropod dinosaurs *Giraffatitan* and *Apatosaurus*. https://core.ac.uk/download/29026919.pdf (accessed on 18th July 2025).
31. Tucker, K. (2012). "Whence this severance of the head?": The osteology and archaeology of human decapitation in Britain. https://core.ac.uk/download/427402624.pdf (accessed on 18th July 2025).

THORAX – RIBS AND STERNUM

7

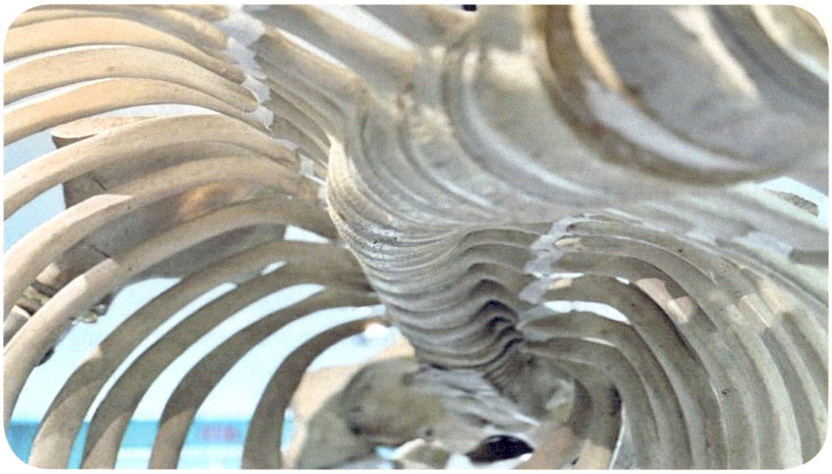

LEARNING OBJECTIVES

After studying this chapter, you will be able to:

1. Discuss the anatomy of the thorax
2. Describe the structure of the ribs
3. Focus on the sternum
4. Learn about rib articulation
5. Know muscles associated with the thorax
6. Focus on common injuries and disorders

Introduction

The thorax, as a crucial constituent of the human frame, performs various functions critical to structural support and physiological processes. Comprising ribs, sternum, and attached musculature, the thorax contains key organs such as the heart and lungs, thereby facilitating crucial functions such as respiration and circulation. The ribs, typically 12 pairs in number, attach to the thoracic vertebrae and constitute a movable but firm structure containing internal organs. Furthermore, the sternum, subdivided into the manubrium, body, and xiphoid process, acts as a rib anchor and facilitates the maintenance of the thoracic cavity's shape and volume. Understanding the intricacies of relationships and mechanics of the thoracic structure plays a fundamental role in an understanding and appreciation of human anatomy and functioning since abnormalities in this system translate to severe health implications. Thoracic complexity extends beyond its structural composition; it is also a central component of respiratory mechanics. Coordination of rib movements and diaphragm contractions with breathing in and out is very important in airflow regulation. The ribs expand and contract rhythmically during every respiration, expanding thoracic cavity volume and hence clearing space for lung inflation. This coordination highlights the coordinated function of thoracic structures in effective respiration. Experiments have revealed that comparative investigations across other mammals show that thoracic structures are typically specialized for specific locomotor and respiratory requirements, such as in bottlenose dolphins, which have specialized systems for successful breathing while in motion (Cotten et al., 2009). Such comparative data emphasize the specializations of the thorax according to evolution, illustrating the versatility and efficacy of this body region. Secondly, the experiential aspect of studying thoracic anatomy has come into the spotlight in medical education, with an emphasis on the need for practical experience alongside book knowledge. Dissection courses, for instance, provide excellent opportunities for students to gain firsthand experience of the anatomical structures, bridging the gap between text and actual applications (Busard et al., 2017). This hands-on learning enhances basic anatomical knowledge and enhances skills essential to clinical practice. By dissecting the ribs and sternum, not only do students gain anatomical knowledge but also learn about human physiology in all its intricacies. The thorax is thus a significant focus in both structural and functional aspects of learning about the human body, further reinforcing the importance of composite education in medical school.

Definition of the Thorax

Thorax is a vital anatomical region in the human body, protecting essential organs and physiological functions. This region of the structure comprises the rib cage, sternum, and thoracic vertebrae, forming a bony framework that supports the vital organs of the chest cavity, including the heart and lungs. The ribs, which are shared with the thoracic vertebrae in a strong but loosely connected system, allow the dynamic expansion and contraction of the thoracic cavity during respiration. This three-dimensional mobility of the thorax is crucial, maintaining with it an associated mechanical motion that supports effective practical respiratory function and the full structural integrity needed to protect the internal organs from damage and external stress. As thoracic injury has such catastrophic consequences, the thorax's anatomical definition is critical in medical sciences, particularly trauma care and car safety engineering. The significance of the thorax is even more pronounced given that thoracic injury is one of the leading causes of mortality in automobile accidents. Thoracic injuries can be caused by sudden deceleration forces, such as rib and sternal fractures. There are specific anatomical features, including age and sex, that can affect the risk of incurring such injuries, making it possible for models like the SAFER human body model (SHBM) to be used in the prediction and prevention of risks that may result from rib fractures in crash situations. Thus, the thorax needs to be understood not just structurally but also in relation to its implications for injury prediction and prevention strategies (Larsson et al., 2023). Properly defining the thorax involves an analysis of its physical composition in addition to its functional value in various situations. For instance, the sternum, which lies in the center of the thoracic cavity, serves as an anchor point for the ribs and increases stability in the thoracic system as a whole. It is essential that thoracic injuries be understood, as fractures of the sternum are common in frontal crashes, where modern evaluation methods may be unable to capture the complexity of injury mechanisms. Existing designs, such as the Hybrid III dummy, fail to come to terms with the sophisticated biomechanics of the thorax, particularly in elderly age groups whose injury risk profile may be very different from that of younger age groups. More biologically accurate human body models are needed to improve injury outcome prediction and enhance trauma preparedness, enabling automotive safety systems to more effectively mitigate thoracic injury risks (Novoa et al., 2018) (Figure 7.1).

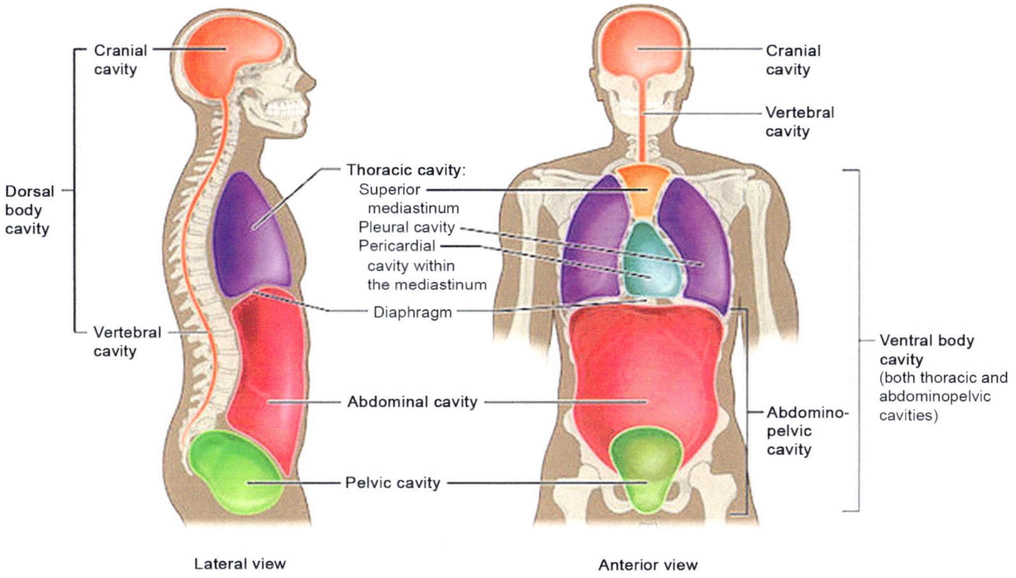

Figure 7.1. The thorax serves as a vital anatomical region within the human body.

Source: https://external-content.duckduckgo.com/iu/?u=https%3A%2F%2Fstudy.com%2Fcimages%2Fmultimages%2F16%2Fdiagrambodycavitiesthoraciccavity.jpg&f=1&nofb=1&ipt=cd030696ee0480c4fc25ae8131e57b7f419e9a102becb709a5b4104a0b941e48.

Importance of the Thorax in Human Anatomy

The thorax is a fundamental structure and functional unit of human anatomy, characterized mainly by the ribs and sternum. Not only does this region protect critical organs, such as the heart and lungs, but it is also primarily responsible for respiratory mechanics. The rib cage, composed of 12 pairs of ribs and the costal cartilages, is a flexible but firm covering that expands and contracts during respiration. This outward expansion facilitates inhalation, while the recoil sustains exhalation, demonstrating the double role of the thorax in defense and respiration. In addition, the fusion of the sternum to the rib cage sustains the support of this body component even further, demonstrating how all of its structures collaborate not just to secure the physical integrity of the thorax but its body function within the human body as well. Understanding the geometry of the developing and growing thoracic cage is important for both clinical and biomechanical reasons. The recent studies concerning the 3D geometry of a child's rib cage revealed extensive morphological changes occurring between infancy and late adolescence. They suggest that with increasing age, the relative proportions of cartilage to rib length change, and that one can use the costal index, the interpretation of which aids in understanding normal thoracic growth. For instance, a progressive change is seen in the costal index, where the decline is followed by an increase, demonstrating a complex interaction between rib and cartilage development. These findings lend credence to the role of the thorax not only in adult life but also during growth stages, providing important information for clinicians seeking to diagnose and treat thoracic abnormalities in pediatric populations (Badina et al., 2013).

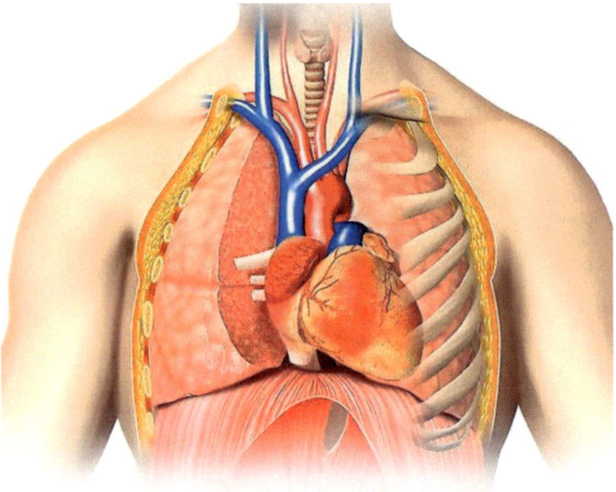

Figure 7.2. The thorax in human anatomy.

Source: https://external-content.duckduckgo.com/iu/?u=https%3A%2F%2Fimages.squarespace-cdn.com%2Fcontent%2Fv1%2F5ed09f01ab927132aa1d3370%2F1da871e7-d08f-4411-90ce-bc394cd01096%2Fthorax.jpg&f=1&nofb=1&ipt=6c77475cc91c5744137a32c447e7d3df68689c74cb69bc2d1838082cda40d218.

Moreover, the thoracic structural design influences other states of disease, such as pectus carinatum, providing a model for understanding the potential for thoracic deformities arising from unbalanced development of its components. Pectus carinatum is produced by hypertrophy of the costal cartilages with associated abnormal protrusion of the sternum. Surgical corrections, e.g., reversed Nuss procedure, illustrate that an understanding of thoracic structure underlies optimal treatment planning. The stresses induced upon the thoracic cage during corrective procedures also underscore the importance of precise anatomical knowledge, as variable positioning of corrective hardware can influence both stress distribution and potential future complications, including scoliosis. Thus, a deep understanding of thoracic anatomy is critical not only for surgical intervention but also for maximizing overall treatment (Coelho et al., 2015) (Figure 7.2).

Overview of Ribs and Sternum

The rib cage, being an intrinsic component of the thoracic cavity, consists of 12 pairs of ribs that posteriorly articulate with the thoracic vertebrae. A rib belongs to three categories: true ribs, false ribs, and floating ribs, based on their connection to the sternum. True ribs (ribs 1–7) connect to the sternum via their own costal cartilages and provide structural support and elasticity. False ribs (ribs 8–10) share a common cartilaginous connection to the sternum, which helps in the distribution of force during movement. Floating ribs (ribs 11–12), lacking sternal attachment, cover the lower organs. This unique configuration allows the rib cage to expand during inspiration and contract during expiration, illustrating the subtle interplay between structural design and the respiratory process in the thorax. The breastbone, or sternum, plays a highly significant role to the overall function and stability of the thorax. It has three major parts: the manubrium, the body, and the xiphoid process. The manubrium articulates with the first rib and clavicle to serve as a solid area of attachment for the upper part of the chest. This region is important in the maintenance of postural position and the function of respiration. The sternum's flat and elongated body serves as an attachment point for the true ribs through costal cartilage. Finally, the xiphoid process, short and cartilaginous in infants, unites and ossifies with advancing age and serves as a reference point for various anatomical landmarks. As a result of its articulated contacts with the ribs, the sternum not only protects the critical organs but also participates in the respiratory mechanics by operating along with the rib cage during ventilation. The evolutionary significance of the rib cage and the sternum is further evidenced by their modularity and versatility. The vertebral constraints in the series present in mammals, their cervical and lumbosacral counts, are indicative of their specific evolutionary course. The muscularization of the diaphragm, an outgrowth of the cervical somites, signifies the unification of the respiratory and locomotor apparatus in mammals, rendering them more effective at respiration and locomotion. These adaptations demonstrate the remarkable capacity of ribs and the sternum to be modified, accommodating the specific respiratory needs of various species. The ability of different muscles to govern thoracic volume, as shown by experiments in animals such as bottlenose dolphins, illustrates how anatomical features may influence physiological function, an interesting interaction of anatomy and function through evolutionary time (Cotten et al., 2009; Buchholtz et al., 2025) (Figure 7.3).

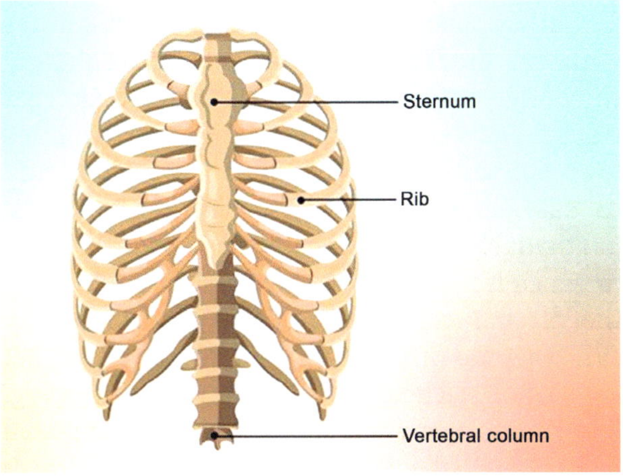

Figure 7.3. The rib cage, an integral component of the thoracic cavity.

Source: https://external-content.duckduckgo.com/iu/?u=https%3A%2F%2Ftse1.mm.bing.net%2Fth%3Fid %3DOIP.sMOlFJrIRnvcLuIp3hQscQHaFg%26pid%3DApi&f=1&ipt=ba 75a706f7d903b9a1 bd5010d 716b18c 176c76d69ceed25c8a27c78de5dc04ba.

7.1. Anatomy of the Thorax

Learning Outcome

1. Definition of the thoracic cavity
2. Structures comprising the thorax
3. Function of the thorax in respiration

The thoracic cavity, shielded by the rib cage and sternum, is an enclosing chamber for critical organs, including the heart and lungs. This anatomical configuration not only offers corporeal protection against external trauma but also plays a critical role in respiration mechanics. The ribcage, made up of 12 pairs of ribs and the breast, forms joints and costal cartilages through which it articulates, allowing for flexibility upon respiration. The three-dimensional configuration of the thoracic cavity is unique, as it changes significantly from infancy through adolescence. Research indicates that from 4 months to 15 years, children's rib cages exhibit geometric changes, including a fall and subsequent increase in the costal index, reflecting a changing cartilage-to-rib length ratio during growth (Badina et al., 2013). This makes the intricate relationship between structural form and function in the thorax even more complex. It is crucial to understand the biomechanics of the ribs to assess their vulnerability to injury, especially because they enclose vital thoracic organs. The rib cage is susceptible to fracture due to the presence of microfractures, which are mainly due to cyclic loading during breathing. Post-Mortem Human Surrogate research has provided insight into the strains the ribs experience during ordinary breathing. These researches indicate that regions of the ribs are able to tolerate specific patterns of strain, allowing tension and compression that have the ability to create microfracture (Stemmer et al., 2016). These strain responses are valuable to identify because a good thoracic biomechanics model helps us better understand the physical stress that ribs undergo. By defining these mechanical variables, researchers are better able to predict fracture risk and further contribute to clinical procedures for thoracic injury.

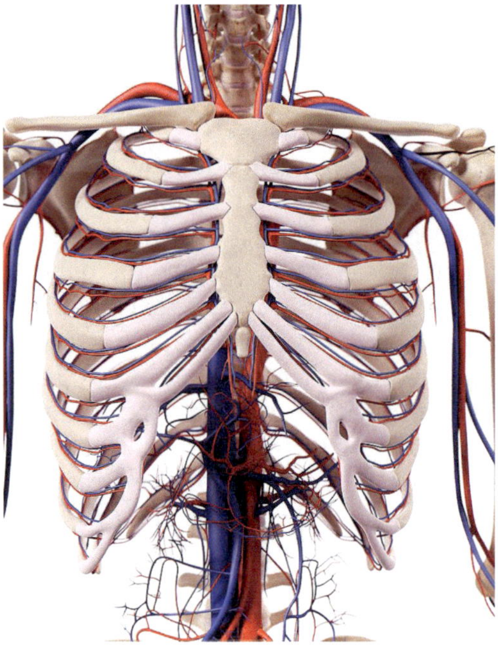

Figure 7.4. Anatomy of the thorax.

Source: https://external-content.duckduckgo.com/iu/?u=https%3A%2F%2Fimages.fineartamerica.com%2Fimages-medium-large-5%2F2-human-thoracic-anatomy-sebastian-kaulitzkiscience-photo-library.jpg&f=1&nofb=1&ipt=abf8d02971bbe40dbdf85bb7305c0bbff53dfba1b3ef67ca7ff29e0e34899ead.

Additionally, the anatomy of the thorax is not limited to mere structural components; it includes the complex arrangement of muscles, nerve tissue, and connective tissue that facilitate breathing and support cardiovascular function. The intercostal muscles lying between the ribs are also responsible for opening and closing the thoracic cavity during inhalation and exhalation, thereby influencing airway pressure and airflow. The muscles assist the diaphragm in forming a coordinated team, an essential component of effective respiration. On top of that, neurovascular bundles, which lie within the rib cage, are responsible for sensory and motor functions of the thoracic cavity, further contributing to its anatomical sophistication. The continual adaptation of rib cage structure in response to environmental demands—whether it is enlargement in children or adaptation to physical load—reflects the dynamic nature of thoracic anatomy and its essential role in ensuring the efficacy of the respiratory and circulatory systems (Figure 7.4).

7.1.1. Description of the Thoracic Cavity

The thoracic cavity is a vital anatomical structure in the human body that shelters critical organs such as the lungs and heart. It is bounded by the ribs, vertebral column, sternum, and diaphragm, and plays not only a protective role for these critical organs but also a role in respiration. The ribcage is a critical component of this dynamic function, providing structural support while allowing for breathing flexibility. Each rib subsequently articulates with the thoracic vertebrae and curves along the body, providing protection against external trauma. This sophisticated mechanism explains that the thoracic cavity must be constructed to safeguard the integrity of its contents, particularly under the physiological stresses to which it is regularly subjected. Understanding the mechanical aspects of the thoracic cavity can provide insight into factors that affect respiratory efficiency and overall well-being. The thoracic cavity is defined by its distinctive anatomical characteristics, which maximize respiratory mechanics. The diaphragm, a dome-shaped muscle that constitutes the base of the thoracic cavity, is a central player in ventilation. During inspiration, as the diaphragm contracts, it moves downward, increasing the volume of the thoracic cavity and thus allowing air to enter the lungs. The coordination of the intercostal muscles and ribs further enhances this process, allowing the rib cage to expand and contract rhythmically. Research indicates that microfractures in ribs under normal ventilation conditions can affect their integrity and their loading response during intense exercise. This highlights the delicate balance within the thoracic cavity, where structural strength must coexist with functional requirements (Stemmer et al., 2016). The precise integration of these anatomical structures illustrates the complexity of respiratory physiology. Moreover, the thoracic cavity's role is not merely protection and ventilation; it is actively engaged in linking respiration with locomotion. In other mammals, the thoracic cavity assists in coordinating motion with respiration, such as in the bottlenose dolphin. These aquatic mammals exhibit a characteristic decoupling of the respiratory and locomotor systems, underscoring the potential for variation in thoracic mechanics across species. Study of their muscular anatomy reveals adaptations for maintaining fast ventilation during surfacing, emphasizing the functional versatility of the thoracic cavity (Cotten et al., 2009). Such versatility not only facilitates efficient gas exchange but also illustrates how evolutionary pressures have shaped the thoracic structures in distinct environments. These conclusions highlight the significance of the thoracic cavity, reporting its multifaceted participation in respiratory as opposed to locomotor activities.

7.1.2. Components of the Thorax

The thorax, an essential structure of the human skeletal system, consists of the ribcage and sternum, which together surround vital organs such as the heart and lungs. The ribcage consists of 12 pairs of ribs, which vary in their structure and functionality and are divided into true ribs, false ribs, and floating ribs. True ribs, the first seven pairs, are in direct contact with the sternum by costal cartilage, allowing adequate expansion of the thorax during respiration. The remaining ribs are less directly connected to the sternum, which allows elasticity and mobility of the thoracic space. This intricate structure enables the thorax to support respiratory mechanics and provides structural support that maintains the integrity of thoracic organs, illustrating the importance of these elements in human physiology. Rib morphology is developed considerably from infancy to adulthood through a process that is typified by uneven allometric changes. There is indication that complex changes in rib curvature and inclination facilitate the transformation from the pyramidal infant thorax to the adult barrel-shaped thorax. These are structural and functional with respect to the capacity of the thorax, or more specifically, the respiratory efficiency. The segment of the thoracic spine registers an increase in medio-lateral dimensions, reflecting developmental modifications to adapt to the maturation of respiratory and overall body mechanics. Moreover, studies using geometric morphometrics found that variation in ribcage anatomy is influenced by age, sex, and race, demonstrating the dynamic interaction between form and function across populations (Barash et al., 2013). The sternum, often overshadowed by the much-documented ribcage, is important in the thoracic skeleton. It is divided into three identifiable parts: the manubrium, body, and xiphoid process, each playing its own role in the overall support and attachment of the thoracic skeleton. As a site of attachment for the ribs and the clavicles, the sternum contributes to the integrity of the thoracic wall but also allows for the necessary movement of breathing. Changes in the position of the sternum and the angular positions in relation to the ribs have been determined to impact respiratory patterns, particularly with increasing age. Studies show that when thoracic size changes with age, the breathing mechanism also changes correspondingly, underscoring the importance of recognizing age-related changes in thoracic anatomy to differentiate normal developmental variations from possible pathological states (Joshua et al., 2014) (Figure 7.5).

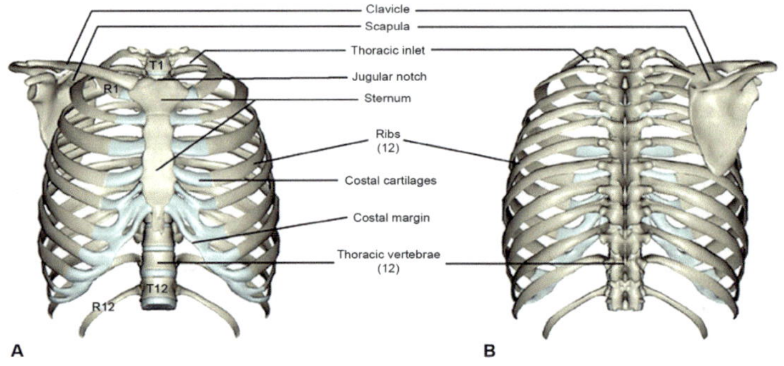

Figure 7.5. Components of the thorax.

Source: https://pocketdentistry.com/wp-content/uploads/285/B978032306807900003X_gr1.jpg.

7.1.3. Role of the Thorax in Respiratory Function

The thorax plays a crucial role in the respiratory process, as it protects vital organs such as the heart and lungs. The composition of the thorax, comprising the sternum and ribs, makes it possible for the chest cavity to open and close during respiration. Specifically, the ribs, which articulate with the thoracic vertebrae and sternum, form a dynamic, elastic structure that can adapt to changes in volume. When the diaphragm becomes contracted and the intercostal muscles elevate the ribs, the thoracic cavity expands, generating a negative pressure that sucks air into the lungs. The mechanical connection is essential for efficient gas exchange, underscoring the significance of the thorax in respiration. Understanding the anatomy and dynamics of the thoracic complex is crucial for appreciating how these physiological mechanisms operate in concert with respiratory needs. Moreover, the development of the thorax is closely related to respiratory efficiency at different stages of life, as evidenced by studies showing that the thorax undergoes remarkable morphological changes from infancy to adulthood.

For example, the pyramidal shape of the thorax in infants develops into a barrel shape in adults, enhancing respiratory capacity and efficiency. All changes in the dimensions of the thorax, both antero-posterior and medio-lateral diameters, point towards adaptations required to accommodate enlarging lungs and other thoracic organs. These variations in growth are influenced by both genetic and environmental factors, highlighting the significance of the thorax's geometry in preserving respiratory function throughout a person's life. Recognition of such developmental trajectories is important for understanding potential respiratory problems associated with abnormal thoracic morphology, especially in children (Badina et al., 2013). In addition to its structural characteristics, the functional significance of the thorax is further revealed by its complex biomechanical properties. The movements of the ribs, sternum, and breathing muscles determine the mechanics of breathing and influence overall respiratory function. Specifically, the costal cartilage between the sternum and ribs facilitates mobility through smooth motion with inspiration and expiration. Changes in the costal index with increasing age reflect the relative cartilage volume-to-rib length ratio and, consequently, exert a significant effect on thoracic mobility and subsequent breathing patterns (Badina et al., 2013). This association highlights the importance of thoracic biomechanics to clinical applications, particularly in determining abnormalities that have the potential to disrupt normal respiratory function. Also, analysis of thoracic growth from a biomechanical perspective enlightens us about physical growth and its relationship to respiratory performance, leading to specific intervention strategies in pediatric and adult populations (Figure 7.6).

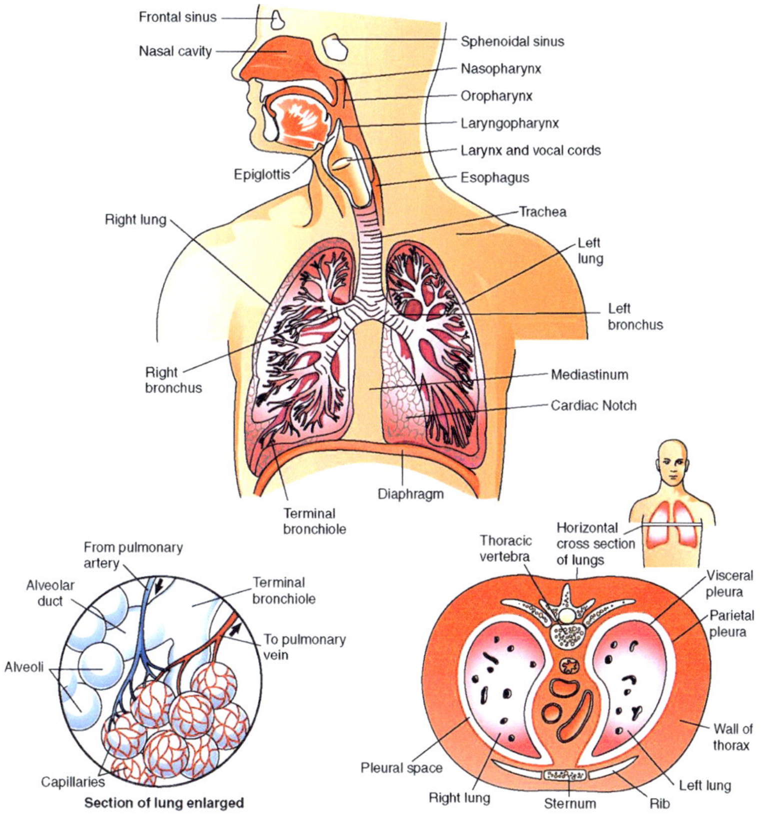

Figure 7.6. The thorax plays a critical role in respiratory function.

Source: https://external-content.duckduckgo.com/iu/?u=https%3A%2F%2Fi.pinimg.com%2F736x%2Fef%2Fda%2F46%2Fefda46d8fd21a0600cb8ade1d1170241.jpg&f=1&nofb=1&ipt=44ccbfa4a92dfa82c2d852551c8061880c1dfba94467aa8875ea05f9bdccbf21.

Test Your Knowledge

1. What are the main components of the thorax, and how do they protect vital organs like the heart and lungs?
2. How does the thoracic skeleton support respiration and maintain the structural integrity of the chest?

7.2. Structure of the Ribs

Learning Outcome

1. Ribs types: true, false, and floating
2. Rib anatomy: components and characteristics
3. Role of ribs in support and protection

The structure of the ribs plays a significant role in shaping the overall thoracic chamber and its consequences for respiratory mechanics and protective functions. Comprising 12 pairs of ribs, the ribs exhibit a layered structure that enhances the thorax's capacity to resist deformation during body movements. All the ribs are posteriorly fixed to the thoracic vertebrae and project forward, where they either directly join the sternum or indirectly via costal cartilage. The anatomical structure not only facilitates respiratory movement but also provides strong yet flexible support for critical organs such as the heart and lungs. Geometrical studies of the rib cage have yielded valuable insights into developmental change, particularly in children. Data gathered in the form of three-dimensional reconstructions of 960 ribs illustrate how the rib structures evolve with age, providing a reference for thoracic anatomy across different populations (Badina et al., 2013). As development occurs within the rib cage, its morphology changes significantly, particularly during early childhood. The overall adult thoracic shape can be determined by the age of two, but rib patterns are more complex. The ribs gradually slope forward with advancing age, and their relative proportions change considerably, leading to a transition from the cylindrical thoracic shape of infancy to the more oval shape of the adult. These changes are more than merely cosmetic; they reflect the functional changes at the underlying level necessary for proper ventilation and pulmonary health. Geometric morphometric analysis of recent growth patterns revealed that allometric growth between the upper and lower thoracic parts is differentiated and that independent developmental paths contribute to adult rib morphology. Such information underscores the intricacies of rib development and the manner in which aging influences thoracic configuration (Barash et al., 2013). The importance of rib morphology extends beyond mere anatomy; it involves close relationships with respiratory physiology and clinical results. In children, rib shape is critical for normal lung function and respiratory health.

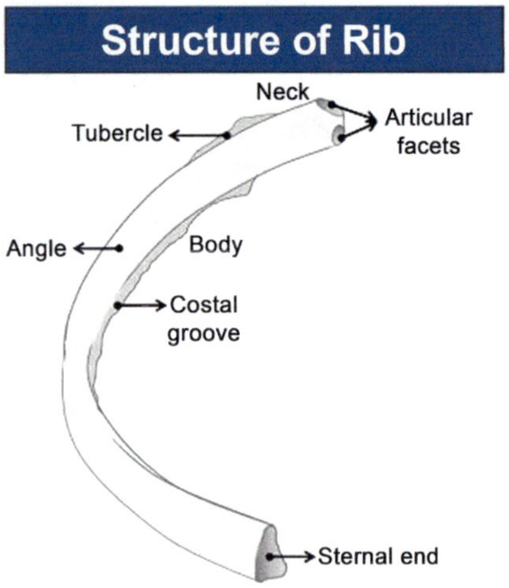

Figure 7.7. The structure of the ribs.

Source: https://external-content.duckduckgo.com/iu/?u=https%3A%2F%2Fbiologyreader.com%2Fwp-content%2Fuploads%2F2021%2F12%2Fstructure-of-rib.jpg&f=1&nofb=1&ipt=84f508af559e53c85d56637d880671713d4f1293291826e0be54f72af99b67ea.

Abnormalities of chest wall development can lead to pathology such as restrictive lung disease; therefore, a morphologic understanding of ribs is important. With the development of parameters such as the costal index, which measures the ratio of cartilage length to rib length, clinicians can efficiently assess thoracic development in children. The index can help detect deviations from standard growth and enable early intervention to address any impending conditions affecting health.

Expanding knowledge of rib structure not only informs practice but also underpins a greater understanding of human thoracic anatomy, evolutionary adaptations, and the nuances that exist within our development and function (Badina et al., 2013) (Figure 7.7).

7.2.1. Types of Ribs: True, False, and Floating

The human ribcage comprises different types of ribs, which are classified by their anatomical structure and attachment to the sternum. Vertebrosternal ribs or true ribs are the first seven pairs, which are connected to the sternum via costal cartilage. The direct attachment provides stability and support to the thoracic cavity, which offers adequate protection to vital organs such as the heart and lungs. True ribs are not only required for the protection of such organs but also play a significant role in respiratory mechanics, enabling the rib cage to expand and contract during respiration, underscoring their essential role in both skeletal support and respiration. Knowledge of true ribs enables one to comprehend the overall biomechanical activity of the thoracic skeleton and could lead to improved techniques in medical imaging and intervention for thoracic trauma. False ribs, which include pairs eight, nine, and ten of the ribs, are categorized based on their indirect fixation to the sternum. Instead of attaching directly to it, they are attached to a common cartilage that is united to the costal cartilage of the next higher rib. This provides some flexibility to the rib cage, which is necessary for encasing respiratory motion without compromising structural integrity. The increased mobility of false ribs, on the other hand, is in juxtaposition with the rigidity of true ribs, demonstrating the diversity of functional designs within the thoracic structure. Anatomical variation between true and false ribs is of concern in the evaluation of thoracic trauma because individuals may experience varying effects depending on the types of ribs involved, underscoring the need to consider such variations in clinical diagnoses of rib trauma (Holcombe et al., 2025). Finally, floating ribs, which consist of the 11th and 12th sets of ribs, are another category necessary to know about thoracic anatomy. As opposed to true and false ribs, floating ribs possess no anterior attachment to the sternum or to any other costal cartilages and terminate separately in the posterior abdominal wall muscles. This anatomical feature not only contributes to the greater range of motion of the lower rib cage but also is an evolutionary adaptation of the rib framework. Even though floating ribs provide less abdominal organ protection compared to other ribs, the mobility of floating ribs serves to contribute to many body movements and provides flexibility during bending and twisting. Interestingly, the presence of floating ribs highlights the complexity of rib structure and function, as they represent an intermediate biomechanical model balancing protection and mobility, particularly when considering age- and sex-differentiated variances in rib structure (Paulson et al., 2023) (Figure 7.8).

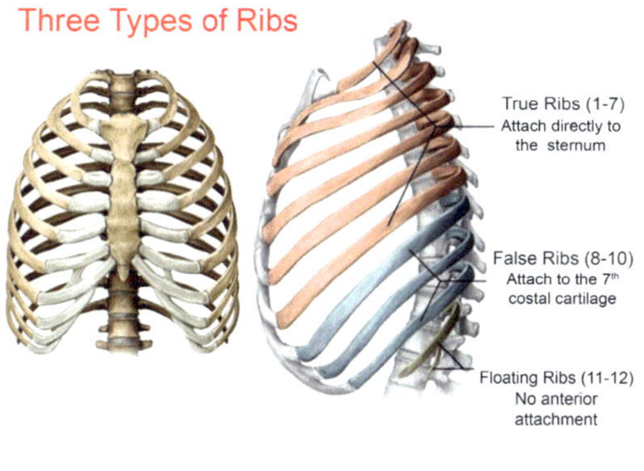

Figure 7.8. Types of ribs: true, false, and floating.

Source: https://external-content.duckduckgo.com/iu/?u=https%3A%2F%2Fi.pinimg.com%2Foriginals%2F16%2F8f%2F4d%2F168f4d47120502fffe736f12425d2a1d.png&f=1&nofb=1&ipt=126dcd1016f8173ff25e6ace040200e72e7ce00ffde17ce9b23d239fbe8e9dad.

7.2.2. Rib Anatomy: Parts and Features

The ribcage, which is an elementary component of the thorax, consists of 12 pairs of ribs, whose functions are essential in shielding thoracic organs and the respiratory process. Every rib possesses a bony feature with various characteristics, classified into three categories: true ribs, false ribs, and floating ribs. True ribs, consisting of the first seven pairs, link directly to the sternum via costal cartilage, providing flexibility and movement during breathing. On the other hand, the lower five pairs are the false ribs, either indirectly connected to the sternum or not connected to the sternum at all. The floating ribs, especially the last two pairs, are unique in that they lack anterior attachments, demonstrating the diversity of ribs and their important functions in the human body, particularly in providing structural strength while still allowing for respiratory efficiency. The anatomical arrangement of ribs exhibits distinctive features, including the head, neck, tubercle, and body, each serving a particular purpose in the function and interaction of the rib with surrounding structures. The head forms a joint with the thoracic vertebrae, enabling flexibility in respiration and upper-body movements. The neck is an intermediary link between the head and the tubercle that articulates with the respective transverse process of the vertebra. The body, or shaft of the rib, is important in defining the ribcage angle, impacting not only the form of the thorax but also the mechanics of ventilation. These anatomical features need to be understood because the growth of thoracic structure during development, from childhood through adulthood, depicts extraordinary developmental changes that are involved in respiratory mechanics as well as body shapes throughout life, highlighting adaptations for survival (Barash et al., 2013). Moreover, the intricate relationship between rib anatomy and overall thoracic morphology is significant to locomotion as well as respiratory efficacy in general among species, particularly hominoids. Variations in thorax shape and size provide windows on its specializations during evolution, demonstrating how variation in anatomy can influence consequences in function. For instance, the broader thorax in hominoids is not merely a mechanical adaptation but also denotes adaptations supporting greater scapular mobility and respiratory mechanics, particularly when considering compensations such as the larger dorsoventral diameter to offset the effects of orthograde posture. These adaptations also underscore the importance of rib anatomy to the evolutionary history of many species, demonstrating how structural modifications can optimize respiration while adapting to diverse locomotor modes (Chan et al., 2014).

7.2.3. Function of Ribs in Protection and Support

The ribs play a crucial role in protecting and supporting the thoracic cavity. They form a structural part of the rib cage that contains vital organs such as the lungs and heart. Not only does it offer physical protection from the outside, but this bony structure also maintains the rigidity of the thoracic and spinal regions overall. Their placement in the body allows them to transmit external forces, which is crucial during activities that expose the body to potential impact. Additionally, their flexibility, together with the intercostal muscles, allows breathing to occur such that expansion and constriction of the thoracic cavity occur without interrupting the structure of the spinal and ribcage. Besides protection, the ribs also help in providing structural support necessary in upholding posture as well as to facilitate movement of the body. The thoracic structure formed by the ribs also provides attachment sites for breathing and upper limb movements, in addition to their mechanical support. Thorax maturity and the adult thoracic shape, a result of developmental change from an infant pyramidal structure to an adult barrel shape, demonstrate rib adaptation to functional stress through the passage of time. This growth is not merely physical, but also the complex interplay of anatomical factors during development, as evidenced by rib-morphology research across varied phases of ontogeny (Barash et al., 2013). Also, the functional relevance of ribs in preventing injury during high-impact events, such as road accidents, is reflected in the biomechanics literature. Research on rib fractures reveals the mechanism by which ribs deflect trauma through force absorption and dispersal, preventing it from piercing protective sheaths that protect vital organs (Havránek, 2020). By defining biomechanical measures to assess rib injury and its impact, this research highlights the role of the ribcage in preserving life and in improving vehicle construction and safety components. Hence, the ribs are a key skeletal component that exemplifies the subtle balance of support and protection and accommodates the varying pressures one experiences throughout a lifetime.

Test Your Knowledge

1. What are the different types of ribs, and how are they classified based on their attachment and structure?
2. How do the features of the ribs, such as costal cartilages and curvature, contribute to thoracic flexibility and respiration?

7.3. The Sternum

Learning Outcome

1. Anatomy of the sternum: manubrium, body, and xiphoid process
2. Role of the sternum in the rib cage
3. Clinical significance of the sternum

The breastbone is still a key spot in the thoracic skeleton that serves as a point of anchorage for the ribcage. The flattened and elongated bone consists of three middle parts: the manubrium, the body, and the xiphoid process. Not only does it provide structural support to the ribs, but it also protects vital organs such as the heart and lungs. During breathing, the sternum helps move the thoracic cavity, thereby facilitating the expansion and contraction necessary for effective breathing. Furthermore, its attachment to the clavicles and the costal cartilages of the ribs highlights its contribution towards thoracic stability. An in-depth understanding of the sternum's anatomy is vital for health professionals, particularly in cases involving trauma or surgery of the thoracic region. In addition, the evolutionary history of the sternum provides insights into the morphological patterns found across various vertebrate clades. Surprisingly, the modern mammal has a distinctive segmented sternum, in contrast to the monoelementary sternum of paleosynapsids. The transition reflects an intricate evolutionary pathway, as the sternum became progressively regionalized to meet the functional demands of avian flight, terrestrial locomotion, and mammalian respiration. Discoveries of multipartite ossified sternum among the ancient synapsids, such as the gorgonopsian, indicate that the mammalian sternum-related traits have deeper evolutionary roots than they were previously known to. These discoveries provide essential context for understanding the evolution of skeletal morphologies to meet shifting biomechanical and environmental demands, and thus for understanding their posture and locomotion over time (Bendel et al., 2022).

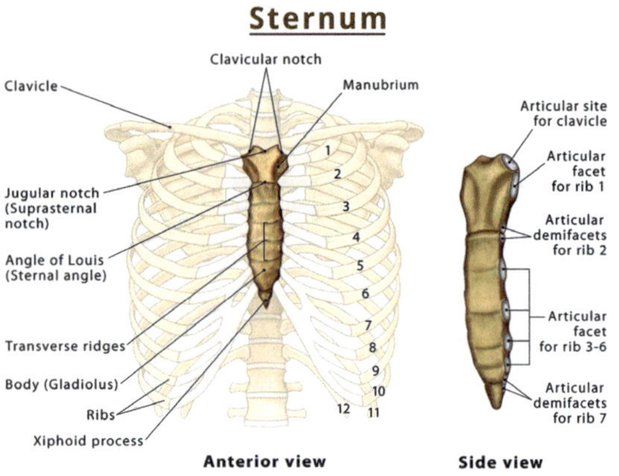

Figure 7.9. The sternum.

Source: https://external-content.duckduckgo.com/iu/?u=https%3A%2F%2Fwww.theskeletalsystem.net%2Fwp-content%2Fuploads%2F2021%2F12%2FSternum-Parts-Anatomy-Labeled.jpg&f=1&nofb=1&ipt=ee4cf1c7a36afcededc8ec3042162d44e05519904c850530f05398fbc553e718.

Experimental procedures, such as anatomical dissections, have significantly contributed to our understanding of the sternum and its role as a functional unit of the human body. Through experimental procedures, anatomy students can visualize and palpate the sternum, learn about its relationships with adjacent structures, and observe its function in thoracic mechanics. Importantly, these training programs bridge the gap between theory and practice, offering students unique insight into the complexities of human anatomy (Busard\uf2 et al., 2017). Experiential learning in this regard not only consolidates the basic concepts of sternal anatomy but also sets the stage for future advances in surgical interventions and medical practice. Lastly, an expanded understanding of the sternum's structure and history is added to our knowledge of the human body and its functional capabilities as part of the more general vertebrate biology (Figure 7.9).

7.3.1. Anatomy of the Sternum: Manubrium, Body, and Xiphoid Process

The sternum, as an important component of the thoracic skeleton, comprises primarily three components: the manubrium, body, and xiphoid process. The superior-most structure is the manubrium, which articulates laterally with the first pair of clavicles and ribs and possesses the sternal notch on its superior edge. This section is not only vital for structural support but also for enabling movement and flexibility within the thoracic cavity. The region of intersection between the manubrium and the body is referred to as the sternal angle and is a significant anatomical landmark used in clinical diagnostics to assess the alignment of the thorax and rib cage.

As a result, the area is crucial to the structural integrity and also to the dynamic function of the thoracic skeleton, and this emphasizes the importance of its anatomy in numerous medical tests. The body of the sternum constitutes the longest component of the sternum, lying directly on the manubrium and tapering to join onto the xiphoid process. This medial portion contains costal notches for the attachment of ribs two through seven to increase strength and anchorage to the ribcage to facilitate respiration. The body itself is very strong, supporting both the protection of the sensitive organs, such as the heart and lungs, as well as room to accommodate the respiratory motions necessary in inhalation and exhalation. Moreover, trauma or abnormality in this region can have significant effects on thoracic function and may compromise respiratory efficiency and cardiovascular status. Anatomical understanding of the sternum is significant, especially in clinical contexts of thoracic trauma and robotic surgery. The xiphoid process, being the most variable and smallest part of the sternum, is often underrated despite its anatomical importance. Functionally, it is an area of muscle attachment that supports the diaphragm, abdominal muscles, and rectus abdominis, all of which help stabilize the core and thoracic cavity. Curiously, while the xiphoid is primarily cartilaginous in youth, it ossifies with age, which can have implications for many medical evaluations and interventions, such as thoracic surgery. Further, xiphoid process anomalies such as xiphoid syndrome emphasize the clinical significance of familiarity with this entity in clinical practice. Both clinical significance and anatomical features of the xiphoid process depict its role in maintaining the thoracic cavity overall healthy and functional.

7.3.2. Role of the Sternum in the Rib Cage

The breastbone, or sternum, is a fundamental component of the rib cage's structural support. Found on the anterior midline of the thorax, the sternum facilitates a central point for the attachment of the ribs, particularly the true ribs, which attach directly to the sternum by costal cartilages. This point of attachment not only provides stability to the rib cage but also enables its dynamic motion during respiration. Mandibular sternum shape supports contraction and expansion that serve to aid proper lung ventilation. Its positioning also supports the thoracic cavity shape, an aspect that plays a key role in protecting key organs, including the heart and lungs, from harm caused by external shocks or trauma. The sternum has three key parts anatomically: the manubrium, body, and xiphoid process. All segments possess varying articulatory movements, along with acting as sites of attachment for massive respiratory muscles such as the pectoralis major and the diaphragm. These muscles provide aid in the changes in thoracic volume during inhalation and exhalation. The geometric position of the sternum and its articulation with adjacent ribs govern the effectiveness of the respiration process during various stages of life. Thoracic size differences, determined from the position of the sternum, reflect evolutionary adaptations of the rib cage to support respiratory mechanics across populations, reinforcing the importance of the sternum in maintaining respiratory health (Joshua et al., 2014).

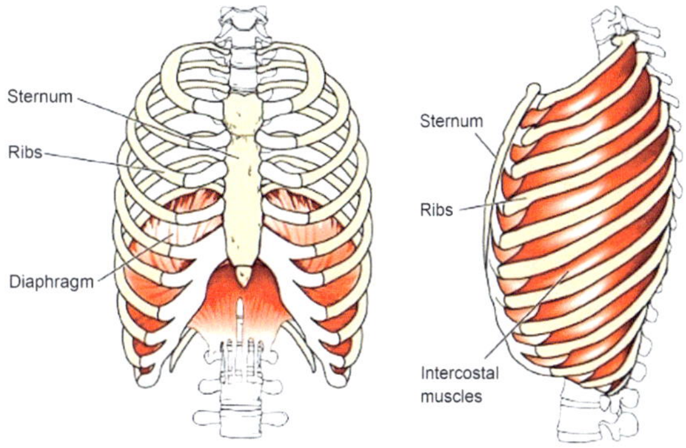

Figure 7.10. Sternum in the Rib Cage

Source: https://external-content.duckduckgo.com/iu/?u=https%3A%2F%2Fa-z-animals.com%2Fmedia%2F2023%2F03%2Fshutterstock_23857276.jpg&f=1&nofb=1&ipt=4956f051302c005750e843c33e81f88198f123bc8b3983e20d99753dd532bd44.

In addition to its functional and structural importance, the sternum is also important in thoracic growth and anthropometry studies. Changes in sternal morphology throughout growth phases influence the thoracic cage's shape and function as a whole. Research indicates that the early formation of adult-type thoracic shapes is encouraged by changes in the sternum and rib inclination as youngsters grow into adults. Since thoracic size varies during development, including expansion of the respiratory and alimentary tracts, the position and orientation of the sternum assume significance in achieving an optimum compromise between respiratory economy and structural stability. Therefore, understanding the role of the sternum in the rib cage not only sheds light on its significance from an anatomical point of view but also enhances thoracic development dynamics and disease and health implications (Barash et al., 2013) (Figure 7.10).

7.3.3. Clinical Significance of the Sternum

The clinical significance of the sternum extends beyond heart and lung protection; it is the foundation for numerous medical assessments and treatments. The sternum is an important landmark in thoracic surgery and procedures, including routine median sternotomy for cardiac surgeries. Familiarity with the morphology and development of the sternum is relevant for effective surgical planning and minimizing complications. For instance, the 3D geometry of the sternum will influence how surgery is performed to correct congenital heart anomalies or to perform transplant operations. This information is complemented by research on children's 3D sternum geometry, which shows that abnormalities in the sternum can have implications for diagnosing and treating thoracic complaints among pediatric patients (Badina et al., 2013). Additionally, the clinical evaluation of the sternum is important for diagnosing and treating other pathologic entities. Sternum abnormalities, such as pectus excavatum or pectus carinatum, can lead to respiratory and cardiovascular complications. The anomalies must be carefully evaluated, typically with imaging tests to determine their severity and the best therapeutic approach. Knowledge of the growth and development of sternal morphology from infancy to adulthood is integral; evidence suggests that sternal shape varies dramatically throughout growth, with a significant influence on overall thoracic shape and function (Barash et al., 2013). Clinicians must therefore be aware of such growth patterns to appropriately inform their management strategies, tailoring interventions to age and physical maturity. Besides, the relationship with other thoracic components enhances its importance within the overall clinical framework. Research has also shown that the anatomy of the sternum has been directly related to the growth and placement of adjacent ribs and costal cartilages. These relationships enhance the importance of the function of the sternum as a structure, but also as an impetus of the biomechanical function of the thorax. Sternal pathology can disrupt this equilibrium, and only with a full understanding can intervention be effective. As further research further enriches our understanding in the areas of sternal geometry and associated thoracic anomalies, clinical diagnostic accuracy and surgical interventions will be more precise, resulting in improved outcomes for patients undergoing thoracic intervention, emphasizing the clinical importance of sternums in contemporary medicine (Badina et al., 2013; Barash et al., 2013).

Test Your Knowledge

1. What are the anatomical regions of the sternum, and what is their functional significance in thoracic anatomy?
2. How does the sternum serve as an attachment point for ribs and muscles of the chest?

7.4. Rib Articulation

Learning Outcome

1. Costovertebral joints
2. Costochondral joints
3. Sternocostal joints

The rib joint is the most important feature of the thoracic skeleton, providing both structural support and flexibility to the trunk during breathing. Each rib articulates with the adjacent vertebrae at the costovertebral joint, allowing a dynamic range of motion essential for normal breathing patterns. This articulation allows the thoracic cavity to expand and contract on exhalation and inhalation, demonstrating the central role of the ribs in respiratory physiology. Furthermore, a greater understanding of rib articulations encourages an appreciation of evolutionary progress; rib forms have co-evolved alongside mammalian breathing mechanisms. The evolutionary alterations observed in the ribs demonstrate their functionally significant transformation from early tetrapods to modern mammals, thereby establishing a correlation between respiratory efficiency and skeletal structure. While examining the various forms of rib articulations, it is important to note the differences among true ribs, false ribs, and floating ribs, as each plays an important role in the thoracic structure. True ribs (ribs 1–7) are attached to the sternum directly by costal cartilage and give maximum support and protection to the organs inside. False ribs (ribs 8–10) attach indirectly to the sternum, which gives more flexibility to the thoracic cage and the capacity for respiratory expansion. Floating ribs (ribs 11–12) lack an anterior attachment and reduce weight but enhance mobility in the lower thorax. This differentiation of rib articulation types highlights the evolution towards a light yet strong skeletal system, optimizing protection and mobility in line with environmental needs.

These differences highlight the complexity of rib articulation, rendering it an area of research for the thoracic skeleton. Recent research using advanced imaging methods has uncovered complex patterns of growth of the rib cage, significantly impacting our current understanding of rib articulation's developmental characteristics. Three-dimensional morphology analysis of ribs shows that the adult thoracic form is attained earlier than previously believed, progressing from the newborn circular form to an ovoid in adults. Notably, the orientation of ribs changes throughout development, with the anterior edges descending below the posterior boundaries, indicating the complex interaction of growth mechanisms with function. Such a shift not only accounts for the required spatial relationships among the components of ribs but also examines the impact of differential rates of development of many thoracic systems. The larger adult thoracic dimensions provide important insights into how rib articulation improves breathing and muscular function across lifespan development (Barash et al., 2013; Bendel et al., 2022) (Figure 7.11).

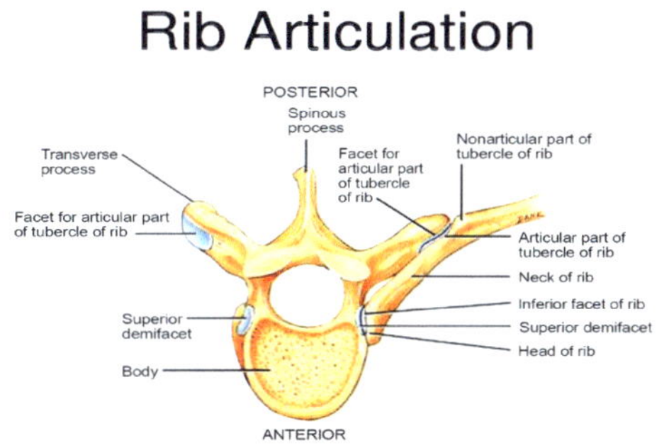

Figure 7.11. The rib articulation is a fundamental aspect of the thoracic skeleton.

Source: https://external-content.duckduckgo.com/iu/?u=http%3A%2F%2Fimage.slideserve.com%2F176541%2Frib-articulation-l.jpg&f=1&nofb=1&ipt=6893f49f692542c04bebcba586734c09c61552f94be52e76e68e54f6c85a0751.

7.4.1. Costovertebral Joints

The costovertebral joints, located within the thorax, are an element of the thoracic structure and function of the ribcage. These synovial joints articulate the thoracic vertebrae bodies and the rib heads to provide a dynamic range of motion through respiration. The joint comprises facets on the vertebral bodies and matching intervertebral discs, providing important stability and facilitating torsional movements important for lung inflation. Apart from holding the ribcage, the structure is essential in protecting vital thoracic organs. It is significant to learn the mechanics of these joints in the analysis of respiratory function as they give space for expansion and contraction of the thoracic cavity during exhalation and inhalation, thereby highlighting their significance in this anatomy and also in clinical work. Apart from their anatomical role in respiration, the costovertebral joints are significant in various pathological conditions, particularly those associated with spinal deformities such as scoliosis. A priori, studies emphasize the need to model such joints realistically when developing surgical solutions to correct these deformities. As an example, finite element models (FEM) have been designed to simulate the mechanical behavior of the thoracic spine and ribcage and thereby enable engineers and clinicians to make predictions about the outcomes of treatment such as bracing or surgery. These models examine clinical indices, such as rib hump and Cobb angles, in order to offer patient-specific solutions, thereby improving the precision of surgery and patient care.

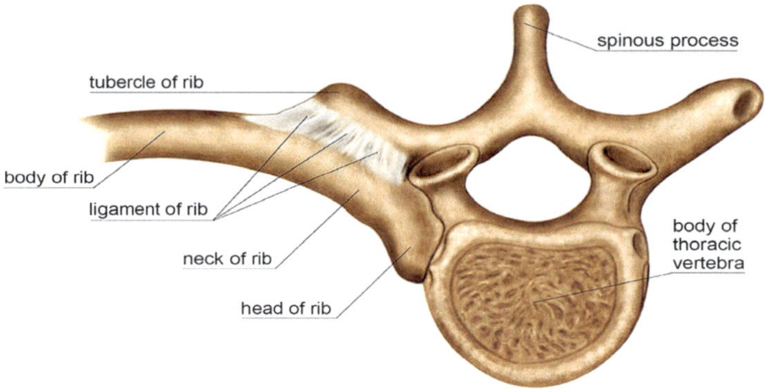

Figure 7.12. The costovertebral joints.

Source: https://external-content.duckduckgo.com/iu/?u=https%3A%2F%2Fimages.fineartamerica.com%2Fimages-medium-large-5%2Fcostovertebral-joint-asklepios-medical-atlas.jpg&f=1&nofb=1&ipt=2b77c9964a214fe68279e5ed3ee909cf33000cd5d5bed9f056eff1335cc42642.

These advances highlight the necessity of integrating anatomical data and biomechanical analysis to improve surgical outcomes and better understand the effects of thoracic deformity (Abelin-Genevois et al., 2016). Moreover, interaction between the costovertebral joints and surrounding soft tissues is essential for maintaining spinal function and integrity. Interposed between these joints are stabilizing intervertebral discs and enveloping ligaments, which contribute to stability and mobility with dynamic motion of the spine. Clinical assessment of how such structures respond to external load during motion—i.e., during lifting or torsion—is important for providing key input into rehabilitation programs after injury or surgical intervention. The biomechanical consequences of disrupted biomechanics, as seen in scoliosis, make it more difficult to relate to and lead to decreased range of motion and functional impairment. As highlighted by recent research, the accurate characterization of the stiffness properties in spinal finite element models can significantly influence the mechanical responses of the joints and consequently the surgery planning and surgical outcome after surgery (Polanco et al., 2022) (Figure 7.12).

7.4.2. Costochondral Joints

The costochondral joints, which are the articulations between the ribs and the costal cartilages, are important to the thoracic anatomy and have an impact on both respiratory mechanics and stability. These are not synovial joints in the classical sense but are cartilaginous joints, and while limited motion is present, it is necessary for the expansion and contraction of the thoracic cavity that occurs during the process of breathing. The flexibility of the costochondral joints enables the intercostal muscles and diaphragm to move effectively, which is essential for adequate ventilation. Moreover, the integrity of these joints is vital; any disease of these joints can affect mobility and respiratory status, hence it is of significant clinical importance in thoracic health and disease. Pathological joint disorders of the costochondral joints can result in severe pain and complications, and thus, a knowledge of them is essential in clinical practice. Among the common disorders of the joints are Costochondritis, Tietze syndrome, Slipping Rib Syndrome, and Rib Tip Syndrome. These conditions all share a unique clinical challenge due to the anatomical proximity of the costochondral joints to critical organs such as the lungs and heart, which can lead to symptoms that mimic far more serious conditions. This mimicry can lead to misdiagnosis or delayed treatment, underscoring the importance of proper clinical diagnosis and evaluation. Appropriate management strategies for these disorders are critical, aimed at inhibiting inflammation and alleviating pain while preserving joint function and overall thoracic mobility (Samimi et al., 2022). In addition, the biomechanical characteristics of the thorax, including the costochondral joints, are critical to understanding thoracic trauma, especially traumatic. The commonality with which thoracic injuries appear in scenarios such as road traffic accidents underlines the necessity of robust protective mechanisms within these regions, as recent evidence has highlighted. In line with these studies, costochondral trauma, despite often being underestimated, could be implicated in more complex thoracic traumas, of which sternal fractures are prominent in scenarios involving frontal impact. Their interaction with adjacent structures plays a pivotal role in understanding injury mechanisms and in the design of more effective restraint systems for automobiles that reduce the risk of such injuries (Novoa et al., 2018). Increasing knowledge about these joints will guide both therapeutic and preventive interventions in thoracic medicine.

7.4.3. Sternocostal Joints

The sternocostal joints, the cartilaginous joints of the costal cartilages of the first seven ribs with the sternum, are highly significant in the structure and function of the thorax. They are synovial joints with restricted movement, primarily respiration, and facilitate expansion and reduction of the thoracic cavity. All joints contribute to the overall elasticity and mobility of the rib cage required for normal breathing. The initial sternocostal joint, which directly connects the first rib with the manubrium, is a synchondrosis and is not very mobile. However, the remainder of the joints do permit infinitesimal gliding movements, which are essential for the mechanism of breathing and expiration. Understanding the anatomy and function of joints is important for understanding the biomechanics of breathing, especially across various physiological states (Piatsko et al., 2021). As the thorax dynamically changes with each respiratory cycle, it is essential that the function and integrity of the sternocostal joints remain unimpaired to maintain normal pulmonary function. Mobility of the joints not only enables augmented thoracic capacity during inspiration but also assists in the efficient expulsion of air during exhalation.

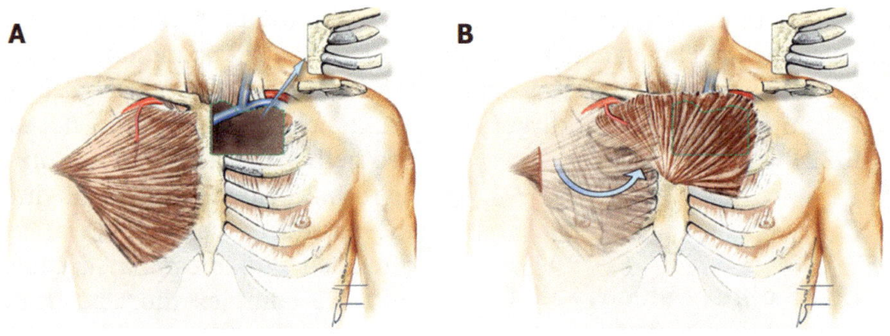

Figure 7.13. The sternocostal joints.

Source: https://external-content.duckduckgo.com/iu/?u=https%3A%2F%2Foaepublishstorage.blob.core.windows.net%2Fa5a6166f-ac1c-4f9a-b113-f529bcc7bbd6%2F2764.fig.1.png&f=1&nofb=1&ipt=53f0c86395d06f0bb505f56d8a48cf0d72b906c7a305528858a6defc06f16632.

Dysfunction or injury of the joints may result in restricted thoracic mobility and lead to pulmonary issues. Moreover, conditions such as costochondritis, an inflammatory condition of the cartilage of these joints, can significantly affect quality of life by causing pain and discomfort during breathing. Hence, assessment of sternocostal joints and nearby tissues could gain insight into bigger thoracic disorders, and hence, acquiring detailed knowledge of their anatomical and physiological aspects is important (Sposato et al., 2024). The clinical relevance of the sternocostal joints extends beyond mere respiratory mechanics; they also play a part in numerous musculoskeletal disorders. Patients with cystic fibrosis (CF), for instance, may exhibit abnormal thoracic mobility and musculoskeletal pain resulting from long-term alteration of thorax structure. Research indicates that decreased thoracic expansion and increased tender points are common in CF patients and may be associated with sternocostal joint dysfunction (Sposato et al., 2024). Manual therapy techniques be effective in pain reduction and the enhancement of thoracic mobility. Therefore, careful evaluation and treatment of these joints can be an important aspect of managing thoracic symptoms, particularly among groups with compromised respiratory function (Piatsko et al., 2021) (Figure 7.13).

Test Your Knowledge

1. How do ribs articulate with the thoracic vertebrae and sternum, and what types of joints are involved?
2. What is the significance of the costovertebral and costosternal joints in respiratory movements?

7.5. Muscles Associated with the Thorax

Learning Outcome

1. Intercostal muscles
2. Diaphragm
3. Accessory muscles of respiration

The thorax, which houses the ribs and sternum, is more than a protective cover for vital organs; it is also the site of significant muscular attachments to permit respiration and movement of the upper limbs. The major muscles of interest associated with the thorax include the intercostal muscles, the diaphragm, and some accessory muscles. The intercostal muscles, between the ribs, consist of external, internal, and innermost layers that play important roles in expanding and constricting the thoracic cavity to facilitate breathing. The external intercostals assist inhalation by elevating the ribs, whereas the internal intercostals assist forced exhalation by depressing the rib cage. Together, these muscles alter the size of the thorax, working in conjunction with the diaphragm, the primary muscle of inspiration, as it contracts to enlarge the vertical diameter of the thorax, thus drawing air into the lungs. In addition to the intercostal muscles and diaphragm, a few accessory muscles of respiration are called upon in more taxing exercise or respiratory distress. Among them are the sternocleidomastoid and scalene muscles, which elevate the first and second ribs to create additional space for inhalation. The functional competence of these muscles will become impaired with advancing age, leading to altered breathing patterns and thoracic dimensions. Such anemic decline is usually expressed as other anatomical changes that influence respiratory capacity, as studies have shown that thoracic cage dimensions differ significantly across age and body composition. Knowledge of these age-related changes in the thoracic wall and musculature is important for health professionals to distinguish normal aging processes from possible pathological conditions, providing insight into respiratory health throughout life (Joshua et al., 2014). Research of postnatal development and growth of the thoracic cage also sheds light on muscular adaptations observed across a lifetime. It is known that the thoracic shape undergoes striking alterations from infancy to maturity, with changes across anatomical regions driven by the development of respiratory and other systemic processes (Barash et al., 2013). Far from being merely structural, such alterations have significant impacts on respiratory mechanics. For example, the development from a pyramidal infant thorax to an adult barrel-shaped thorax shows how the muscles develop to meet increasing respiratory demands over time, particularly as activity patterns vary. By studying the ontogenetic growth of the thoracic skeleton, researchers can better understand how the relationship between muscular and skeletal growth affects respiratory efficiency, emphasizing the overall significance of muscular integrity to thoracic function and general health.

7.5.1. Intercostal Muscles

Of all the structures of the thorax, the intercostal muscles are most importantly central to the accommodation of respiratory motion and preservation of the rib cage's structural integrity. These muscles, between two succeeding ribs, are divided into external, internal, and innermost layers, each with different functions. The external intercostals are primarily involved during inspiration by elevating the ribs and expanding the volume of the thoracic cavity and hence the lungs. On the other hand, the internal intercostals are primarily involved in forced expiration, lowering the ribs and reducing thoracic volume. This interactive mechanism not only highlights the vital functional characteristics of intercostal muscles during respiration but also demonstrates their significance for thoracic stability during various physical exercises. Histochemical staining reveals that intercostal muscles have a heterogeneous profile of muscle fibers, which is proportional to their breathing functions. In a study of the cat intercostal muscles, three fiber types were characterized based on enzymatic activity, and their functional capabilities were described. Interestingly enough, the cranial and caudal parts of the thorax, with a larger proportion of red fibers, are primarily engaged in passive breathing movements. In contrast, those in the central thorax with more white fibers are best suited for muscle contraction during forced breathing.

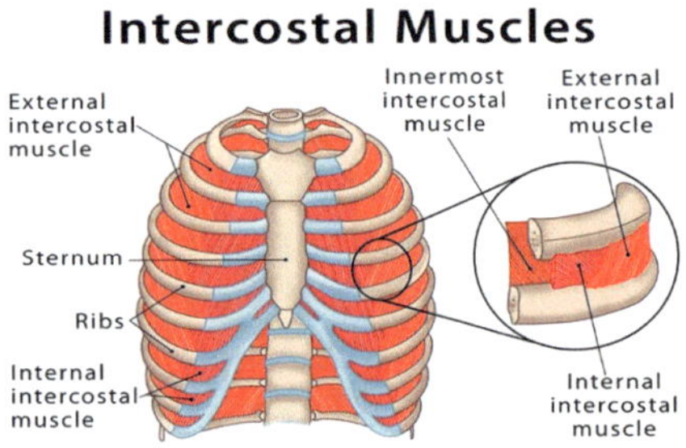

Figure 7.14. The intercostal muscles.

Source: https://external-content.duckduckgo.com/iu/?u=https%3A%2F%2Fi.pinimg.com%2F736x%2F18%2Fdb%2Fbf%2F18dbbf5fbad92f986453c956ae941520.jpg&f=1&nofb=1&ipt=4b5517d689d30be4fe9678cdd5fb649136e23d6d61f782fd349d109523218b1a.

This muscle fiber type difference underscores the unique functions of intercostal muscles during breathing and exercise, thereby influencing thoracic mechanics and overall pulmonary function (Nishiyama et al., 1965). Moreover, intercostal muscles are important for coordinating locomotion and respiration, particularly in species such as bottlenose dolphins. There is evidence that although these marine mammals have learned to relate ventilatory activity to swimming, intercostal muscles are still involved in airflow management. The anatomy of muscles allows rapid changes in the volume of the thoracic cavity, making possible explosive inhalation—the activity critical for surfacing and effective oxygen acquisition (Cotten et al., 2009). Consequently, the functional anatomy of intercostal muscles has applications beyond locomotion on land, as illustrated across species and environments. In all, such observations testify to the intercostal muscles' significant role in thoracic respiratory mechanics as well as their adaptive role in a range of physiological conditions (Figure 7.14).

7.5.2. Diaphragm

The diaphragm is arguably the most significant of the thoracic cavity muscles and plays the role of respiration, in addition to marking the separation between the thoracic and abdominal cavities. In the shape of an inverted dome, during contraction upon inhaling, the diaphragm flattens to create negative pressure that sucks air into the lungs. Apart from facilitating easier respiration, this process is also responsible for delivering air within the lungs' alveoli to facilitate gas exchange. The interaction between the diaphragm and ribcage is intricate; whereas, during inspiration, the ribs expand outward, the diaphragm acts in synchronism to increase thoracic capacity. There is a need to understand the intricate interactions, as imbalances can lead to respiratory disease. Morphological or functional diaphragmatic defects can significantly affect the stability and respiratory efficiency of the overall thorax, underscoring their implications for thoracic anatomy and physiology. In thoracic skeletal developmental research, diaphragm growth and function have been of significant interest, so that it has enlightened how the morphology of the thorax is formed. The study indicates that an adult-like thorax shape emerges early in infancy, yet the diaphragm remains dynamic to variations in the growth patterns of the upper and lower thoracic regions. Changes in the curvature and orientation of the ribs, as described in previous studies, are a function of changes in the diaphragm's response to airflow and pressure differences (Barash et al., 2013). Not only do these changes facilitate efficient respiratory movement, but they also increase the mechanical efficiency of the thorax when fully grown.

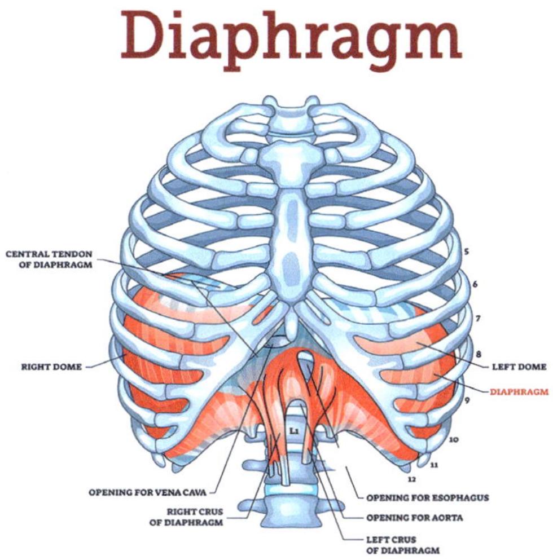

Figure 7.15. The diaphragm is a crucial muscle within the thoracic cavity.

Source: https://external-content.duckduckgo.com/iu/?u=https%3A%2F%2Fassets.lybrate.com%2Ff_auto%2Cc_limit%2Cw_3840%2Cq_auto%2Fimgs%2Ftic%2Fenadp%2Fimage-of-the-diaphragm.jpg&f=1&nofb=1&ipt=a9367f2f5dd79d05fd0d89f3872b7a0a951eae9daf7940f05c79ecf97d6ebd54.

Thus, the evolution of the diaphragm is closely linked to broader anatomical development, further solidifying its role within the larger context of thoracic structure and respiratory function. Beyond its direct respiratory function, the diaphragm is also significant in terms of postural maintenance and stability within the thoracic cavity. The diaphragm is coordinated with the muscles connecting to the ribs and sternum to create the overall posture of the thorax and to influence locomotion patterns. With the evolution of mammals, the function of the diaphragm increased, as this was followed by alterations in ribcage mechanisms and sternum structures (Bendel et al., 2022). The diaphragm facilitates proper force transfer during breathing and upper-body movement. This interaction also has broad implications for mammalian physiology and evolutionary biology since the diaphragm not only aids in breathing but also enables sophisticated motor function and postural adjustments essential for survival (Figure 7.15).

7.5.3. Accessory Muscles of Respiration

Accessory muscles of respiration play a vital role in amplifying the efficiency of breathing, particularly during increased respiratory demand, such as physical activity or respiratory distress. These muscles are mainly located in the thoracic cavity and include the sternocleidomastoid, the scalene group, and the pectoralis major and minor. These muscles assist immensely by elevating the rib cage and the thoracic cavity during inspiration. Their action becomes particularly critical when the diaphragm is insufficient to meet the body's oxygen requirements, underscoring their critical role in respiratory physiology. An understanding of the specific anatomical position and functional capabilities of these muscles sheds light on the complexity of thoracic movement and respiration and provides a heightened appreciation of the thorax's role in respiratory health and efficacy. As far as thoracic anatomy is concerned, the accessory muscles are coupled with the ribs and sternum, thereby giving them a mechanical advantage during respiration. Upon contraction and expansion of the rib cage, the points of attachment of these accessory muscles facilitate the movement of the ribs such that the volume of the lung is increased and gas exchange is more efficient. The ribs, particularly the superior true ribs, provide attachment sites for these muscles, which then have the strength needed for active inspiration. Also, during effortful expiration, the muscles contribute to thoracic compression, demonstrating their multimodal role in both inspiration and expiration. Thus, coordination between the ribs, sternum, and accessory muscles constitutes a dynamic support system which is crucial to effective respiratory performance, particularly during conditions of physiological stress. New technological advances in respiratory monitoring also highlight the importance of being familiar with the accessory muscles of respiration. Wearable device systems, for instance, based on accelerometric signals for monitoring rib movement enable more active involvement in respiratory examination and rehabilitation (Ambrogi et al., 2022). These technologies offer a new understanding of the role of accessory muscles in total respiratory mechanics, underscoring their importance in both sporting and clinical settings. Functional use of such devices is based on a complete understanding of thoracic structure and function. Therefore, ongoing research on the monitoring and evaluation of such muscles is needed, not only to maximize sports performance but also to facilitate recovery for individuals with impaired or diseased breathing, underscoring the imperative interdependency among the anatomical elements of the thorax during breathing (Flack et al., 1921).

Test Your Knowledge

1. Which muscles are primarily involved in respiration, and how do they facilitate inspiration and expiration?
2. How do accessory thoracic muscles contribute to movements of the rib cage during forced breathing?

7.6. Common Injuries and Disorders

Learning Outcome

1. Rib fracture
2. Costochondritis
3. Sternum injury

Thoracic injuries, particularly of the ribs and sternum, are regularly encountered in both clinical and sporting situations. Blunt trauma-induced fractures of the ribs are one of the most frequent blunt trauma-induced injuries, such as those resulting from falls or car accidents. These fractures can potentially lead to serious complications, such as pneumothorax or hemothorax, which significantly affect respiratory function. Moreover, the pain of rib fractures usually inhibits a patient from taking deep breaths, leading to secondary complications like atelectasis or pneumonia from reduced lung expansion. Rib fracture diagnosis typically requires imaging modalities such as chest X-rays or CT scans to assess the extent of the fracture and rule out associated thoracic organ injuries, demonstrating the significance of careful clinical examination in cases of chest trauma. In addition to fractures, several disorders can affect the rib cage and sternum to produce chronic pain and functional limitation. One of the more significant disorders is costochondritis, characterized by inflammation of the costal cartilage connecting the ribs to the sternum. It most commonly occurs as localized anterior chest pain with the risk of mimicking more significant cardiac problems, so correct diagnosis is crucial. Treatment is generally aimed at measures controlling pain, including anti-inflammatory medications and physical therapy to rectify associated musculoskeletal imbalances. Of particular interest is to consider muscular factors, such as the role of the pectoralis minor muscle; tension in this muscle has been linked with altering scapular motion and possibly exacerbating symptoms of pain associated with the shoulder, secondarily impacting thoracic conditions as well (Cruz et al., 2016). Furthermore, forensic analysis has further valued the function of imaging in assessing injury to the thorax, particularly in cases of sharp force trauma. PMCT studies have revealed that even though soft tissue lesions are more prevalent, thoracic bone trauma is frequently seen and can indicate the cause of death, i.e., suicide or homicide (Braun et al., 2022). The addition of cutting-edge imaging modalities to forensic anthropology not only enhances the identification of sharp force trauma but also enhances injury pattern knowledge regarding various circumstances of death. With changing curricula of health care professional education, training in the use of imaging for assessing trauma becomes a must, so that forensic professionals can assess correctly the complexity of thoracic trauma and its bearing in the medical and legal fields.

7.6.1. Rib Fractures

Rib fractures, the most common manifestation of thoracic trauma, typically occur from direct trauma or from excessive force against the chest wall. Such fractures are most prevalent under conditions such as automobile accidents, when the rib cages' structural integrity is compromised due to blunt trauma. The biomechanics of ribs and their protective sheath for vital organs highlight the clinical importance of such injuries. Rib fractures also most frequently occur concomitantly with other traumas of the thorax, such as pneumothorax or hemothorax, which can significantly enhance their clinical severity. Understanding the mechanics of rib injury is important in maximizing prevention techniques and treatment procedures in trauma care to enable medical personnel to effectively deal with the intricacies involved in these kinds of injuries and their potential complications. A rib fracture classification typically entails a simple fracture where a single crack appears on the rib and a complex fracture where multiple ribs may be involved or lead to a complication like flail chest. A dramatic example is the presentation of severe chest wall trauma from high-energy impacts, such as complete bony disruption of the thoracic cage, as in the case of all-terrain vehicle injuries. They will often demand multidisciplinary treatment. A good evaluation of rib fractures can be achieved by having uniform criteria, such as the Abbreviated Injury Scale (AIS), to help clinicians grade the severity and impact of injury as a whole.

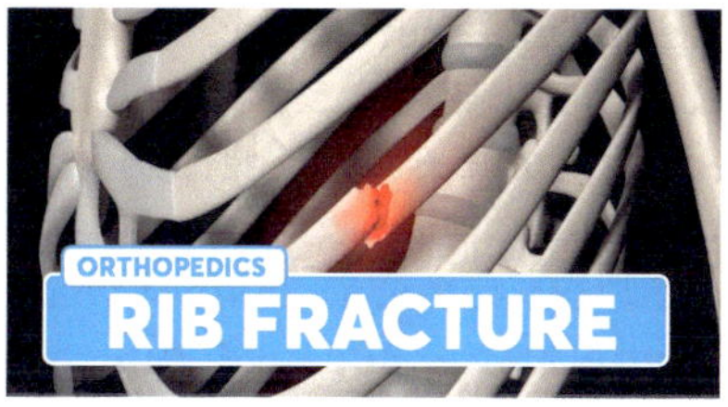

Figure 7.16. Rib fractures.

Source: https://external-content.duckduckgo.com/iu/?u=https%3A%2F%2Fimage.prepladder.com%2Fprepladder%2F2024%2F03%2F05071541%2FRib-Fracture.webp&f=1&nofb=1&ipt=ab97ad38d8b046d1e77cf9d66191e153b58a663d2b149b7b1816472eabe03016.

The requirement for detailed imaging and classification cannot be overstated, as the results directly correlate with prognosis and recovery. More recent biomechanical models are being developed to comprehend rib fractures and associated injuries further. Research has indicated that impact on present criteria can be improved by altering the model to account for personal morphologies and particular loading conditions. The development of mathematical models that account for soft-tissue effects and are not constrained by other criteria provides a more accurate representation of injury mechanisms. As highlighted by recent studies, translating these biomechanical factors into clinical practice can improve injury management. The dynamic nature of thoracic injury evaluation fosters ongoing development of approaches to rib fractures, ultimately culminating in improved patient care and outcomes across different clinical settings (Burlew et al., 2012; Havr Mánek, 2020) (Figure 7.16).

7.6.2. Costochondritis

Costochondritis, defined as a frequent inflammation of the cartilage that links the ribs to the sternum, is a common thoracic disorder. Costochondritis can be extremely painful and annoying in the chest region, which is also referred to for serious conditions such as cardiac events, and therefore requires extensive diagnostic workups. Tenderness in costosternal, costochondral, or costovertebral joints is also the patient's frequent complaint, difficulties exacerbated by motion, deep breathing, or special maneuvers. Because questioning of the junction of structures of rib and sternum and of powerful mechanics occurring there is valuable to general knowledge of the thorax, knowledge of costochondritis is valuable as well in its illustration of musculoskeletal health's complex interdependence in this area. It emphasizes accurate diagnosis and management, encouraging early intervention to maximize symptom relief and patient quality of life. The etiological factors of costochondritis remain multifactorial, including possible acute trauma, repetitive trauma, or even strain from physical exertion. In the majority of cases, the direct etiology may be elusive, complicating treatment options. Alternatively, etiologies such as infection or arthritis can also cause the inflammation, broadening the differential diagnosis. Also, the lack of definitive diagnostic tests further underscores the need for judicious clinical evaluation and patient history to exclude other thoracic diseases in cases of costochondritis. Conservative treatment is usually the treatment of choice, comprising NSAIDs and targeted physical therapy. However, understanding the biomechanics of the rib cage, as outlined in the literature on thoracic structures, can enhance treatment outcomes and enable clinicians to develop personalized, effective rehabilitation programs for affected individuals. Regarding prevalence and consequences, costochondritis most commonly occurs in individuals aged 20–40. Its implications extend well beyond simple discomfort, as it can significantly limit daily functioning and overall quality of life. This thoracic dysfunction may be a cause of psychological distress and anxiety, often secondary to fear of cardiac illness with the onset of chest pain. Education and awareness of costochondritis are thus important both for patients and health professionals. Knowing that this condition is frequently self-limiting enables patients to seek appropriate care and to understand the importance of thoracic function within the sphere of musculoskeletal fitness. This perception engenders an assertive approach to health, the emphasis here being on the necessity of interventional intervention, maintaining functional capability and relieving suffering as a result of this pervasive thoracic injury.

7.6.3. Sternum Injuries

Sternal injuries, though comparatively infrequent in incidence when compared with rib fractures, are a significant problem in thoracic trauma owing to the sternum's position as a central defense organ. The breastbone, or sternum, is a vital part of the thoracic skeleton, securing the ribs and providing structural integrity to the chest wall. Such injuries often happen due to high-impact trauma, i.e., road traffic accidents or sports trauma, leading to sternal fractures or contusions.

The clinical importance may be substantial; a fracture will induce complications, which include chest pain, difficulty in breathing, or even cardiogenic damage. A knowledge of mechanisms of such injuries is therefore important in effective diagnosis and management in clinical practice so that practitioners can avoid morbidity due to such trauma. Diagnosis of sternal injury is usually made by careful clinical evaluation supported by imaging studies. Physical examination may be positive for localized deformity, tenderness, or even swelling, depending upon the extent of injury. Diagnostic imaging, such as chest X-rays or CT scans, may provide invaluable insight into the extent of damage to the sternum and the structures involved. Appropriate diagnosis is necessary since inadequate treatment may lead to chronic pain or respiratory issues. Interestingly, the assessment can also encompass variables such as the incidence of a rib injury underlying the sternal wound and the possibility of concomitant vascular or lung injury, which might complicate the clinical picture. In treating sternal trauma, a general picture that considers the general condition of the patient's thorax is paramount in providing the best possible recovery.

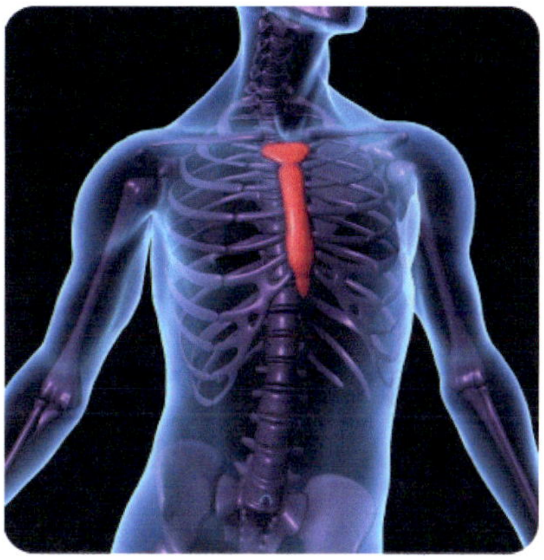

Figure 7.17. Sternum injuries.

Source: https://lirp.cdn-website.com/1b4eeb64/dms3rep/multi/opt/sternum-injury-attorney-640w.png.

Treatment for sternum injuries is based on the severity and nature of the injury. In uncomplicated sternal fractures that are simple, conservative treatment through relief of pain and restriction of activity is most commonly sufficient. Severer fractures, particularly those with displacement or complications, can be surgically treated, however. Rehabilitation is important in the recovery process, with the goal of achieving functional mobility and strength of the thoracic region. This is typically multimodal and incorporates physiotherapy to treat associated impairments of the shoulder girdle. For instance, adaptive shortening or tightening of the pectoralis minor muscle (PMm) may influence thoracic function, underscoring the need for precise stretching interventions, as discussed in studies on shoulder movement-related impairments (Cruz et al., 2016; Wilkinson et al., 2019). By understanding the intricate nature of sternum injuries, medical clinicians can contribute to better patient outcomes through effective treatment and rehabilitation strategies (Figure 7.17).

Test Your Knowledge

1. What are the most common injuries of the thorax, including rib fractures, and how do they affect respiration?
2. How do pathological conditions like scoliosis, flail chest, or thoracic deformities impact the function of the thoracic cavity?

SUMMARY

Overall, the thoracic skeleton and rib cage, comprising ribs and sternum, play a significant role in the thorax's overall structural stability and function. Not only does the thoracic skeleton protect vital organs such as the heart and lungs, but it also provides an important anchor point for respiratory and upper limb movement muscles. The linkage of the ribs to the thoracic vertebrae and the sternum facilitates dynamic expansion and contraction of the thoracic cavity, enabling efficient breathing. This advanced structure indicates the adaptability that has enabled mammals to attain maximum respiratory modes to cater to the varying demands in metabolism. The necessity of such body structures becomes apparent when attempting to explain the sophisticated problems organisms face in different environments, thereby increasing the value of the thoracic skeleton as the pillar of life. In addition, an anatomical understanding of the thorax provides deeper insight into pathological defects that may impede respiratory processes. Pathological states such as fractures of the ribs or injuries of the sternum immediately influence the ability of the thoracic cavity to enlarge. This is to highlight the importance of rib cage stability and functionality in ensuring respiratory efficiency. The interconnection of the thoracic musculatures with the ribs also illustrates the interconnection between structural form and functional ability. It has been proven that muscle structures, such as the intercostals, play an important role in modulating respiratory function. Thus, an exploration of these relations not only enhances knowledge of thoracic function in the intact state but also advances understanding of thoracic injury rehabilitation strategies and, by extension, the broader field of medical education and practice. A comparison of thoracic anatomy across species reveals significant evolutionary patterns that enhance understanding of respiratory adaptation. For instance, in bottlenose dolphins, the coordination of respiratory and locomotory systems exhibits a remarkable adaptation for breath-hold swimming. The morphological and functional characteristics of thoracic muscles in aquatic mammals, as discussed in studies, indicate that the systems have been shaped by evolutionary forces to make optimal performance in water. These findings provoke further research of thoracic skeleton evolution in other taxa and result in new lines of research in anatomy and physiology. By expanding the knowledge of the evolutionary significance of the thorax, we may possibly find new directions in vertebrate biology studies, which eventually help support the relevance of the ribs and sternum in various aspects of biology, e.g., those indicated by Busard et al. (2017) and Cotten et al. (2009).

The thorax, encompassing the ribs and sternum, is a pivotal part of the human skeleton, protecting the respiratory system and defending vital organs such as the heart and lungs. Understanding rib morphology in detail is important, especially considering the variations of rib shapes in different populations. Current research has explained that age, sex, and body morphology contribute significantly to rib characteristics. Specifically, older populations exhibit less steep-cut and more flat rib contours, with an increase in rib span and aspect ratio. These parameters directly influence the biomechanical behavior of ribs, i.e., their resistance to deformation, highlighting the need for age-based models that can accommodate demographic variations in the population (Holcombe et al., 2025). In addition to age-related alterations in rib geometry, mechanisms of injury in thoracic impacts have also attracted increasing attention, particularly in car crashes. Side-impact crashes pose a unique challenge due to the proximity of the torso to inflating side airbags, which may result in severe thoracoabdominal injuries. It is crucial to understand the biomechanical response of the rib cage to such impacts, from which useful occupant safety designs can be engineered. Recent research indicates that injury to the posterolateral thorax is highly correlated with close-proximity airbag deployment (Hallman et al., 2010). This necessitates an immediate re-evaluation of current injury measures and occupant surrogate design to detect these delicate biomechanical correlations. Generally, findings on thoracic anatomy and injury biomechanics emphasize the intricate interactions among rib structure, age, and susceptibility to injury. Researchers are now employing advanced modelling techniques that incorporate population-specific parameters to enhance the precision of simulations used in safety assessments. Addressing biomechanical differences across populations, computational models can provide critical insights to prevent injuries in clinical and automotive safety contexts. Illustrating the need for continuous research, such studies create space for more expansive protective systems, ensuring that all populations' health and well-being are protected within the health care system and transportation safety systems (Hallman et al., 2010; Holcombe et al., 2025).

KEY TERMS FROM THIS CHAPTER

- Body of Sternum
- Costal Groove
- False Ribs
- Head of Rib
- Jugular Notch
- Ribs
- Sternal Angle (Angle of Louis)
- Costal Cartilage
- Costovertebral Joint
- Floating Ribs
- Intercostal Space
- Manubrium
- Shaft of Rib
- Sternum

CRITICAL THINKING QUESTIONS

1. **There are how many pairs of ribs in the human body?**
   a. 10
   b. 12
   c. 14
   d. 16
2. **What type of ribs are directly connected to the sternum?**
   a. Floating ribs
   b. True ribs
   c. False ribs
   d. Sesamoid ribs
3. **Which ribs are "floating ribs"?**
   a. Ribs 1-7
   b. Ribs 8-10
   c. Ribs 11-12
   d. Ribs 1-5
4. **What is the manubrium?**
   a. The topmost part of the sternum
   b. The middle section of the sternum
   c. A bone within the rib cage
   d. A joint between the ribs
5. **Which rib joins the manubrium and the body of the sternum?**
   a. First rib
   b. Second rib
   c. Third rib
   d. Tenth rib

Short Answer Questions

1. How many ribs does the human body contain, and what groups are they in?
2. Explain the structures of an average rib.
3. Discuss the function played by the intercostal spaces.
4. Explain the articulation of the ribs with the thoracic vertebrae.
5. Explain the use of the term "thoracic inlet" and why it is significant.
6. Explain the difference between the anterior and posterior ends of a rib.

Answers to Critical Thinking Questions

1. (b); 2. (b); 3. (c); 4. (a); 5. (b)

REFERENCES

1. Vergari C, Ribes G, Aubert B, Adam C, Miladi L, Ilharreborde B, Abelin-Genevois K, Rouch P, Skalli W. Evaluation of a Patient-Specific Finite-Element Model to Simulate Conservative Treatment in Adolescent Idiopathic Scoliosis. *Spine Deform.* 2015 Jan;3(1):4-11. doi: 10.1016/j.jspd.2014.06.014.Ambrogi, V., Ceccarelli, M., Papuc, P. E., et al. (2022). An analysis of respiration with the smart sensor SENSIRIB in patients undergoing thoracic surgery. https://core.ac.uk/download/553871737.pdf (accessed on 18th July 2025).
2. Badina, A., Lambot, K., Laporte, S., et al. (2013). Quantitative geometric analysis of rib, costal cartilage and sternum from childhood to teenagehood. https://core.ac.uk/download/29137508.pdf (accessed on 18th July 2025).
3. Barash, A., Bastir, M., Coquerelle, M., et al. (2013). Differential growth and development of the upper and lower human thorax. https://core.ac.uk/download/19025308.pdf (accessed on 18th July 2025).
4. Bendel, E. M., Fröbisch, J., Kammerer, C. F., et al. (2022). The earliest segmental sternum in a Permian synapsid and its implications for the evolution of mammalian locomotion and ventilation. https://core.ac.uk/download/611857947.pdf (accessed on 18th July 2025).
5. Braun, S., Indra, L., Lösch, S., et al. (2022). Perimortem skeletal sharp force trauma: Detection reliability on CT data, demographics and anatomical patterns from a forensic dataset. https://core.ac.uk/download/527936833.pdf (accessed on 18th July 2025).
6. Buchholtz, E. A. (2025). Crossing the frontier: A hypothesis for the origins of meristic constraint in mammalian axial patterning. https://core.ac.uk/download/pdf/217014198.pdf (accessed on 18th July 2025).
7. Burlew, C., Moore, E. E., Bailey, J., Jordan, J., Stahel, P. F., Pinski-Sibbel, S., & VanderHeiden, T. (2012). Thoracic hyperextension injury with complete "bony disruption" of the thoracic cage: Case report of a potentially life-threatening injury. https://core.ac.uk/download/pdf/81615493.pdf (accessed on 18th July 2025).
8. Busard, F., Capitummino, R., Carini, F., et al. (2017). Experiences that "reach the heart": Taking part in a whole-body dissection course at the University of Malta. https://core.ac.uk/download/127501248.pdf (accessed on 18th July 2025).
9. Chan, L. K. (2014). The thoracic shape of hominoids. https://core.ac.uk/download/38047959.pdf (accessed on 18th July 2025).
10. Coelho, T. H., Fonseca, J. C., Neves, S. C., et al. (2015). Finite element analysis of pectus carinatum surgical correction via a minimally invasive approach. https://core.ac.uk/download/55633679.pdf (accessed on 18th July 2025).
11. Cotten, P. B., NC DOCKS at The University of North Carolina Wilmington. (2009). The gross morphology and histochemistry of respiratory muscles in bottlenose dolphins (*Tursiops truncatus*). https://core.ac.uk/download/149230384.pdf (accessed on 18th July 2025).
12. Cruz, J., & Morais, N. (2016). The pectoralis minor muscle and shoulder movement-related impairments and pain: Rationale, assessment and management. https://core.ac.uk/download/160796671.pdf (accessed on 18th July 2025).
13. Flack, M. (1921). The Milroy lectures on respiratory efficiency in relation to health and disease. https://core.ac.uk/download/pdf/211978526.pdf (accessed on 18th July 2025).

14. Hallman, J. J. (2010). Detrimental thoracoabdominal interaction with lateral airbag restraints. https://core.ac.uk/download/67759458.pdf (accessed on 18th July 2025).

15. Havránek, M. (2020). The biomechanics of thoracic trauma. https://core.ac.uk/download/333594828.pdf (accessed on 18th July 2025).

16. Holcombe, S. (2025). The development of population-wide descriptions of human rib and rib cage geometry. http://deepblue.lib.umich.edu/bitstream/2027.42/135879/1/svenho_1.pdf (accessed on 18th July 2025).

17. Joshua, A., Pare, V., & Shetty, L. (2014). Variations in dimensions and shape of thoracic cage with aging: An anatomical review. https://core.ac.uk/download/478454162.pdf (accessed on 18th July 2025).

18. Larsson, K. J. (2023). Human body model morphing for assessment of crash rib fracture risk for the population of car occupants. https://core.ac.uk/download/571661922.pdf (accessed on 18th July 2025).

19. N/A. (2025). ICD-10-CM Tabular list of diseases and injuries. https://core.ac.uk/download/619625079.pdf (accessed on 18th July 2025).

20. Nishiyama, A. (1965). Histochemical studies on the red, white, and intermediate muscle fibers of some skeletal muscles. I. Succinic dehydrogenase activity and physiological function of intercostal muscle fibers. https://core.ac.uk/download/12548216.pdf (accessed on 18th July 2025).

21. Paulson, M. M. (2023). Comparison of male and female rib sternal ends and the effects of aging using elliptical Fourier analysis. https://core.ac.uk/download/578419555.pdf (accessed on 18th July 2025).

22. Piatsko, I. A., Tolyaronok, D. A., Usovich, A. K., et al. (2021). Work book in human anatomy. Locomotion apparatus. https://core.ac.uk/download/427551151.pdf (accessed on 18th July 2025).

23. Polanco, M. A. (2022). Utilization of finite element analysis techniques for adolescent idiopathic scoliosis surgical planning. https://core.ac.uk/download/534831653.pdf (accessed on 18th July 2025).

24. Samimi, K. (2022). An overview of costochondral disorders. https://open.bu.edu/bitstream/2144/43727/8/Samimi_bu_0017N_16150.pdf (accessed on 18th July 2025).

25. Schowalter, S., Le, B., Creps, J., & McInnis, K. C. (2022). Rib fractures in professional baseball pitchers: Mechanics, epidemiology, and management. *Open Access Journal of Sports Medicine, 13*, 89–105. https://doi.org/10.2147/oajsm.s288882 (accessed on 18th July 2025).

26. Segura Novoa, R. D. (2018). Occupant protection design with FE human body models. https://core.ac.uk/download/216096500.pdf (accessed on 18th July 2025).

27. Sinderholm Sposato, N. (2024). Thoracic mobility in cystic fibrosis care. https://core.ac.uk/download/620664403.pdf (accessed on 18th July 2025).

28. Stemmer, K. (2016). Characterization of loading environment on human ribs during ventilation. https://core.ac.uk/download/159557922.pdf (accessed on 18th July 2025).

29. van den Broek, D. H. N., Vester, S. C., Tobón Restrepo, M., & Veraa, S. (2023). Sternal abnormalities on thoracic radiographs of dogs and cats. *Animals, 13*(1233). https://doi.org/10.3390/ani13071233 (accessed on 18th July 2025).

30. Whittingham, L. (1248174). (2016). Biomechanical assessment of sports bra performance. https://core.ac.uk/download/288370873.pdf (accessed on 18th July 2025).

31. Wilkinson, A. E. (2019). Injuries of the chest. https://core.ac.uk/download/478315987.pdf (accessed on 18th July 2025).

THE SHOULDER GIRDLE AND UPPER LIMB IN HUMAN OSTEOLOGY

8

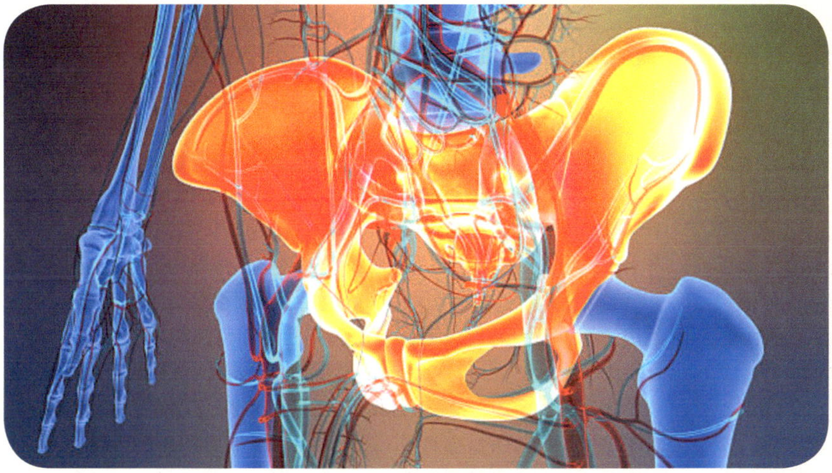

LEARNING OBJECTIVES

After studying this chapter, you will be able to:

1. Discuss the anatomy of the shoulder girdle
2. Focus on the bones of the upper limb
3. Explain the muscles associated with the shoulder girdle
4. Focus on the development and growth of the shoulder girdle
5. Know common injuries and disorders
6. Know the evolutionary perspective

Introduction

Human osteology is of paramount importance in determining the anatomical and functional complexities of the upper limb and shoulder girdle. These aspects are necessary for facilitating varied modes of movement and skilled functions, which are vital for life and social interaction across various environments. An understanding of the intricate biomechanics of the shoulder girdle, and particularly its joints and muscles, allows us to appreciate how human anatomical wholeness has been shaped by evolutionary accommodation. As discussed under Archosauria, limb morphology changes directly affect joint function and muscle activity, further enhancing our understanding of the evolution of the shoulder and upper limb apparatus in humans (Allen et al., 2017). Furthermore, the significance of haptic learning in osteology education underscores the need for experiential learning in studying these anatomical features. Online pedagogies, particularly highlighted during the COVID-19 pandemic, posed unique challenges in biological anthropology courses, e.g., Human Osteology (Gamble et al., 2024). Such conventional methods of learning through physical contact with skeletons are crucial in mastering skills such as bone recognition and age or sex estimation. The use of sensory materials, i.e., plastic model skeletons, in distance learning enabled students to achieve basic osteological objectives comparable to those of students who learned in conventional laboratory settings. This accommodation illustrates how modern pedagogical approaches intersect with the quest for ancient learning, offering a comprehensive foundation of knowledge in human skeletal anatomy. The significance of the study of the shoulder girdle and upper limb goes beyond basic anatomical knowledge; it reveals information regarding functional adaptation and evolutionary history. Locomotor strategy evolution, as seen across different lineages of Archosauria, helps illustrate how limb-structure adaptations have impacted physiological ability over time (Allen et al., 2017). In human beings, the characteristic anatomy of the shoulder girdle and its muscles promotes not only bipedalism but also enhances fine motor skills inherent in everyday activities. A study of these systems in detail illustrates the complexity of transmission of forces and joint dynamics, essential to both old and new anthropological research. Identification of the fundamental features of the shoulder girdle and upper limb is thus essential, as they form the basis for subsequent study of human evolution and mechanical function in broader osteological terms.

Definition of the Shoulder Girdle and Upper Limb

The shoulder girdle and upper limb are a highly evolved anatomical system that provides a vast array of movements and functional capabilities in human individuals. The pectoral girdle, or shoulder girdle, consists of the scapula and clavicle that connect with the sternum and permit upper limb mobility and stability. This configuration is the master key for not only locomotion but also , delicate tasks like manipulation and tool use, and hence its significance in evolution. The upper limb itself consists of the humerus, radius, ulna, carpals, metacarpals, and phalanges. All of these components play a vital role in facilitating upper limb function, including reaching, grasping, and fine motor activity, and they reflect the synergy of anatomy and function in human evolution. Moreover, the shoulder girdle is also accountable for the increased range of upper limb motion due to its unique ball-and-socket joint formed by the humeral head articulating with the glenoid cavity of the scapula. This configuration supports several movements, including flexion, extension, abduction, adduction, and rotation of the action. Unlike other joint configurations in the body that may focus on stability, the shoulder girdle focuses on mobility, a compromise that enables human adaptability across varying environments. Furthermore, the shoulder girdle's musculature, the rotator cuff, and other stabilizing muscles underscore the fine, delicate balance between strength and flexibility necessary for upper limb function. This structural arrangement emphasizes the importance of understanding the shoulder girdle and upper limb in human osteology, as they form the basis for physical action and interaction with the environment. As a prolongation of the shoulder girdle, the upper limbs' developmental and evolutionary characteristics reveal something about functional adaptation between species. For instance, homology among human, primate, and even some non-primate upper limb elements underscores the evolutionary pathways that have led to the present anatomy. Comparative human osteology focuses on how shoulder girdle and upper-limb differences can reflect adaptive solutions to ecological challenges. These investigations outline how the morphology of the upper limb and shoulder girdle in various lineages has been shaped by bone elements, such as adaptations for arboreal locomotion or bipedalism. Through this interaction, learning about the shoulder girdle and upper limb is not only about human anatomy but also about evolutionary biology and adaptation, with the groundwork laid by the principles of functional morphology in comparative osteology and human osteology (Figure 8.1).

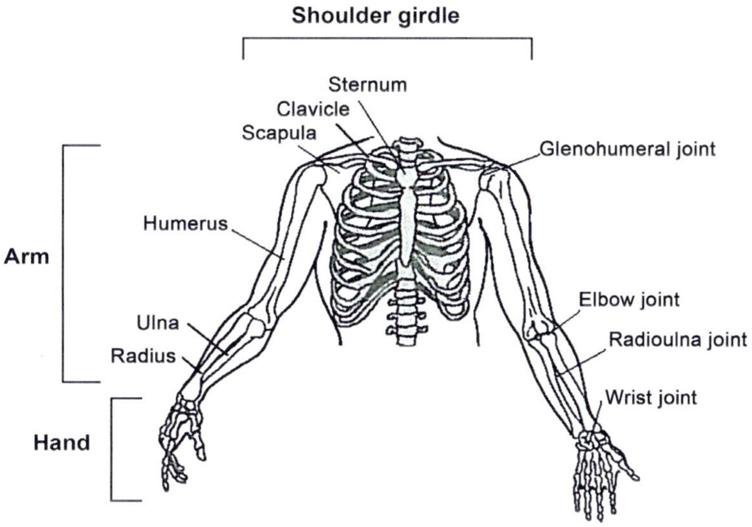

Figure 8.1. The shoulder girdle and upper limb.

Source: https://www.researchgate.net/profile/Jonathan-Tapson/publication/38958341/figure/fig1/AS:669540220428308@1536642236849/Human-upper-limb-shoulder-girdle-arm-and-hand-showing-bones-and-joints-of-the-arm-and.jpg.

Importance of Studying Human Osteology

Human osteology is crucial for understanding the intricate anatomy and functioning of the human body, particularly for the shoulder girdle and upper limb. The skeletal system not only serves as a framework that supports the body but also delivers the primary function of movement as well as stability. By learning about the shoulder girdle and upper limb osteologically, students and clinicians can appreciate the biomechanical basis of human movement. This is particularly relevant in areas of study such as orthopedics, physical therapy, and sports science, as it will enable clinicians to develop more effective treatment and rehabilitation strategies for a range of musculoskeletal disorders. As such, learning from osteological studies is inherently related to enhancing functional ability and rehabilitation in patients with upper limb trauma. Further, human osteology has practical implications beyond anatomical knowledge; it also develops hands-on skills relevant to competence. Competence within techniques like bone identification and estimation of age and sex from skeletons are core to competence within this field. The value of haptic learning—engaging with physical models, as seen in the recent shift to virtual learning due to the COVID-19 pandemic—is an example of how touch-based interaction can foster deeper understanding of complex osteological concepts. Research in schools indicates that students who participated in physical model interaction demonstrated competence comparable to those who took conventional face-to-face laboratory classes. This means that, within a distance-learning environment, the relevance of learning human osteology remains significant, reinforcing the value of employing innovative learning techniques in biological anthropology (Gamble et al., 2024). Secondly, advances in osteological research have broader impacts in society and medicine by informing effective public health interventions and forensic applications. A proper understanding of human skeletal diversity through osteological data can help solve health inequalities and enable more tailored health care and rehabilitation. Furthermore, forensic applications of osteology are critical in legal cases, where osteological analysis can aid in the identification of remains, the estimation of post-mortem interval, and the determination of ancestry. The intersection of osteology and anthropology, as presented in the accompanying learning materials Piatsko et al. (2021), reinforces the necessity for integrated learning that bridges both clinical practices and anthropological discovery. By doing so, rigorous study of human osteology not only enriches academic scholarship but also makes critical contributions to a broad array of professional fields that demand rigorous knowledge of the human body.

8.1. Anatomy of the Shoulder Girdle

Learning Outcome

1. Shoulder girdle components
2. Joints and articulations involved
3. Shoulder girdle functions

The shoulder girdle is a fundamental component of human osteology, composed of a system of complex bones, joints, and muscles that enable it to accommodate a great degree of movement. The shoulder girdle is made up of the clavicle, scapula, and the proximal humerus and connects the upper limb to the axial skeleton. The unique orientation of the scapula provides high arm freedom and flexibility, required for the versatility of arm movements. This is because of the superficial glenoid cavity that articulates with the head of the humerus and is supported by a wide variety of muscles, ligaments, and tendons, which provide stability to the joint. The functional relevance of this anatomy is profound, as the shoulder girdle enables both forceful and precise motion required for activities of daily living and athletic performance. Knowledge of the biomechanics of the shoulder girdle is pertinent, particularly when considering its susceptibility to injury, especially in sports requiring repetitive overhead motion. Volleyball and other sports players are at risk of shoulder injuries due to the rapid forces and movements they generate, such as spiking and serving. Mechanisms of shoulder injury demonstrate a complex interplay between joint stability and muscular leverage, and they show an appreciation for evolutionary adaptations that have been shaping the shoulder anatomy throughout history. For instance, during the transition from sprawling to more erect limb postures in higher vertebrates, modifications in the mechanics of shoulder joint movements increase the risk of injury with some loads and movements. This evolutionist perspective emphasizes the need for specific interventions and preventive measures in athletic training to offset these risks, especially in high-shoulder-use sports, and underscores the importance of valuing (Bahrambeigy et al., 2024) the distinctive demands placed on the shoulder girdle. Muscle action is vital for shoulder stability, being central to both mobility and injury prevention. The shoulder girdle is supported by a complex system of muscles, such as the rotator cuff and the deltoids, which ensure dynamic stability during motion. Variation in muscle length, orientation, and leverage can profoundly influence the efficiency of these muscles, thereby affecting overall shoulder function. In fact, biomechanical models have shown that evolutionary changes in forelimb posture across taxa can alter muscle actions at the shoulder joint and highlight the delicate balance between mobility and stability (Allen et al., 2017). In contemporary physical therapy and sports training, it is imperative to have a keen understanding of this muscle's anatomy and function. This knowledge not only prevents injury but also enhances performance by informing rehabilitation programs and conditioning routines tailored to the unique demands placed on the shoulder girdle during various tasks (Figure 8.2).

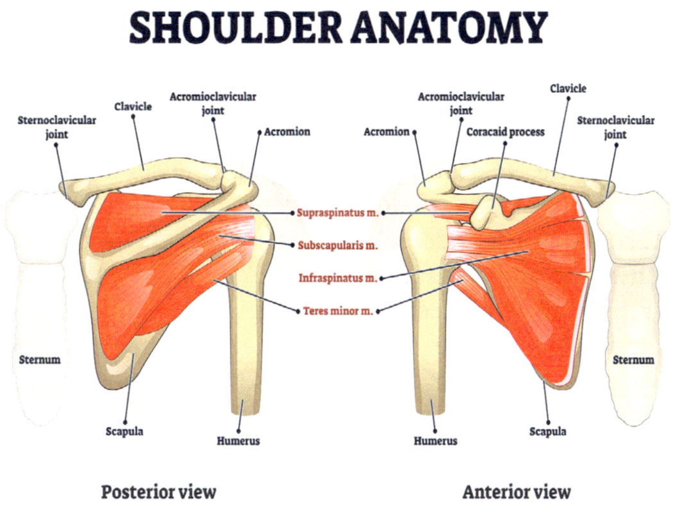

Figure 8.2. The anatomy of the shoulder girdle.

Source: https://cdn-kahjp.nitrocdn.com/nQiQVjalCQBPcHUqLospPRxcCRFSaITk/assets/images/optimized/rev-1c471b8/edmontonboneandjoint.ca/wp-content/uploads/2021/06/Updated-Shoulder-Anatomy-Photo.png.

8.1.1. Components of the Shoulder Girdle

The pectoral girdle, or the shoulder girdle, is an intricate musculoskeletal system of bones and their concomitant musculature that enables the vast variety of movements of the upper limb. Essentially, the shoulder girdle is constituted by two significant bones: the clavicle and the scapula. The collarbone, or clavicle, acts as an important link between the axial skeleton and the upper limb through its articulation with the scapula at the acromial end and the sternum at the sternal end. Simultaneously, the scapula, a triangular, flat bone, provides attachment sites for many muscles that govern shoulder stability and movement. These bones work together to allow dynamic movements of the upper limb for activities ranging from lifting to throwing, which are crucial not only for day-to-day life but also for specific sports. One of the significant aspects of the shoulder girdle is its reliance on a complex association of movement-regulating and stabilizing muscles. Muscles such as the trapezius, deltoid, and rotator cuff muscles maintain the normal functioning of the shoulder girdle. The rotator cuff, in general, is made up of four muscles—supraspinatus, infraspinatus, teres minor, and subscapularis—that work synergistically to stabilize the glenohumeral joint, allowing for a wide range of motion while at the same time preventing dislocation during shoulder movements. The shoulder girdle musculature contributes to overall shoulder girdle flexibility, enabling the limb to execute fine motor activities as well as powerful explosive movements. Therefore, the intricate relationship between the bones and muscles in the shoulder girdle is most important in both functional anatomy and biomechanics of the upper limb. An understanding of the components of the shoulder girdle is important in human osteology, particularly for the prevention and rehabilitation of injury. Shoulder injuries, for example, like rotator cuff tears or shoulder impingement syndrome, generally occur due to overload or abuse of the shoulder girdle complex. Awareness of the anatomical relationships among the clavicle, scapula, and their attendant musculature can guide medical treatment and physical therapy interventions. Aside from this, analyzing these elements across varying populations can improve our understanding of evolutionary adaptations and functional variation, as noted by Abdala et al. (2016) and Gamble et al. (2024). By evaluating the shoulder girdle's anatomical complexity, scientists are also able to enhance further their understanding of its significant role in the overall mechanics of the upper limb and of human movement overall (Figure 8.3).

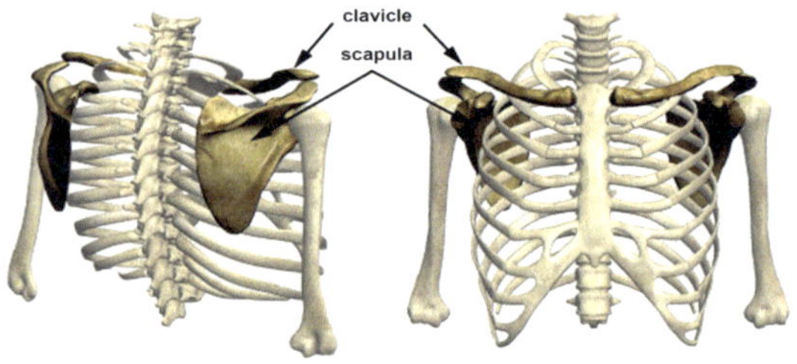

Figure 8.3. The shoulder girdle, also known as the pectoral girdle.

Source: https://ars.els-cdn.com/content/image/3-s2.0-B9780128040218000012-f01-043-9780128040218.jpg.

8.1.2. Articulations and Joints Involved

The shoulder girdle comprises a series of key articulations and joints essential to the mobility and functioning of the upper limb. The most basic joint implicated is the glenohumeral joint, formed through the articulation of the humeral head and glenoid cavity of the scapula. This ball-and-socket joint is characterized by the extensive motion it permits, including flexion, extension, abduction, adduction, and rotation. This mobility is needed for activities that require overhead reach or complex arm movements. The acromioclavicular joint also connects the scapula's acromion to the clavicle, stabilizing and enabling movement of the shoulder girdle during dynamic movement. The coordination of these joints is vital to the coordination of the upper limb, highlighting the anatomic subtleties supporting the extensive flexibility necessary for functional and sports activities. In addition to the glenohumeral and acromioclavicular joints, the scapulothoracic articulation is also a major contributor to shoulder girdle mechanics. This mechanism is not a synovial joint per se, but rather a functional connection between the scapula and thoracic rib cage that accommodates gliding movements that supplement the dynamic motions of the upper limb. The ability of the scapula to slide down the thoracic wall is crucial to position the glenohumeral joint in an optimal position for the range of movements, for instance, reaching and throwing. Furthermore, alterations in scapular orientation can significantly influence shoulder joint function and, consequently, muscular force production and joint stability, particularly in an environment of repetitive stress or risk of injury. Scapulothoracic joint biomechanics need to be understood to diagnose and prevent shoulder injuries, which are prevalent in sports that require overhead movements or high-speed arm actions. The biomechanical features of the shoulder girdle joint also have a complex relationship with evolutionary adaptation. Comparative anatomy research reveals extreme differences in joint mobility and muscle leverage between species, particularly between more sprawling species, such as crocodilians, and more erect, bipedal species, such as certain dinosaurs. The joint range and the analysis of muscle action illustrate how adaptation to several modes of locomotion can alter functional competence of the forelimb, influencing how species experience and interact with the environment. Such an evolutionist paradigm is particularly relevant when considering mechanisms of injury in modern sporting environments, such as volleyball. High-magnitude actions, including serving and spiking, place significant stress on shoulder joints, underscoring the need for prevention and training programs to incorporate these biomechanics (Bahrambeigy et al., 2024). Understanding these articulations and their evolutionary history can be used to design effective rehabilitation protocols and enhance athletic function (Figure 8.4).

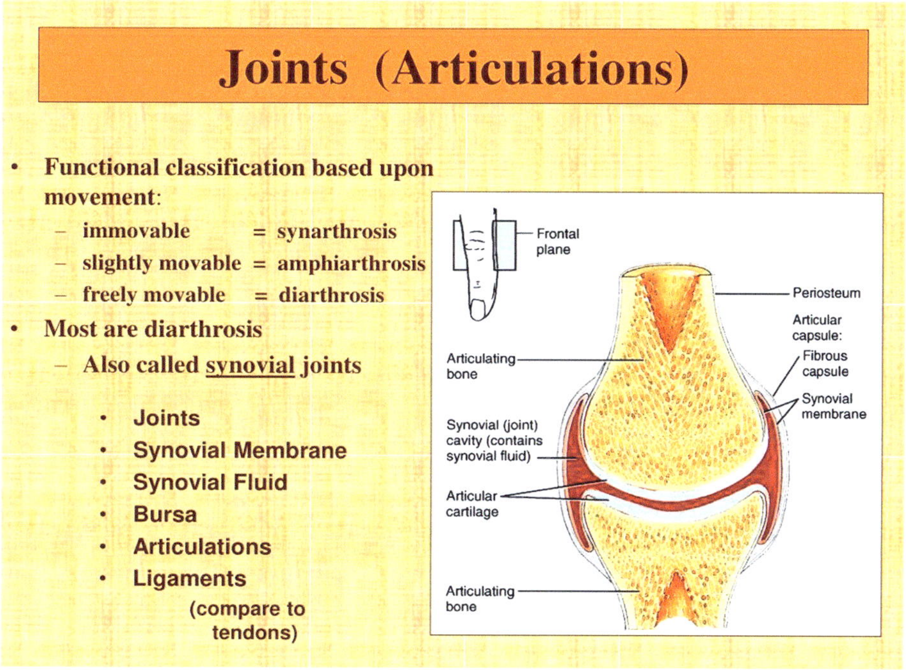

Figure 8.4. Articulations and joints involved.

Source: https://external-content.duckduckgo.com/iu/?u=https%3A%2F%2Fimage.slideserve.com%2F1099849%2Fjoints-articulations-l.jpg&f=1&nofb=1&ipt=b81c1f8e83ea72e322ccb1ccd6f8a9085df89fdaefaeac2f8344446101f08640.

8.1.3. Functions of the Shoulder Girdle

The shoulder girdle is a significant interface between the upper limb and the axial skeleton, which has a fundamental purpose to enable a wide range of movements necessary in normal,regular activity. The shoulder girdle consists of the clavicle and scapula, which they support the shoulder joint and provide points of origin for numerous muscles. The shoulder girdle's unique anatomy provides for a wide range of motion, supporting actions like flexion, extension, abduction, adduction, and rotation of the arm. These are not merely functions necessary for simple actions like reaching and lifting, but also for specialized sporting movements, where strength and accuracy are critical. The dynamic interaction between the tendons, ligaments, and attachment muscles of the shoulder girdle enables the upper limb to move without compromising the level of stability required in most physical activities essential to the functioning of humans. In addition, the shoulder girdle becomes crucial for the biomechanical effectiveness of upper limb movement in most activities, like those encountered in sport and manual labor. The orientation of the scapula plays a key role in providing the muscles with maximum leverage, which becomes even more pronounced in movements requiring high rates of acceleration, such as throwing or spiking in volleyball. Muscles originating on the shoulder girdle and inserting on the humerus are essential for the execution of strong movements with minimal possibilities of getting injured. A review of biomechanical models indicates that postural changes, particularly in the articulation of the shoulder joints and the functioning of muscles, have a substantial impact on performance and vulnerability to injury. This conflict between mobility and stability leads to the fine balance that the shoulder girdle must maintain, not only impacting sport performance but also daily function (Allen et al., 2017). Lastly, understanding the mechanics of the shoulder girdle also involves noting how shoulder injury can affect its effective mechanics. The commonality of shoulder injuries among athletes, particularly those who play overhead sports like volleyball, also points to preventive measures and targeted rehabilitation protocols (Bahrambeigy et al., 2024). Therefore, physiotherapy students and professionals should establish a thorough knowledge of the shoulder's biomechanical structure and the prevalent risks involved in particular sports activities. Such knowledge is crucial for establishing effective injury-prevention strategies and improving athletes' performance. By prioritizing the importance of education on shoulder girdle function and associated biomechanics, prospective professionals can serve people more effectively, maximizing their shoulder health and performance and enhancing athletic productivity and quality of life.

Test Your Knowledge

1. What are the primary bones and joints of the shoulder girdle, and how do they contribute to upper limb mobility?
2. How does the articulation of the clavicle and scapula enable a wide range of arm movements?

8.2. Bones of the Upper Limb

Learning Outcome

1. Principal bones: humerus, radius, and ulna
2. Role of the carpals in wrist movement
3. Phalanges and their contribution to hand movement

Understanding the anatomy of the upper limb is crucial in human osteology, particularly concerning the shoulder girdle. The shoulder girdle, formed by the scapula and clavicle, is the fundamental connection between the upper limb and the axial skeleton. Its unusual shape provides a wide range of motion, enabling functions such as reaching, lifting, and throwing. The S-shaped curve of the clavicle, which is its most characteristic feature, is mainly responsible for stabilizing the shoulder area as well as for facilitating mobility. Unlike the clavicle, the broad, triangular scapula is involved in the articulation of the humerus in the glenohumeral joint. Notably, the relationship of these bones not only allows for upper limb function but also serves as an excellent example of evolutionary adaptation for bipedalism and diverse manipulative activity, which indicates the anatomical significance of the bones in the upper limb. In the investigation of the humerus, the upper limb's longest bone, its intrinsic role in allowing upper limb function becomes readily apparent. The humerus articulates with the scapula and also the bones of the forearm, and therefore is the primary bone for the movement of the arm. Its proximal end consists of a rounded head that lies in the glenoid cavity of the scapula, giving an extensive range of motion in the shoulder joint. In addition, the anatomical neck and the greater and lesser tubercles of the humerus are sites of attachment for muscles important for rotational and lifting movements. With scientists studying the biomechanical properties of the humerus, differences in movement patterns and muscle leverage are observed, particularly in the context of evolution from sprawling to more erect limb postures, demonstrating the adaptation of this bone for upright human walking and altered functional demands (Allen et al., 2017). The forearm bones, the radius and the ulna, are further indicative of the intricacy of the skeletal system of the upper limbs. These two bones work together to facilitate intricate forearm movements, such as supination and pronation. The radius on the lateral side of the forearm has a significant contribution to wrist movement and works with the carpal bones to facilitate varying hand positions. Conversely, the ulna, located medially, serves as the hinge for elbow flexion and extension. Awareness of the individual and conjoint actions of the ulna and radius sheds light on the evolutionary forces that enable and facilitate the use and manipulation of tools, a requirement for human survival. Recent studies have also emphasized the importance of haptic learning devices in the education of osteology to reinforce these anatomical rules, suggesting that physical models can be used to gain insights into the complex relationships among these bones (Gamble et al., 2024) (Figure 8.5).

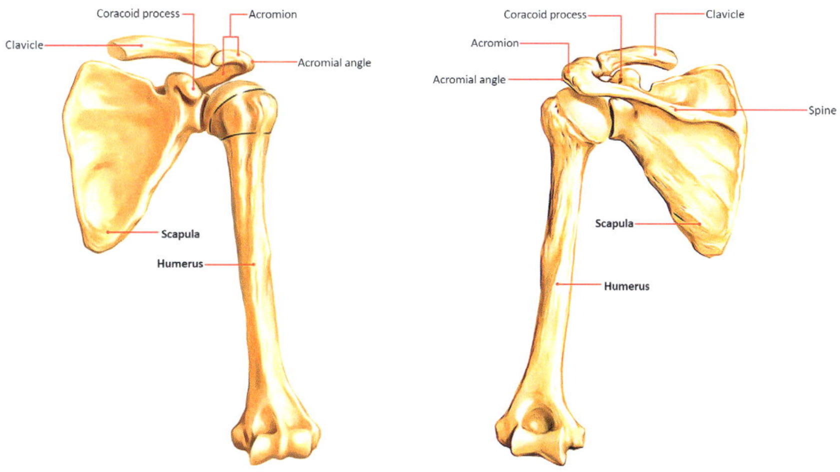

Figure 8.5. Bones of the upper limb.

Source: https://external-content.duckduckgo.com/iu/?u=https%3A%2F%2Fwww.earthslab.com%2Fwp-content%2Fuploads%2F2017%2F07%2FScapula-intro-front-1.jpg&f=1&nofb=1&ipt=5761a2d757cc1204ffa0ad4faca2255b1cae5ff3d77ef4624d92b58676932532.

8.2.1. Major Bones: Humerus, Radius, and Ulna

The structure of the upper limbs is primarily influenced by the humerus, ulna, and radius, all of which collectively produce dexterity and mobility. The humerus, being the longest bone in the upper arm, extends from the shoulder joint all the way down to the elbow and is a key part of upper limb articulation. Its rounded head rotates within the shallow glenoid cavity of the scapula to offer a high level of freedom in the glenohumeral joint. The humeral neck supplements the rotatory movement, and sites for the attachment of the rotator cuff muscles on the greater and lesser tubercles are utilized to provide stabilization and support to the movements of the shoulder. The humerus' interaction with surrounding soft tissue structures underscores its importance in upper-limb biomechanics, as envisioned in evolutionary studies delineating limb-anatomy adaptations across various vertebrate lineages (Allen et al., 2017). With the humerus, the radius and ulna form the forearm with definite but synergistic functions.

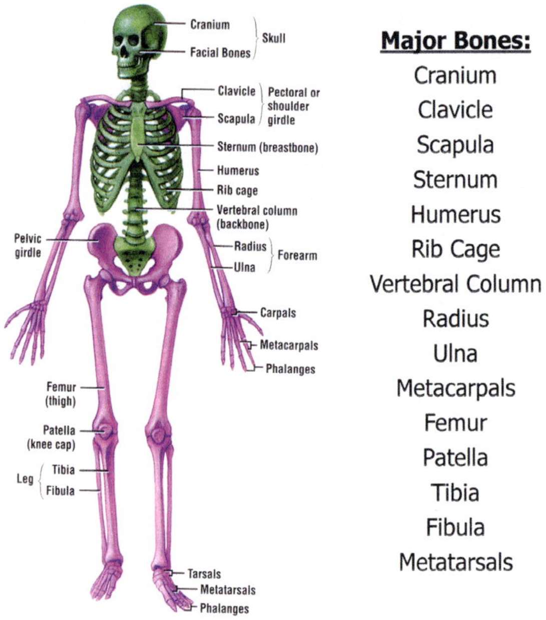

Figure 8.6. The upper limbs framework is significantly forged by the humerus.

Source: https://external-content.duckduckgo.com/iu/?u=https%3A%2F%2Fslideplayer.com%2Fslide%2F12937962%2F78%2Fimages%2F6%2FMajor%2BBones%3A%2BCranium.%2BClavicle.%2BScapula.%2BSternum.%2BHumerus.%2BRib%2BCage.%2BVertebral%2BColumn.%2BRadius..jpg&f=1&nofb=1&ipt=e5d49c781b1b7e9dfe6086eb9e8bed861877bd2793dabc24a9d7e06dc9e98a97.

The ulna, which is longer and not as mobile, joins with the humerus at the elbow in a hinge joint to allow for flexion and extension of the arm. The radius, however, is anatomically configured to rotate upon the ulna so that pronation and supination of the hand and wrist are enabled. This allows for many complex motions required for fine motor activity tasks. Understanding the biomechanics of bone interaction is significant, especially in light of evolutionary progress from rudimentary quadrupedal constructions to more advanced bipedalism in man, where the function of the forelimbs has evolved beyond mere locomotion to encompass intricate manipulative motions (Allen et al., 2019). The integration of the humerus, radius, and ulna reflects a sophisticated system of bony support that functions as a core factor in upper limb function. Each bone makes a definite contribution to the overall biomechanics of motion: the humerus provides strength and stability, while the radius and ulna provide flexibility and range.

This triad of bones not only impinges upon limb movement but is also extremely important for postural stability and overall upper limb coordination. As osteological and biomechanical research increasingly illuminates these structures, it is increasingly evident that their study provides us with significant insight into human evolutionary history. The comparative analysis of these anatomical features across different species continues to inform theories of the evolution of locomotion and grasping ability in our lineage, bearing witness to the ongoing fusion of form and function in the study of human osteology (Allen et al., 2017) (Figure 8.6).

8.2.2. Role of the Carpals in Wrist Function

The carpals are of prime importance in wrist movement, serving as the structural components that provide the hand with movement and stability. With two rows of eight bones, the carpals form a complex structure that unites the forearm to the hand. Through such a structure, there is widespread movement in the wrist with structural uniformity. The distal row of carpals, comprising the scaphoid, lunate, triquetrum, and pisiform, articulates directly with the radius, providing essential stability. Contrariwise, the distal row, the trapezium, trapezoid, capitate, and hamate, articulates with the metacarpals, enabling dexterous movements required for grasping and manipulation. The intricate coordination of these bones significantly contributes to accomplishing tasks ranging from the most delicate fine motor actions to forceful grip motions. Thus, the functional and anatomical significance of the carpals is significant in human osteology. The carpals also significantly contribute to wrist movement through their support of intricate movements and varied ranges of motion. A considerable amount of this flexibility is maintained through the unique articulations between the carpal bones themselves, which not only allow flexion and extension but also radial and ulnar deviations.

Such movements are required for precision tasks, for example, writing or playing a musical instrument. Furthermore, carpals' alignment provides stability for the transmission of forces around the wrist, maximizing shock absorption and minimizing the risk of damage. As seen in studies of archosaur locomotor shifts, in which limb structure changed to accommodate multiple modes of locomotion, the carpal architecture of humans illustrates how evolutionary refinement has improved wrist biomechanics for complex functions and survival. The carpals thus demonstrate an evolutionary shift that enhances our understanding of human anatomy. Furthermore, the health of the carpals is essential to prevent conditions such as carpal tunnel syndrome, which can significantly affect wrist functionality.

Carpal tunnel syndrome arises when the median nerve at the wrist is compressed, typically due to repetitive movement or improper wrist posture. The treatment relies on working with the underlying anatomy, and thus, carpals are essential in pathology and rehabilitation. Similar to the modifications in early archosaur locomotor modes, wrist mechanics can have a profound impact on limb function as a whole. Therefore, the study of the function of the carpals not only educates us about their anatomical diversity and mechanical advantages but also underscores their importance in clinical settings. Combined, these observations substantiate the fundamental role the carpals play in wrist function and explain their relevance to the broader context of human osteology (Figure 8.7).

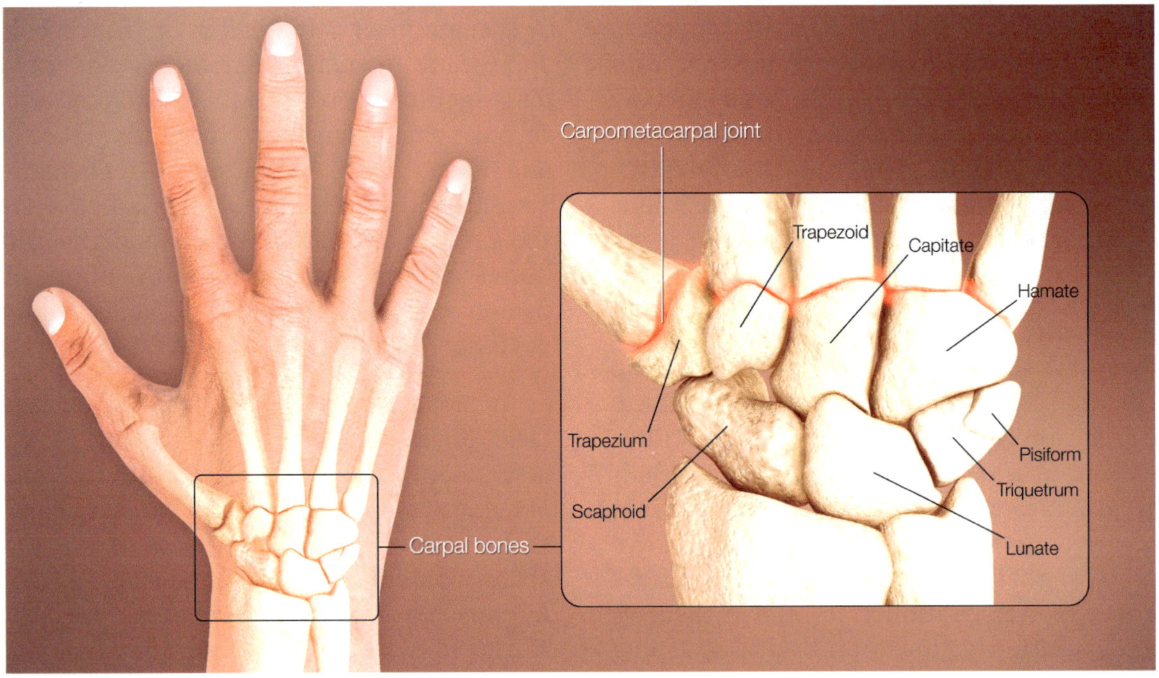

Figure 8.7. Role of the carpals in wrist function.

Source: https://upload.wikimedia.org/wikipedia/commons/a/a1/3D_Medical_Animation_Human_Wrist.jpg.

8.2.3. Phalanges and Their Significance in Hand Movement

The phalanges, the digital bones of the fingers, play a fundamental role in facilitating complex hand movement required for various tasks. Every hand contains 14 phalanges separated into three sections for every finger—proximal, middle, and distal phalanges—apart from the thumb, which only possesses two. Such a unique pattern allows us to have a lot of flexibility and dexterity, enabling us to perform fine-motor tasks such as writing, typing, and playing music. The phalangeal pattern is not just responsible for gross motor function but is also crucial for fine motor control in terms of the cooperative action of the fingers. The phalanges are thus significant not only from a skeletal perspective but also in their functional capacity to enable human interaction with the environment.

The biomechanical features of the phalanges, including their articulation with the metacarpals at the metacarpophalangeal joints, also reflect their significance in hand motion. The joints permit multiple motions, such as flexion, extension, abduction, and adduction, to facilitate a range of grip patterns and motions.

The phalanges also assist with the opposability of the thumb, a characteristic feature of human hands with significant evolutionary advantages. This opposability enables fine pinching and grasping, enhancing object-handling ability. Such advanced interaction among phalanges and other components of the hand testifies to the evolutionary significance of the upper limbs' bony structure in enabling occupational function, directly associated with the origins of tool use in early hominins. In addition to their mechanical role, the phalanges play a very important function in human osteology: they are implicated in overall hand structure and function. Variations in phalangeal structure, both in length and curvature, can reveal a person's habitual hand manipulation, which may mirror occupational requirements or cultural use. Furthermore, the anatomy of phalanges is significant in the diagnosis and treatment of injuries or conditions of the hands, such as fractures or arthritis. The significance of the phalanges goes beyond being a simple anatomical structure; they have a central role to play in furthering our knowledge of human evolutionary biology and functional adaptations that led to our lineage. Lastly, phalanges are not mere bones but part and parcel of the grand ballet of hand movements that define human ability and creativity.

Test Your Knowledge

1. What are the major bones of the upper limb, and how are they arranged from the shoulder to the hand?
2. How do structural differences between the humerus, radius, and ulna support specific functions of the upper limb?

8.3. Muscles Associated with the Shoulder Girdle

Learning Outcome

1. Primary muscle groups: deltoids and rotator cuff
2. Role of muscles in maintaining shoulder stability
3. Impact of muscle activity on the mobility of the upper limb

The shoulder girdle, a highly advanced structure upon which upper limb movement depends, is composed of a group of main muscles that enable an extensive array of movements. These muscles include the trapezius, rhomboids, and serratus anterior, which have varying functions in moving and stabilizing the scapula. The trapezius, from the base of the skull to midspine and sideway to the acromion, elevates and rotates the scapula. The rhomboids, below the trapezius, retract the scapula, providing stability during a number of upper-limb activities. The serratus anterior, which surrounds the thoracic wall, is responsible for scapular protraction and upward rotation. This combined action is significant in facilitating movement, such as reaching overhead or lifting, and highlights the significance of these muscles in the shoulder girdle (Allen et al., 2017). Understanding the biomechanics of muscles becomes more relevant in light of their evolutionary heritage. Research on locomotor changes in Archosauria shows that differences in limb posture between sprawling and vertical modes of locomotion directly affect muscle leverage and performance (Allen et al., 2017). Due to the necessity of the shoulder girdle for a variety of activities, ranging from locomotion to fine-motor dexterity, protracting and retracting shoulder girdle muscle adaptations underscore their importance during evolution. These changes in muscles not only enhance mobility but also indicate the biomechanical stress placed on the shoulder as organisms developed more vertical postures. Such comparative-anatomy notes on these muscles in other animals provide richer insight into the work they performed in human osteology. The utility of the shoulder girdle muscles is relevant in applied fields such as sports medicine and physical therapy, too. The prevalence of shoulder injuries, for instance, is greatly enhanced in overhead sporting individuals like those engaging in volleyball, where sudden movement puts extreme stress on shoulder musculature. Understanding typical muscle activities and each muscle's contribution to stabilizing and mobilizing the shoulder is paramount for effective injury prevention and rehabilitation.

Through a focus on strengthening these vital muscles, physiotherapists can develop specific interventions that address vulnerability in the shoulder girdle. This realization not only reduces the incidence of injury among athletes but also maximizes performance by enhancing shoulder function, illustrating the significant relationship between muscular anatomy and sporting biomechanics (Figure 8.8).

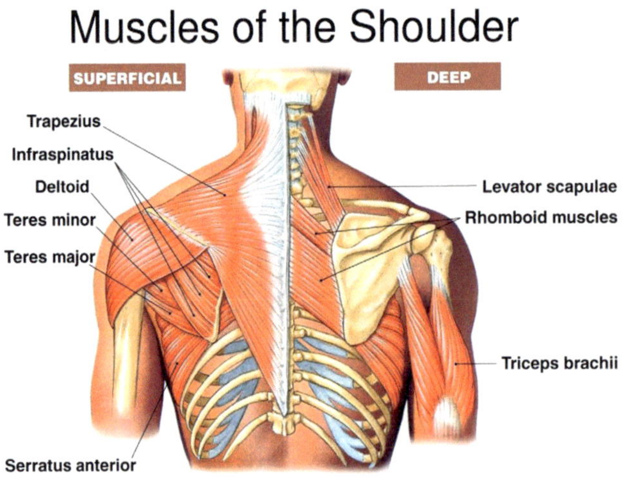

Figure 8.8. Muscles associated with the shoulder girdle.

Source: https://external-content.duckduckgo.com/iu/?u=https%3A%2F%2Fimage1.slideserve.com%2F2370144%2Fmuscles-of-the-shoulder-l.jpg&f=1&nofb=1&ipt=9edf50c105f23447efafc73876008fec0943c33eb03596cf653d58ae880b8de1.

8.3.1. Major Muscle Groups: Rotator Cuff and Deltoids

The shoulder girdle, a complex unit composed of the clavicle, scapula, and humerus, provides the foundation for upper-limb mobility. Centering this dynamic system are the rotator cuff and deltoids, which permit a wide range of movement and stabilize the glenohumeral joint. The rotator cuff has four muscles—supraspinatus, infraspinatus, teres minor, and subscapularis—each with a specific function in the movement of the shoulder. These muscles combined stabilize the humeral head within the glenoid cavity to enable compound movements such as arm elevation and rotation. Their roles are crucial in most sporting activities, and this leads to a better understanding of shoulder biomechanics and injury susceptibility, particularly in high-impact activities such as volleyball, where repetitive movement compromises shoulder integrity (Bahrambeigy et al., 2024). The deltoid muscle, traditionally recognized triangular appearance, is the key to shoulder abduction, flexion, and extension. Composed of three distinct muscle fibers, anterior, middle, and posterior, the deltoid muscle facilitates a range of movements of the upper limb while contributing to the shoulder's stability. Different fibers perform different roles: anterior fibers help in flexion and medial rotation, middle fibers help in abduction primarily, and posterior fibers take part in extension and lateral rotation of the arm.

With this flexibility, smooth, dynamic movements necessary for everyday tasks and sports are made possible (Ferguson et al., 2023). Understanding of the intricate interaction between the rotator cuff and deltoid is required by practitioners who are looking to avoid shoulder injury, particularly in those participating in repetitive overhead sports and similar exercises. Injuring the deltoid and rotator cuff muscles can potentially drastically impair shoulder function, and understanding their biomechanics is thus paramount. Large unreparable rotator cuff tears, for example, are a common source of pain and functional impairment, particularly in young active patients. Multiple surgical alternatives exist to restore shoulder mechanics, yet outcomes may be unpredictable (Ferguson et al., 2023). Adequate understanding of shoulder biomechanics, including the effects of specific movements on muscle dynamics, is required for successful rehabilitation and injury-prevention strategies. Conditioning exercises that physiotherapists and sports medicine practitioners can prescribe should be used to strengthen the rotator cuff and deltoids to minimize the risk of injury and maximize sports performance. Total awareness of these large muscle groups is ultimately critical for maintaining shoulder health and maximizing the overall functionality of the upper limb in sport and daily activities (Figure 8.9).

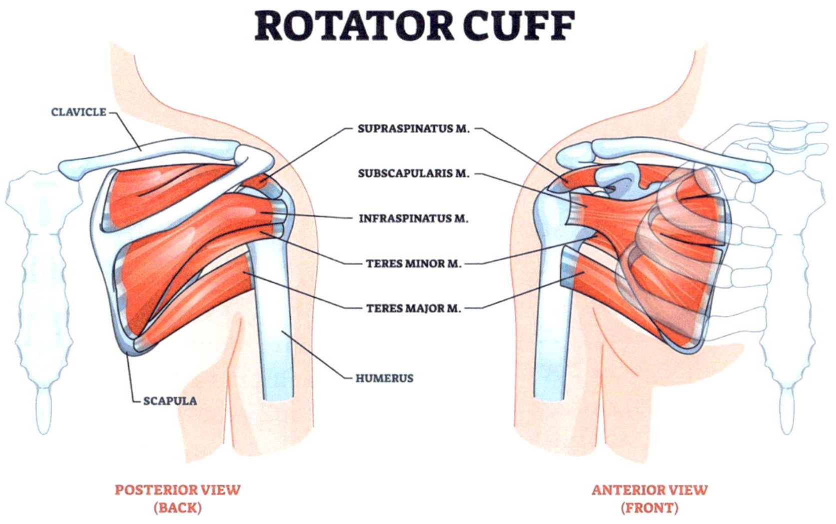

Figure 8.9. The shoulder girdle, a complex structure that includes the clavicle.

Source: https://cdn-degmb.nitrocdn.com/ttfRdoaCkYdYriFDAQYzsXWjIyYFFwdP/assets/images/optimized/rev-b9904d4/3dmusclelab.com/wp-content/uploads/2023/08/rotator-cuff.jpg.

8.3.2. Role of Muscles in Shoulder Stability

The stability of the shoulders is crucial for optimal upper limb function, particularly in sports that are activity-based. The intricate group of muscles surrounding the glenohumeral joint plays a pivotal role in guaranteeing this stability. The four main muscles of the rotator cuff—supraspinatus, infraspinatus, teres minor, and subscapularis—support and stabilize the head of the humerus onto the shallow glenoid cavity. This muscular stabilization is significant as the shoulder joint anatomy lacks intrinsic bony stability and relies on muscular stabilization to a large extent. Also, the dynamic balance among these muscles allows for maximum motion without dislocation, a risk compounded in highly stressful sports like volleyball, where fast, repetitive movement requires strong stabilization mechanisms to minimize the danger of injury resulting from an improper amount of shoulder musculature strain (Bahrambeigy et al., 2024). Further, muscle tone and coordinated contractions are also paramount for shoulder stability. Muscles must be active even in passive conditions to ensure joint stability, a phenomenon termed dynamic stabilization. The ability of muscles to respond to rapid position changes or sudden forces is crucial, especially in movements involving overhead movement. This dynamism provides shoulder stability while still allowing flexible movements. When establishing balance in muscle forces, injury risk is heightened. This is particularly relevant for athletic players who engage in repetitive overhead movements. Understanding how the biomechanics of shoulder stability work allows physiotherapists and coaches to develop specific conditioning programs that will prevent injury. Improving muscular coordination and strength is often how this is done (Bahrambeigy et al., 2024). In discussing the adaptation and evolution of the human upper limb's musculature, consideration must also be given to the influence of past physical activities on the shoulder joint's integrity. Research on osteological evidence has found that specific repetitive movements, such as climbing or canoeing, lead to characteristic cortical defects in the bones associated with the shoulder joint. These flaws reflect the biomechanical forces exerted on the region by repetitive physical activity. As seen from human skeletal evidence, avulsion injuries provide considerable insight into the nature of activities that result in long-term muscle adaptation. This historical perspective emphasizes the importance of both intrinsic muscular stability and the extrinsic influences on shoulder function, and thereby enhances our understanding of the shoulder girdle's evolutionary factors about human activity and biomechanics (Figure 8.10).

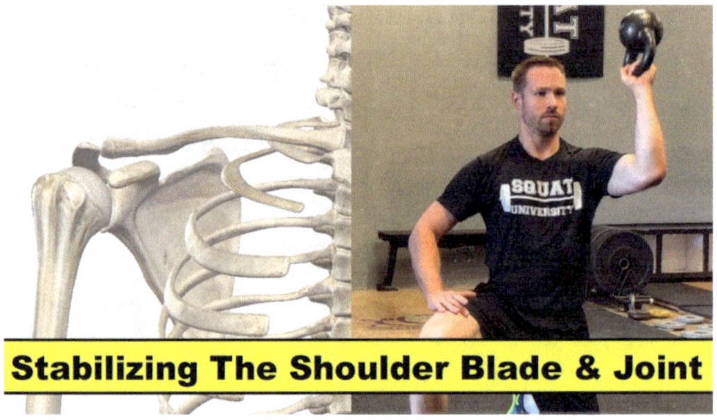

Figure 8.10. Role of muscles in shoulder stability.

Source: https://external-content.duckduckgo.com/iu/?u=https%3A%2F%2Fsquatuniversity.com%2Fwp-content%2Fuploads%2F2018%2F10%2Fblog-covers.jpg%3Fis-pending-load%3D1&f=1&nofb=1&ipt=6a8210bf7062f30f93a27a16ffe6e294aacea0c16beb4c4dad48a72586d95b14.

8.3.3. Impact of Muscle Function on Upper Limb Mobility

Shoulder girdle musculature function is vital in determining upper limb mobility. The shoulder girdle comprises of key structures, such as the scapula, clavicle, and their respective musculature, that affect the upper limb range of motion. Muscle actions around the shoulder joint, such as flexion, extension, and rotary movements, are significantly dictated by the anatomy and position of the scapula. For example, muscle-leverage-enhancing adaptations can have a large impact on how well the arm can be moved in space. These anatomical nuances are valuable to recognize, particularly when explaining how various evolutionary stresses have driven muscle performance and limb motion in various groups, recording key locomotory transitions from sprawling to more upright postures, as highlighted in research on Archosauria, which investigates muscle activity in terms of joint mobility and body form-induced changes (Allen et al., 2017). In comparison to shoulder mobility, muscle function and joint dynamics become increasingly complex as we look at the shoulder girdle in its evolutionary context. The extreme variations in muscle actions and forces across movements underscore the need for muscle synergies and the value of integrated training programs for optimizing function. For example, in volleyball players, repetitive overhead motion activates specific shoulder muscles that, if not properly conditioned, may be the site of fatigue or injury. Biomechanical knowledge is crucial in this case because certain activities predispose the person to shoulder injury from overuse. Effective prevention and management of such injuries depend on a general knowledge of shoulder dynamics and targeted conditioning procedures that maximize the muscle function involved in upper limb mobility, thereby facilitating optimal performance and injury protection (Bahrambeigy et al., 2024). Moreover, muscle function is not confined solely to sporting environments but also has relevance in clinical settings and recovery. Functional impairment of the shoulder girdle can significantly restrict upper limb movement with resultant effect on daily function. Effective rehabilitation protocols must hence address restoration of muscle strength and flexibility of the shoulder complex. This is not just a matter of management of the symptomatic issue, but also the generation of awareness of the biomechanical rationale to muscle function. An integrated approach, grounded in musculoskeletal anatomy, biomechanics, and injury-prevention mechanisms, can play a significant role in enhancing the success of rehabilitation programs. With persistent advancements in our understanding of the shoulder girdle's function among human osteology, it is progressively clear that muscle function plays an important role in dictating upper limb mobility, influencing both health gain and overall quality of life among different populations (Bahrambeigy et al., 2024).

Test Your Knowledge

1. Which muscles stabilize the shoulder girdle and facilitate movements such as abduction, adduction, and rotation?
2. How do the coordinated actions of the rotator cuff muscles contribute to shoulder stability and mobility?

8.4. Development and Growth of the Shoulder Girdle

Learning Outcome

1. Embryological development of shoulder bones
2. Childhood and adolescent growth processes
3. Growth and development determinants

The shoulder girdle, made up of the clavicle and scapula, plays a significant role in human skeletal growth and supports a wide range of upper limb movement. The collarbone, or clavicle, is one of the first bones to ossify in human fetuses and undergoes a unique intramembranous ossification. This is not only used as a support structure but is also required to bridge the appendicular and axial skeletons. Shoulder girdle maturity is assisted by the positioning and integrity of these bones so that the upper limb gets a sound base to lie on. Just as significant is the co-ordinated growth of the scapula and clavicle because any divergences would lead to altered biomechanics and potential shoulder area pathologies. Shoulder girdle formation is not a unitary process either; it is intimately linked with the structures attached and functional loads at various developmental stages.

During infancy and childhood, the shoulder girdle's relatively high plasticity enables adaptation to functional movements such as crawling and reaching. During children's growth and development, the morphology of the shoulder girdle allows a greater range of motion and mobility. This flexibility brings to the fore the application of the shoulder girdle to everyday movement and demonstrates how it develops through interaction with the environment and motor experience. This growth may give feedback to early childhood assessments of physical status and motor function, underlining the importance of the shoulder girdle in coordinated development and growth. Lastly, the development of the shoulder girdle is more important in anthropology and osteology. For instance, studies of fossilized skeletal material from early humans can provide data on the biomechanical implications of shoulder girdle evolution, including changes in lifestyle and environmental stress. Analysis of burial rituals, as observed in certain archaeological excavations, might show correlations between historic population activity patterns and shoulder girdle morphology. In addition, modern osteology courses, such as the use of plastic model skeletons in online learning, emphasize the importance of haptic learning exercises for understanding complex anatomical frameworks. Together, these factors provide insight into the dynamic relationship of shoulder girdle formation with its significance within the broader context of human skeletal evolution and anthropology, as determined by Dockall et al. (1994) and Gamble et al. (2024) (Figure 8.11).

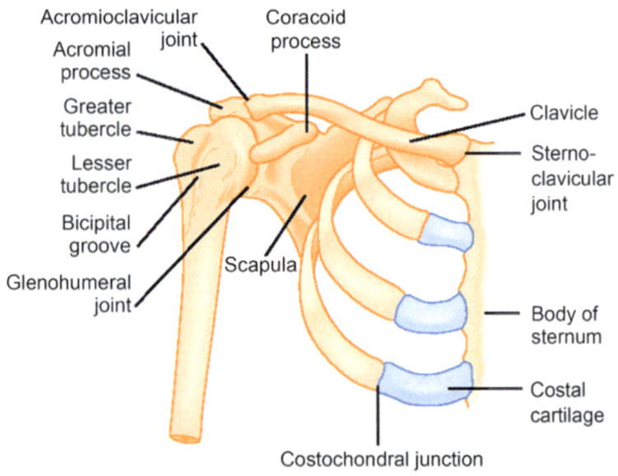

Figure 8.11. Development and growth of the shoulder girdle.

Source: https://external-content.duckduckgo.com/iu/?u=https%3A%2F%2Fai2-s2-public.s3.amazonaws.com%2Ffigures%2F2017-08-08%2F616bb149dbee27fa7a6602472ab0fc2571ac028a%2F2-Figure87.1-1.png&f=1&nofb=1&ipt=b2d88a63a5c1520b9925f1ced4469e278aa7bb65544563ac5bbbf93658cfe3815.

8.4.1. Embryological Development of Shoulder Bones

Embryonic development of shoulder bones plays a crucial role in the assembly of the skull girdle, with profound consequences for the function of the upper limb. Skeletal components necessary to accommodate limb movement are supplied by the contribution of mesodermal tissues during the early stages of embryogenesis. Specifically, the lateral plate mesoderm gives rise to the bones that comprise the pectoral girdle, including the scapula and clavicle. Furthermore, differential expression of key developmental genes, such as Tbx5, plays a role in guiding the morphogenesis of such structures. A defect in sternum development can lead to abnormalities in the shoulder girdle, ultimately affecting the biomechanics of the arm. The evolutionary significance of these processes further underscores their pivotal role in establishing the anatomical foundations for terrestrial locomotion, reflecting the intricate dynamics between genetic and environmental forces (Bickley et al., 2013). The coordination of the muscular and skeletal systems is observed in the simultaneous development of shoulder bones and their corresponding musculature. As the shoulder girdle forms, the musculature responsible for moving these bones begins to differentiate and organize. Embryonic precursor cells, under the influence of local signaling molecules, migrate and differentiate to form the various muscles that stabilize and enable motion of the shoulder joint. Muscles such as the deltoid and rotator cuff form in concert with the scapula and clavicle, indicating the interrelated nature of these structures during embryonic life. The cooperative formation of both muscle and skeletal systems ensures adequate support for the shoulder girdle to enable the limbs extensive range of motion. Aberrancies of development in either of these systems—either due to genetic mutations or interference from the environment—can lead to significant loss-of-function characteristics seen in various clinical conditions, highlighting the importance of studying embryological mechanisms (Sefton et al., 2018). As development proceeds, sophisticated genetic pathways control the formation of bones in the pectoral girdles, highlighting common evolutionary features among vertebrates. An interspecies comparison sheds light on the evolutionary conservation of embryological processes pivotal to shoulder bone formation. For instance, the same genetic markers applied in limb formation across species reflect common ancestry that has necessitated the evolution of the shoulder girdle. This knowledge provides details on the evolutionary adaptations of the human shoulder that have made it more mobile and powerful for walking upright. Further, examining the embryological origin of these bones shows that they are adapted for functional needs, for example, the need for a robust structure that can resist many activities, from mechanical loading to skilled manipulation. These developmental processes need to be appreciated in both evolutionary biology and clinical practice, guiding the medical management of musculoskeletal conditions (Bickley et al., 2013).

8.4.2. Growth Patterns During Childhood and Adolescence

It is necessary to have a good understanding of growth patterns during childhood and adolescence to investigate the anatomical growth of the shoulder girdle and upper limb. Growth is not linear but is characterized by distinct phases under the control of genetic, environmental, and hormonal influences. In the early years of life, the musculoskeletal system, including the shoulder girdle, undergoes enhanced growth that sets the stage for future physical development. Studies highlight that significant changes begin at puberty, with the onset of growth spurts and alterations in body composition, which have significant effects on upper-limb size. During this period, epiphyseal closure and skeletal maturation contribute significantly to adult shape determination, ultimately affecting functional capabilities such as coordination and strength. The interaction between sex differences in growth patterns complicates the interpretation of shoulder girdle and upper limb development. Since development research emphasizes, boys and girls have differing growth rates and timeframes for their growth spurts, which often lead to individualized skeletal features regarding upper limb strength and size. For instance, boys show greater increases in muscle mass, while girls tend to exhibit greater increases in limb length. This difference is important when interpreting anthropometric measurements or posture tests, as sex differences can affect the interpretation of osteological results. Further, structural changes in the shoulder girdle during these growth phases reflect the biomechanical forces acting on it during various physical activities. Research on lower-limb growth, such as patterns of femoral and tibial growth, can also inform upper-limb growth, with bilateral skeletal development playing an important role. Research on developmental patterns from early childhood to adolescence has produced evidence of certain adaptations in the femur and tibia, with implications for identifying similar mechanisms in the shoulder girdle. During phases of key growth, especially during puberty, bone morphology and density change. As discussed in the existing literature, variations in the upper limb skeleton across populations amplify the significance of growth patterns, with functional implications for activity and sports-related functioning. To better appreciate the human osteological implications, it is important to incorporate these findings within a comprehensive framework encompassing both upper and lower limb development, again underlining the importance of multidisciplinary approaches to biological anthropology (Figure 8.12).

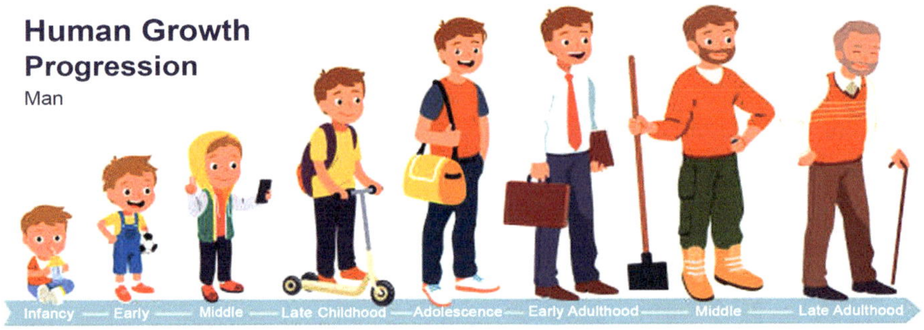

Figure 8.12. An in-depth understanding of growth patterns during childhood and adolescence.

Source: https://www.shutterstock.com/image-vector/generations-set-newborn-child-old-600nw-1933085348.jpg.

8.4.3. Factors Influencing Growth and Development

Understanding of growth and development factors as applied to human osteology, particularly the shoulder girdle and upper limb, is pivotal to comprehension. The patterns of growth of the skeletal elements are closely associated with a complex combination of genetic, environmental, and developmental factors. Genetic determination establishes the potential size and shape, as determined through various traits related to the skeleton. The acromial shape, for instance, can be pretty varied across populations and constitutes both genetic traits and biomechanical loads accumulated over a lifetime. The interplay of genetic factors and environmental stressors underscores the need for an interdisciplinary understanding of such phenomena in the field of osteology. Environmental factors such as diet and bodily exercise play significant roles in bone development. Inadequate nutrient availability may lead to skeletal malformations, as exhibited through the maturity and functionality of the upper limb and shoulder girdle. Conversely, those who are exposed to chronic physical stress, particularly in labor-intensive occupations, may possess skeletal modifications reflecting underlying patterns of growth. This realignment usually yields characteristics previously thought to be exclusively genetic, as in studies that show the prevalence of os acromiale does not reflect solely genetic factors but also the collective influence of stress and lifestyle. The ability to study these characteristics on a broader scope reveals bountiful information about human development. As research on such factors continues, haptic learning in osteology teaching cannot be overstressed. Students invited to engage in tactile learning processes, such as bone model handling, reinforce their understanding of skeletal features and improve their ability to identify developmental disorders and variations. Recent studies show that distance learning models that incorporate hands-on experiments have the ability to achieve the same mastery in students, and this highlights the importance of hands-on learning methods in biological anthropology. This adds weight to instructional practice's ability to accommodate diverse learning settings, highlighting that experience and education are central to developing one's understanding of the skeletal system and its development (Gamble et al., 2024). Moreover, with improvements in the accuracy of information on genetic and biomechanical factors, researchers can develop more advanced educational systems tailored to the diverse needs of students in osteological education (Villao et al., 2007).

Test Your Knowledge

1. How does the shoulder girdle develop from embryonic stages to full skeletal maturity?
2. What factors, including genetic and mechanical influences, affect the growth and morphology of the shoulder girdle?

8.5. Common Injuries and Disorders

Learning Outcome

1. Types of shoulder injuries (e.g., fractures, dislocations);
2. General upper limb disorders (e.g., carpal tunnel syndrome);
3. Treatment and rehabilitation processes.

The shoulder girdle and upper limb are particularly prone to a variety of injuries and conditions, most of which are secondary to the area's delicate anatomy and biomechanics. A great example of this is shoulder impingement syndrome, in which the rotator cuff tendons are pinched during arm movement. This is an illness that causes pain and a limited range of motion in both patients and athletes. In athletes, particularly in overhead sports such as volleyball, cumulative stresses on the shoulder significantly increase the risk of injury. Volleyball players, for example, are under a high compressive and rotational force during activities like spiking and serving, and thus have an increased rate of shoulder injuries. As has been demonstrated in recent studies, targeted injury prevention can significantly reduce these risks, ensuring a healthier sporting tradition and lower injury levels in high-risk sports (Bahrambeigy et al., 2024). Another common disorder that takes place in the shoulder girdle is a rotator cuff tear, which may be acute or chronic. The rotator cuff is a group of muscles and tendons that support the shoulder joint and enable wide arm movements. Acute injury due to falls or forceful lifting may lead to tears, while chronic degenerative tears result from aging or cumulative trauma. Older individuals are particularly prone to chronic tears and subsequently present with chronic pain and restriction of function. The analysis of skeletal remains found in archaeological sites has also provided evidence about the prevalence and nature of such injuries in past populations. For instance, observations from Late Woodland skeletons show widespread reactive changes at specific rotator cuff sites, suggesting that injuries have been prevalent in the past and are most commonly found with activities involving widespread shoulder use, much like current patterns observed in clinic environments (Neidich et al., 2020). Apart from traumatic damage, overuse syndromes are a significant problem in the context of shoulder disorders. Bursitis and tendonitis can be acquired as a result of recurrent stress imposed on the shoulder by certain occupations or sporting activities. For instance, sports that involve repetitive overhead arm movement, such as swimming and tennis, can over time enhance wear and tear on shoulder structures. Education and awareness of these injuries of overuse are critical to prevent and treat. The literature now advocates incorporating proper biomechanics and movement principles into training regimens to minimize excessive stress on the shoulder girdle. With greater awareness of these common injuries and disorders, health professionals can use improved rehabilitation protocols, optimizing return to function and avoiding repeated injury across various sports and work environments (Bahrambeigy et al., 2024) (Figure 8.13).

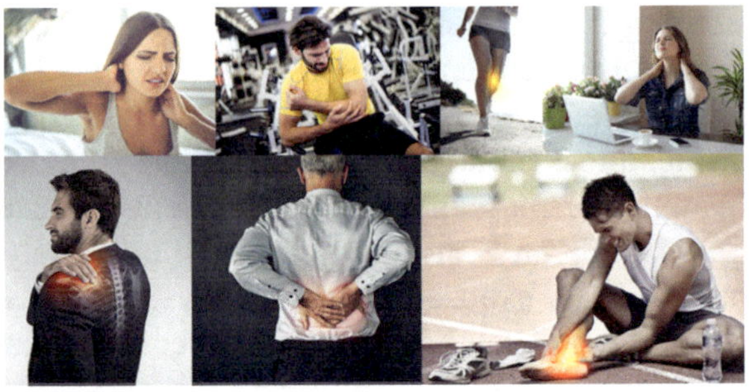

Figure 8.13. Common injuries and disorders.

Source: https://images.ctfassets.net/f8wkf96k66ir/1DPUh3isPq6i2EgcOE6MUi/18bc31f622b894581a879e758f763304/Musculoskeletal-disorder.jpg?fm=jpg&fl=progressive&q=90&w=1200.

8.5.1. Types of Shoulder Injuries (e.g., Dislocations and Fractures)

The shoulder joint, a structurally intricate device composed of the humerus, scapula, and clavicle, is susceptible to numerous injuries characterized by specific mechanisms and complications. Among them, the most frequent are dislocations, typically caused by traumatic events such as falls or blows. In anterior dislocation, the head of the humerus moves forward, resulting in sharp pain and mobility impairment. The concomitant ligamentous and muscular injuries have a substantial effect on the stability of the joints, necessitating an emergent medical therapy to restore function. This type of injury not only impairs athletic function but also causes chronic complications, such as recurrent dislocations or degenerative changes in the shoulder joint, highlighting the importance of appropriate rehabilitation and prevention in risk groups (Domić Kunić et al., 2018). Fractures of the shoulder girdle represent a common type of injury, typically resulting from high-energy impact or falls, particularly in older patients. The most frequent fractures involve the proximal humerus, clavicle, and scapula. Fractures of the proximal humerus, in particular, can compromise shoulder joint stability and are associated with inherent osteoporotic changes in older patients. Treatment of their severity and displacement is dependent in others, while surgery is required to enable maximal recovery and return to function. Understanding the biomechanical origins of such injuries, including repetitive stress and physical loading, also helps develop intervention strategies to prevent their occurrence and enhance recovery outcomes among affected individuals (Marinho et al., 2013). Within human osteology, shoulder injury analysis provides valuable information about the occupational hazards and lifestyles that have influenced different populations over time. Bone remains analysis reveals that various pathologies of the shoulder, such as healed fractures and chronic dislocation marks, which are generally indicative of manual labor or engagement in physical combat, are typical among historical groups that served in armies. These findings highlight the association between activity patterns and injury prevalence, offering a glimpse of the physical demands placed on humans across different sociocultural settings. By exploring these patterns, scientists are able to draw conclusions about health, lifestyle choices, and the adaptive musculoskeletal system's reaction to environmental pressures, underlining the importance of the shoulder girdle in the contemporary as well as in ancient times (Domić Kunić et al., 2018) (Figure 8.14).

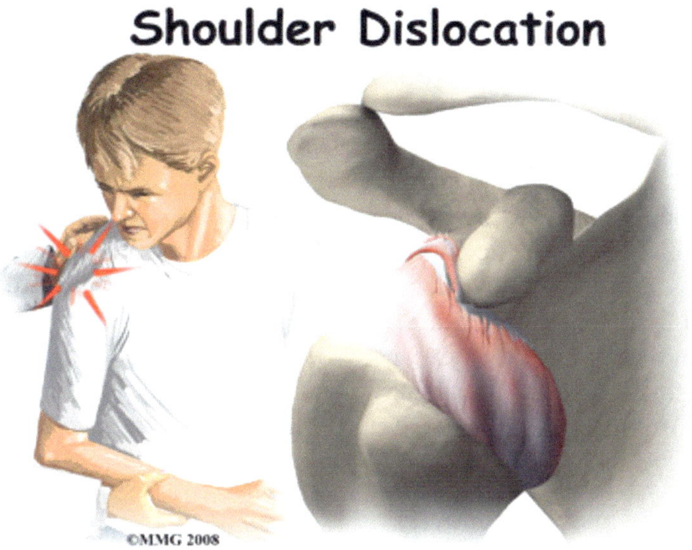

Figure 8.14. Types of shoulder injuries.

Source: https://www.advancedorthopedic.net/media/img/345550/shoulder_dislocation_intro01.jpg.

8.5.2. Common Upper Limb Disorders (e.g., Carpal Tunnel Syndrome (CTS))

An example of a widespread upper limb condition is CTS, a syndrome caused by compression of the median nerve as it traverses the carpal tunnel of the wrist. This neuropathy is usually seen in individuals who perform repetitive wrist motions, such as those involved in certain occupational activities, e.g., typing and assembly. The clinical presentation typically includes numbness, paresthesia, and weakness of the hand, particularly the thumb, index, and middle fingers. If the median nerve is severely compressed, patients experience severe discomfort, which impairs daily activities and work output. Ergonomics educational campaigns and proper wrist placement may decrease the incidence of CTS, underscoring the need for workplace design education to prevent such conditions (Venning et al., 2008). In addition to carpal tunnel syndrome, other upper limb disorders affecting people are tendinitis and rotator cuff injuries, which primarily affect the shoulder girdle. Tendinitis, specifically rotator cuff tendinitis, results from repetitive motion and inflammation of the tendons and is found among athletes and individuals with physically demanding work. Symptoms may include localized pain, diminished range of motion, and weakness in shoulder movement. The pathology of these entities underscores the anatomical significance of the shoulder girdle in producing a wide range of upper limb mobility.

A proper understanding of the musculoskeletal structure is crucial for preventing injury and guiding rehabilitation. Incorporation of specialized exercises and adaptive techniques can be employed for optimal function and recovery for affected individuals, provided that healthcare practitioners are proactive in prevention and management within their practice (Atkinson et al., 2015). Furthermore, the impact of common upper limb disorders, including carpal tunnel syndrome and rotator cuff injuries, is not limited to overt physical symptomatology but also affects psychological functioning and overall quality of life.

Chronic pain and related functional impairment can result in frustration, lost productivity, and even depression or anxiety in affected individuals. Management of these disorders requires an interdisciplinary approach, balancing orthopedic assessment and physical therapy with psychological counseling. Educational interventions to promote awareness of risk factors and prevention strategies may stimulate healthier lifestyle choices and support early intervention. By understanding the interactions among the shoulder girdle, upper limb function, and the prevention of disorders, clinicians can achieve better health outcomes for patients (Venning et al., 2008).

8.5.3. Treatment and Rehabilitation Options

Management and rehabilitation of shoulder girdle injuries should be multidisciplinary, with a focus on restoring function and relieving pain. In the event of severe injury to the glenoid or humeral head, surgery is warranted. The Latarjet coracoid transfer is a surgical technique used to treat recurrent anterior shoulder instability. It has gained popularity for its effectiveness in stabilizing the shoulder, particularly among patients with associated bony defects. While it has been promising in surpassing other stabilization methods, it is also critical to note that the Latarjet procedure can lead to increased superior translation of the shoulder, a factor clinicians must consider during rehabilitation. Thus, effective rehabilitation protocols after surgery should be tailored to enable recovery while preventing potential complications arising from the altered biomechanics (Degen et al., 2013). Rehabilitation following shoulder surgery is often focused on a formal exercise program to enhance strength and mobility. Passive range-of-motion exercises are typically added first to prevent stiffness and promote healing. Active range-of-motion and strengthening exercises may be gradually added as the patient progresses. This staged approach is essential for guarding against placing unwarranted stress on the shoulder structures—you can call them ligaments, tendons, and bones—early in the recovery process. Interestingly, rehabilitation must also consider anatomical variations, as studies indicate that variations in scapular anatomy influence rehabilitation. For instance, the positioning of the glenoid baseplate in reconstructive surgery is a direct consequence of the scapular anatomy underlying it, underscoring the importance of rehabilitation protocols individualized to each patient's shoulder girdle anatomy (Gupta et al., 2016). Additionally, incorporation of modalities such as manual therapy, electrical stimulation, and ice will contribute to healing post-surgery or trauma. These alternative modalities can assist in managing pain and swelling, thereby making rehabilitation more effective. Patient education is also involved, as knowledge of the mechanics of the shoulder girdle allows for recovery. By educating patients about their condition and rehabilitation goals, clinicians can enhance compliance with rehabilitation programs, ultimately leading to improved functional outcomes. Overall, successful rehabilitation and treatment of the shoulder girdle must be multimodal, integrating surgical, rehabilitative, and educational components, tailored to each patient's needs and anatomical considerations, thereby maximizing the potential for recovery and restoration of function in the setting of injury or surgery (Figure 8.15).

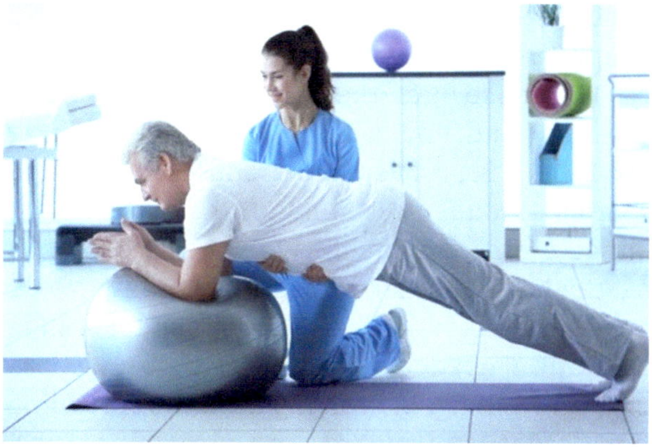

Figure 8.15. The treatment and rehabilitation of shoulder girdle injuries necessitate a multifaceted approach.

Source: https://cdn2.hubspot.net/hubfs/281126/rehab%20therapy.jpg.

Test Your Knowledge

1. What are the most frequent injuries of the shoulder girdle, and how do they impact range of motion and function?
2. How do degenerative conditions like osteoarthritis or rotator cuff tears affect the shoulder girdle?

8.6. Evolutionary Perspective

Learning Outcome

1. Comparative anatomy of the primates' shoulder girdle
2. Evolution of human upper limb function
3. Implications for interpreting human evolution

The evolutionary perspective on the shoulder girdle and upper limb is important for understanding the functional adaptations that facilitated the transition from arboreal environments to terrestrial locomotion in hominins. This transition is highlighted by extreme morphological development, especially of the scapula and humerus, and reflects changes in mechanical demands. For instance, the initial archosaurs possessed sprawling limb postures, which enabled a range of locomotor strategies. While some lineages, however, became more adapted to erect postures, e.g., the sauropodomorph dinosaurs, their forelimbs achieved greater mobility and stability for ground locomotion. These changes reveal how evolutionary pressures shape skeletal morphology to optimize posture control and muscle activity around the shoulder joint, showing a distinct progression from early quadrupedal structures to highly specialized adaptations in subsequent forms. This gives us a glimpse into the interrelation between anatomy and environmental needs (Allen et al., 2019). Moreover, the trend toward more complex modes of locomotion had substantial impacts on joint mobility and it leverage. In particular, shoulder girdle development was a critical factor allowing an expanded range of motion needed for brachiation as well as bipedal walking. In evolving from the sprawling limb posture toward the erect posture, changes in scapular orientation resulted in fundamental modifications in the action of major muscles surrounding the shoulder joint. The biomechanical differences observed in early sauropodomorphs relative to their predecessors illustrate the functional importance of these morphological changes. Through evaluation of the anatomical changes from a comparative point of view, it is evident that the evolutionary development of the upper limb is not simply a matter of shape but is directly tied to locomotor efficiency and flexibility within different ecological niches, therefore maintaining the relevance of evolutionary adaptations in human osteology (Allen et al., 2019). In addition to locomotor adaptations, an understanding of early man's difficulties also assists in the evolutionary history of the shoulder girdle and upper limb. Osteoarchaeological data, such as the Juan Primo burial site, indicate the risks of parturition during prehistoric times. Skeleton remains in place are very significant to what has been understood regarding maternal health and selection forces that might have had an influence on upper limb functionality with regards to childbearing and childcare. Developing musculoskeletal structures not only signify movement adaptations but also other survival aspects, such as childcare and protection. Thus, the evolution of the upper limb and shoulder girdle must be understood in a broader context that considers reproductive strategy and social behavior, underscoring the intricacy of human origins and the multidimensional functions of these anatomical structures for survival and social interaction.

8.6.1. Comparative Anatomy of the Shoulder Girdle in Primates

The shoulder girdle of primates is characterized by extensive anatomical diversity, which is critical for the study of their locomotion and evolutionary history. This is reflected in variations in the shape and position of the scapula, clavicle, and humerus among primate groups. Hominoids, for instance, which include both humans and apes, have a relatively posteriorly positioned scapula compared to other primates. This has enabled greater shoulder motion during activities involving elevation and abduction. Anatomical structure is used to delimit functional homologies among extant hominoids, ultimately to propose selective pressures that constructed this anatomy over primate evolution. Shoulder girdle comparative studies across primate groups also indicate potential lines of evolution from common ancestors versus convergent adaptation to identical environmental pressures. Large skeletal characters such as scapular breadth and orientation of the glenoid cavity represent significant morphological features to be related to specific locomotion modes. Skeletal dimensions in six hominoid species and macaques have revealed significant differences in shoulder anatomy, indicating ontogenetic development as well as phylogenetic history. This variation points to the impact of evolution on shoulder girdle structure and reveals how different species have adapted their anatomical templates to meet their individual locomotor requirements (Osborn et al., 2008). The functional relationships between bones and muscles in the shoulder complex also teach us about the mechanics of upper-limb movement in primates. Studies have shown that coordination among the clavicle, trapezius, and sternocleidomastoid muscles is critical for stabilizing the shoulders and head during movement, enabling efficient use of movement patterns. The presumption that the muscles are used in load-carrying functions is yet another demonstration of the evolutionary significance of the shoulder girdle anatomy. Multiple skeletal measurements have shown bilateral asymmetries related to muscle activations in terms of load bearing, extending the idea of adaptation under functional pressure over time. This structure-function relationship is relevant when considering evolutionary shoulder girdle development within the broader context of human osteology (Osborn et al., 2008) (Figure 8.16).

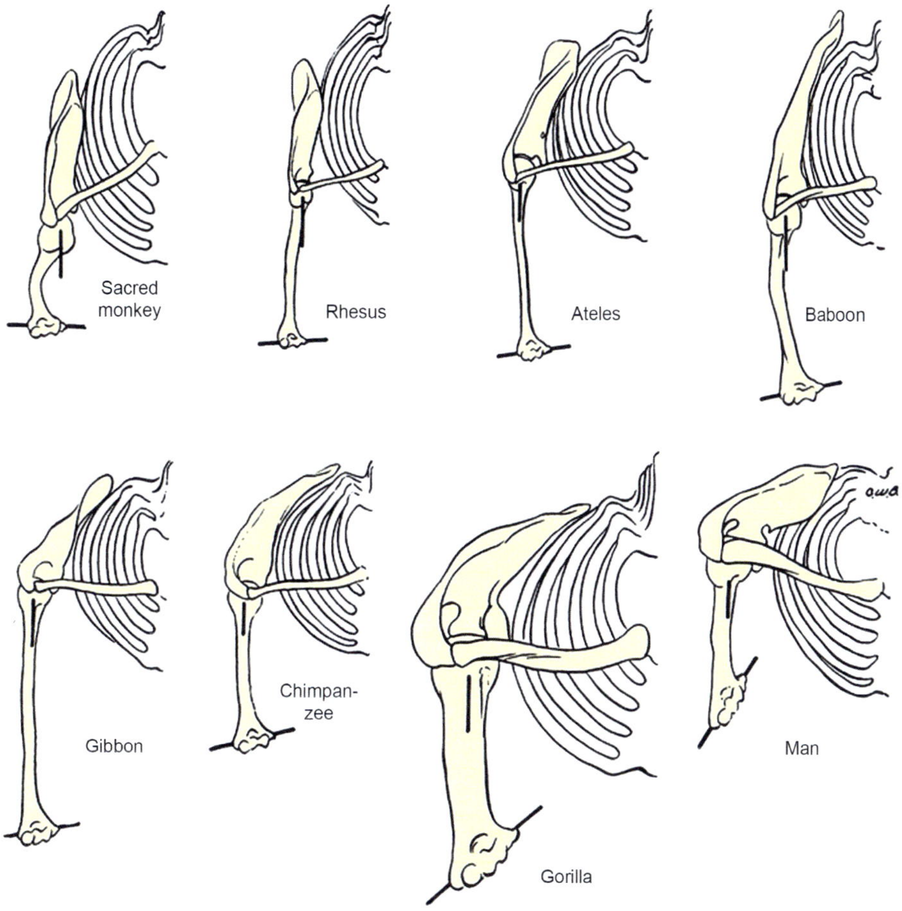

Figure 8.16. Comparative anatomy of the shoulder girdle in primates.

Source: https://media.springernature.com/lw685/springer-static/image/chp%3A10.1007%2F978-3-662-45719-1_1/MediaObjects/324233_1_En_1_Fig6_HTML.gif.

8.6.2. Evolution of Upper Limb Function in Humans

Upper limb development in humans is a complex interaction of anatomical and biomechanical development provoked by environmental forces and behavioral adaptation. The upper limbs of early hominins were adopted initially for arboreal travel, primarily devoted to climbing and gripping. However, the adaptation for bipedalism revolutionized these functions because efficient two-legged locomotion progressively eliminated the need for upper limb locomotion. In contrast, the creation of tools and the manipulation of objects came to predominate the use of the upper limbs. Such a change required modifications in the musculoskeletal anatomy to enable greater dexterity and finesse in finger and hand movement, which eventually paralleled the cognitive development of early humans. In the study of comparative models of locomotor transitions in vertebrate lineages, e.g., those concerning upper limbs, one can find striking parallels with human evolution. The biomechanical models that were formulated from studies of other archosaurs' limb function, and more directly the transition to erect postures, shed light on the evolutionary path of the human arm and shoulder girdle. In biomechanical accounts, analyses of joint range of motion and muscle leverage showed that alterations in limb orientation had a major influence on muscle action, thereby redefining upper limb capability. For example, the evolution of the glenohumeral joint in early hominids reflected the evolutionary innovations observed in other animals when moving from one locomotor strategy to another, enabling better manipulation and tool use and, at the same time, affecting how the shoulder joint works when switching between activities like climbing and walking (Allen et al., 2017). More studies of these evolutionary advancements highlight not just an increase in the functioning of the upper limb but also a reduction in its reliance on basic locomotory activities. As human ancestors established themselves, the frequency and pattern of physical activity imposed selective pressures on the upper limb, necessitating specific adaptations in the shoulder girdle and arm anatomy. For instance, with the emergence of bipedalism as the dominant form of locomotion, the shoulder joint musculature evolved to support both load lifting and the complex motion involved in tool use. These changes involved a trend towards columnar posture in the forelimb, increasing flexion movements during work. Thus, such adjustments not only favored manipulation within the terrestrial environment but also highlighted the strong correlation between evolutionary adaptations and functional needs across the full primate and human evolutionary scenario (Allen et al., 2019).

8.6.3. Implications for Understanding Human Evolution

An understanding of the shoulder girdle and upper limbs' evolutionary implications is critical in understanding the intrigues of human evolution. Comparative studies of the shoulder anatomy of non-human hominoids and humans identify most Homo-specific adaptations. The shoulder anatomy of non-human hominoids is geared toward arboreal movement, suggesting they are better suited to horizontal and vertical climbing, both of which may require arm-lowering mechanisms. By contrast, the human shoulder evolved toward greater motion-permitting flexibility and greater manipulative capacity, particularly in tool use and bipedal activity. The shoulder morphology biomechanics represent an evolutionary trade-off, with apes adapting for climbing efficiency and humans capitalizing on dexterity and reaching, with differences in evolutionary pathways established by behavioral and environmental factors (van Beesel et al., 2022). The increased use of haptic learning in education in biological anthropology has also demonstrated that experiential learning is key to understanding osteological characteristics that correspond to evolutionary processes. Experiments conducted amidst the COVID-19 pandemic validated the efficiency of using plastic model skeletons to advance remote learning in Human Osteology. The models allow students to actively engage with skeletal forms, enhancing their ability to identify bones and comprehend their functional properties. The ability to correctly identify skeletal forms and their implications for locomotion and behavior is essential, as it forms a foundation for understanding evolutionary adaptations. Therefore, incorporating tactile learning into the curriculum can help close gaps in traditional education and provide students with a more profound understanding of the evolutionary background of human anatomy (Gamble et al., 2024). Analysis of the evolutionary significance of shoulder girdle adjustments provides insight into the behavioral and ecological techniques used by early hominins. Analysis of glenohumeral biomechanics highlights the impact of muscle attachment differences on movement efficiency. Greater arm-lowering ability in non-human apes suggests that their evolutionary trajectories prioritized particular locomotor adaptations, which could help explain how early humans likely traveled through their habitats. By thoroughly examining these adaptations, scientists can infer the ecological challenges early hominins encountered and how they responded to them through anatomical changes. This finer-grained appreciation not only enriches the field of human osteology but also our understanding of the broader human evolutionary narrative, with a focus on the intricate interrelationship between form, function, and adaptation throughout our evolutionary history (van Beesel et al., 2022).

Test Your Knowledge

1. How has the evolution of the shoulder girdle facilitated tool use and manipulation in humans compared to other primates?
2. What anatomical changes in the shoulder girdle reflect adaptations for increased upper limb mobility and dexterity?

SUMMARY

It is crucial to value the intricate interrelationship between anatomical structure and functional performance. The shoulder girdle, which consists of the clavicle, scapula, and associated musculature, provides extensive motion necessary for a variety of activities. The anatomy provides substantial support for a range of locomotor and manipulative activities, emphasizing the evolutionary significance of the shoulders' ability to adapt. Of particular interest is the relevance of the division of adaptation through limb structure for understanding ancient and contemporary human activity and its biomechanics. The interplay of these factors underscores the need for an integrative strategy in studying the function of the shoulder girdles in human evolution and function. Furthermore, the application of shoulder biomechanics has implications that extend beyond anatomy to include injury prevention and rehabilitation. For instance, in athletic contexts, the shoulder joint is particularly susceptible to injury due to the high stresses involved in actions such as serving and spiking in volleyball. Understanding the mechanics of these movements provides a foundation for designing interventions that can reduce injury risk, as supported by biomechanics studies. As evolved in physical therapy centers, an acute comprehension of joint biomechanics combined with knowledge of common injuries is vital to effective prevention and rehabilitation programs. Integrating anatomical knowledge and functional application provides a rich understanding of maintaining shoulder health, particularly for overhead sport athletes (Bahrambeigy et al., 2024). Finally, the evolutionary history of humeral morphology and glenohumeral function increases our understanding of the adaptations that have shaped the human shoulder. For example, as outlined in biomechanical studies of limb movement across various archosaurian clades, changes in forelimb posture and muscle leverage are closely tied to changes in locomotor strategies. This data provides background knowledge that can be utilized to assess contemporary human shoulder dynamics and shows the importance of ongoing research in this area. By combining knowledge from the fields of evolutionary biology and biomechanics, we have a deeper appreciation of the shoulders' complex function and its effects on health, performance, and rehabilitation within contemporary society. The results of this study not only highlight the importance of the shoulder girdle in osteology but also suggest the need for continued research into its multiple functions (Allen et al., 2017).

Given the complexity of the shoulder girdle and upper limb in human osteology, several salient points are highlighted that suggest the adaptability of these structures during evolution. The intricate interaction between limb anatomy and locomotor function is most clearly expressed in the evolution from quadruped to biped, as seen within the clade Archosauria. This transition involved extensive alterations in joint architecture and muscle action, particularly in the shoulder joint, where complex movements such as elevation and protraction are governed by the orientation of the scapula and other contacting surfaces. The biomechanical explanation provided by researchers accounts for dramatic variations in muscle leverage and joint mobility across species and their implications for how such evolutionary modifications enable diverse locomotor modes and physiologic functions within the vertebrate clade (Allen et al., 2017). Teaching strategies in human osteology, particularly amid the COVID-19 pandemic, also highlight the critical importance of hands-on, experiential learning. Remote learning methods using plastic model skeletons provided a window to bridge the experience gap caused by the unavailability of conventional laboratory facilities. Research comparing remotely tutored undergraduates with traditional learners shows that students achieved satisfactory results in bone recognition, but the use of advanced skills, such as sex and age estimation, was highly limited. This accentuates the fundamental importance of haptic learning in making a holistic contribution to understanding osteological principles, suggesting that practical experience remains essential to mastering such a skill within the discipline (Gamble et al., 2024). The synergistic application of biomechanical analyses and innovative teaching strategies is a satisfying context in which to better understand the evolution and application of the shoulder girdle and upper limbs in human osteology. Identifying disparities between erect and sprawling limb postures not only highlights the adaptive value of musculoskeletal change but also underscores the importance of effective pedagogy that supports diverse learning environments. Outcomes from both biomechanics studies and instructional measures collectively corroborate the use of a multifaceted methodology in the field, one that integrates empirical investigation and practical teaching methods to enhance learning outcomes. Such a synthesis enhances the value of the dynamic relationship between structure and function in human skeletal anatomy, which is of high significance to prospective osteologists and anthropologists (Allen et al., 2017; Gamble et al., 2024).

KEY TERMS FROM THIS CHAPTER

- Acromioclavicular Joint
- Acromion
- Carpals
- Clavicle
- Coracoid Process
- Deltoid Tuberosity
- Glenoid Cavity
- Greater Tubercle
- Head of Humerus
- Humerus
- Lesser Tubercle
- Metacarpals
- Olecranon Process
- Phalanges
- Radial Tuberosity
- Radius
- Rotator Cuff
- Scapula

CRITICAL THINKING QUESTIONS

1. **Which bones form the shoulder girdle?**
   a. Scapula and clavicle
   b. Clavicle and humerus
   c. Scapula and humerus
   d. Sternum and clavicle
2. **Which bone is also known as the collarbone?**
   a. Scapula
   b. Clavicle
   c. Humerus
   d. Sternum
3. **What is the function of the glenoid cavity?**
   a. Attachment site for muscles
   b. Forms with the humeral head to form the shoulder joint
   c. Supports the scapula
   d. Forms with the clavicle
4. **Which scapular process forms the highest point of the shoulder?**
   a. Coracoid process
   b. Acromion
   c. Glenoid cavity
   d. Spine of the scapula
5. **The humerus distally articulates with which bones?**
   a. Clavicle and scapula
   b. Radius and ulna
   c. Scapula and clavicle
   d. Carpal bones

Short Answer Questions

1. What is the structure of the shoulder girdle?
2. Describe the function of the clavicle in the shoulder girdle.
3. How does the clavicle join the scapula and sternum?
4. Describe the structure and function of the humeral head.
5. Describe the articulation of the humerus and scapula at the shoulder joint.
6. Describe the functional significance of the muscles of the rotator cuff in the shoulder girdle.

Answers to Critical Thinking Questions

1. (a); 2. (b); 3. (b); 4. (b); 5. (b)

REFERENCES

1. Abdala, A., Abdala, A., Adams, A., Allin, E. F., Allin, C., Anthwal, N., Barghusen, H., et al. (2016). Morphological evolution of the mammalian jaw adductor complex. https://core.ac.uk/download/151161615.pdf (accessed on 18th July 2025).
2. Santana-Cabrera J, Alamón-Núñez M, Alberto-Barroso V, Delgado-Darias T. Exploring the risks accompanying child-bearing in aboriginal society on Gran Canaria (Canary Islands, 13th-15th cal. CE): death of a pregnant woman during her third trimester. *Homo.* 2019 Aug 29;70(1):45-56. doi: 10.1127/homo/2019/1011. PMID: 31475291.Allen, V., Hutchinson, J. R., Otero, A., et al. (2019). Forelimb muscle and joint actions in Archosauria: Insights from *Crocodylus johnstoni* (Pseudosuchia) and *Mussaurus patagonicus* (Sauropodomorpha). https://core.ac.uk/download/pdf/296426869.pdf (accessed on 18th July 2025).
3. Atkinson, M. A., Davies, D. C., Dyball, R., et al. (2015). The Anatomical Society core regional anatomy syllabus for undergraduate medicine. https://core.ac.uk/download/161126464.pdf (accessed on 18th July 2025).
4. Bahrambeigy, N. (2024). Common shoulder injuries and preventative approaches in volleyball workshop for physiotherapy students Satakunta University of Applied Sciences. https://core.ac.uk/download/638722739.pdf (accessed on 18th July 2025).
5. Barros, A. P. (2014). Ontogeny, phylogeny, and functional morphology of the hominoid shoulder girdle. https://core.ac.uk/download/29141528.pdf (accessed on 18th July 2025).
6. Bickley, S. R. B. (2013). The gene Tbx5 links development, evolution, and adaptation of the sternum in terrestrial vertebrates. https://core.ac.uk/download/19777091.pdf (accessed on 18th July 2025).
7. Bonsall, C., Boroneant, A., Bălăşescu, A., et al. (2019). Early Neolithic burials from Grumăzeşti-Deleni (Neamţ County, Romania). https://core.ac.uk/download/322484094.pdf (accessed on 18th July 2025).
8. Carroll, R. L. (1977). Permo-Triassic "lizards" from the Karoo System. Part II: A gliding reptile from the upper Permian of Madagascar. https://core.ac.uk/download/39674856.pdf (accessed on 18th July 2025).
9. Degen, R. (2013). Complex shoulder instability: The role of the Latarjet coracoid transfer. https://core.ac.uk/download/61639641.pdf (accessed on 18th July 2025).
10. Dockall, H. D. (1994). Human skeletal remains from the Tyson site (41SY92). https://core.ac.uk/download/215496487.pdf (accessed on 18th July 2025).
11. Domić Kunić, A., Šlaus, M., & Pivac, T. (2018). Reconstructing the life of a Roman soldier buried in Resnik near Split, based on the anthropological analysis of his skeleton. https://core.ac.uk/download/212496299.pdf (accessed on 18th July 2025).
12. Ferguson, D. (2023). A biomechanical comparison of a subacromial balloon spacer, superior capsular reconstruction, and a rigid subacromial spacer in a massive irreparable rotator cuff cadaveric model. https://core.ac.uk/download/571283687.pdf (accessed on 18th July 2025).
13. Foster, A. E. (2015). Characterization of a cortical defect of the ulna found in the Fernvale archaeological population (40WM51) of the South Harpeth River Valley in Middle Tennessee. https://core.ac.uk/download/647350885.pdf (accessed on 18th July 2025).

14. Gamble, J. A., & Gilmour, R. J. (2024). Bones at home supporting haptic learning and universal design beyond the biological anthropology laboratory. https://core.ac.uk/download/644028705.pdf (accessed on 18th July 2025).
15. Gupta, A. (2016). The role of scapular morphology in reverse shoulder arthroplasty. https://core.ac.uk/download/76075550.pdf (accessed on 18th July 2025).
16. Heckert, A. B., NC DOCKS at Appalachian State University. (2016). Rotten Hill: A Late Triassic bonebed in the Texas Panhandle, USA. https://core.ac.uk/download/345085403.pdf (accessed on 18th July 2025).
17. Jenkins, F. A. (1971). The postcranial skeleton of African cynodonts: Problems in the early evolution of the mammalian postcranial skeleton. https://core.ac.uk/download/552115050.pdf (accessed on 18th July 2025).
18. Marinho, L. M. O. (2013). Perimortem blunt force trauma analysis: On the reconstruction of the circumstances of death of human skeletal remains. https://core.ac.uk/download/43586847.pdf (accessed on 18th July 2025).
19. Neidich, D. L., & Ostendorf Smith, M. (2020). Major questions about teres minor: The pattern of reactive changes in a precolumbian human skeletal sample from Illinois. https://core.ac.uk/download/346347875.pdf (accessed on 18th July 2025).
20. Osborn, M. L. (2008). Effects of handedness on the skull and shoulder bones. https://core.ac.uk/download/217399619.pdf (accessed on 18th July 2025).
21. Piatsko, I. A., Tolyaronok, D. A., Usovich, A. K., et al. (2021). Work book in human anatomy. Locomotion apparatus. https://core.ac.uk/download/427551151.pdf (accessed on 18th July 2025).
22. Pujol Bayona, A. (2016). Ontogénesis postnatal de la extremidad inferior basada en telemetrías y morfometría geométrica. Aplicación en paleoantropología y antropología forense. https://core.ac.uk/download/43555181.pdf (accessed on 18th July 2025).
23. Sefton, E. M. (2018). Evolution of the amphibian head and neck: Fate and patterning of cranial mesoderm in the axolotl (*Ambystoma mexicanum*). https://core.ac.uk/download/154872963.pdf (accessed on 18th July 2025).
24. van Beesel, J. (2022). Biomechanical consequences of variation in shoulder morphology in the Hominoidea. https://core.ac.uk/download/523372727.pdf (accessed on 18th July 2025).
25. Venning, G. (2008). A pilot study of the profile of injuries that presented to the student chiropractic sports council at the Pick 'n Pay 94.7 cycle challenge from 2002 to 2004. https://core.ac.uk/download/18215246.pdf (accessed on 18th July 2025).
26. Villao, L. (2007). Modern frequency and the significance of acromial shape in the etiological debate of os acromiale. https://core.ac.uk/download/268806316.pdf (accessed on 18th July 2025).

THE PELVIC GIRDLE AND LOWER LIMB IN HUMAN OSTEOLOGY

9

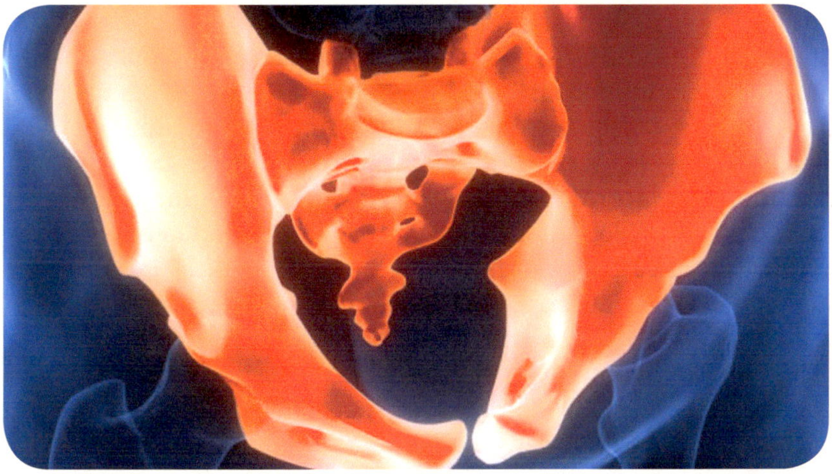

LEARNING OBJECTIVES

After studying this chapter, you will be able to:

1. Discuss the anatomy of the pelvic girdle
2. Explain the structure of the lower limb
3. Understand the development of the pelvic girdle
4. Know the biomechanics of the lower limb
5. Evaluate pathologies of the pelvic girdle
6. Focus on the evolutionary perspective

Introduction

The study of the pelvic girdle and lower limb of human osteology ranks top in importance while studying the evolutionary history of hominins as well as their functional anatomy. The pelvic girdle acts as a center of stability and mobility, carries the upper body load, and aids in bipedal locomotion. This specific adaptation is the result of evolutionary forces that have operated over millions of years to shape human physiology. By observing structural variations in the pelvic girdle across species, researchers can infer the locomotor habits that defined our early evolutionary line. Exploring biomechanical and morphological transformations not only assists in understanding modern human anatomy but also builds towards more universal discourse on evolutionary biology, especially locomotion adjustments from quadrupedality to bipedality in other vertebrates, as explored in the biomechanics of archosaurs that describe evolving locomotor strategies (Allen et al., 2017). The lower limb, outside of the pelvic girdle, also provides fundamental insight into human development and adaptation. The lower limb, made up of the femur, tibia, fibula, and the associated joints, is a critical structure to support running and walking on two legs. This limb structure results from complex interactions among muscle, bone, and joint tissues, sculpted by environmental and genetic factors. Understanding the anatomical elements of the lower limb and how they function in conjunction with the pelvic girdle is essential, particularly in professions like forensic anthropology, where accurate determination of age, sex, and ancestry can be determined through skeletal remains. New developments, such as the use of remote learning techniques and haptic learning with models, highlight the critical role of active and experiential learning in understanding these anatomical complexities, as evidenced in human osteology education research (Gamble et al., 2024). In addition to their relevance to anatomical study, the pelvic girdle and lower limbs transcend anatomical discussion into a broader context of human adaptation and survival. These skeletons not only reflect evolutionary developments but are also engaged in activities such as locomotion, balance, and giving birth. The diversity observed in pelvic girdle morphology across populations can provide evidence of adaptations to different environmental stresses and lifestyles. With further investigation in these fields, the adoption of modern methodologies and techniques, such as biomechanical modeling and comparative analysis with other animals, serves as the basis for osteological understanding. Ultimately, this foray into the pelvic girdle and lower limb will foster a greater appreciation for human evolutionary biology and the intricate relationship between anatomy and function in our species.

Definition of Osteology

Osteology, as a scientific discipline, is dedicated to the study of bones, their structure, function, and development in vertebrates. Primarily, it concerns the extensive study of the skeletal system, i.e., the intricacies of bone formation, growth, and regeneration. Osteology is not merely concerned with classifying and naming various bones but also with studying how bony tissues respond to various biological and environmental stimuli. By examining the pelvic girdle and lower limbs, osteologists can uncover vital information about locomotion, load distribution, and evolutionary adaptation over time. Further, the understanding of osteological principles enlightens us on basic concepts of human anatomy and physiology that are central to medical occupations, anthropology, and forensic examination. The study of human osteology exceeds the elementary anatomical categorization because it also highly benefits interdisciplinary inquiries. For instance, biological anthropology employs osteology to address questions of human evolution and variation. Interdisciplinarity in this case often draws on the analysis of skeletal remains to estimate demographic trends, health status, and the lifestyles of their ancient occupants. Additionally, the emergence of remote education through the COVID-19 pandemic has forced innovative pedagogical action within the field. Studies demonstrated that distance students were able to effectively attain central human osteology learning objectives using tactile, take-home skeletal models, highlighting the importance of hands-on skills to acquire proficiency in identification and quantitative skills in Gamble et al. (2024). Understanding the importance of osteology to vertebrate evolution reveals that adaptations in bone types reflect general adaptive strategies. As seen across various vertebrate groups, losses or reductions of appendages are the result of changes in gene expression rather than in coding sequences, illustrating the complexity of evolutionary pathways. The multifaceted interactions among osteological consequences, developmental biology, and environmental stress warrant the pelvic girdle and lower limb as a functional anatomy and evolutionary research focus. By interpreting the molecular mechanisms underpinning these adaptations, osteology integrates genetic information with morphological observation, thereby deepening our knowledge of vertebrate phylogeny and the evolutionary significance of bony components in diverse taxa, as illustrated in studies comparing appendage reduction across vertebrate lineages (Sanger et al., 2021) (Figure 9.1).

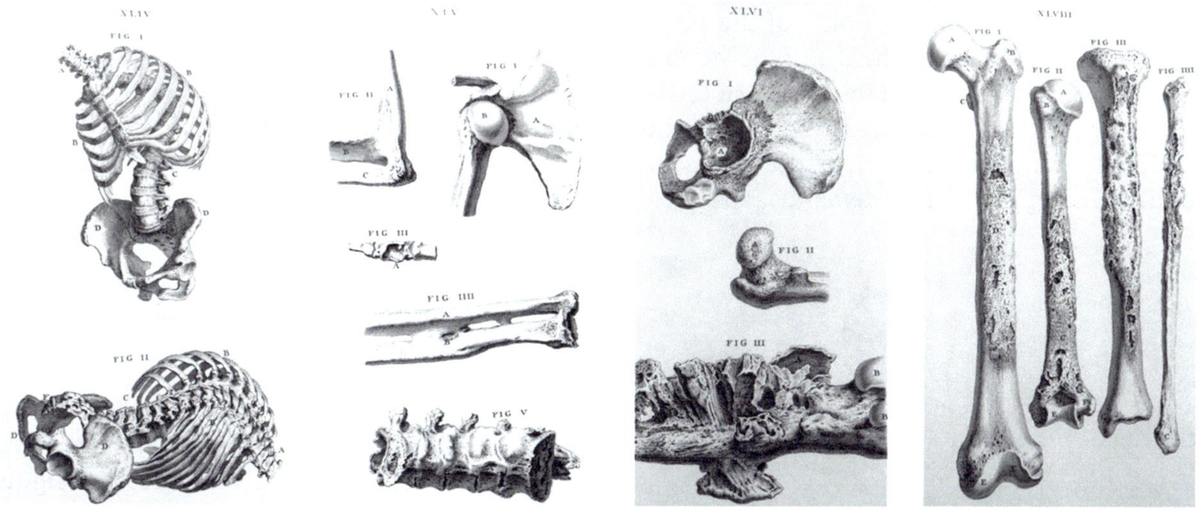

Figure 9.1. Osteology, as a scientific discipline.

Source: https://external-content.duckduckgo.com/iu/?u=https%3A%2F%2Fboneandjoint.org.uk%2Fapi%2Fasset%2F2048-0105.16.360093%2F360093-galleyfig4.jpeg&f=1&nofb=1&ipt=6240a073a7b755641b5ae13762228a6b7d2d0124ca23f8f54b41714b1623cb0d.

Significance of the Pelvic Girdle and Lower Limb

The pelvic girdle is a fundamental structure of human osteology, effectively specializing the human body for bipedal locomotion. Comprising the fused ilium, ischium, and pubis, the girdle supports the weight of the upper limb when sitting and standing and transmits the weight to the lower limbs during movement. Its design not only supports bipedalism but also enables a variety of sophisticated movements, such as squatting, running, and climbing, demonstrating an evolutionary advantage that has facilitated human survival and mobility. Moreover, the pelvic girdle houses significant anatomical features, such as the acetabulum, which articulates the femur to form the hip joint. This joint's structural support is crucial in the balance and resistance to dynamic forces that happen during walking, making the pelvic girdle's role of structural support and functional mobility in human anatomy prominent. The lower limb complements the pelvic girdle's role by being crucial in efficient walking, providing the outputs necessary for walking and weight-bearing. Comprised of the femur, tibia, fibula, and foot bones, the lower limb is aesthetically beautiful and capable of agility and strength. The proximal femur itself has adaptations for walking and running on two legs, including its angle and its dense structure, which can withstand the stress of locomotion. Also, the muscles that encircle the lower extremity, such as the quadriceps and hamstrings, work synergistically to produce powerful, coordinated movements required for activities ranging from walking to athletics. This musculoskeletal complex allows humans to move across different landscapes and climates, thereby underscoring the lower limb's role in providing flexibility to adapt and survive in numerous environments. Lower limb and pelvic girdle both have a huge role to play in reproductive health and stability. In females, the architectural plan of the pelvis adjusts to give birth, with changes in pelvic inlet and outlet dimensions from those of men to suit this major process. These variations reflect the dual functionality of the pelvic girdle, balancing mobility and reproductive demands.

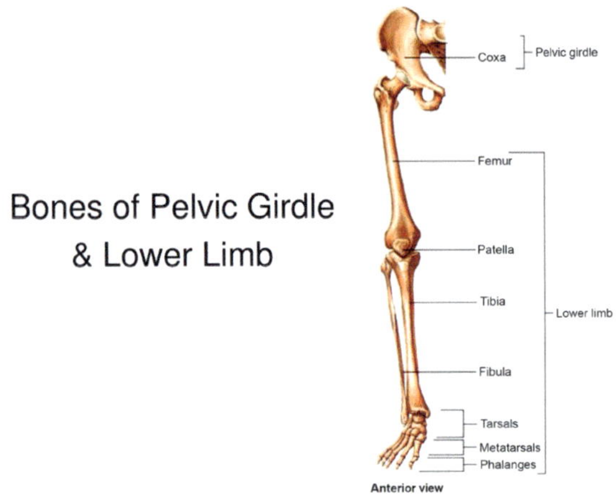

Figure 9.2. The pelvic girdle serves as a pivotal structure in human osteology.

Source: https://external-content.duckduckgo.com/iu/?u=https%3A%2F%2Fimage.slideserve.com%2F354864%2Fbones-of-pelvic-girdle-lower-limb-l.jpg&f=1&nofb=1&ipt=a06d715e271c916eba4590de3a04625922282bbbfebaa4169924f2dd5f040ea9.

In addition, earlier work focuses on the incorporation of hip joint morphology into overall locomotor function, suggesting an internal morphofunctional cue that may provide insights into evolutionary habits in hominoids. The evolution of these structures has enabled immense diversity in locomotor activity, highlighting the importance of pelvic girdle and lower limb anatomy in understanding human evolution and contemporary biomechanics. Overall, an appreciation for the pelvic girdle and lower limbs extends well beyond structure to reveal profound evolutionary changes that affect our species' locomotion and physical interaction with the world around us (Figure 9.2).

9.1. Anatomy of the Pelvic Girdle

Learning Outcome

1. Structures of the pelvic girdle
2. Functions of the pelvic girdle
3. Sex differences in the pelvic girdles of males and females

The pelvic girdle is a vital component of the human skeletal system, delicately designed to support the body's weight while enabling movement and mobility. The three bones that unite to form the acetabulum, the socket of the femur, and thus the hip joint are the ilium, ischium, and pubis. The bony structure of the pelvic girdle not only provides a firm foundation for the lower limb but also protects vital organs located within the pelvic cavity, such as the bladder and reproductive systems. This dual function of support and protection highlights the evolutionary significance of pelvic girdles, which have progressively developed over time to facilitate bipedal mobility in humans, altering the way our predecessors traversed varied topographies. Appreciation of such anatomical complexities contributes to our knowledge about their role in biomechanics and human evolution. Apart from its structural role, the pelvic girdle provides stability and equilibrium during locomotion. The sacroiliac joint, which forms a union between the ilium and the sacrum, provides this in that it allows locomotion and also provides shock absorption from the top portion of the body during movement. This coupling permits force transfer between the upper and lower body, essential for running and bipedal gait. Moreover, the shape and direction of the pelvic inlet, as determined by sex-specific anatomical characteristics, play an important role in gait economy and dynamics. For instance, the larger female pelvic inlet is tailored to childbirth and demonstrates a functional compromise between two competing biological functions—reproduction and locomotion. These anatomical characteristics reflect the intricate relationship between the form and function of the pelvic girdle. The muscular attachments of the pelvic girdle further underscore its importance in human osteology, as they provide powerful movement and support during various physical activities.

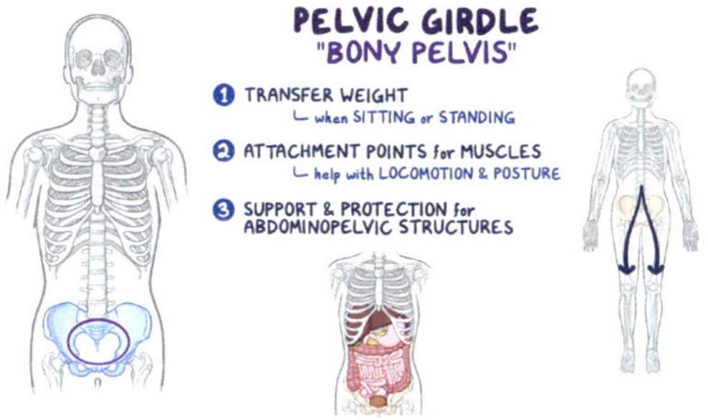

Figure 9.3. The pelvic girdle represents a critical component of the human skeletal system.

Source: https://external-content.duckduckgo.com/iu/?u=https%3A%2F%2Fd16qt3wv6xm098.cloudfront.net%2F5UjBTOLnQOOL5uApOANh4sWsQh6RnICh%2F_.jpg&f=1&nofb=1&ipt=45102fa18c3df538b7fe1d4a919f98078e45dba6b657c8a6130d76a306701eff.

Muscles such as the gluteus maximus, iliopsoas, and pelvic floor musculature directly affect not only movement but also posture and core stability. The multifunctional roles of these muscles in walking to complex athletic maneuvers illustrate the pelvic girdle's vital position in functional physiology. Additionally, anatomical variations of the pelvis can affect athletic performance, underscoring the significance of biomechanical investigation in this subject. Collectively, the anatomical and functional complexities of the pelvic girdle mirror its central role in the broader context of the lower limbs' osteology and biomechanics, confirming that the evolutionary development of this structure has far-reaching implications for human mobility and health throughout the lifespan (Figure 9.3).

9.1.1. Components of the Pelvic Girdle

The pelvic girdle is a complex anatomical framework composed of several significant elements responsible for determining human locomotor roles and structural support. The most central and primary component of the pelvic girdle is the os coxae, comprising the two hip bones connected to the sacrum at the sacroiliac joints. The individual os coxae is also further divided into three primary sections: ilium, ischium, and pubis. The ilium is the superior and largest segment with broad surfaces for attachments of muscles, while the ischium forms the posterior surface of the pelvis for bearing weight when sitting. The pubis contributes to the anterior part of the pelvic girdle, where the two halves coalesce at the pubic symphysis, allowing for limited movement, which is essential in parturition and other forms of physical exercise. Understanding these aspects brings a better comprehension of the evolutionary suitability of the human pelvic girdle, particularly for bipedal movement. Further, the pelvic girdle's architectural design also yields to significant function in addition to weight-bearing and locomotion. The pelvic cavity of the os coxae protects vital organs in the lower abdomen and plays a key role in reproductive health. In females, the pelvic girdle exhibits specialized morphological characteristics such as a wide subpubic angle and a wider pelvic inlet, which are crucial for giving birth. While men have a narrower pelvis width and greater depth, the specialized features highlight the functional specialization of the female pelvis to accommodate the passage of a child during birth. This dimorphism is significant in understanding not only anatomical variation for sex but also the concomitants for biomechanical function and potential childbirth complications, so a general approach to the study of human osteology on the basis of sex difference and reproductive health is required.

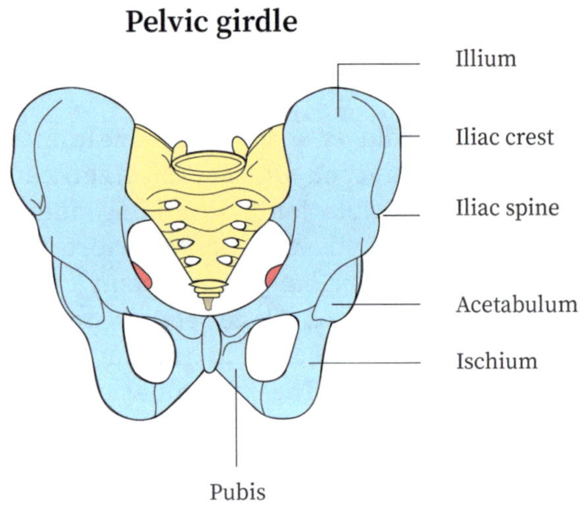

Figure 9.4. The pelvic girdle.

Source: https://external-content.duckduckgo.com/iu/?u=https%3A%2F%2Fcms-media.bartleby.com%2Fwp-content%2Fuploads%2Fsites%2F2%2F2021%2F06%2F07142553%2FBones-Of-The-Pelvic-Girdle-1-1024x877.jpg&f=1&nofb=1&ipt=b695e889559996026c7376527 5efc5a90b35ede5e2c9197f7b34dfd150baaf53.

Finally, in addition to its anatomical elements, the pelvic girdle is deeply involved in muscular dynamics through its roles in motion and stability. Various muscles, such as the iliopsoas, gluteals, and pelvic floor muscles, originate or insert onto the os coxae and create the intricate movements of hip flexion, extension, abduction, and rotation. The sequence and size of these groups of muscles can vary in individuals, usually due to ethnoracial differences, as discussed in research that determined various musculature characteristics in populations (Synstelien et al., 2001). These differences remind one to seek out and acknowledge individual and group differences in clinical practice and anthropological inquiry. A consideration of the components of the pelvic girdle, along with these muscle attachments, gives profound insights into human locomotion, athletic potential, and the evolutionary developments that have shaped the functions of the lower limb in humans (Figure 9.4).

9.1.2. Functions of the Pelvic Girdle

The pelvic girdle supports several functions critical to the efficient locomotion and stability of bipedal animals. Most critically, it sustains the upper body's weight during varying activities such as walking, standing, and running. The structure of the pelvic girdle, comprising the ilium, ischium, and pubis, is a broad, basin-shaped structure that is effective in transmitting mechanical loads. This anatomical design not only accommodates symmetrical weight transmission during movement but also allows attachment of significant muscle groups, such as those associated with hip flexion and extension. As such, the pelvic girdle facilitates efficient energy expenditure during locomotion, enabling adjustment to the changing environmental demands encountered by humans and their ancestors throughout their evolutionary history. The second critical function of the pelvic girdle is to guard the internal organs within the pelvic cavity. The closeness of the pelvic girdle to organs such as the bladder, reproductive organs, and lower gastrointestinal tract serves as a natural safeguard against damage. The encasing furnished by the pelvic girdle not only supports the structural stability of such organs but also plays a functional role, including in giving birth. The femoral and axillary dimensions of the pelvis can change during labor, underscoring their importance for reproductive success from an evolutionary standpoint. Further, pelvic shape changes, which vary with factors such as ethnicity or sex, could affect both ancestral fitness and biomechanical function, suggesting the evolution of adaptive traits under environmental influence (Synstelien et al., 2001). Lastly, the pelvic girdle assists in locomotion by stabilizing the lower limbs, providing the foundation for bipedal walking. This connection is important since it allows the coordination of the leg's muscular forces with those of the pelvic girdle in order to create effective movement patterns. The biomechanics of bipedalism is typified by a complex coupling of joint motion and muscle leverage, necessary for propulsive and balancing functions. Homologous structures observed in evolutionary forebears, such as the evolution of quadrupedal to bipedal locomotion in archosaurs, illustrate how pelvic anatomical modifications relate to locomotor functional adaptation. Enhanced muscle activity in the vicinity of the hip joint enables robust, versatile motion, illustrating the co-evolution of structural change and biomechanical effectiveness in human osteology (Allen et al., 2017).

9.1.3. Differences Between Male and Female Pelvic Girdles

The variation between the male and female pelvis girdles is largely influenced by biological and evolutionary changes, primarily associated with reproduction. The female pelvis is usually broader and more circular to accommodate childbirth. The structure has a wider pelvic inlet and larger pelvic canal measurements, which are needed for the fetus during childbirth. In contrast to the female, the male pelvis is usually narrower and taller to maximize bipedal movement and body strength. The differences are most apparent when comparing the size of the outlines of the pelvic inlet and outlet; females possess wider transverse diameters, whereas males exhibit wider anteroposterior measurements.

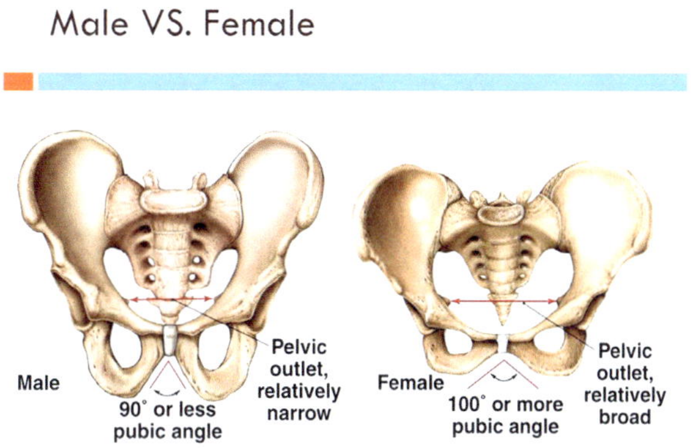

Figure 9.5. Differences between male and female pelvic girdles.

Source: https://external-content.duckduckgo.com/iu/?u=https%3A%2F%2Fthemasterpiecemom.com%2F800%2F600%2Fhttp%2Fimages.slideplayer.com%2F31%2F9794071%2Fslides%2Fslide_12.jpg&f=1&nofb=1&ipt=d8ab7865674536298f2470817b08270526c609b01d8561066c2e4048ec4c1814.

These differences in structure emphasize the adaptive significance of the pelvis for reproductive biology and underscore the value of noting them to fields such as anthropology and medicine. In increasing attention, it is found that such structural differences in pelvic girdles also extend to the regional composition and architectural structure of the pelvic bones. For instance, the femoral morphology provides insight into differences: males have a deeper, wider sciatic notch than females, again in connection with the functional needs of giving birth. Furthermore, the ischial tuberosity size is significantly different, as they are wider apart in female pelves to allow for giving birth. A comparative human osseous structure study found that the pelvic girdles of males tend to be wider, with measures such as the outlet anteroposterior diameter significantly larger in males than in females, supporting the hypothesis of a stronger, more functionally adapted girdle (Nwoha et al., 2000). Differences in anatomy such as this not only play a part in an explanation of human skeletal biology but also inform broader implications for evolutionary development. Recent research has focused on the impact of environmental and genetic factors on the morphology of the pelvis across different populations. Comparing pelvic girdles among modern and medieval men, researchers found glaring disparities in dimensions such as interspinous and intercristal distances, which were higher in modern men than in their ancient counterparts (Czwojdziński et al., 2019). These findings address the evolutionary consequences of lifestyle change, variation in body mass, and the overall mechanical loading of the pelvis over time. Such data show that while basic anatomical variation between male and female pelves has been consistent, ongoing changes in societal behavior and physical requirements will ultimately drive the evolution of pelvic architecture. Therefore, the interaction between biological adaptation and environmental considerations emphasizes the dynamic nature of human osteology and the significance of the interdisciplinary nature of investigations into these anatomical variations (Figure 9.5).

Test Your Knowledge

1. What are the main bones and joints that form the pelvic girdle, and how do they support the trunk and protect internal organs?
2. How do structural differences between the male and female pelvic girdles relate to function and reproduction?

9.2. The Structure of the Lower Limb

Learning Outcome

1. Major bones of the lower limb
2. Lower limb-related joints
3. Muscles and their role in lower limb movement

The lower limb, as a component of human locomotion and support, comprises several major structures that work together to facilitate movement. Centered to this anatomical region is the pelvic girdle, a solid structure formed as a result of the convergence of the ilium, ischium, and pubis. This girdle, besides supporting the weight of the head and arms when standing and walking, also plays a role in load transfer between the lower limbs and the axial skeleton. The pelvic girdle is structured to possess a deep acetabulum that offers stable articulation with the femur, allowing a variety of movements associated with locomotion. Furthermore, the complex interaction between the bones and their respective musculature highlights the lower limb's ability to respond to varying activities, making it a focal point in human osteology. Outside of the pelvic girdle, the femur is the longest and most powerful bone in the human skeleton and acts as the main connection to the knee and, therefore, impacts the function of the entire lower limb. Supported by its unique proximal features, such as the head and neck of the femur, this bone facilitates great movement at the hip joint, crucial for running, jumping, and ascending. The distal end of the femur divides into the medial and lateral condyles, which terminate in the tibia to form the knee joint.

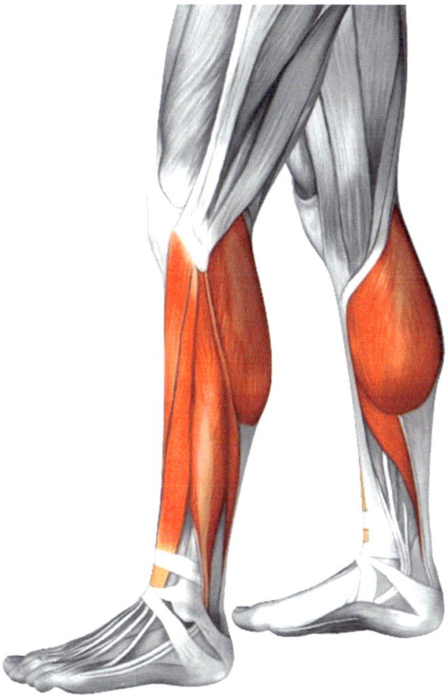

Figure 9.6. The structure of the lower limb.

Source: https://external-content.duckduckgo.com/iu/?u=https%3A%2F%2Fknowledge.carolina.com%2Fwp-content%2Fuploads%2F2021%2F11%2Fshutterstock_674183425.jpg&f=1&nofb=1&ipt=e9ac0acf7c699d6f093cecae4f505e73aad98e6c550600d52a3885b9da2a9f48.

This joint is critical for weight-bearing activities because it allows extension and flexion, the necessary motions of locomotion. The femur's structure, combined with its stabilizing cartilage and ligaments, is a prime example of evolutionary adaptation to bipedalism, a fundamental aspect of human anatomy that sets our species apart from all other vertebrates. Lastly, the lower limb contains the intricate form of the tibia and fibula, which are responsible for providing movement and stability. The tibia is larger and stronger of the two bones, responsible mostly for bearing weight and forming an integral part of ankle joint function, while the fibula mainly provides attachment points for muscles and stabilizes. The structural formation of these bones offers effective shock absorption and force transmission during activities such as running and jumping. Furthermore, the jointed connections between the tibia, fibula, and a few of the tarsal bones of the foot, and the arches formed due to the foot's structure, offer a dynamic and rigid platform for movement. This complex interplay of bones and muscle joints highlights the structural significance of the lower limb in human osteology, as it not only displays functional adaptations but also evolutionary principles displayed in species, as seen in comparative studies such as those on Megalancosaurus (Renesto et al., 2023). Continued findings of these anatomical structures continue to provide additional information on human locomotion as well as the bone adaptations that enable it (Figure 9.6).

9.2.1. Major Bones of the Lower Limb

The structure of the lower limb is primarily defined by a series of major bones that serve crucial roles in locomotion and bearing weight. The pelvis, which includes the ilium, ischium, and pubis, is the structural support connecting the lower limbs with the axial skeleton. This arrangement stabilizes not only the body during various activities but also the pelvic organs. The combined shape of the pelvic girdle provides both flexibility and stability, which absorbs the complex movements of walking and running. This adaptation is essential to upright bipedal gait, showing the evolutionary alteration that has occurred in humans. Moreover, the morphology of the girdle influences the biomechanics of walking, which may be informative of human evolutionary history and quadruped-bipedal transition, according to studies of Archosauria evolution (Allen et al., 2017).

The femur, or thigh bone, is the longest and strongest bone of the human skeleton and forms a significant part of the lower limb. Its unique shape, with a spherical head and acetabular articulation, allows tremendous mobility at the hip joint. The femur endures heavy loading and provides the leverage necessary for effective locomotion. The distal femur articulates with the tibia and fibula at the knee joint, underscoring its key role in lower extremity mechanics. Understanding the femurs function and morphology sheds light on how it is connected to the adjacent muscles and ligaments in terms of motion. Such a connection reveals the complexity of the human body's structure and the importance of the femur in stabilizing the system and facilitating various physical activities performed in daily life (Synstelien et al., 2001). The two large bones of the lower leg that offer stability and mobility, along with the femur, are the tibia and fibula. The greater tibia, or shinbone, bears most of the weight passed from the femur through the knee joint. Its solid construction is critical for weight-bearing activity, as it serves as the base for the mechanical demands imposed on the lower limb during locomotion.

The fibula, although considerably narrower and not directly responsible for weight-bearing, plays a critical role in lateral support of the ankle and attachment of muscles. The relationship between the tibia and fibula during use is important for the integrity of the ankle joint and for stance or gait balance. Collectively, these bones exhibit remarkable adaptations that enable diverse locomotor activity, bearing testimony to the sophisticated design that is an intrinsic part of human osteology and the evolutionary history of the lower limb (Allen et al., 2017) (Figure 9.7).

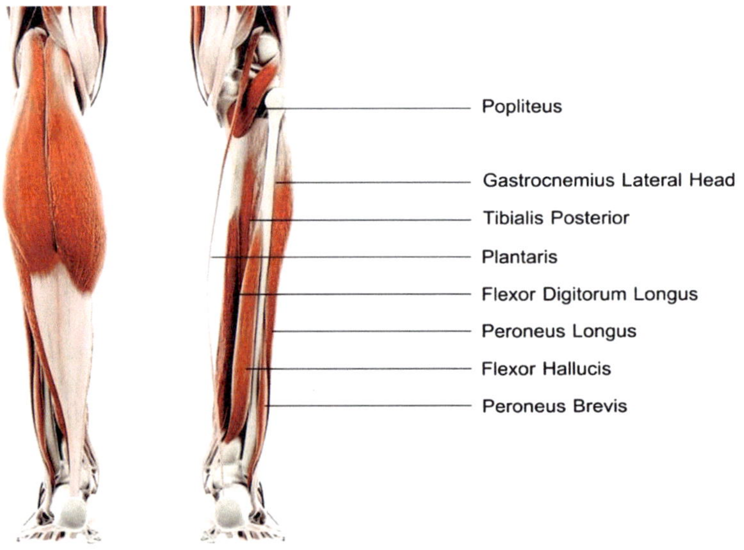

Figure 9.7. Major bones of the lower limb.

Source: https://external-content.duckduckgo.com/iu/?u=https%3A%2F%2Fmblexguide.com%2Fwp-content%2Fuploads%2F2022%2F07%2FPosterior-lower-leg-muscles-e1658874415183.jpg&f=1&nofb=1&ipt=b4c629f1ad5c155935789e6c8d7c9bb4550927642759814ld6de04c0727f5ae2.

9.2.2. Joints Associated with the Lower Limb

The osseous framework of the lower limb comprises many important joints that provide an extensive range of movement and facilitate bipedal walking. The ball-and-socket hip joint connects the femur to the pelvis, providing for flexion, extension, abduction, adduction, and rotation. The depth of the socket, provided by the shape of the acetabulum, maximizes stability while providing excellent mobility. The hip joint illustrates how anatomical specializations, such as the femoral head and the orientation of the related ligaments, facilitate human bipedal efficiency. Also, the knee joint that is formed by the femur, tibia, and patella articulation exists mainly as a hinge joint. It receives flexion and extension movements, as well as limited rotational movement, which are necessary for activities of locomotion such as walking, running, and jumping.

These attributes are what display the complexity of joints within the lower limb and their evolutionary implications for human mobility. Additionally, the ankle joint constitutes a critical anatomical interface allowing complex motions for productive gait and stability. Comprising the tibia, fibula, and talus, the ankle joint allows dorsiflexion and plantarflexion, enabling forward movement and stability during various activities. The structural anatomy of the ankle, in addition to the ligaments and joint capsule, provides protection and mobility, making it distinct from other joints. In addition, the subtalar joint, located below the ankle, is pivotal in enabling foot inversion and eversion, providing flexibility for walking on uneven surfaces. With human movement across different landscapes, the subtalar and ankle joints' flexibility allows not only locomotion but also shock absorption, emphasizing the lower limb's biomechanical economy in evolutionary terms, as discussed in the analysis of changes in locomotion in Archosauria (Allen et al., 2017). Finally, the joints of the lower limb are supplemented by the intricate system of foot articulations. They are the metatarsophalangeal and interphalangeal joints, which contribute to the foot's overall movement and flexibility. The metatarsophalangeal joints allow for flexion and extension of the toes for balance and push-off while traveling.

The interphalangeal joints also allow for other support to toe articulation. The coordination between these joints and the muscles that drive them is vital for maintaining an appropriate walking pattern, which mirrors the evolutionary advantages conferred by bipedalism. The common action of the joints of the lower limb illustrates evolutionary forces that have shaped the human musculoskeletal structure to provide greater mobility, stability, and rapid responsiveness across various environments, as seen in the broader functional morphology comparisons among locomotor types (N/A, 2017) (Figure 9.8).

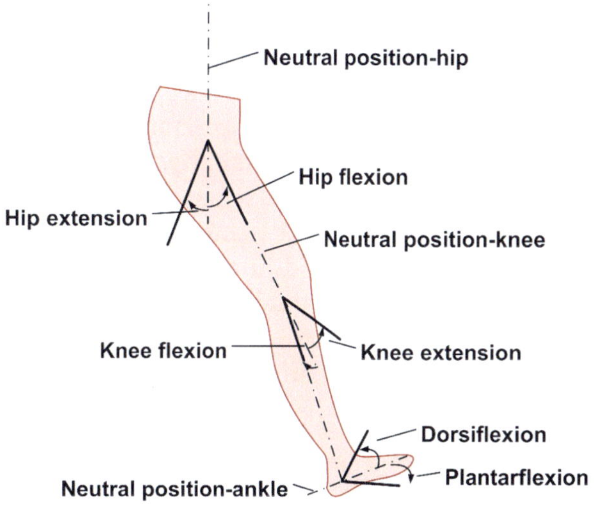

Figure 9.8. Joints associated with the lower limb.

Source: https://www.researchgate.net/profile/Hayder-Al-Shuka/publication/330917511/figure/fig12/AS:779420835016756@1562839816961/Lower-limb-joints-positions-50.png.

9.2.3. Muscles and Their Roles in Lower Limb Movement

The muscles of the lower limb play important roles in movement and stabilization, depending on their orientation and anatomical arrangement around the pelvic girdle and its associated joints. Gluteal muscles, located in the back of the pelvis, are primary movers in hip extension and abduction and are major contributory bipedal walking structures. As a case in point, the gluteus maximus not only aids running and climbing but also stabilizes the hip joint during these movements, preventing lateral movement. Moreover, synergistic action among the gluteal muscles, particularly during balance or turning tasks, highlights the intricate coordination required for efficient lower limb movement. Observation of muscular interactions along the pelvic girdle provides further perspective on how human osteology facilitates movement, particularly by considering the evolutionary trade-offs that render bipedal animals dissimilar from their quadruped ancestors. The comprehensive muscle anatomy of the lower limb also encompasses the quadriceps group and hamstring muscles, which are primarily involved in knee joint mobility and stability. Quadriceps, which consist of four muscular components, play a primary role in knee extension, essential in walking, running, and jumping activities. In conjunction with the quadriceps, hamstrings that induce knee flexion plays an equally essential role in the gait cycle by controlling the braking of the leg movement, particularly in a stride's follow-through. This dynamic coactivation between flexors and extensors underscores the importance of muscle balance in maintaining joint integrity and mobility. By analyzing the biomechanical function of these muscle groups, we can better appreciate how muscular efficiency and coordination serve as a foundation for locomotor strategy and, subsequently, inform rehabilitative treatments for lower limb injuries and conditions related to muscle weakness or imbalance. In addition, the calf muscles, gastrocnemius and soleus, are primarily responsible for walking, running, and jumping through their effects on the ankle joint. They are primarily responsible for plantarflexion, which allows individuals to rise onto their toes during gait, enhancing propulsion and stability. The activation of calf muscles is also crucial for shock absorption during footstrike, underscoring their role in attenuating impact force. As lower limb musculature adapts to varying demands for posture and activity, muscle activation and coordination are determined by gravitational forces and surface conditions. Understanding these mechanisms brings with it a necessary understanding of the adaptive alterations that occurred in the lower limb form and function, which once more throws light upon the complexity present in the subject of human osteology, specifically regarding how muscles facilitate locomotion and postural changes (Allen et al., 2017; N/A, 2017).

Test Your Knowledge

1. What are the major bones, joints, and muscle groups of the lower limb involved in locomotion?
2. How does the anatomical structure of the lower limb enable weight bearing and efficient movement?

9.3. Development of the Pelvic Girdle

Learning Outcome

1. Embryological development of the pelvic girdle
2. Growth patterns and alterations throughout life
3. Normal developmental abnormalities

Pelvic girdle formation is a polyfactorial process regulated by many genetic, environmental, and mechanical factors throughout human evolution. The pelvic girdle, composed of the ilium, ischium, and pubis, is a critical connector between the trunk and lower limb for locomotion and bipedalism. In embryonic development, the mesodermal tissues differentiate to form the bones of the pelvis, which not only serve as the structural foundation for the pelvic girdle but also influence the organization of contiguous musculature. Through their interaction with developing muscles and ligaments, the shapes of these bones are determined, which are required for both locomotion and stability. Over time, selective pressures, such as the need for efficient bipedalism, have continued to refine the evolution of the pelvic girdle, resulting in obvious anatomical specializations that differentiate Homo sapiens from other primates. Morphological characteristics of the pelvic girdle yield clues regarding the hominin evolutionary lineage. Research has established that pelvic shape varies among races, with consequences concerning the utilization of pelvic environments at a muscular level. Research discovered increased cross-sectional area of specific muscles in certain populations, indicating significant differences in the os coxae morphology. This has led to speculation about the size and shape differences the pelvic girdle might exhibit based upon racial and ethnic origins, particularly regarding the integration of the iliopsoas muscles over the pelvic brim. As explained in the outcomes of this research, statistical analysis found differential size variations in the os coxae between white and black males, calling for consideration of such variations when researching pelvic girdle growth and its functional implications in organic systems of movement and exercise, which would have applicability in fields like sports science and physical anthropology (Synstelien et al., 2001). Also, the academic importance of accurate skeletal modeling in learning pelvic girdle anatomy has emerged, particularly in online learning settings. In instruction in biological anthropology, model skeletons and hands-on experience enhance students' ability to identify and dissect anatomical structures effectively.

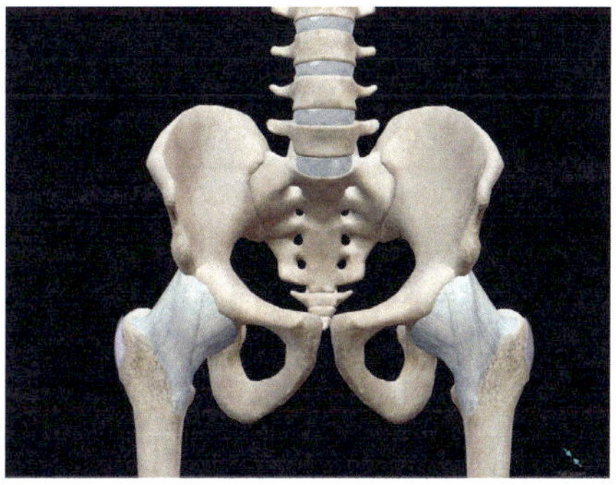

Figure 9.9. The development of the pelvic girdle.

Source: https://external-content.duckduckgo.com/iu/?u=https%3A%2F%2Fwww.visiblebody.com%2Fhubfs%2FBlog_Images%2Fpelvic-girdle-front-hips.png&f=1&nofb=1&ipt=563bf68fd7da766d1438145d5457158b0095929c2e28f82cd40c924325138395.

Recent studies have used plastic model skeletons to achieve learning outcomes in human osteology, where haptic learning is a critical component for studying complex anatomical details. Results show that remote-educated undergraduates could achieve equal competency in bone identification when incorporating comparative, hands-on techniques compared to students who had typical digital methods. This supports the value of hands-on learning devices that allow examination of skeletal details, thereby enhancing comprehension of pelvic girdle development. These approaches are not merely significant for academic growth but also for cementing the role of osteological training across a variety of anthropology lab courses as we adapt to new educational challenges (Gamble et al., 2024) (Figure 9.9).

9.3.1. Embryological Development of the Pelvic Girdle

The embryological development of the pelvic girdle is a complex process that begins very early during gestation, eventually forming the foundation for human walking. The pelvic girdle is developed initially from the lateral plate mesoderm, which plays a role in the formation of the embryonic skeleton. Concurrently, somatic mesoderm develops into the paired bones of the pelvis, namely the ilium, ischium, and pubis. This skeletogenic development is a series of stringently controlled morphogenetic events that lead to chondrification and subsequently ossification. Understanding these processes in human osteology is crucial because embryonic developmental failure can lead to congenital conditions that affect pelvic morphology and function. Therefore, a complete examination of such an early development forms the basis for an understanding of normal and pathological anatomy of the pelvic girdle throughout a person's life. The development of the pelvic girdle continues, undergoing significant changes that optimally increase its functional capacities, particularly in the lower limbs. Turning points for development are related to the fusion of the pelvic bone and joint articulations with the sacrum and femur. These support considerable loads, particularly during bipedal locomotion, and therefore evolved to achieve stability and mobility. The acetabulum, a key component of the articulation, is created by the coming together of the ilium, ischium, and pubis, reflecting the delicate coordination exercised during embryonic life. Any disruption in this coordination can cause joint malformations, underscoring the importance of familiarizing oneself with normal embryological patterns and their potential clinical equivalents. This information is particularly relevant to orthopedic and rehabilitative management of pelvic and lower limb function. In addition, the continuity between the pelvic girdle and the lower limb is emphasized during embryonic and postnatal development. Proper alignment and integration of the pelvic girdle are necessary for ensuring proper gait patterns and overall body mechanics. During initial development, pelvic bone alignment is set by a combination of genes and biomechanical tension from surrounding musculature. More varied functions of ligaments, tendons, and muscles become more evident in the developing fetus, actively molding the pelvic region as it adapts to changing posture and movement. The longitudinal development of plastic embryonic form to rigid adult shape reveals the fine adaptations for human walking. Appreciation of these finer developmental details becomes essential for grasping not just anatomy but also the functional importance of the pelvis within human osteology, as suggested in studies highlighting postural responses that are possible as a result of deviations in the development of the pelvis (Carlini et al., 2022; Ernst et al., 2012).

9.3.2. Growth Patterns and Changes Through Life

The formation of the pelvic girdle is directly associated with the general patterns of growth that can be seen throughout human life, with varying stages from embryonic formation to full maturity. The pelvic girdle first forms from mesenchymal precursor cells, which are involved in both chondrification and subsequent ossification. This timeline begins in utero, as primary ossification centers form, producing an identifiable pelvic structure that will further develop through childhood into adulthood. Of particular interest is that the pelvis is composed of three primary bones—the ilium, ischium, and pubis—that fuse over time, delineating a complex developmental process. The unique growth patterns of the pelvic girdle not only pertain to individual biological factors, but also external considerations, such as fetal movement, which have been identified to affect the general development of the pelvis and which can vary significantly between individuals, leading to further understanding of human osteology (Abel et al., 2016). The pelvic girdle undergoes numerous changes throughout life under the influence of factors such as age, sex, and exercise. During puberty and childhood, the pelvis is formed as pubertal hormonal changes lead to major changes in bone density and morphology. For instance, during development, a woman has a broader subpubic angle and alterations in acetabular depth, adaptations that facilitate birth. During adulthood, life and health variations, such as physical activity levels and the occurrence of injury, influence the development and modification of pelvic architecture. These variations also emphasize the dynamic nature of skeletal development, demonstrating how genetic and environmental influences mold the development and health of the pelvic girdle and lower limb structure throughout life (Abel et al., 2016). In exploring the outcome of patterns of pelvic girdle growth to reproduction and maternal well-being, archaeological studies of skeletal groups can inform us about the historical challenges of childbirth. As an example, evidence within the Juan Primo necropolis shows dystocia complications that may arise due to pelvic morphological variation and result in the level of maternal mortality of pre-industrial populations. The skeletal record from these settings indicates that stressors related to pregnancy, including eclampsia or placental issues, may have had a significant impact on the health of both mother and child. Looking at these examples demonstrates not only the bony alterations of the pelvic girdle across life stages but also the highly significant role it plays in childbirth outcomes, underscoring its importance in human osteology and the evolutionary perspective on growth stages (Figure 9.10).

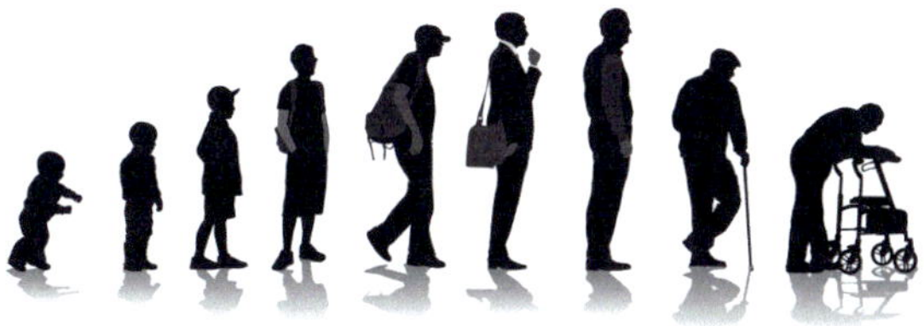

Figure 9.10. The pelvic girdles development is intricately tied to the broader growth patterns observed throughout human life.

Source: https://external-content.duckduckgo.com/iu/?u=https%3A%2F%2Fpsychhelp.com.au%2Fwp-content%2Fuploads%2F2020%2F06%2FiStock-682424594-1.jpg&f=1&nofb=1&ipt=de8379ae3c4fd361a6209589060c0d39939648a89247bfd7e5de25dd19aaf705.

9.3.3. Common Developmental Disorders

It is important to study common developmental disorders to understand their impact on the human skeletal system, particularly the pelvic girdle and lower limbs. Disorders such as developmental dysplasia of the hip (DDH) entail abnormal joint development in the hip, and it could lead to malposition and functional impairment. DDH typically occurs due to a combination of genetic and environmental factors in infancy and pregnancy. Left untreated, the long-term effects of DDH can be seen in the form of osteoarthritis and reduced mobility, underlining the importance of early diagnosis and treatment. Knowledge of the interaction between developmental disorders and skeletal anatomy reveals how anatomical differences affect the overall health and mobility of an individual and, therefore, the significance of active orthopedic evaluation in vulnerable populations. Besides hip dysplasia, other developmental disorders, such as clubfoot, have profound effects on the morphology and function of the lower extremities. Clubfoot, or congenital talipes equinovarus, is a deformation of the foot, causing an inward rotation and disrupting the normal alignment of the pelvic girdle. Clubfoot is caused by a multifactorial etiology, including both genetic predispositions and intrauterine positioning dynamics. Early intervention with methods such as the Ponseti technique will restore the foot's position and prevent long-term disability. This treatment emphasizes the overlap between osteological studies and treatment procedures, as developmental anatomy analysis drives treatment protocol. For every clubfoot, there is an obvious disruption of anatomical distortions to the lower limb's functional competency, further underscoring the necessity for in-depth clinical evaluations from birth. Obstetric complications, as attested in archaeological contexts, also have a role of paramount importance in comprehending developmental disorders since they could be connected to the pelvic girdle. For example, evidence from the pre-Hispanic necropolis at Juan Primo provides insight into how the health of the mother could influence fetal development, particularly regarding disorders that can occur in the process of giving birth. Maternal disorders such as eclampsia or dystocia are likely to result in significant stressors that can be detrimental to mother and child, leading to increased maternal mortality and developmental disorders in offspring. These ancient cases echo today's realities and show how developmental disorder prevalence is influenced by historical and socio-environmental factors. By synthesizing osteoarchaeological data with contemporary research, scientists can develop a more accurate model of the relationship between maternal health, developmental disorders, and skeletal well-being, particularly involving the pelvic girdle and lower limb function (Synstelien et al., 2001; Alamón-Núñez et al., 2019) (Figure 9.11).

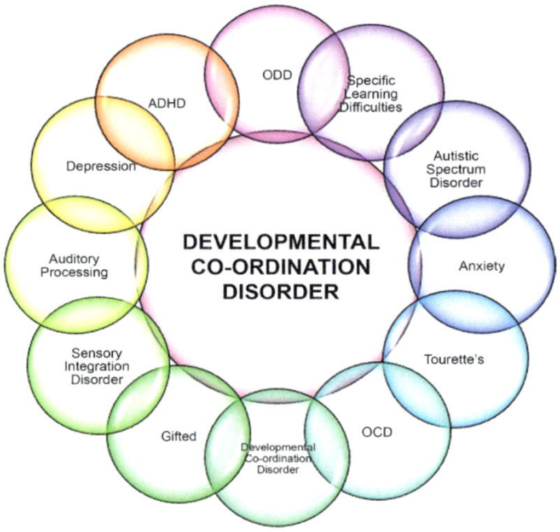

Figure 9.11. The study of common developmental disorders.

Source: https://external-content.duckduckgo.com/iu/?u=https%3A%2F%2Fwww.lanc.org.uk%2Fwp-content%2Fuploads%2F2012%2F10%2FDCD.png&f=1&nofb=1&ipt=2676255018189366f4c08e413e1c0dcb2cf27964a6da73ab5f6ddecad7c4bb18.

Test Your Knowledge

1. How does the pelvic girdle develop from embryonic stages to adulthood?
2. What genetic and hormonal factors influence the growth and maturation of the pelvic girdle?

9.4. Biomechanics of the Lower Limb

Learning Outcome

1. Gait analysis and its significance
2. Forces acting on the lower limb when moving
3. Biomechanical influence on sporting performance

Lower limb biomechanics plays an important role in human gait appreciation, particularly in the framework of the pelvic girdles structural and functional adaptations. At the intersection of bipedalism and anatomical sophistication, the lower limb undergoes dynamic changes during motion, underscoring the importance of joint biomechanics and the interactions among muscular forces. The pelvis and lower limb ensemble reflects an evolutionary shift from quadrupedal to bipedal locomotion, profoundly influencing the anatomical organization of the elements. Biomechanical models, described in a chapter on locomotor extremes in Archosauria, show that changes in limb anatomy directly influence motion capabilities, muscle moment arms, and joint ranges. These findings shed light on the intricate relationship between pelvic positioning and limb function, highlighting the need for in-depth analysis in human osteology rather than mere anatomical explanations (Allen et al., 2017).

In addition, the pelvic girdle's unique structure enables load distribution and support during movement, underscoring its biomechanical importance. With the ischium, ilium, and pubis forming the hip bones, the human pelvis has evolved to support bipedal walking as well as the intricate interplay of various groups of muscles. The adaptation occurs not just in stationary forms but also in dynamic biomechanical processes, where muscular action near the hip joint is used to enhance mobility and walking power. Evidence indicates that the musculature here takes up and transfers forces generated during locomotion, with greater gait pattern flexibility. This function of the pelvic girdle in humanity's movement is a milestone in the optimization of form and function and a critical element of osteological studies of human mobility (Abel et al., 2016).

Finally, biomechanical analysis of the lower limb provides valuable insight into the ontogeny of the pelvic girdle and its broader influence on locomotion. Pelvic structure underlies developmental processes that highlight the significance of genetic and environmental factors, including fetal movement as a potential structural determinant.

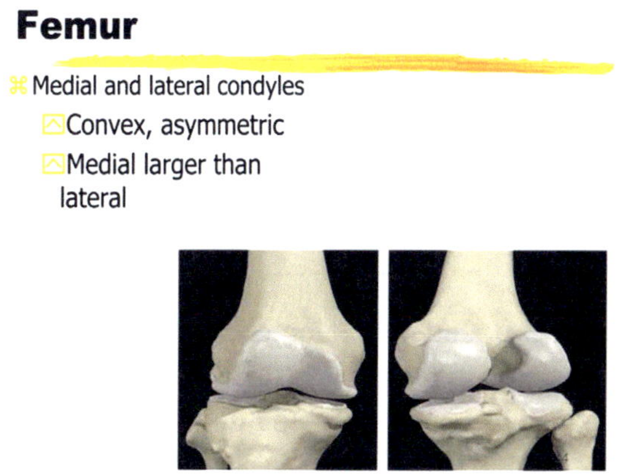

Figure 9.12. The biomechanics of the lower limb.

Source: https://external-content.duckduckgo.com/iu/?u=https%3A%2F%2Fimage.slidesharecdn.com%2Fbiomechanicsofle-200330171244%2F85%2FBiomechanics-of-lower-Limb-34-638.jpg&f=1&nofb=1&ipt=62d5c873c99887f7d98e0d559146fadce3fadc883489e22af407802cac49b638.

This area of research encourages exploration of how variation in pelvic morphology may determine locomotor efficiency and adaptability throughout life. Secondly, this type of research offers a window to understanding pelvis and lower limb pathologies that arise as a result of poor development, with the emphasis upon the interconnectedness of biomechanical theory and clinical concerns. With the demystification of lower limb biomechanics, researchers are increasingly able to make contributions to enhanced understanding of human evolution and functional anatomy and, as a result, to human osteology as a body of knowledge in general (Abel et al., 2016) (Figure 9.12).

9.4.1. Gait Analysis and Its Significance

It is crucial to learn gait analysis to examine the mechanism of human walking, particularly in relation to the pelvic girdle and lower limbs in human osteology. Gait refers to the manner in which individuals walk or run, and it is composed of many elements such as joint movement, balance, and muscular activity. Analysis of gait requires accurate biomechanical measurements that yield information on both the normal patterned movement and deviations due to injury or disease.

Using advanced technologies such as force plates and motion capture systems, scientists quantify gait parameters, including joint angles, cadence, and stride length. This three-dimensional analysis is crucial for physical rehabilitation, sports science, and ergonomics because it enables the specification of areas of concern that guide interventions to enhance mobility and function. Gait analysis has importance extending beyond its clinical relevance, as it also provides evolutionary knowledge of human gait. It can be evaluated how biomechanical conditions were fundamentally changed through evolutionary development to gain an overall impression about the evolution of human gait from our primate lineage. Quadruped to biped transitions show significant advances in lower limb morphology and pelvic girdle structure. Transitions involving changes in muscle leverage and joint mobility, for instance, emphasize the interplay between structural trade-offs and functional demands acting on the musculoskeletal apparatus. These results underscore the survival stress that must have given rise to modern gait patterns and pelvic morphology, illustrating how such anatomical differences enabled efficient bipedal locomotion in a variety of settings to enhance survival and exploration. Additionally, gait analysis helps facilitate understanding of specific pathologies that may restrict locomotion, underscoring its value in research and clinical practice. Ailments such as arthritis, stroke, and neurological disorders can impact gait dramatically and yield distinctive patterns, which clinicians read to organize rehabilitation strategies.

Reading gait deviations, for example, can enable therapy toward restoring mobility and enhancing quality of life. Moreover, gait analysis is particularly relevant in sports, where awareness of an athlete's gait can guide performance optimization while minimizing injury. Therefore, integrating gait analysis into human osteology's consideration of the pelvic girdle and lower limb not only enhances our understanding of biomechanics but also facilitates the development of tailored solutions for rehabilitation and enhanced performance across diverse populations.

9.4.2. Forces Acting on the Lower Limb During Movement

The human lower limb is subjected to continuous forces during movement, which are essential for stability and locomotion. They are the gravitational, inertial, and muscle forces, all three of which are critical in biomechanics. When the body moves, the gravitational force is always in the downward direction, and thus it influences the pattern of bone and joint loading in the lower limb. Muscles contract to generate movement, producing forces that must counteract gravity and other reaction forces during activities such as running or jumping. Such dynamics are relevant to understand because the interaction between forces determines the mechanical efficiency of the lower limb, with implications for performance during physical tasks and for susceptibility to injury. In locomotion, the transmission of forces through the lower limb and pelvic girdle must be examined to understand the intricacies of human movement. When individuals shift from standing to walking, the lower limb undergoes a series of force applications that differ across joints, such as the hip, knee, and ankle. These forces are associated with the anatomy of the pelvis and lower limbs, which have evolved for efficient bipedalism.

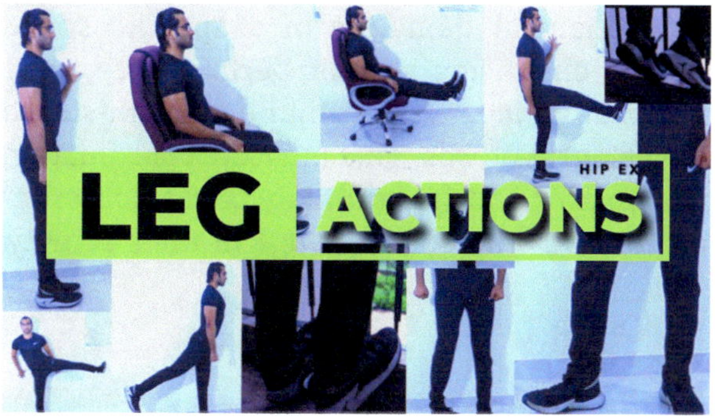

Figure 9.13. Forces acting on the lower limb during movement.

Source: https://external-content.duckduckgo.com/iu/?u=https%3A%2F%2Fi.ytimg.com%2Fvi%2FX_CxHj3xA2Y%2Fmaxresdefault.jpg&f=1&nofb=1&ipt=694fb5fdb7543524f2ffab5974992cf0282f08a1543973aaa7292c937c6c41eb.

The pelvis is a stable base that enables sharing between forces created by muscle activation and ground reaction forces along the lower limb. Further, limb postural alterations strongly influence joint mobility and muscle leverage, demonstrating biomechanical modifications in compensation for shifting postural demands across varying physical activities, as described in Allen et al. (2017). Even the assessment of forces on the lower limb has to do with anatomical variation and its functional implications. Variation in the size and distribution of musculature between groups has been found in recent studies, which may influence locomotion mechanics. For instance, a study demonstrated that the psoas major, a significant muscle area variation, is linked to pelvic anatomy variation, as in Synstelien et al. (2001).

Such findings support the idea that the os coxae of an individual may have specific morphologies that influence muscle function and overall locomotor performance. These anatomical factors were employed to develop a more advanced model of the modulation of biomechanical forces during movement and, by extension, to expand our knowledge of evolutionary adaptations and recent variation in human osteology (Figure 9.13).

9.4.3. Impact of Biomechanics on Athletic Performance

The field of biomechanics has revolutionized our understanding of athletic performance, particularly in the case of the pelvic girdle and lower limb mechanics. By evaluating the relationships among muscle attachments, joint motion, and body weight, researchers can assess the coordination and efficiency of athletes' movements across different disciplines. The design of the pelvic girdle and lower limbs is crucial for enabling movements that demand agility, power, and velocity. Here, the history of agility estimates across a variety of species, including extinct theropods, has shed light on how body structure influences performance capability.

For example, an estimated agility index for tyrannosaurids preserved not only muscle force but also mechanical advantage, thereby shedding light on the profound impact of anatomy on motion efficiency in both extinct and extant forms (Burns et al., 2019). It is important for the improvement of training techniques and prevention techniques to realize the relationship between anatomical features and sports movement. The relationship between pelvic girdle shape and lower limb mechanics enables sportsmen to maximize performance, for example, in many sports where explosive movements such as sprinting and jumping are imperative. Recent advances in computer modeling, such as geometric morphometrics, have enabled scientists to extrapolate possible muscular configurations in extinct species and their implications for locomotor patterns. Based on a hypothetical musculature of Australopithecus afarensis by considering modern relatives, scientists compare human biomechanics and suggest that learning about evolutionary perspectives can inform contemporary athletic training schemes (Mogg et al., 2018). Such observations underscore the intricate shape of the pelvis and lower limbs, accentuating their significance to the optimization of human performance. As athletes seek optimal performance, biomechanics provides a fundamental basis for investigating and optimizing their physical capabilities. By investigating the mechanical forces related to varied activities, sport scientists are able to characterize techniques that optimize posture, minimize energy expenditure, and optimize propulsive forces. Throughout this exploration of motion, the pelvis is not only a stabilizer but also a dynamic force that directly assists the lower limbs in executing complex motions. By understanding the specific role of the pelvic girdle and lower limb kinematics, practitioners can design training programs that match the biomechanical demands of a specific sport, thereby enhancing athletic performance while minimizing the risk of injury from ill-suited movement patterns. This intricate coordination of structure and function is what is necessary for athletes who seek an edge in their activity.

Test Your Knowledge

1. How do joints and muscles of the lower limb work together during walking and running?
2. What biomechanical principles help reduce stress on the lower limb during weight-bearing activities?

9.5. Pathologies of the Pelvic Girdle

Learning Outcome

1. Common pathologies and injuries
2. Osteoarthritis and its effect
3. Surgical interventions and procedures

The pelvic girdle is a vital anatomical complex for support and locomotion, and is subject to many pathologies that can broadly impact functionality and general health. Among these conditions, pelvic girdle fractures are of concern due to their prevalence in trauma cases, typically caused by motor vehicle accidents or falls. These fractures can have incapacitating consequences, including chronic pain and impaired mobility. Additionally, stress fractures, which most often occur in athletes or those subject to repetitive strain, highlight the importance of familiarizing oneself with the biomechanics of the pelvis. Such injuries have not only physical consequences; they can also elicit psychological responses, causing anxiety and a reduction in overall quality of life. Therefore, the study of pelvic girdle pathologies is most important because it not only encompasses the bodily framework of human osteology but also the various repercussions generated by such disorders. Another significant aspect of pelvic girdle pathologies concerns developmental disorders that can arise during the complex process of ontogeny. The complex formation of the pelvic girdle involves several stages of ossification and is influenced by genetic and environmental factors. For example, conditions such as congenital hip dysplasia may result in hip joint misalignment or instability, necessitating early treatment to prevent further complications. In addition, conditions such as osteoarthritis may affect the pelvic girdle, leading to degenerative changes over time. All these pathologies influence not just the physical stability and activity but also may result in chronic pain syndromes and functional impairments. Research into these issues within the contexts of human osteology is essential for the successful realization of treatment and rehabilitation protocols to improve patient outcomes.

Research into maternal health in pelvic girdle pathologies is also essential as these pathologies directly influence pregnancy outcomes. Historic skeletal analysis, as revealed in the pre-Hispanic necropolis of Juan Primo, provides considerable evidence of the difficulties women faced during childbirth. Evidence suggests maternal and fetal mortality could have been brought about by problems like dystocia or eclampsia, which illustrates the stresses that ancient populations were subjected to. This understanding is not only crucial to the rebuilding of human lives in the past but also to the presentation of modern issues with maternal health. The use of pelvic girdle pathologies extends into the field of public health, where skeletal stability and the success of childbirth are progressively entwined. Therefore, an understanding of these pathologies assists both in learning about the past and in current medical practices, ultimately leading to a better understanding of human osteology (Figure 9.14).

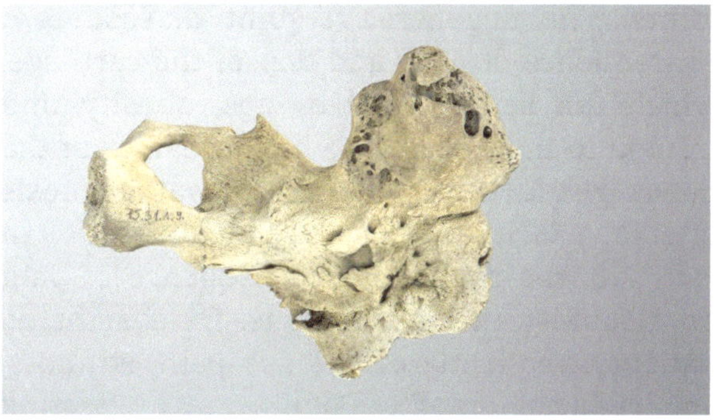

Figure 9.14. Pathologies of the pelvic girdle.

Source: https://external-content.du ckduckgo.com/iu/?u=https%3A%2F%2Fmedia.sketchfab.com%2Fmodels%2F51c 8821ba36a41909ab7c4237c21eb29%2Fthumbnails%2F11960d9064b0481da712d17dd4544cac%2F2456a2a3d19b476b9f4e9ef1e0ccf5bb.jpeg&f=1&nofb=1&ipt=e8bce4c1b852b31e391 5ff83a7a7de78765d74ee394585a3dfbe6f82c4e6f1d1.

9.5.1. Common Injuries and Conditions

Knowledge of common injuries and conditions affecting the pelvic girdle and lower limb is necessary in the study of human osteology to appreciate their anatomical and functional significance. Femur and pelvis fractures are some of the most frequent injuries. They occur as a result of high-impact trauma in the form of motor vehicle accidents or falls, which often lead to significant morbidity. Pelvic fractures are frequently complicated by the intricate nature of the girdle, which supports weight and allows movement.

The complications of the fractures involve hemorrhage and damage to contiguous organs, and therefore, diagnostic and therapeutic approaches need to be effective. Assessment of fracture stability—stable or unstable—has significant implications for treatment planning, rehabilitation, and follow-up. Osteoarthritis is another common condition of the lower limb, particularly involving the hip and knee joints. The degenerative joint disease is a consequence of wear and tear of the cartilage, which can be hastened by age, obesity, and trauma to the region. The biomechanics of the pelvic girdle are crucial in the pathogenesis of osteoarthritis because any abnormalities in gait patterns could be a consequence of pain or disability in such regions. Osteoarthritis patients frequently experience pain, stiffness, and reduced mobility, significantly affecting their quality of life. Osteoarthritis can also lead to compensatory mechanisms over time, increasing the risk of further injury to the involved musculature and joints. Knowledge of these interrelated disorders emphasizes the need for worldwide management methods that take into account not only the symptoms but also the related biomechanical dysfunctions. Lower limb tendinopathy is also a common condition that usually occurs in physically active individuals and athletic populations. Conditions such as Achilles and patellar tendinopathy are chronic overuse injuries.

These injuries not only manifest with pain and inflammation but can also affect the functionality of the lower limb as a whole, ultimately leading to altered biomechanics. Sports medicine has shown heightened interest in preventive interventions and rehabilitation programs designed to counteract and prevent the development of such conditions. It is crucial to understand the basic characteristics of the pelvic girdle and how they interact with the lower limb musculature when devising effective intervention programs. Thus, understanding common conditions and injuries supports an integrated care approach and reduces long-term functional impairments associated with these prevalent conditions.

9.5.2. Osteoarthritis and Its Effects

Osteoarthritis, a degenerative joint condition, involves the pelvic girdle and lower extremity to a considerable extent, leading to pain and functional impairment. Osteoarthritis is characterized by reduced articular cartilage, leading to bone-on-bone contact with movement. This type of wear and tear can lead to pain, stiffness, and swelling, particularly in load-carrying joints such as the hips and knees. In the context of human osteology, an understanding of osteoarthritis expression in bones can reveal the health and lifestyle of individuals in both contemporary and archaeological populations. For instance, the preservation of skeletal remains showing evident osteoarthritic changes can provide information on age-related patterns and social factors that affect joint health, shedding light on the broader implications of osteoarthritis in pre-industrial communities (Alamón-Núñez et al., 2019).

Osteoarthritis effects do not end at osteoarthritic pain; they also impact an individual's quality of life and mobility. In particular, dysfunction of the lower limb and pelvic girdle joints may limit daily activities, increasing dependence on others for assistance. Such a limitation can have broader social consequences, including decreased participation in community life and economic activity. In addition, the psychological burden of chronic pain due to osteoarthritis can result in mental health problems like depression and anxiety. Anthropologically, the study of osteoarthritis in skeletons can elucidate the adaptive responses individuals use to counter such challenges, such as changes in locomotion or lifestyle, which are pivotal to understanding survival among prehistoric populations (Dunn et al., 2016).

In paleopathology, the study of osteoarthritis provides significant evidence of past populations' health. The intensity and prevalence of osteoarthritis in archaeological remains express the influence of environmental factors, diet, and activity on joint condition. For instance, individuals with hard work or repetitive tasks have higher frequencies of osteoarthritic alterations in their pelvic girdle and lower limb bones, whose assumptions propose direct lifestyle influence on joint degeneration. Conversely, a lower prevalence of osteoarthritis in certain groups may indicate a less active lifestyle or variations in dietary habits that positively affect joint health. Therefore, the examination of osteoarthritis skeletal markers not only tells us something about the health of the individual but also leaves room for a broader understanding of biological adaptations and lifestyle variations that shaped human experience in different environmental contexts (Alamón-Núñez et al., 2019) (Figure 9.15).

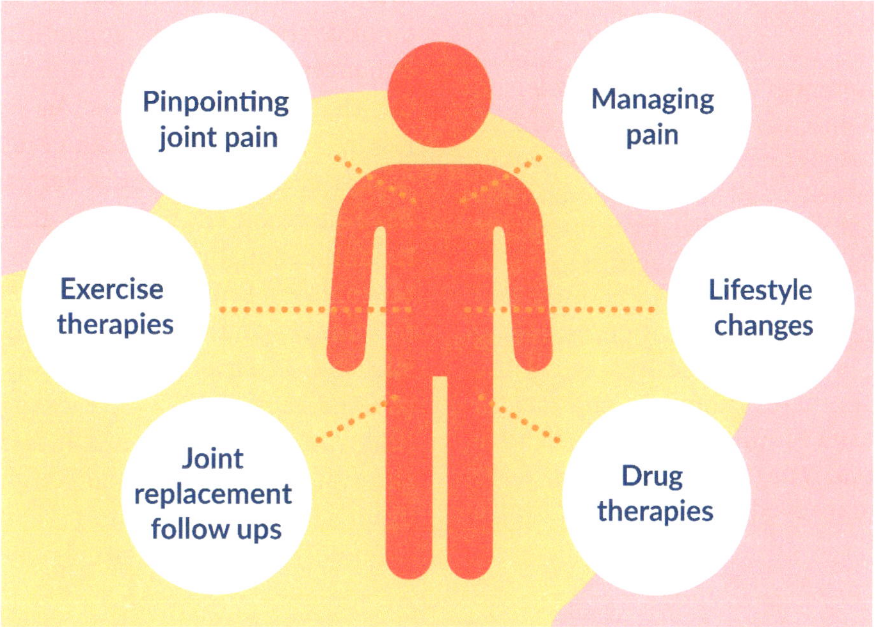

Figure 9.15. Osteoarthritis and its effects.

Source: https://external-content.duckduckgo.com/iu/?u=https%3A%2F%2Fbepartofresearch.nihr.ac.uk%2FdA%2Fc885e485b0%2F001316%2520NIHR%2520Osteoarthritis%2520Infographics_Artboard%25201%2520(1).jpg&f=1&nofb=1&ipt=8806326aba46fe1dd09747301db664abc3ffbf3cd377ec6af6d27ed6c2d58c9d.

9.5.3. Surgical Interventions and Treatments

Surgical interventions play the most critical role in the management of pelvic girdle and lower limb diseases, particularly where there are structural deformities and trauma. The interventions can range from minimal arthroscopic interventions to severe open interventions aimed at realigning bones, stabilizing fractures, or improving joint function. Conditions such as hip osteoarthritis, femoral head necrosis, and complicated fractures often need surgical treatment to restore movement and relief from pain. The intricacy of such procedures demands a thorough understanding of the osteology of the structures involved, as surgeons need to operate in sensitive anatomical areas to achieve the best results.

Additionally, the effectiveness of such interventions depends to some extent on the patient's rehabilitation regime after surgery, hence the need to approach the condition in an integrated manner through both surgery and nonsurgical approaches. In scoliosis, surgery is indicated if nonsurgical management fails to adequately treat the condition. For instance, those with functional scoliosis are candidates for surgery if they present with severe curvature and associated functional impairment. Recent research has shown that both exercise therapy and surgical procedures can be effectively combined to treat spinal deformity, with improvements in curvature and trunk asymmetry. Physical conditions preoperatively may be enhanced not only by an intense program of exercise, but also by postoperative results that could be positively influenced. This places emphasis on interprofessional practice by orthopedic surgeons, rehabilitation specialists, and physical therapists in managing scoliosis and concomitant disorders and thereby guaranteeing a holistic plan of care that addresses all the factors of the patients' function and health (Solberg et al., 1993). Enhanced postoperative management and surgical techniques have tremendously improved prognoses for those undergoing treatment for pelvic and lower limb disorders. Technologies such as robotic-assisted surgery and bioengineered joint replacements are revolutionizing the field, enabling more focused interventions with shorter recovery times. Also critical is the integration of rehabilitation protocols post-operatively; successful rehabilitation not only enhances functional recovery but also reduces the risk of complications. As research in this regard continues, evidence-based practice remains a central concern. For example, studies have increasingly indicated that personalized rehabilitation protocols can support surgical outcomes in scoliosis disease, hence increasing the understanding of the interaction between surgical intervention and physical therapy (Collins et al., 2020). This changing landscape illustrates the dynamic interplay between surgical advancement and comprehensive care in orthopedic treatment.

Test Your Knowledge

1. What are common disorders affecting the pelvic girdle, and how do they impact mobility and posture?
2. How can trauma, degenerative diseases, or congenital abnormalities affect pelvic girdle function?

9.6. Evolutionary Perspective

Learning Outcome

1. Evolution of the hominin pelvic girdle
2. Adaptations for bipedalism
3. Comparative anatomy with other primates

The evolutionary setting of the lower limb and the pelvic girdle is paramount for understanding human osteology, particularly the adaptation that led to bipedal gait. Standing on two legs enables mobility and more efficient energy expenditure, which is essential for early hominins living in diverse habitats. Over time, the pressures of selection have reorganized the human pelvis into the unique form that enables locomotion and reproduction. The complexities of this compromise can be appreciated from the shape of the pelvic inlet and the dimensions of the pelvic canal, both of which are of crucial significance during parturition. As observed in recent research, not only has pelvic morphology been influenced by evolutionary forces but also by secular change in nutrition and general health, signifying an active evolutionary process based on environmental influences that affect skeletal form (Driscoll et al., 2010). Further knowledge of evolutionary modifications requires an emphasis on current morphological variation in the pelvis across populations. Recent research examining individuals in the United States from 1840 through 1981 emphasizes the significance of environmental influences, such as improved nutrition and reduced heavy labor, which may have contributed to changes in pelvic size. Through these modifications, the birth canal size has been shown to change significantly, indicating a trend toward an elliptical birth canal. This adaptive shift suggests a shift in reproductive modes among modern humans, which may lead to the adoption of new modes of birth that are less energetically costly. Additionally, evidence of secular changes across a number of demographic populations underscores the adaptive process of human evolution, demonstrating how environmental and biological factors intertwine to shape human form (Driscoll et al., 2010). Beneath an appreciation of the evolutionary perspective as it pertains to the pelvic girdle and lower limb is the concept of adaptive morphology. An appreciation of other animals, with examples of functional adaptations in catfishes, can explain the various strategies organisms employ in response to the environments and ecological niches they inhabit. As the family Trichomycteridae possesses specialized traits for living in diverse habitats, so too has the human pelvis evolved to support bipedalism and efficient delivery. The interplay between structural alterations of the pelvis and the forces driving that evolution is itself a multifaceted relationship between functionality and environmental factors. Finally, these evolutionary findings provide an integrated platform for the explanation of the pelvis function in human osteology, both encapsulating the past evolution of our lineage and being relevant to contemporary applications.

9.6.1. Evolution of the Pelvic Girdle in Hominins

Hominin pelvic girdle evolution is a fundamental piece of information in explaining bipedalism and its consequences for reproductive anatomy. As hominins evolved completely upright, significant pelvis morphological changes developed to allow for this new pattern of locomotion. The pelvis was developed to support the weight of the upper body and to provide a stable base for the lower limbs. Features included a wider, shorter ilium, which is advantageous for positioning the body mass more centrally over the legs. These changes enhance stability and equilibrium in bipedal walking, illustrating the intricate interaction between pelvic structure and locomotion. This adaptive adjustment is an expression not only of the demands of terrestrial ambulation but also of forces of energy efficiency in locomotion that became increasingly significant as hominins diversified their environments and behaviors. Structural adjustments of the pelvic girdle also overlap with those of early hominin reproductive strategy. The morphological characteristics of the pelvis must accommodate the demands of bipedalism and facilitate childbirth. Determined in Australopithecus afarensis-associated discoveries, the pelvic morphology of early hominins like Lucy contained adaptations for bipedalism as well as birth. Discoveries show that Australopith pelvic inlets were more circular than those of their quadrupedal ancestors, thus facilitating a different mechanism of birth from that of modern humans. This is not easy of delivery, however, since the tightness of fit of the neonate's head in the birth canal indicates an obstacle-ridden delivery process. The modification of the pelvic girdle therefore exhibits a delicate balance between movement and reproductive efficiency, and it is among the determinants of the evolutionary trajectory of the hominin lineage (Desilva et al., 2017). Moreover, the evolution of the pelvic girdle is not just about locomotion and giving birth. Its muscularity and associated pelvis morphology are also involved in overall balance and stability during walking. Hominin adaptations involving gluteal muscle realignment, better mechanics in favor of bipedal locomotion, and stride economy were present. As with other mesodermally derived structures, the evolution of hominin pelvic girdles in response to diverse ecological demands implies an interaction between anatomical evolution and ecological demands. This evolution is similarly reflected in the evolution of bipedality in other animals, albeit with specific specialization in hominins based on their unique lifestyle and survival needs (N/A, 2020). Thus, the evolution of the pelvic girdle not only enhances our understanding of the anatomy of humans but also reveals the hominid-dominant process of form, function, and evolutionary strategy in the hominin lineage (Figure 9.16).

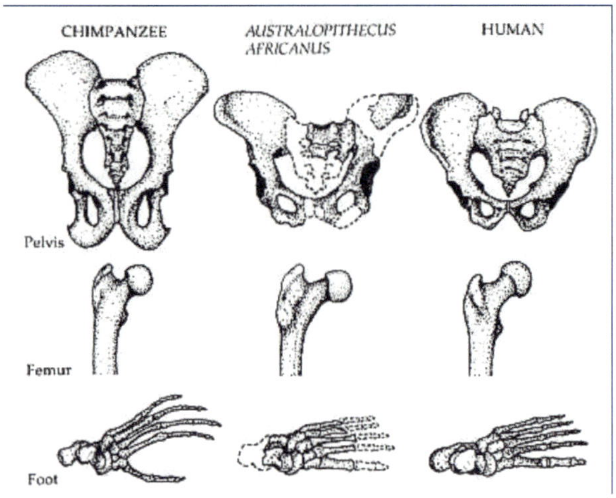

Figure 9.16. The evolution of the pelvic girdle in hominins.

Source: https://external-content.duckduckgo.com/iu/?u=https%3A%2F%2Fimage2.slideserve.com%2F4807813%2Fhominin-pelvis-structure-l.jpg&f=1&nofb=1&ipt=d7699e96325af4125b508b8950c74cc6b5b3c583182 09327ccabea947836f5fe.

9.6.2. Adaptations for Bipedalism

The evolution of bipedalism in humans is a complex process, regulated by a myriad of anatomical adaptations that support walking in a standing posture. One of the significant changes lies in the structure of the pelvic girdle, which has adapted to accommodate the needs of bipedal walking. The human pelvis is shorter and broader compared to the quadrupedal ancestors, supporting balance and stability. Such a morphological shift effectively shifts the weight of the upper part to the lower extremities during ambulation. Also, the shifting of the hip joints relative to the vertebral column is crucial in maintaining proper balance during walking or running, to allow for a more conservative gait. Combined, these changes in the pelvic girdle illustrate the intricate interplay between anatomy and mechanics in the instance of bipedalism and how evolutionary pressures have altered our body structures to enable upright walking. The changes also involve significant alterations in the shape and function of the lower limb. The thigh bone, or femur, has also been altered to provide greater leverage and support for ambulating on two legs. The angle of the femur, or the angle of inclination, is sharper and allows for the most efficient distribution of weight while walking. This reduces lateral forces at the knee and enhances stability when it supports weight, a crucial characteristic for human beings who walk through the use of their lower limbs. The foot, too, evolved to have arches that dissipate shock and function like a spring in action. These anatomical adaptations of the lower limb—particularly the femur and foot—accentuate the direction of evolution toward effective bipedal walking, underscoring an evolved process of adaptation specific to the demands of terrestrial walking. The impact of bipedalism upon reproductive biology also underscores the subtleties of human evolution, with a particular focus upon pelvic girdle shape and function. The human bony pelvis illustrates a compromise between parturition's biological requirements and locomotion's mechanical needs. As explained in a chapter on secular pelvic changes in morphology, the dimensions of the pelvic canal have evolved to provide space for the larger-headed baby without compromising the functionality required for walking upright.

The narrowing of the pelvic inlet, in addition to the lengthening of certain diameters, has influenced the childbirth process to facilitate the rotational birth mechanism prevalent in modern humans. The multidimensional accommodations accentuate the role played by evolutionary forces towards shaping the human body, with the pelvis being a classic example of how locomotion and reproductive modes come together to create a distinctive human form (Driscoll et al., 2010).

9.6.3. Comparative Anatomy with Other Primates

Comparing with other primates is important for understanding evolutionary modifications in the anatomy of the pelvic girdle and lower limb. The structural differences between humans and their closest relatives, such as chimpanzees and gorillas, are clear. Of great importance, the human pelvis has been specialized for bipedalism, with an increase in a more bowl-shaped structure supporting walking upright (N/A, 2020). On the contrary, the pelvis of non-human primates is constructed to support both bipedalism and quadrupedalism, a pointer to their diverse locomotor strategies. The adaptations of the human pelvis are not just a response to modifying locomotor demands but also have substantial functional implications, e.g., modifications in the location of muscles in the pelvis to facilitate stability and equilibrium. Further, the differences between non-human primate and human femoral structure underscore the evolutionary trajectory toward efficient bipedal walking. While non-human primate lower limbs are adapted for brachiation and climbing, the human femur is characterized by a unique angle of inclination and a robust diaphysis specialized for weight-bearing activities (Garrison et al., 2024). This anatomical distinction allows for a more effective center of gravity when walking and running, reducing the energetic cost of locomotion. Comparative analysis indicates that limb segment proportions and form, particularly those of the femur and tibia, directly relate to dynamic movement patterns, illustrating how evolutionary forces favored human adaptation to life on land. In addition to structural variation, integrating functional anatomy into studies of the lower limb and pelvic girdle reveals the complexity of primate locomotor evolution. Research on the auricular surface of the ilium has provided a new angle for viewing and comparing age estimation in human beings and chimpanzees, which reflects the evolutionary relationship between the two species (Garrison et al., 2024). This comparative approach highlights the shared anatomical features while outlining specialized adaptations that arise from differing habitat use and locomotor behaviors. Based on an understanding of these anatomical differences, scientists can better appreciate the biomechanical importance of pelvic and limb anatomy, explaining the evolutionary forces that shape not just human form but also that of our primate relatives.

Test Your Knowledge

1. How has the evolution of bipedalism influenced the structure of the pelvic girdle and lower limb?
2. What differences between human and primate pelvic anatomy reflect evolutionary adaptations for upright walking?

SUMMARY

By bringing together the complexities of the pelvic girdle and lower limb within the framework of human osteology, it is evident that these elements are not only anatomical structures but are inextricably part of the context of locomotor evolutionary stories. The evolution of the pelvic girdle and the adaptations of the lower limbs demonstrate the significant transformation from earlier forms to modern humans. This trajectory highlights the importance of identifying these skeletal elements not only on their own, but also as part of larger systems influenced by biomechanical needs and external forces. These perceptions are essential for understanding how human mobility evolved and how its alteration influenced the patterns of activity that were imperative for survival and adaptation. In addition, the science of human osteology, particularly that of the pelvic girdle and lower limbs, has profound pedagogical implications. As demonstrated in recent efforts to maximize remote education during the COVID-19 pandemic, the haptic experience is critical when perceiving complex anatomical relationships. The provision of plastic model skeletons in isolated settings, as underscored by the research, enabled broader bone identification and the competence required for sex and age estimation, though with some limitations. Such a process underscores the significance of revolutionary research approaches in anthropology instruction, reiterating that effective learning processes must align with our understanding of osteological fundamentals, particularly in practical training and sensory learning. Finally, the learning and comprehension objectives of the pelvic girdle and lower limb extend beyond the classroom into practical applications. Increased knowledge of osteology equips medical, anthropological, and forensic practitioners with the tools they need to evaluate skeletal remains correctly. Moreover, as the evolutionary context presented in Allen et al. (2017) is emphasized, the variations documented in lower limb function inform us about bipedalism and its evolutionary significance, linking biomechanical efficiency to survival. Last but not least, an in-depth examination of the lower limb and pelvic girdle in human osteology is essential to grasping not only the evolutionary history of early hominins but also the pedagogical approaches necessary to prepare prospective anthropologists for the daunting challenge of reading human skeletal remains.

The pelvic girdle is a fundamental structural foundation for the lower limbs and is central to human locomotion and stability. It is made up of the ilium, ischium, and pubis, which collectively form the innominate bone on either side of the body that, in addition to supporting the upper body weight when standing or sitting, enables transmission of forces from the trunk to the lower limbs when the body is walking or running. The pelvic girdle morphology has evolved uniquely compared to that of other vertebrates, particularly in its bipedal adaptations, which have potential implications for walking and balance. Understanding the pelvic architecture provides insight into how these adaptations were significant for human success as an evolutionary entity, as well as the biomechanical efficiency they imbue for upright stance during activity, thereby providing a fundamental appreciation of lower limb function in human osteology. When examining the lower limb, one recognizes its complex structure, comprising the femur, patella, tibia, fibula, and numerous joints that allow movement. The femur, the longest and strongest bone, connects the pelvis to the lower leg, the tibia and fibula providing a robust framework for weight-bearing and movement. All the bones have structural and functional significance, demonstrating the evolutionary adaptations required for walking on two legs. For instance, individual joint surface alignment, and the articulation of the knee and ankle joints, provide the necessary range of motion for running and jumping. In addition, the lower limb musculature, guided by anatomy, aids in stabilization and power generation, further enhancing human ability. Understanding of the complexity of the lower limb allows academics to appreciate the physiological load on these muscles and bones and their important role in general human movement. The use of technology and innovative pedagogic methods in teaching anthropology has also influenced the understanding of human osteology. COVID-19 remote learning adaptations required the use of tangible resources, such as plastic model skeletons, that significantly enhanced the students' comprehension of osteological principles. One study compared the knowledge of remotely taught undergraduates with that of their traditionally instructed peers. Results showed that distance learners performed well in bone identification compared with procedures for sex and age estimation, underscoring the role of haptic learning in osteological skill development. This result supports the need for sound course design in biological anthropology by demonstrating that hands-on experience directly improves students' skills in skeletal analysis. As such, pedagogical approaches address the multifaceted nature of learning human osteology, aligning fundamental anatomical knowledge with practical application and ultimately increasing educational worth for future anthropologists (Allen et al., 2017; Gamble et al., 2024).

KEY TERMS FROM THIS CHAPTER

- Acetabulum
- Femur
- Fibula
- Greater Trochanter
- Head of Femur
- Hip Joint
- Ilium
- Ischium
- Lateral Malleolus
- Lesser Trochanter
- Medial Malleolus
- Metatarsals
- Patella
- Pelvis
- Phalanges
- Pubis
- Sacrum
- Tarsals

CRITICAL THINKING QUESTIONS

1. **Which bones form the pelvic girdle?**
   a. Sacrum and coccyx
   b. Ilium, ischium, and pubis
   c. Femur and tibia
   d. Sacrum and femur
2. **What is the largest bone in the human body?**
   a. Tibia
   b. Femur
   c. Fibula
   d. Ilium
3. **Which part of the pelvic girdle articulates with the femur?**
   a. Acetabulum
   b. Pubic symphysis
   c. Iliac crest
   d. Ischial tuberosity
4. **What is the function of the obturator foramen in the pelvis?**
   a. Articulation with the sacrum
   b. Passage for nerves and blood vessels
   c. Support for the abdominal organs
   d. Attachment site for the femoral head
5. **Which bone is the weight-bearing bone of the lower leg?**
   a. Femur
   b. Fibula
   c. Tibia
   d. Patella

Short Answer Questions

1. What bones constitute the pelvic girdle?
2. Describe the three parts of the hip bone.
3. What is the function of the acetabulum?
4. Describe the location and significance of the ischial tuberosity.
5. Explain the function of the iliac crest in the pelvic girdle.
6. Describe the articulation between the talus and the tibia in the ankle joint.

Answers to Critical Thinking Questions

1. (b); 2. (b); 3. (a); 4. (b); 5. (c)

REFERENCES

1. Verbruggen, S. W., & Nowlan, N. C. (2017). Ontogeny of the human pelvis. *The Anatomical Record, 300*(4), 643–652. https://doi.org/10.1002/ar.23541Adriaens, D., Baskin, J. N., & Coppens, H. (2010). Evolutionary morphology of trichomycterid catfishes: About hanging on and digging in. https://core.ac.uk/download/55867718.pdf (accessed on 18th July 2025).
2. Alamón-Núñez, M., Alberto-Barroso, V., Delgado-Darias, T., et al. (2019). Exploring the risks accompanying child-bearing in aboriginal society on Gran Canaria (Canary Islands, 13th–15th cal. CE): Death of a pregnant woman during her third trimester. https://core.ac.uk/download/578100786.pdf (accessed on 18th July 2025).
3. Allen, V., Hutchinson, J. R., Otero, A., et al. (2017). Forelimb muscle and joint actions in Archosauria: Insights from *Crocodylus johnstoni* (Pseudosuchia) and *Mussaurus patagonicus* (Sauropodomorpha). https://core.ac.uk/download/141887609.pdf (accessed on 18th July 2025).
4. Arias-Martorell, J. (2018). The morphology and evolutionary history of the glenohumeral joint of hominoids: A review. *Ecology and Evolution, 9*, 703–722. https://doi.org/10.1002/ece3.4392 (accessed on 18th July 2025).
5. Atkinson, M. A., Davies, D. C., Dyball, R., et al. (2015). The Anatomical Society core regional anatomy syllabus for undergraduate medicine. https://core.ac.uk/download/161126464.pdf (accessed on 18th July 2025).
6. Burns, M. E., Cotton, J. R., Currie, P. J., et al. (2019). Lower rotational inertia and larger leg muscles indicate more rapid turns in tyrannosaurids than in other large theropods. https://core.ac.uk/download/480409847.pdf (accessed on 18th July 2025).
7. Carlini, A. A., Galliari, F. C., & Sánchez-Villagra, M. R. (2022). Evolution of the axial skeleton in armadillos (*Mammalia, Dasypodidae*). https://core.ac.uk/download/543233869.pdf (accessed on 18th July 2025).
8. Collins, M. J., Deviese, T., Higham, T., et al. (2020). Saving bones: A direct comparison of FTIR-ATR, whole bone percent nitrogen, and NIR. https://core.ac.uk/download/322819450.pdf (accessed on 18th July 2025).
9. Czwojdziński, A., Grzegorzewski, A., Kubicka, A. M., Musielak, B., Czubak, J., Jóźwiak, M., & Rychlik, M. (2019). Variation in pelvic shape and size in Eastern European males: A computed tomography comparative study. https://core.ac.uk/download/201279538.pdf (accessed on 18th July 2025).
10. Desilva, J. M., Laudicina, N. M., Rosenberg, K. R., et al. (2017). Neonatal shoulder width suggests a semirotational, oblique birth mechanism in *Australopithecus afarensis*. https://core.ac.uk/download/482689516.pdf (accessed on 18th July 2025).
11. Driscoll, K. R. D. (2010). Secular change of the modern human bony pelvis: Examining morphology in the United States using metrics and geometric morphometry. https://core.ac.uk/download/268764452.pdf (accessed on 18th July 2025).
12. Dunn, T. E. (2016). Estimation of body mass index from the metrics of the first metatarsal. https://open.bu.edu/bitstream/2144/15301/1/Dunn_bu_0017N_10728.pdf (accessed on 18th July 2025).

13. Ernst, C. H., & Seidel, M. E. (2012). *Trachemys.* https://core.ac.uk/download/211340408.pdf (accessed on 18th July 2025).
14. Gamble, J. A., & Gilmour, R. J. (2024). Bones at home supporting haptic learning and universal design beyond the biological anthropology laboratory. https://core.ac.uk/download/644028705.pdf (accessed on 18th July 2025).
15. Garrison, K. (2024). The auricular surface of chimpanzees (*Pan troglodytes*) as an indicator of age. https://core.ac.uk/download/646797243.pdf (accessed on 18th July 2025).
16. Marques, M. P., Ceríaco, L. M. P., Stanley, E. L., Bandeira, S., Agarwal, I., & Bauer, A. M. (2019). A new species of girdled lizard (Squamata: Cordylidae) from the Serra da Neve Inselberg, Namibe Province, southwestern Angola. *Zootaxa, 4668*(4), 4. https://doi.org/10.11646/zootaxa.4668.4.4 (accessed on 18th July 2025).
17. Mogg, J. A. (2018). Refining locomotory style in the fossil record through use of 3D geometric morphometrics and muscle attachment sites in the fossil species *Australopithecus afarensis.* https://core.ac.uk/download/231840931.pdf (accessed on 18th July 2025).
18. N/A. (2020). The ecomorphology of facultative bipedality in *Lepidosauria*: Implications for the evolution of reptilian bipedality. https://core.ac.uk/download/328720136.pdf (accessed on 18th July 2025).
19. Nwoha, P. U. (2000). Sex differences in the bony pelvis of the fruit-eating bat, *Eidolon helvum.* https://core.ac.uk/download/268450850.pdf (accessed on 18th July 2025).
20. Renesto, S., & Saller, F. (2023). Differences in the hindlimb anatomy in the two species of the late Triassic drepanosauromorph diapsid *Megalancosaurus* indicate habitat partitioning within the arboreal environment. https://core.ac.uk/download/572923623.pdf (accessed on 18th July 2025).
21. Sanger, T., Stuart, Y. E., & Swank, S. (2021). (Non)parallel developmental mechanisms in vertebrate appendage reduction and loss. https://core.ac.uk/download/591045398.pdf (accessed on 18th July 2025).
22. Solberg, G. (1993). Plastic changes in spinal function of pre-pubescent scoliotic children engaged in an exercise therapy programmed. https://core.ac.uk/download/145042987.pdf (accessed on 18th July 2025).
23. Synstelien, J. A. (2001). Differences in the os coxae between blacks and whites: A musculoskeletal approach to human variation. https://core.ac.uk/download/588287985.pdf (accessed on 18th July 2025).
24. Zug, G. R. (1971). Buoyancy, locomotion, morphology of the pelvic girdle and hindlimb, and systematics of cryptodiran turtles. http://deepblue.lib.umich.edu/bitstream/2027.42/56386/1/MP142.pdf (accessed on 18th July 2025).

THE HANDS AND FEET IN HUMAN OSTEOLOGY

10

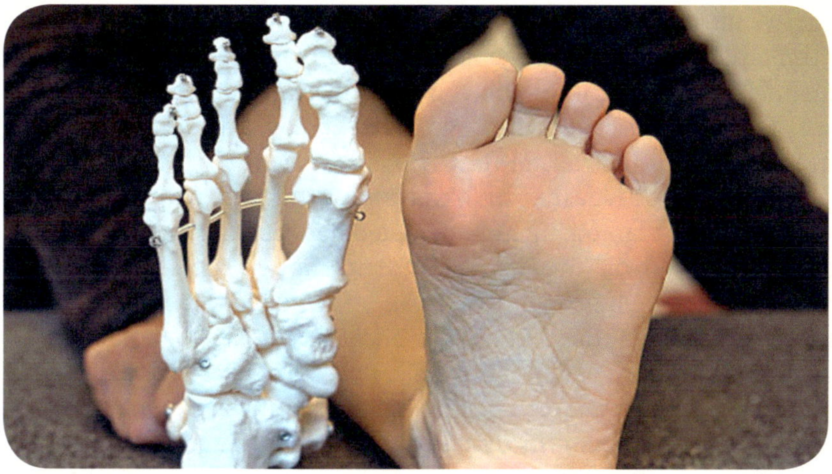

LEARNING OBJECTIVES

After studying this chapter, you will be able to:

1. Explain the anatomy of the human hand
2. Evaluate the anatomy of the human foot
3. Understand the development of the hands and feet
4. Discuss the functional significance of the hands
5. Know the functional significance of the feet
6. Focus on common hand and foot pathologies

Introduction

The examination of human osteology, particularly of the hands and feet, is an important part of studying human anatomy in its evolutionary context. As hands and feet are the primary devices for manipulation and locomotion, these appendages have evolved intricate structures to perform numerous tasks. Osteological analysis of these appendages not only informs us about physical development but also provides us with insight into the lives of individuals of another culture. This study enhances our understanding of how environmental factors and social practices have a bearing on skeletal disease and morphology. In an archaeological setting, the knowledge of hands and feet helps scholars reconstruct past lives, health status, and even social status between populations. Burials also provide significant information about past societies, including how people were treated based on their physical or health status. The excavation of human skeletons, for instance, at the Tyson site, reveals demographic patterns and health experiences among early communities. For instance, excavation at the site yielded several subadult skeletons that highlight children's vulnerability to high mortality in earlier times, when mortality was high due to numerous social and environmental stresses. These analyses not only inform us about the individuals in question but also about broader cultural views of childhood, death, and burial practice. Moreover, the state of well-preserved skeletal material allows detailed osteological analysis, enabling the researcher to discuss implications for health, morbidity, and the impact of communal practice on skeletal integrity. In more severe cases, the condition of the remains of bones can signal violence and punishment practices or social histories of violence. Perimortem amputations, for instance, as indicated in medieval Portuguese necropolis skeletal remains, illustrate how forensic osteology bridges the gap between historical reports and medical science. These findings emphasize the value of physical integrity and trauma in cultural practice, often bringing to light unpleasant facts of people's lives, especially in legal procedures. Analysis of such cases through an osteological approach enriches the discussion of human behavior and social norms, illustrating the coexistence of physical structure and societal values. This interdisciplinary research on the hands and feet of osteology offers broad scope for interpreting human existence across various periods, emphasizing these limbs' functional and cultural importance.

Definition of Osteology

Osteology is the scientific examination of bones and one of the fundamental sciences in biological anthropology. Osteology analyzes the structure, function, development, and variability of skeletal systems across populations and species. This area of research is particularly relevant when studying portions of the human body, such as the hands and feet, that are integral to movement and manipulation. On a larger scale, osteology provides insight into health, disease, and anthropological history and provides valuable data for archaeology, medicine, and forensic science. By understanding the form and structure of bones, scientists can make inferences about cultural practices, dietary practices, and environmental adaptation, furthering our knowledge of the human experience from an anatomical perspective. Moreover, osteology has become increasingly pertinent through applied applications, specifically in the classroom, such as anthropology lab courses. The instant shift to distance education ushered in by the COVID-19 pandemic validated the need for haptic engagement with osteological specimens to achieve the required learning outcomes. As observed in studies conducted at institutions such as Mount Royal University and the University of Manitoba, students who were trained in human osteology benefited greatly from the use of plastic model skeletons in distance education. This new technique not only facilitated bone identification but also enhanced core osteological skills necessary for sex and age estimation, underlining the significance of haptic learning in osteology education. Such findings underline ongoing efforts to adapt teaching practices within the discipline so that students remain proficient in necessary osteological techniques regardless of the learning context (Gamble et al., 2024). The individual study of bones in the hands and the feet also underscores the significance of osteology in human anatomy and function. These parts of the body have many distinctive bones, whose combined functionality and versatility are necessary for the entire body's functioning and movement. The hands, for example, have a complex arrangement that enables a range of movement and flexibility. At the same time, the feet support the entire body's weight, allowing walking on two legs. The examination of trauma and pathological conditions in these areas provides insights into anthropological health and activity patterns, as seen through studies of excavated groups, such as those at Akhetaten. The study of skeletal remains, based on injuries or illnesses, can reconstruct the lived lives of human beings and, as a result, the dynamics involved during a given period of history, thereby underscoring the importance of osteology in understanding the human past (Hodgin et al., 2012) (Figure 10.1).

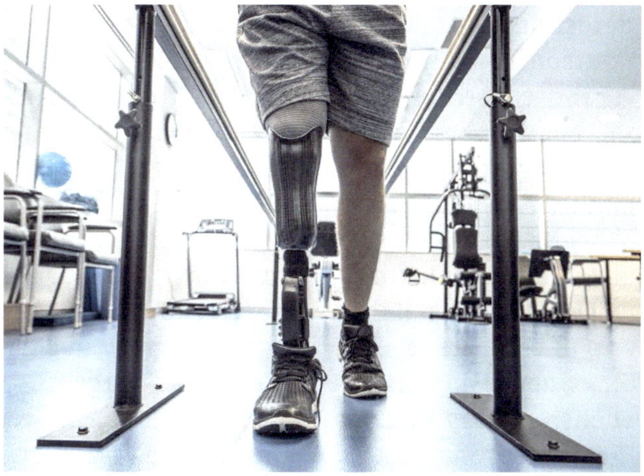

Figure 10.1. Definition of osteology.

Source: https://external-content.duckduckgo.com/iu/?u=https%3A%2F%2Fwww.thoughtco.com%2Fthmb%2FFn-TdLjtcOepJ6KhfXAfhualF1Q%3D%2F1250x0%2Ffilters%3Ano_upscale()%3Amax_bytes(150000)%3Astrip_icc()%2Fprostheticlimbs-5c77140346e0fb0001edc77d.jpg&f=1&nofb=1&ipt=b391dd65bf2e5a190d706c869a766c7f41de33d75cefb3a9ae1721d8a112ff62.

Importance of Studying Hands and Feet

The study of hands and feet in the context of human osteology provides important insights into the anatomical and functional elements of the human body. Hands, composed of a high-level network of bones, tendons, and ligaments, are pivotal in dexterity and manipulation. The same goes for the feet, which are responsible for bipedal locomotion and for bearing weight and supporting movement. With this understanding of the distinct skeletal structures of these extremities, more intricate applications are now being made in medicine, anthropology, and rehabilitation. For instance, data on bone structure differences can be used to diagnose injury and deformity, so it is important that a thorough study of the hands and feet be conducted in osteological analyses. These intricate finer aspects of these skeletal systems provide not only personal physiological variations but also broader evolutionary paths pertinent to human evolution. In educational settings, the importance of engaging with the anatomy of the hands and feet becomes increasingly pertinent. As recent studies have shown, remote teaching has brought to light issues in osteology education, particularly regarding tactile learning experiences. The use of take-home models, as demonstrated in studies with Mount Royal University and the University of Manitoba undergraduate student populations, illustrates the impact of experiential learning on osteological information retention. Results indicated that students who participated in activities relevant to bone identification were at the same level of competency as other students receiving face-to-face education, underscoring the pivotal role of haptic learning in this field. Thus, including hands-on experiences in osteology courses not only improves students' academic skills but also promotes an increased appreciation for the complexities of hand and foot skeletal anatomy (Gamble et al., 2024). Understanding the anatomy and functional significance of the hands and feet is relevant to other medical disciplines as well. Knowledge of skeletal frameworks is highly significant in clinical practice, particularly in identifying anatomical landmarks necessary for injection and pulse detection. One study explained that learning outcomes could be improved with interactive and constructivist approaches to education, emphasizing the maintenance of knowledge for long bone anatomy, present in the hands and feet as well (Tynes et al., 2014). By applying several teaching approaches, lecturers can enhance learning retention and student engagement, ultimately contributing to higher levels of competency in clinical practice. The findings above highlight that not only is a comprehensive grasp of the anatomy of the foot and hand theoretical, but it is also essential in empowering students to be successful healthcare and medical career professionals whose work demands accuracy and anatomical proficiency.

10.1. Anatomy of the Human Hand

Learning Outcome

1. Principal bones of the hand
2. Joint structure and function
3. Hand muscles and tendons

The anatomy of the hand is highly significant in human osteology due to its complex structure and functional importance. The hand consists of 27 bones and is separated into three distinct segments: the metacarpals, carpal bones, and phalanges. The eight carpal bones are arranged in two rows, forming the wrist's underlying structure, which allows the range of motion needed for manipulation and grasping. The metacarpals connect the carpal bones to the phalanges, supplying a stabilizing skeleton for the fingers. There are three phalanges in each digit, but the thumb has two. This complexity not only assists the hand's agility but is also vital for activities such as tool usage, which has been a key determinant in human evolution. Awareness of this anatomical complexity is vital for doctors treating conditions affecting the function and growth of the hands. The functional attributes of the hand's anatomy are directly linked to its anatomical attributes, especially in osteology. The unique arrangement of the bones allows for a diverse array of movement, characterized by the intricate joint structures, including the carpometacarpal joints and metacarpophalangeal joints. These are critical in many grip mechanisms, including power and precision grips, which primarily rely on the coordinated movement of multiple bones and muscles. In particular, thumb opposition is a feature that identifies us and enables us to enhance our manipulation skill and separate humans from the majority of other animals. Investigation into these functional features informs clinical practice, particularly in rehab settings, where hand function rehabilitation is central. As highlighted by existing learning campaigns, the use of osteology modules focused on these areas can enhance understanding and practice in clinical settings, underscoring the importance of a solid anatomical foundation in practice (Eckel et al., 2021). The foot is also anatomically analogous to the hand, further supporting the crucial role of extremities in human osteology. Even though anatomical configuration is employed for numerous reasons, both appendages are this sophisticated and specialized. Forensic science now recognizes the importance of the foot in human identification, particularly when remains are so fragmented that only lower limbs are found. This refers to the need for extensive research on the use of the foot in human identification, given the relative dearth of published literature on this topic. The unique anatomy of the foot, including the various bones, ligaments, and tendons, enables locomotion and balance. With continued research in human remains, attention to the skeletal foot parameters will interpret the biological profile and the identity of the individual in fragmentary remains more effectively (Barrett et al., 2014) (Figure 10.2).

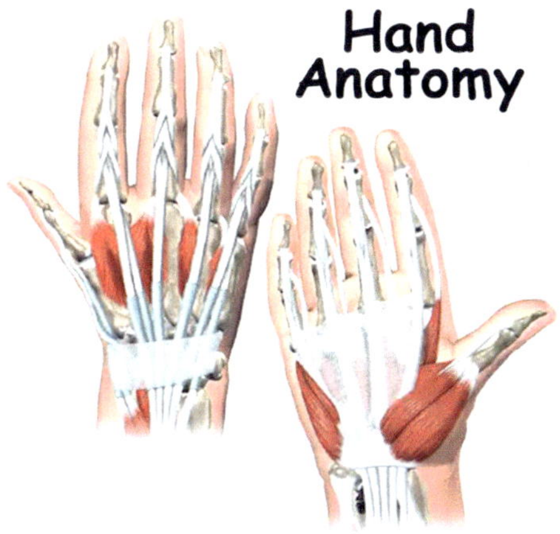

Figure 10.2. The anatomy of the hand plays a significant role due to its complex structure and functional importance.

Source: https://www.southmountainpt.com/media/img/376/hand_anatomy_intro01.jpg.

10.1.1. Major Bones in the Hand

A look at the important bones of the hand reveals a complex, intricate structure that is the backbone of human dexterity. The hand consists of 27 bones, classified into three broad categories: carpal bones, metacarpals, and phalanges. The eight carpal bones form two quadruplets, providing stability and flexibility to the wrist. The carpal bones, which include the scaphoid, lunate, and trapezium, play an important part in the hand's range of motion and use. Five long bones situated between the fingers and the wrist, referred to as the metacarpals, connect to the carpal bones and create the support base of the palm. All these bones work together to enable grasping, manipulation, and other fine motor functions, underscoring the importance of each bone in the hand's anatomy and functional capacity. Additionally, naming the phalanges, which comprise 14 bones, underscores their specialization in supporting intricate finger movements. There are three phalanges for each of the fingers, the proximal, middle, and distal. The thumb possesses two phalanges: the proximal and the distal. This structure allows for easy demonstration of a wide variety of motions, ranging from firm grips to delicate pinches. All the phalanges are constrained by joints for flexion and extension, which are required for performing various activities throughout the day. Moreover, the arrangement of muscles, ligaments, and tendons around the bones enhances mobility and tactile sensitivity, rendering the hand highly versatile. Knowledge of the structural organization of the phalanges is crucial when taking into account the hands biomechanical functionality under normal and pathological conditions. Their formation and age-related variations also complement the functioning of these important bones in the hand. Techniques such as histomorphometry, quantitative analysis of histological architecture, can provide valuable information on the aging process of bones as well as their morphological characteristics. The implications of such work are significant, particularly in paleodemographic models and forensic identifications, where understanding bone remodeling and pattern of growth is of essential importance. Even as the clavicle is studied separately, comparative research with hand bones can reveal similarities in developmental patterns and age-estimation methods, and contribute to the diversity of human osteology. More research into the anatomy of the hand using advanced research tools underscores the importance of hand bones in examining skeletal health at the individual and population levels (Paulman PhD et al., 2001; Inthasan et al., 2017).

10.1.2. Joint Structure and Function

The intricate joint structure is crucial to the functional dexterity of hands and feet, which are necessary instruments of movement and interaction. Joint structure consists of many parts, including cartilage, synovial fluid, ligaments, and connective tissues, all of which enhance agility and stability. For instance, the synovial joints' capacity for wide range of motion provides space for dexterous activities such as manipulation and grasping objects.

The functional effectiveness afforded by these joints' evolutionary design is not only advantageous for function but also exhibits an excellent harmony between mobility and strength, mainly as observed in metacarpophalangeal and interphalangeal joints of the fingers. This versatility underscores the importance of joint structure in the coordination of complex movements, which are fundamental to survival and social interaction across a vast variety of ecosystems. Joint function studies often cross species boundaries to explore evolutionary mechanisms, shedding light on the biomechanical trade-offs that govern joint form. A case in point is the aye-aye (*Daubentonia madagascariensis*), with remarkable adaptations in its fingers for arboreal climbing.

The elongated fingers of the aye-ayes enable foraging in challenging environments that necessitate specialized joint mechanics to manage forces during climbing and descent (Ancrenaz et al., 2010). This is a typical theme in joint function across different species, where different species have specialized adaptations to deal with environmental pressures. The emphasis on joint function across a variety of primate species underscores the significance of adaptive strategies, revealing the intimate connections between form and function in ensuring biomechanical efficiency across diverse environments. The isomorphism between anatomy and function in joints reveals a major characteristic of human osteology: variation within structural forms while maintaining basic similarity across species. The new mix of primitive features and novel adaptations in primate hands enhances their overall biomechanical effectiveness in both manipulation and locomotion (Kivell et al., 2016). Furthermore, an extensive study of the morphology of specific joint types can yield insights into evolutionary pressures that shape skeletal adaptation over time. As the intricacies of joint structure and function are continually elucidated through research, a more nuanced understanding of the evolutionary history of the hands and feet emerges. This information not only adds to current knowledge of human osteology but also lays the groundwork for future research in comparative anatomy and biomechanics across various taxa, thereby furthering understanding of joint function (Figure 10.3).

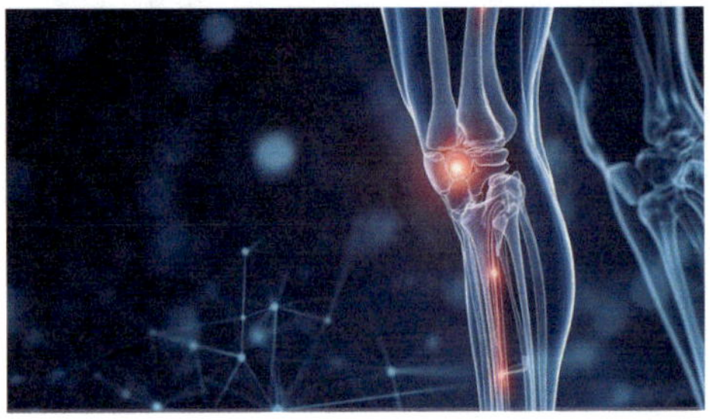

Figure 10.3. The intricate design of human joints.

Source: https://t4.ftcdn.net/jpg/13/38/06/11/360_F_1338061118_W90cpqe2PDuKOkqiOAfZ5Ei9kzSSCnfZ.jpg.

10.1.3. Muscles and Tendons Associated with Hand Movement

The muscles and tendons concerned with hand motion are exceptionally developed and well organized, a result of the hand's vital association with fine motor skills as well as gross motion. The muscles involved in hand motion are divided into intrinsic and extrinsic muscles. The extrinsic muscles are located in the forearm, with tendons extending to the hand. These are responsible for achieving strong grips, such as grip and lift. The intrinsic muscles are found within the hands themselves, performing fine work like small-object manipulation and intricate hand movements. This anatomical variation not only depicts the adaptive evolution of the hand towards various functions but also emphasizes the crucial role of muscle and tendon coordination in achieving the specific movements required for day-to-day activities. Muscles like the flexor digitorum profundus and flexor digitorum superficialis are key in finger flexion.

These muscles originate in the forearm and insert onto the digital phalanges, allowing flexion of the fingers at several joints. The extensor muscles, however, such as extensor digitorum, are involved in finger extension and in enabling activities, such as releasing objects. Conversely, muscle tension differs across these groups, allowing for varied motion. This is more prevalent in activities that involve grip strength and precision, such as writing or playing an instrument. This study shows how interactions and equilibria among these muscle groups, mediated by their respective tendons, shape the intricacies of hand movement biomechanics and their significance in human osteological formation. Moreover, the mechanical function of muscles and tendons in controlling hand movement is defined by their anatomical integration with the hand skeleton. Tendons are not merely linkages between bones and muscles; they also facilitate kinetic energy transfer during movement. The cellular and molecular basis of tendon development that has been researched provides hints towards their adaptability and evolutionary significance. As it has been explained in research on the amniote jaw complex, the same principles can be applied to explaining the functions of mechanical forces in the development of hand musculature and tendon anatomy over time. The ability to coordinate tendons, muscles, and bones effectively is necessary for enhancing dexterity and strength, leading to functional diversity in human hand use (Taylor et al., 2012; Abzhanov et al., 2019).

Test Your Knowledge

1. What are the major bones, joints, and muscle groups that make up the human hand?
2. How do the structure and arrangement of the hand bones contribute to fine motor skills and precision grip?

10.2. Anatomy of the Human Foot

Learning Outcome

1. Large foot bones;
2. Joints' structure and function;
3. Foot movement-related muscles and tendons.

The human foot is a highly intricate structure composed of numerous bones, ligaments, tendons, and muscles that collectively assist movement and stabilization. The foot contains 26 bones, grouped into three categories: tarsal, metatarsal, and phalangeal. The tarsal bones consist of seven distinct bones, including the calcaneus and talus, which play significant weight-bearing and movement roles to enable the foot to adapt to varying surfaces. The phalanges and metatarsals provide flexibility and rigidity to enable propulsion and balance required during walking and running. Recognition of this complex anatomy is central to the fields of osteology and podiatry, as any alteration or destruction of this system can result in severe functional impairment and pain. The ligaments of the foot also contribute to overall function by stabilizing with a degree of flexibility. In the foot, there are intrinsic and extrinsic ligaments, which connect bones but also allow necessary movement. The arches of the foot are supported by intrinsic ligaments, necessary for shock absorption during walking, supplemented by support from beneath the leg by extrinsic ligaments.

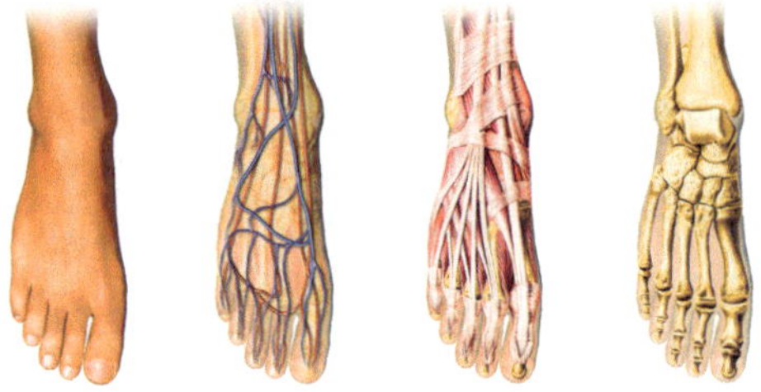

Figure 10.4. The human foot is an intricate structure composed of numerous bones.

Source: https://www.palmettostatepodiatry.com/wp-content/uploads/2023/08/Depositphotos_25639401_XL-scaled.jpg.

Understanding the role these ligaments have to play in complications like flatfoot or pronation disorder, which occur because of inadequate support or trauma, is part of studying the anatomy of the foot. Research has demonstrated that educational interventions, such as dissection, help students to understand the anatomy structures better, ultimately leading to enhanced performance in practical exams and general mastery of the subject (Paulman PhD et al., 2001). Clinically, the intricacy of foot anatomy plays a vital role in the management of day-to-day pathologies. For example, conditions like plantar fasciitis, bunion, and Achilles tendinitis are all closely related to the anatomy and biomechanical function of the foot. By learning about the distinctive structure and function of each component of the foot, health professionals can devise individualized treatment programs. This is also used in the interpretation of archaeological skeletal remains, such as Caddo subadult burials, which provide information on the health status and activity levels of ancient populations through skeletal morphology and evidence of pathologies (Dockall et al., 1994). Thus, the human foot anatomy not only shows an excellent evolutionary adaptation but is also a prime thematic field in the osteology and related fields (Figure 10.4).

10.2.1. Major Bones in the Foot

The human foot is a complex organ composed of numerous bones that work together to provide support, stability, and mobility. The tarsal bones are the base of the foot's anatomy and include the talus, calcaneus, navicular, cuboid, and the medial, intermediate, and lateral cuneiform bones. The talus is the keystone, articulating with both the fibula and the tibia, thereby permitting ankle motion.

The heel bone, or calcaneus, supports the weight of the foot when standing and walking. Together, these tarsal bones form the foundation upon which the other foot bones are sustained, enabling an advanced range of motion that is required for locomotion as well as equilibrium. Understanding of this fundamental architecture is central to the biomechanics of the human foot and its application to movement and posture.

The rest of the foot, excluding tarsal bones, consists of five metatarsal bones that connect tarsals to the phalanges, or toe bones. Each of these five metatarsals is characterized by a head, shaft, and base and functions to support and push off during a walk or run. The first metatarsal, of both functional and size significance, plays a vital role in maintaining balance and supporting body weight during two-legged walking. Also, the alignment of metatarsals makes possible the formation of the longitudinal arch and the transverse arch of the foot, which are focal points of the foot's structure and function. Through their actions with both the tarsals and the phalanges, the metatarsal bones play a major role in the mechanics of foot motion, enabling efficient locomotion on various surfaces. Finally, the phalanges, consisting of 14 bones that form the toes, contribute to the agility and functional ability of the foot. The toes consist of three phalanges (distal, middle, and proximal), except for the big toe, which consists of two.

The phalanges allow for refinement of balance and accommodation in gait pattern, characteristics necessary for a broad spectrum of activities, including walking, running, and jumping. In addition, the intricate organization of the ligaments and tendons of these bones allows for flexion and extension, necessary for effective foot motion and stability. Analyzing the roles of both phalanges and metatarsals not only underscores their importance in human anatomy but also underscores that aberrations in these bones result in functional deficiencies, thereby impacting mobility and overall quality of life.

10.2.2. Joint Structure and Function

The intricate structure of joints is at the heart of the functional capability of the hands and feet, which are critical in human osteology. The human skeleton consists predominantly of synovial joints, which are lubricated by synovial fluid that facilitates frictionless movement and reduces friction between articulating surfaces. The joints of the hands enable the extensive mobility required for grasping, handling objects, and performing complex tasks.

The complexity of joint structures, such as ligaments, tendons, and cartilage, should facilitate effective damping of dynamic forces during various functions. For example, during grasping, the integrity and alignment of the joint components stabilize while allowing flexibility. This unison of mobility and stability is crucial, as a malfunction in joint structure can significantly impair dexterity and overall function in both hands and feet. Functionally, the foot joints are a remarkable adaptation to bipedal locomotion, supporting and facilitating mobility, a fundamental requirement of human existence. The tarsal, metatarsal, and phalangeal joints of the foot work together to withstand shock, travel complex terrain, and provide for a smooth gait. The advanced mechanics of events such as walking, running, and jumping rely heavily on the structural organization of these joints.

In addition, the joint mobility of the foot allows for adaptation to varied surfaces and stability under varied conditions. As an example, the foot arches, supported by complex joint interactions, are significant in supporting the body weight and reducing stress when the body is moving. Accordingly, any change in the structure of the joints, regardless of whether it is brought about by injury or degenerative diseases, has profound implications for movement and overall biomechanical function. Scholarly, the investigation of joint structure and function goes beyond mere anatomical description to encompass biomechanical factors and evolutionary insight. Comparative observations, such as those in non-human primates, illustrate the adaptive strategies used to address joint pressures during locomotion across varying environments.

For instance, research on the aye-aye indicates that digit morphology and joint function changes are associated with varying locomotor strategies and produce specialized biomechanical trade-offs in order to meet environmental demands (Ancrenaz et al., 2010). This study is crucial not only for the study of human bipedalism but also for understanding the evolutionary pressures that have shaped current hand and foot morphology. As highlighted by the literature, a deeper study of the structure-function interface of primate joints can offer useful insights into evolutionary biology and clinical application (Kivell et al., 2016). The interdisciplinary approach highlights the importance of interdisciplinary studies in further advancing our knowledge of joint mechanics within the broader context of osteology (Figure 10.5).

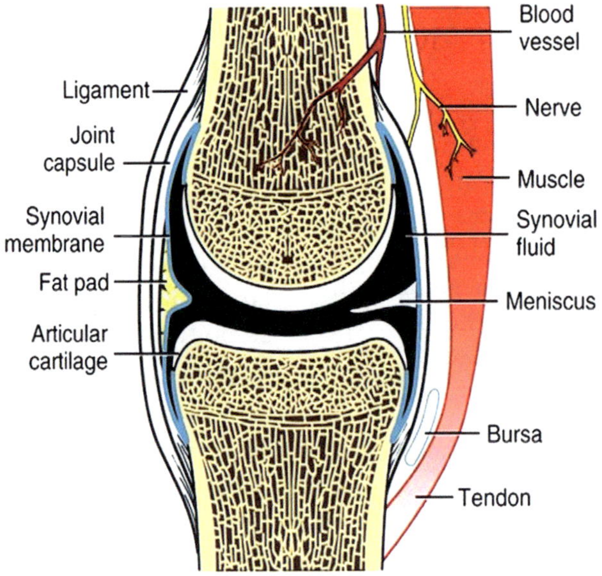

Figure 10.5. The intricate design of joints.

Source: https://musculoskeletalkey.com/wp-content/uploads/2016/12/B9780323089449000022_f002-007-9780323089449.jpg.

10.2.3. Muscles and Tendons Associated with Foot Movement

It is crucial to have an idea about the tendons and muscles used in foot movement when studying human osteology, since they are both key to locomotion as well as balance. The foot musculature can be broadly categorized into intrinsic and extrinsic muscles. Intrinsic muscles, which are located inside the foot, play a specific role in fine motor control, support of the arch, and toe movement. These are the abductor hallucis and the flexor digitorum brevis, which stabilize the foot during activities such as walking and running.

The extrinsic muscles, however, that have their origin in the lower leg, govern the foot through the long tendons that run from the ankle joint and influence movements such as dorsiflexion and plantarflexion. This double classification highlights the complex interactions required for effective gait mechanics and overall mobility. Tendons linking such muscles to bone share equal significance during locomotion in the foot, as they transmit force supplied by muscle contraction.

The Achilles tendon is an excellent example, linking calf muscles to the calcaneus and facilitating powerful plantarflexion. The tendon is instrumental in activities requiring explosive action, such as sprinting and jumping, underscoring its role in sports performance. Furthermore, tendons like the peroneus longus and tibialis anterior stabilize the foot's arch and assist inversion and eversion, respectively. These functions also highlight the tendons' function in structural support and mechanical load distribution, essential for effective locomotion. These contributions are significant to learn in the context of physical therapy and athletic training, in which muscle and tendon injury repair has a significant impact on mobility and performance. The relationship between muscles and tendons is not only central to human locomotion in modern humans but also sets the stage for identifying evolutionary changes in other animals. For instance, biomechanical analyses of extinct species, e.g., non-avian theropods, illustrate how muscle-tendon configurations influence locomotion dynamics and locomotor efficiency (Abourachid et al., 2018). Similarly, the study of extinct sthenurine kangaroos reveals changes in their anatomical structures that supported unusual locomotion behaviors, illustrating their evolutionary past (Figueirido et al., 2014). These comparative analyses demonstrate how understanding the development of muscle and tendon informs our concept of human foot mechanics and its related evolutionary significance. Examining these relationships, we can establish linkages between current musculoskeletal function and the evolutionary pressures that have shaped it.

Test Your Knowledge

1. What are the main bones and arches of the human foot, and how do they support body weight and movement?
2. How does the anatomical structure of the foot differ from that of the hand in terms of function?

10.3. Development of the Hands and Feet

Learning Outcome

1. Embryological development of the bones of hand and foot
2. Patterns of growth in children
3. Aging changes

Human osteology of the hands and feet is the result of complex evolutionary growth, and it is closely followed by functional adjustments made in response to different environments. During embryonic development, the upper and lower limbs undergo significant modifications, which are controlled by the environment and genes. The hands-and-feet formation shows the relationship between morphogenesis and osteogenesis, resulting in structures that allow a wide range of movements and actions. In humans, the precision grip of the hand and push-off function of the foot permit a wide variety of activities, ranging from tool use to upright walking. Understanding this evolution also sheds light on skeletal development, health, and potential pathology in these critical extremities, and addresses their essential role in everyday function and the total mobility of the human skeleton.

Individual pattern formation is revealed when the sophistication of the bones of the fingers and toes is taken into account. During initial fetal development, the limbs form a collection of undifferentiated mesenchymal condensations that progressively differentiate into bones and joints. This process is regulated by a variety of signaling pathways and transcription factors involved in differentiation and growth. Development of digits on both the hands and feet is significant, as this implies attainment of functional dexterity and balance. Phalange differentiation, combined with metacarpal and metatarsal articulation, suggests evolutionary adaptations that not only facilitate locomotion but also provide manipulative and balancing functions. Moreover, examinations of fossilized bones have shown variations in these bones that are in accordance with various environments and ways of life, helping to better understand human evolutionary history (Dockall et al., 1994). Additionally, comparisons of fossilized and contemporary skeletal bones help us better understand the evolution of hands and feet among species. Specifically, research on primate relatives, such as the aye-aye, highlights the role of evolutionary stress in shaping limb structure and function.

The arboreal ones require modifications to the bone structure, resulting in hands capable of grasping and manipulating objects precisely and feet capable of providing support on varied terrain. Such findings illustrate the biomechanical compromises that result from environmental niches, shaping the nature of functionally important traits of the hands and feet. From examining such adaptations, anthropologists gain valuable insights into the lines of evolution that gave rise to the modern human skeleton, as well as illustrating anatomical transformation alongside the pressures of survival our ancestors faced in diverse environments (Ancrenaz et al., 2010) (Figure 10.6).

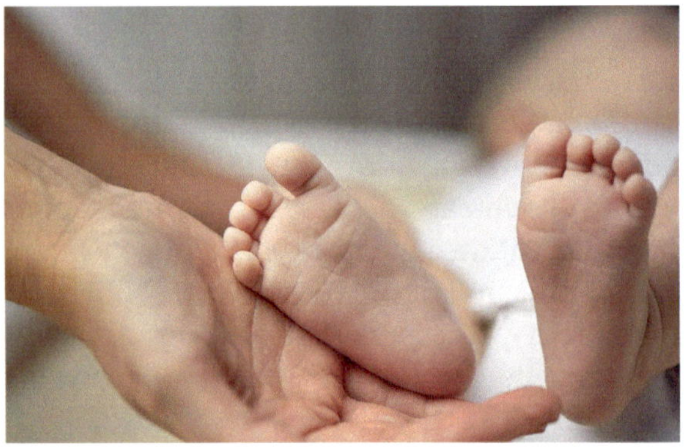

Figure 10.6. Development of the hands and feet.

Source: https://aucklandchildrensphysio.co.nz/wp-content/uploads/2018/05/feet-1200x750.jpg.

10.3.1. Embryological Development of Hand and Foot Bones

The embryologic origin of the bones of the hand and foot is a complex process that occurs at an early stage of human life, predominantly during the first trimester. This begins with the development of the limb bud, which forms from interactions between the ectoderm and the mesoderm. The muscles and bones are created through the contribution of the mesodermal layer, and the skin and nerves are developed from the ectodermal layer. As limb buds extend, they begin to develop more recognizable hand and foot morphologies, marked by the formation of skeletal components that delineate the digits. During this pivotal period, precursor forms of bone also undergo chondrogenesis, during which cartilage models are formed before ossification converts them into hard bone, illustrating the intricate dance between genetic signaling and environmental factors in the development of human dexterity and mobility.

The process of ossification can be divided into a few phases, with primary ossification centers initially appearing in the long bones of the limbs at the seventh week of pregnancy. By this time, cartilaginous models of the metacarpals and phalanges are well developed. It persists as secondary ossification centers emerge, especially in the epiphyses, which are essential for subsequent growth and joint function. Differentiation of the cartilage into bone is also not uniform; it varies between the hand and foot due to variations in the demands of function. The hands, highly specialized for fine motor control and manipulation, undergo a more complex and rapid process of ossification than the foot, in which bone development is oriented toward providing structural stability and support. The embryological development of hand and foot bones thus plays an organizing role in determining their functional potential later in life. Moreover, there can be congenital abnormalities in the development of hand and foot bones during the above-discussed processes. Syndactyly and polydactyly are only a few such conditions related to the number and form of digits. Syndactyly, involving partial or complete fusion of the next phalanges, is prone to alter function and is primarily known to be congenital (Adrian et al., 2011). The etiology of such anomalies is not clearly understood, but it is believed to result from disruptions in signal transduction pathways that control digit development. Investigating such conditions not only provides a better understanding of skeletal embryogenesis but also impacts pediatric surgery and rehabilitation techniques, underscoring the need to treat these anomalies for functional restoration. Aside from that, studies involving fetal remains have demonstrated the importance of accurately assessing skeletal maturity and anomalies, underscoring the role of osteological analysis in both scientific and clinical practice (Sanders et al., 2009).

10.3.2. Growth Patterns in Childhood

Growth patterns in childhood are a significant topic in human osteology, particularly of the hands and feet. During the early years, children's bones experience accelerated growth, similar to their overall development. The growth pattern is therefore a combination of muscular and skeletal growth, which is quite crucial in developing functional independence. The hands and feet, being sites of aggressive development and expansion, are excellent markers of overall health and nutrition during early life. For instance, the development of fine motor skills is closely linked to the maturation of bones in the hands, while the legs are vital for ambulation and other physical activities. Hence, observing such growth patterns can shed ample light on how biological and environmental factors contribute to children's development. Also, the timing of growth spurts across different anatomical regions, including the hands and feet, reflects variations in child growth patterns. Research indicates that while the trunk and extremities can grow at different rates, the hands and feet follow a specific sequence that reflects major developmental milestones.

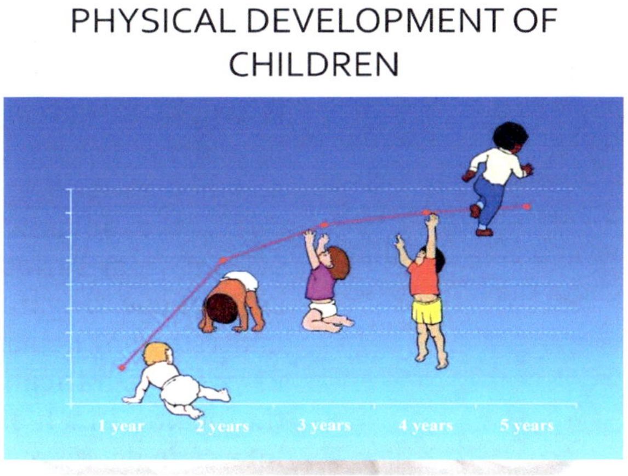

Figure 10.7. The growth patterns observed in childhood.

Source: https://external-content.duckduckgo.com/iu/?u=https%3A%2F%2Fimage1.slideserve.com%2F2194433%2Fphysical-development-of-children-l.jpg&f=1&nofb=1&ipt=68e4e7b693a2e447857ddfa423789d9903acb71df5b47b2329504eb93a5709d6.

During early childhood, the fingers increase significantly, which is important in understanding and manipulation jobs that are established in this stage. As children engage with and learn about the world, the phalanges, metacarpals, and metatarsals of the hands and feet grow in width and length as they adapt to increased dexterity and stability. Identification of such growth patterns is useful to anthropologists and osteologists not just in the analysis of skeletal remains, but also in approximating the modern population's health and lifestyle, because equivalent patterns can point to genetic and nutritional disease.

Comparative analysis of patterns of child growth across different populations can also yield valuable insights into earlier health patterns and living conditions. By analyzing bone remains, as described in excavated work at sites referenced in the literature, scientists can determine the body stresses children endured in different ecological settings. For instance, variations in the proportions of hand and foot bones may suggest differences in environmental factors, such as climate or available nutrients, that directly affect growth rates. In addition, the significance of these growth trajectories can be carried over to medical practice and pediatrics today, where knowledge about normal growth patterns helps diagnose children's illnesses. Accordingly, the investigation of growth patterns during childhood not only increases knowledge of human osteology but also offers a model for examining the interface between biology, health, and cultural practices throughout the life course (Figure 10.7).

10.3.3. Changes with Aging

With aging, extensive changes occur in the bony architecture of the hands and feet, mirroring general physiological changes. The hands, with their intricate bony architecture, begin to show a gradual reduction in bone density and structural strength, leading to osteoarthritis. Remarkably, the articular cartilage lining the joints can become thin, leading to pain and decreased mobility. This degradative process is particularly severe in phalangeal joints, wherein functional limitations can drastically reduce manual dexterity. Further, age-related changes in ligament flexibility and muscle strength can exacerbate these degradative processes, making routine activities more difficult and reducing quality of life. Collectively, these alterations highlight the importance of precise osteological examination in assessing hand-skeleton functionality and aging in human osteology. The morphological alterations of the foot are part of the aging process, thus pointing to the interdependence of skeletal status and mobility. Arch flattening of the feet is among the most pronounced consequences of aging in the foot, which may lead to considerable changes in walking mechanisms and posture. This is primarily due to the natural deterioration of connective tissue and tendons that support the architecture of the foot. Also affected are the toes, with reduced range of motion and increased stiffness, mostly due to arthritis. Not only do these modifications render the individual more susceptible to falls, but they can also lead to secondary disorders such as bunions and plantar fasciitis. Understanding such functional and anatomical modifications is crucial in developing successful strategies to address the issues of the elderly segment, and hence, it is a significant area of study under the domain of human osteology. As evident from various archaeological findings, changes due to aging are a critical component in understanding human osteology, which provides us with significant information regarding the health and lifestyle of past populations. Interestingly, the excavations in the nature of those that have been conducted at graveyards yield useful osteological data that divulges people's status and health across different life stages. For instance, information collected from the Tyson site shows that subadult remains possess certain imprints of developmental stress or health ailments which determine the character of life during early life (Dockall et al., 1994). Similarly, Smith's Fort excavation draws out the importance of the study of skeletal remains in understanding the process of aging and how it impacts mobility and overall vitality (Barrett et al., 2004). Analysis of these trends in historical context further enhances our understanding of human adaptation and resilience, providing an even broader picture of the implications of aging in osteology (Figure 10.8).

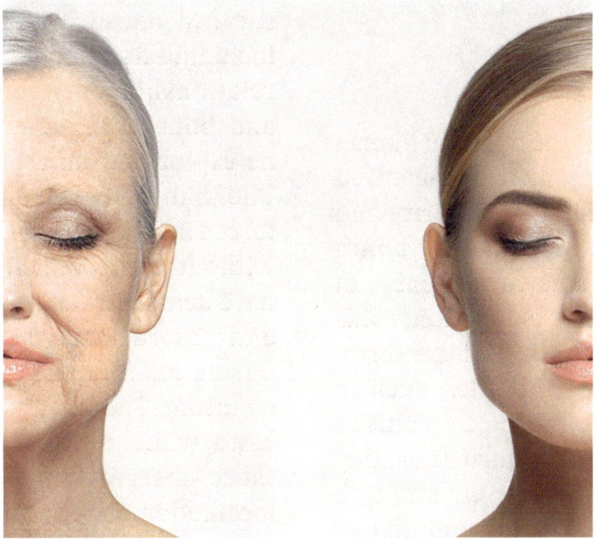

Figure 10.8. Changes with aging.

Source: https://external-content.duckduckgo.com/iu/?u=https%3A%2F%2Fwww.cascadeface.com%2Fwp-content%2Fuploads%2F2022%2F01%2Fshutterstock_1028141644.jpg&f=1&nofb=1&ipt=9add2f479c90f5874dd4df424e4a6db2465567b5bd73557f1f8b42a23b404c3d.

Test Your Knowledge

1. How do the hands and feet develop during embryonic and postnatal stages?
2. What genetic and environmental factors influence the normal development of hands and feet?

10.4. Functional Significance of the Hands

Learning Outcome

1. Function in tool use and manipulation
2. Impact on way of life and daily functioning
3. Evolutionary perspective on hand function

The functional significance of the hands in human osteology is demonstrated by their well-evolved anatomical framework, including dexterity and strength. The human hand contains 27 bones that constitute a unique framework capable of performing an extensive range of functions. This singular allocation of strength and dexterity enables not only gross motor abilities, such as lifting and gripping, but also fine motor abilities required for complex movement, such as writing and crafts. Both the capacity to apply strength and finesse enable people to accomplish a wide range of activities, from tool use to expressive gesture. Moreover, the evolution of the human hand shows an increasing emphasis on manipulation, supporting the notion that hand function is an inseparable component of cultural and technological progress over time. An understanding of morphological traits in the broader context provides significant insight into the role of the hands in human behavior and social life. In the evolutionary history of the primates, the hands are a great illustration of adaptive significance. Looking at primate anatomy, particularly the range of hand structures within different species, reveals variations that match specific ecological niches. Arboreal animals, for instance, require prehensile capacities that demand not just the strength of grasping but also manipulation of objects in three-dimensional space. The aye-aye (*Daubentonia madagascariensis*) is an apt example; its extended fingers have evolved to enhance foraging, allowing it to extract insects from tree bark successfully. These adaptations reveal the extent to which an organism's environment shapes the mechanical properties of skeletal elements, such as the hands. This strength-manipulation balance is a hallmark of the complex evolutionary trade-offs that define functional anatomy, so underlining the fundamental role that hands have in the survival and success of various primate species, including humans (Ancrenaz et al., 2010). The relationship between functional significance and bone architecture in the hands can also be explored from a biomechanical perspective. The hand's form should accommodate the forces involved in performing various functions without compromising dexterity. Researchers have demonstrated that the hands can distribute and absorb loads, reducing the risk of injury during high-impact activities such as climbing or lifting. The pressure distribution across the hand while conducting varied tasks, such as those observed in the aye-ayes' characteristic locomotion patterns, demonstrates how selective pressures have shaped skeletal arrangements for enhanced performance (Kivell et al., 2016). Also, the adaptive features offer insights into the physical boundaries of hand function, including the fact that as humans developed, subtle changes enabled more versatility. In a way, the hands are not only appendages but also vital tools that lay open both the adaptive past and functional pressures experienced by human beings and their primates.

10.4.1. Role in Manipulation and Tool Use

The hands, as manipulation devices, are key to the evolution of human tool use, an identifying feature that marks Homo sapiens from the rest of the animal kingdom. The structure of the opposable thumb of the human hand facilitates a unique repertoire of fine movements required for gripping and manipulating objects. This anatomical feature allows increased hand coordination, a key component of sophisticated processes such as tool production and complex fine-motor activities. The implications of this manipulation extend beyond mere function, as manual specialization has been implicated in the emergence of thought and language. Alternative explanations of the relationship highlight the significance of manual abilities in understanding human prehistory and development, a point reinforced by recent studies examining brain pathways that govern these specialized movements (Steele et al., 2009). Further, the evolutionary record of tool use also indicates a basic association between hand dexterity and survival-adaptive mechanisms. Hominins at a relatively early stage were likely to have been using raw tools for hunting and gathering, which also influenced their bodily adaptations and social structures. Not only did resource availability grow with the capacity to use tools, but social cooperation was also made possible through groups that functioned collaboratively. This collaborative aspect underscores the importance of dexterous hand movements, suggesting that the hands served not only as instruments for survival but also as facilitators of social interaction and cultural transmission. Archaeological record is utilized in the provision of proof of tool forms that establish population-level right-hand bias when undertaking such tasks, with an added emphasis on the significance of handedness and manual role specialization during human evolution (Gamble et al., 2024). In the current research, the role of the hands during manipulation and tool use remains paramount, as evidenced by pedagogical practices in anthropology teaching. Virtual teaching methods adopted during the COVID-19 pandemic revealed a profound understanding of the importance of practice in delivering competency in human osteology and related subjects. Students, while being offered plastic model skeletons for their identification and classification, showcased an impressive ability to acquire foundational osteological capabilities, bridging the theoretical-application gap. While these findings underscore the crucial role of tactile learning, they also suggest the sustained utility of the hand as an instrument for understanding human anatomical form. The study reaffirms that hand dexterity and tool evolution remain a worthwhile topic of research, highlighting the continued utility of exploring the hands in human osteology and beyond (Gamble et al., 2024) (Figure 10.9).

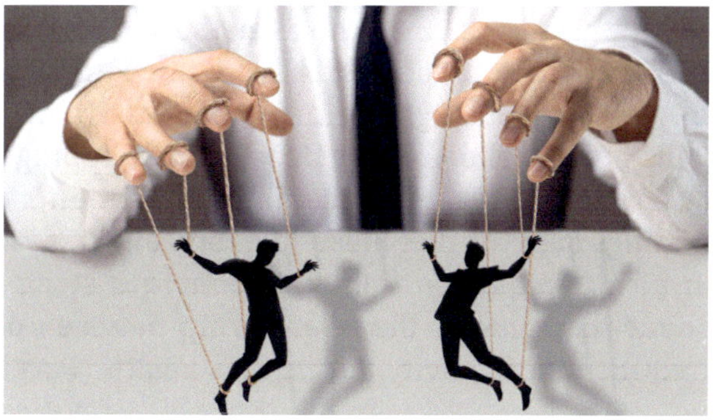

Figure 10.9. Role in manipulation and tool use.

Source: https://jeninesmithinc.co.za/wp-content/uploads/2025/05/dictatorship-oppression-collage-concept-1200x675.jpg.

10.4.2. Impact on Daily Activities and Lifestyle

The intricacy of human osteology, particularly of the hands and feet, has significant impacts on daily activities and lifestyle. The extremities serve not only as limbs but also as key components in the execution of tasks, from basic locomotion to fine manual labor. Abnormalities or injury to the finger and toe bones and joints directly affect an individual's capabilities in performing daily activities. Examples of these conditions include fractures or degenerative joint disease, which can completely restrict mobility and dexterity, rendering individuals unable to pursue activities that improve the quality of life. Consequently, familiarity with these osteological features is vital for understanding how skeletal health can immediately impact labor and social relationships. Analysis of human skeletal remains discovered in Fernvale reveals the biomechanical loading to which bodies were subjected during ordinary labor. The cortical defect observed in the bones indicates that climbing, canoeing, or crossing rough ground was responsible for the specific skeletal adaptations and trauma. These findings demonstrate how lifestyle activities and environmental factors affect the musculoskeletal system over time. By way of illustration, the avulsion injury documented here demonstrates the effects of particular physical stressors on hands and feet. From an understanding of these stressors, researchers are then able to reconstruct historical lifestyles and which they impacted health, making explicit how these physical activities were integral to survival and social engagement in groups (Foster et al., 2015). Furthermore, this analysis of degenerative joint disease among groups such as those at the Poole-Rose ossuary provides insight into the contribution of daily activities to long-term skeletal health. The frequency of degenerative changes in the radii of this group sheds light on the impact of arable food production and other subsistence activities on joint health. The varying frequency of lipping and eburnation on joint surfaces reflects the ways different activities produce different amounts of wear and tear on the skeletal system. Hence, the findings suggest that lifestyle habits affected the functioning and health of the hands and feet and, in turn, the quality of life and activities of daily living. Understanding of these trends informs us about the value of the relationship between our activity and bone health, guiding contemporary treatments of activity advice and health (Parks et al., 2002) (Figure 10.10).

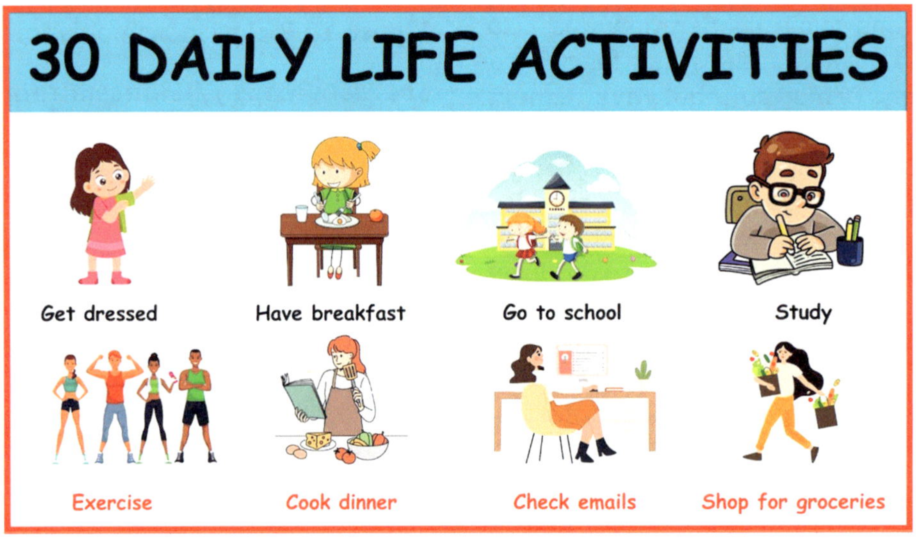

Figure 10.10. Impact on daily activities and lifestyle.

Source: https://external-content.duckduckgo.com/iu/?u=https%3A%2F%2Fi.ytimg.com%2Fvi%2FAOIYjtQLg9U%2Fmaxresdefault.jpg&f=1&nofb=1&ipt=00ed34e38f2d9d3aaca062066c6494bf32676752904a033e32d84a2aec8e81c2.

10.4.3. Evolutionary Perspective on Hand Function

The evolutionary perspective on hand function provides fascinating insights into how human hands have evolved to acquire specialized features that enhance their function. Through millions of years of evolution, structural changes within the hands enabled humans to execute activities requiring sophisticated manipulation and precision, differentiating them from all other tetrapods and primates. These structures, such as the opposable thumb, enable grasping, an essential skill for using tools and performing intricate tasks. On the contrary, other creatures, such as sauropods, have different evolutionary modifications related to their ecological niches, including the elongation of the neck, employed nearly exclusively for feeding. Their unique cervical anatomy shows how evolutionary pressures shape anatomical structures in response to survival needs, providing an interesting frame of reference for understanding specialized human hand adaptations in a broader evolutionary context (Taylor et al., 2012). Moreover, the role of hands is linked with its evolutionary history. The emergence of bipedalism in early hominines necessitated modifications to limb structure that influenced the use and function of the hands. The shift to high-level walking, as good as it was, also influenced the evolution of fine motor activity of the upper limb. Researchers indicate that the integration of the centrale into the scaphoid bone in the hominoid wrist is a unique morphological adaptation of this evolutionary process (Chamberlain et al., 2020). These changes have established a biomechanical platform that supports dexterous behavior, facilitating locomotion and object manipulation. These adaptations are not only structural but also functional, implying a closer evolutionary connection between present-day humans and their ancestors who used various forms of locomotion, such as knuckle-walking, which indicates the flexibility and versatility of the hands. Hand function is also crucial in the context of evolution, as the complex use of the hand has been linked to the evolution of tool-making and problem-solving skills. This aspect adds another layer to the narrative of human evolution, highlighting the coevolution of hand dexterity and mental capabilities. The evolution of tools, from primitive stone tools to advanced machines, is a demonstration of how hand anatomy has influenced human intelligence and creativity. As humans evolved, their hands not only maintained survival but also facilitated complex social interactions and technological development. Understanding of this interface between anatomical complexity and functional evolution is critical to understanding the contribution of the hands in human osteology, as they are central to their meaning beyond being anatomical structures to propelling cultural and technological evolution (Taylor et al., 2012; Chamberlain et al., 2020).

Test Your Knowledge

1. Why are opposable thumbs important for the functional efficiency of the human hand?
2. How do muscles, joints, and sensory feedback work together to enable complex hand movements?

10.5. Functional Significance of the Feet

Learning Outcome

1. Role in locomotion and balance
2. Impact on sporting performance
3. Evolutionary perspective of foot function

The human foot performs a variety of functions critical to successful walking and overall biomechanical stability. Its advanced structure, comprising 26 bones, numerous tendons, numerous ligaments, and scores of muscles, has been optimized to meet the demands of bipedalism. The foot's structural architecture enables efficient energy transfer during walking or running, which is essential for endurance and speed. Further, the foot's three separate arches—the medial longitudinal arch, the lateral longitudinal arch, and the transverse arch—serve the purposes of shock absorption and support. The arches enable the foot to adapt to irregular ground and maintain balance and stability during movement. Therefore, the functional significance of the feet extends beyond locomotion; it involves a whole system that enables complex interactions with the environment during locomotion or during everyday activities. Apart from locomotion, balance and stability, which are integral components of human physical action, are maintained by the feet. The structure of the foot encourages an upright stance, which is important for activities that require accuracy and strength, such as standing, walking, and executing various sports movements. Receptors in the foot, especially in the soles, are important sources of sensory feedback on pressure, texture, and temperature. This sensory feedback is required for well-coordinated movements and motor control. Additionally, the foot's flexibility allows for more than one movement, i.e., dorsiflexion and plantarflexion, which is essential in actions like climbing, jumping, and dancing. Hence, the functional importance of the feet is not confined to balance; it entails intricate coordination between sensory input and motor responses, enabling complex physical functions and adjustments. The functional value of the human foot may also be appreciated by comparing it with other animals' solutions to bipedal locomotion. The transition from quadruped to bipedal locomotion has necessitated a radical change in foot structure. Human feet deviate from those of other locomotory modes in possessing a more rigid metatarsal structure and non-opposable toes. This specialized configuration gives better propulsion and stabilization in walking on two legs. Furthermore, the foot has adapted not only to support body weight but also to facilitate various types of motion, such as running or walking long distances, which may have been vital in human evolution to ensure survival. Hence, the functional significance of the feet lies in evolutionary adaptations rooted in the way human beings walk and in their ability to survive across varying environments (Figure 10.11).

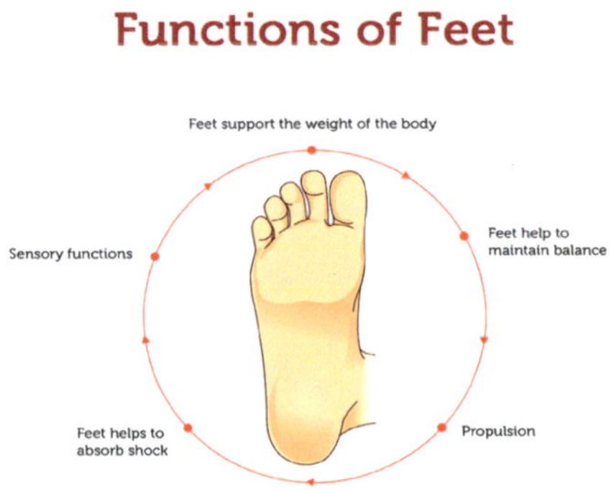

Figure 10.11. Functional significance of the feet.

Source: https://external-content.duckduckgo.com/iu/?u=https%3A%2F%2Fassets.lybrate.com%2Fimgs%2Ftic%2Fenadp%2Ffunction-of-feet.jpg&f=1&nofb=1&ipt=324323effbdbfa32edf86a89aea86e19b0a646f507973fc282fbbe6ed6c1cc94.

10.5.1. Role in Locomotion and Balance

Human hands and feet possess a strongly developed structure that is firmly integrated with locomotion and balance, reflecting their functional needs and evolutionary forces. This involves the hands, which have opposable thumbs and a sophisticated pattern of bones that allow dexterous movements necessary for grasping and handling objects. This flexibility not only makes daily actions easier but also assists with balance in other activities, such as climbing or walking along rough ground. The biomechanical benefit of hand shape allows for the distribution of loading, minimizing stress, as evidenced by studies on aye-aye walking, whereby digit positions are maximized to minimize loads in movement (Ancrenaz et al., 2010). Therefore, the hands serve dual roles during locomotion through supportive and propulsive interaction with the surrounding world, which illustrates the intricacies of human biomechanics. The feet serve not only as supports; they are a sophisticated system developed for efficient bipedalism. Human foot structure, comprised of alignment of tarsal and metatarsal bones, provides an immovable base that supports motion without displacing the body's weight out of balance. This unique architecture allows a range of motions, from running and walking to jumping, each requiring a distinct mechanism to maintain balance. The body solutions of larger extinct kangaroos, particularly those that developed a bipedal striding gait rather than regular hopping, bear witness to the necessity of stability in the process of locomotion (Figueirido et al., 2014). These evolutionary developments show how the foot design affects not only the capacity to run fast but also the ability to stand firm on various surfaces, confirming the interconnected nature of walking and stability. As the interconnected functions of the hands and feet are examined, they are perceived not as independent entities but as an overall system designed for movement as much as for balance. Both limbs coordinate to allow humans to perform complicated activities that require a very delicate sense of balance and coordination. For example, as the feet provide the propulsion and stability for locomotion, the hands come into play in the process of orientation maintenance, such as reaching out for support or manipulating objects during movement. This fusion is necessary for movements that require stability and dexterity, creating ease in interacting with the world. Lastly, the feet and hands illustrate how evolutionary adaptations have led to advanced locomotor capabilities in man, thereby emphasizing the role of these structures in maintaining equilibrium and enabling efficient motion throughout life and during exceptional activities (Figure 10.12).

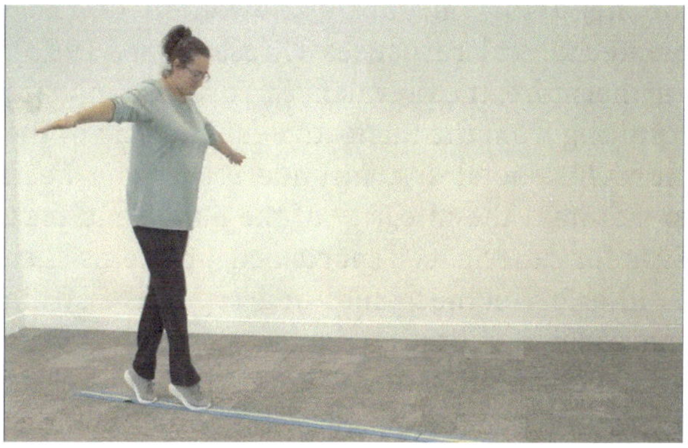

Figure 10.12. Role in locomotion and balance.

Source: https://external-content.duckduckgo.com/iu/?u=https%3A%2F%2Fi.ytimg.com%2Fvi%2Fp5v0zP6FGz8%2Fmaxresdefault.jpg%3Fsqp%3D-oaymwEmCIAKENAF8quKqQMa8AEB-AH-CYAC0AWKAgwIABABGGUgYChVMA8%3D%26rs%3DAOn4CLC3R11B4l5gt_TVqEl8LugDWE7Pbg&f=1&nofb=1&ipt=6c2377bedf1f9a75b5f1896e0cdde259dc97455ddb1586854589b0d0220ad674.

10.5.2. Impact on Athletic Performance

The intricate interplay between human osteology and athletic performance is based on the structural aspects of hands and feet. These limbs provide vital leverage and support for a multitude of athletic motions, from the speed of running to the precision of hand-eye coordination in sport. Bones, joints, and soft tissues in the hand and feet form a complex biomechanical system that enables athletes to perform explosive movements while maintaining balance under load.

Understanding of the mechanical response of these tissues, such as response under impact loading, is critical to maximize athletic performance and avoid injury. The research demonstrates that the composite nature of bone and soft tissue, as outlined in previous work, indicates their adaptation to dynamic loads exerted during sporting activity and the need for improved knowledge of their biomechanical responses (Kress et al., 1996). Furthermore, the prevalence of overuse injuries resulting from the ineffective functioning of the musculoskeletal system underscores the need to maintain the integrity of the hands and feet. Even for experienced sportsmen, problems such as inferior biomechanics and repetitive strain can cause debilitating damage. A study of the acute presentation of overuse injuries in cyclists illustrates the frequency of musculotendinous strains, particularly of the hamstrings and other significant muscle groups involved in lower extremity function (Venning et al., 2008).

The results demonstrated common injury sites that are generally due to suboptimal loading patterns or anatomical misalignments. Thus, the appropriate alignment and strengthening of the hands and feet not only increases performance data but also can significantly reduce the possibility of injury, allowing athletes the potential to achieve their highest levels. Finally, the development of protective devices and training strategies based on principles of human osteology can further enhance athletic performance. By understanding how different parts of the body respond to impact forces and the mechanical parameters involved, athletes and coaches can design strategies that achieve maximum physical output while safeguarding against damage. For example, incorporating functional training that emphasizes the dynamic capabilities of the hands and feet will increase an athlete's performance. Knowledge of the criteria of injury from biomechanical research helps in the development of better gear and training programs to minimize risks from high-impact sporting activity. Transfer of biomechanical data to sport training, thus, is a valuable step towards creating strong athletes who can perform at their level in their sport (Kress et al., 1996) (Figure 10.13).

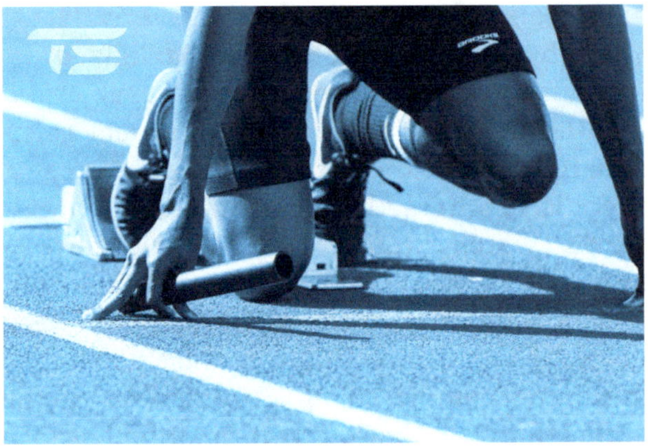

Figure 10.13. Impact on athletic performance.

Source: https://cdn.prod.website-files.com/61791a8b6c568b9710518140/673da658e24af215faa38764_Speed%20Training%20and%20Injury%20Prevention%20Tips%20for%20Sprinters%20(1).jpg.

10.5.3. Evolutionary Perspective on Foot Function

Anatomical function of the foot has been totally revolutionized, as the adaptive needs of human forebears have been satisfied. The most dramatic of these is probably the development of the arch, which facilitates shock absorption and energy economy in bipedalism. The midfoot bones, particularly the tarsals, have been altered to form a complex assembly that allows for body weight distribution while maintaining flexibility and support. This morphological response is a direct response to varying environmental stimuli, i.e., movement across varying landscapes. With the transition of hominins from arboreal existence to terrestrial foraging, foot function development emerged as a component of survival, as a suitably adapted foot facilitated more effective long-distance locomotion and the capacity to withstand, thereby enabling early man to exploit new ecological niches and resources.

Exploring the evolutionary perspective of foot function further highlights the influence of climate and environmental variation upon anatomical adaptation. In Late Pleistocene eras, climatic change would have been conducive to the evolution of highly efficient locomotion to travel long distances in search of food and resources. Such adaptations would have been conducive not only to skeletal change but also to musculature change, which enhances the efficiency of bipedalism. The foot's structural integrity, including alterations of the metatarsals and phalanges, would have been under selective pressure, enabling early man to run and walk for long distances. This athleticism forged a profound connection with nature, which would be essential for survival and for interaction with society in critical moments of human evolution.

The implications of these evolutionary developments extend beyond mere physical function; they encompass a range of cultural and behavioral accommodations as well. As the purpose of the foot changed, so too did the social practice of moving around, making tools, and sharing knowledge for mobility and the use of the landscape. The evolution of some burial traditions, as documented in research such as the VPLF function within ancient Maya cemeteries, reveals the influence anatomical features had on defining social structures and culture. The interconnection of foot morphometrics and its functional optimality with broader biocultural contexts further supports the relevance of osteological studies in identifying the complexity of human evolution. Such examinations, both biological profiles and cultural contexts, highlight the intricate relationship between lived experience and anatomical adaptation in historical populations (Narayan, 2023; Kelmelis et al., 2025).

Test Your Knowledge

1. How do the arches of the foot contribute to balance, shock absorption, and locomotion?
2. What role do the feet play in maintaining posture and efficient bipedal walking?

10.6. Common Pathologies of the Hands and Feet

Learning Outcome

1. Injuries and fractures
2. Degenerative disease (e.g., arthritis)
3. Congenital anomalies

Hands and feet are prone to many pathologies, both congenital and acquired, with significant impacts on mobility and function. Shared pathologies involve osteoarthritis, which usually affects the joints in the hands and feet because of wear and tear over time. The condition presents itself as pain, stiffness, and limited range of motion, causing daily functions to be complex. Rheumatoid arthritis also lays siege to these extremities, as it is described by inflammation of the joints that cause pain and deformity. Identification of these pathologies, in general, is valuable because they provide information on the lifestyles and environmental stressors that affected people's health over time, and thus are highly informative to osteologists studying skeletal groups. Malformations and deformities in the hands and feet will also be very informative concerning historical patterns of health. Polydactyly and syndactyly, both congenital conditions, provide information on genetic variation and its prevalence within populations. Similarly, the presence of conditions like clubfoot may indicate the economic and social flexibility of the people in the past, since the deformities tend to necessitate special interventions and reactions from society. The interpretation of the conditions allows osteologists to construct narratives about the way of life and health beliefs of different cultures, and the manner in which the physically hindered managed to move within their worlds. Additionally, how widespread these pathologies are and what meaning they hold contribute to a broader framework of human health and resiliency over time. Trauma-related pathologies, like dislocations and fractures, are also present on the hands and feet and typically represent the everyday activities of past populations. The nature of the injury will inform researchers about occupational hazards, social ceremonies, and even aggression in a population. For instance, a detailed study of healed fractures can reveal insights into the medical understanding and treatment of various historical periods. Moreover, the study of skeletal remains from archaeological diggings, such as those revealed during the excavation of Smith's Fort, Barrett et al. (2004), provides immediate evidence of physical hardship suffered by people. In the same way, studies at locations like the Anglo-Saxon execution cemetery at Walkington Wold (Allison et al. 2007) give us new information about the prevalence of trauma, expanding our understanding of the way in which such pathologies affected individuals and populations during the past (Figure 10.14).

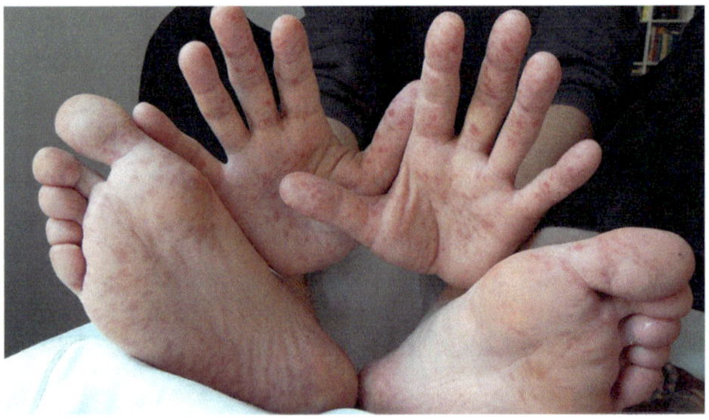

Figure 10.14. Common pathologies of the hands and feet.

Source: https://vitalrecord.tamu.edu/wp-content/uploads/2017/06/hfm-wikicommw.jpg.

10.6.1. Injuries and Fractures

In human osteology, understanding injuries and fractures, particularly those of the hands and feet, provides essential insights into past human activities and social interaction. Bones' presentation of trauma helps explain not only the material circumstances of trauma but also the prevailing social conditions, for instance, violence and lifestyle. For instance, examination of bone remains will show patterns characteristic of interpersonal violence, e.g., defensive injuries. A medieval skeleton found in Gloucester demonstrates this, with cut marks characteristic of weapon use. This observation highlights how fractures can serve as markers not just of personal health but also of community dynamics, cultural practices, and conflict-resolution strategies used during a particular period in history, underscoring the importance of injuries in the study of human osteology. Hand and foot fractures can significantly disable the ability of a person to perform or function, emphasizing the importance of mobility and dexterity in the past. Bone analysis of amputation victims, such as victims in the Estremoz necropolis, can provide an interesting view into the practice of society in trauma or punishment. The discovery of skeletons with their hands and feet amputated shows a commonality in their experiences, and therefore, questions regarding judicial process and community norms in medieval Portugal must be asked. These findings lead to greater insight into how both non-fatal injury and intentional violence, in society's manifestation of purposeful amputations, intersect with the narrative of social stratification and judicial intervention. Each fracture or injury of the skeletal record has a story, one which informs us of the lived experiences of individuals and the productivity of their settings. Furthermore, the significance of hand and foot injuries extends far beyond individual trauma; it also affects the interpretation of broader archaeological evidence. Most notably, those researching patterns of trauma need to consider the cultural meaning of such injuries, including potential rituals relating to death or violence. The Gloucester skeletal material not only represents the results of interpersonal violence but also embodies a mirror of diet and lifestyle factors that may predispose an individual toward specific health issues, for instance, anemia. Thus, analysis of injuries in human osteology involves an interdisciplinary investigation that integrates anthropology, history, and medicine to establish a holistic knowledge of human lives in the past. The types and frequencies of fractures and injuries are strong indicators of past human activity and societal structure, chronicling long-term interactions between physical health and cultural pursuits (Figure 10.15).

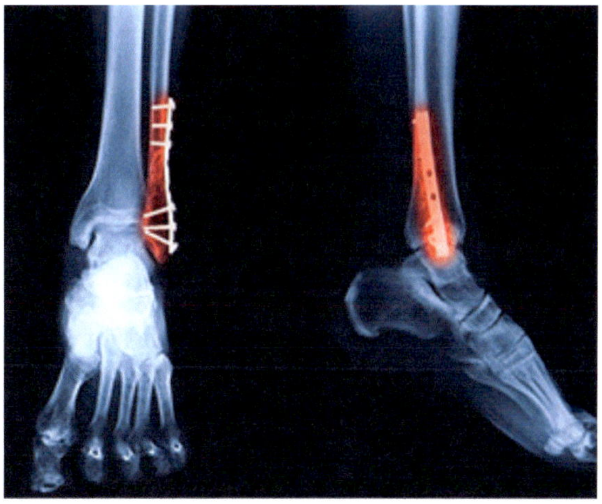

Figure 10.15. Understanding injuries and fractures.

Source: https://www.mytorontophysio.com/wp-content/uploads/2018/11/Traumatic-Injuries.jpg.

10.6.2. Degenerative Diseases (e.g., Arthritis)

The impact of degenerative diseases, particularly arthritis, on human osteology underscores the interplay between environmental and biological factors. Arthritis, which incorporates inflammation and the destruction of joint tissues, significantly affects the skeletal system, particularly in sensitive areas such as the hands and feet. The hands and feet are subjected to various stresses and injuries throughout an individual's life, which may accelerate degenerative changes. For instance, the anatomical conformation of the metatarsals and phalanges renders them very prone to repetitive stress and externally induced wear and tear. Therefore, examination of the skeletal manifestations of arthritis can provide information about past communities and their lifestyle parameters, as well as the incidence and manifestations of such conditions across various ages and geographic regions. Degenerative diseases like arthritis both affect individual morbidity and reflect broader societal trends through archaeological correlates. When osteological remains exhibit degenerative disease, such as osteophyte formation or joint space narrowing, researchers can infer a range of lifestyle parameters, including diet, exercise, and occupation. Especially, soldiers from previous populations would have perhaps manifested a higher incidence of lower reactive arthropathy due to the physical load it placed upon them, as proposed by Avon et al. (2014), that most often, malnutrition, war-related stressors, lower living conditions, and overpopulated housing resulted in adverse health conditions among these populations. These results can be pivotal for understanding how some occupations affected bone health and for getting a glimpse of the lifestyle of individuals who lived centuries ago. In addition, research on degenerative diseases in osteological samples underscores the need for aggressive methods and interdisciplinary approaches. Researchers are increasingly focusing on detailed characterization of osteoarthritis and other degenerative conditions through careful evaluation of skeletal pathology, morphology, and biomechanics (Becker et al., 2019). This small-data approach allows for effective comparison of biologically and culturally related populations, enriching the overall analysis of occupational and environmental etiologic factors contributing to skeletal change. By integrating paleopathological data with biomechanical assessment, scientists aim to build multidimensional accounts of human disease and health in the past. Such a multidimensional understanding is important, not just for interpreting skeletal evidence, but also for understanding the applicability of degenerative diseases today and the potential avenues for future research into this significant area of osteological study (Figure 10.16).

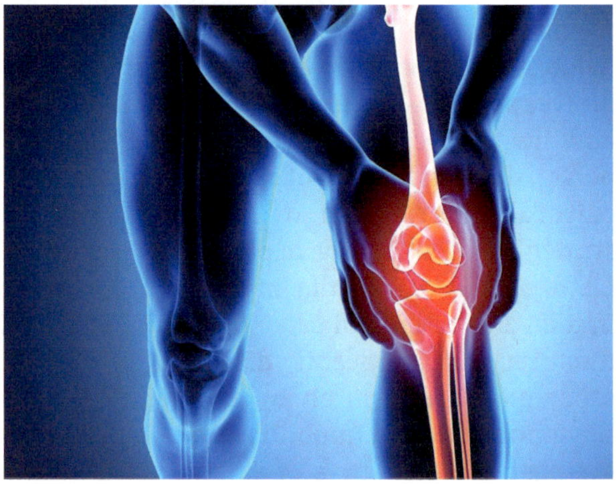

Figure 10.16. The impact of degenerative diseases.

Source: https://www.drashishsuryawanshi.com/wp-content/uploads/2022/09/7_2-1024x770.jpg.

10.6.3. Congenital Anomalies

Congenital anomalies represent one of the most significant areas within human osteology, that is, hands and feet, where developmental irregularities can have significant implications for skeletal form and function. Anomalies typically arise during embryonic life and can be expressed as variations in size, shape, or number. For example, polydactyly and syndactyly, both of which are conditions where there is the additional presence of fingers or toes and the union of the digits, respectively, are direct manifestations of such defects. An understanding of such conditions provides not just insight into developmental biology but also into the evolutionary history of humans. Fossil evidence from bone remains enables scientists to chart the prevalence of such anomalies over time, thereby enhancing our knowledge about the adaptability and resilience of the human race within the context of genetic predispositions.

Excavation and analysis of ancient human bones have greatly advanced the study of osteology, particularly the prevalence of congenital anomalies within a specific population. Studies, including recent findings in Ulaanbulag, Mongolia, report cases of congenital radioulnar synostosis (CRUS), an anomaly in which the radius and ulna bones of the forearm fuse. The discovery of such a condition in archaeological contexts not only sheds light on the health of past populations but also supports the role of genetics in shaping physiological differences among populations. Besides, understanding these congenital anomalies helps develop an understanding of demographic trends and social contexts, revealing how these conditions affected the activities and lives of ancient humans, including their mobility and tool use, which are at the heart of human evolution and cultural history (Bayarsaikhan et al., 2023). No less important are the conclusions drawn from the study of skeletal anomalies, which can inform us about broader health issues among ancient humans. The study of skeletons from the Necropolis of Big Mound revealed instances of cervical vertebrae fusion and abnormalities, which are part of a group of congenital conditions that affect the skeletal system (Russeva et al., 2011). These anomalies not only reveal aspects of past health and lifestyle, but also raise questions about potential lifestyle influences on these individuals. By examining these conditions, congenital anomalies can be linked to environmental factors such as diet and occupational hazards, creating, once again, a finer connection between genetics and external factors in human osteological development. Finally, the examination of congenital anomalies and their application to the hand and foot helps us to better know human history, health, and endurance (Figure 10.17).

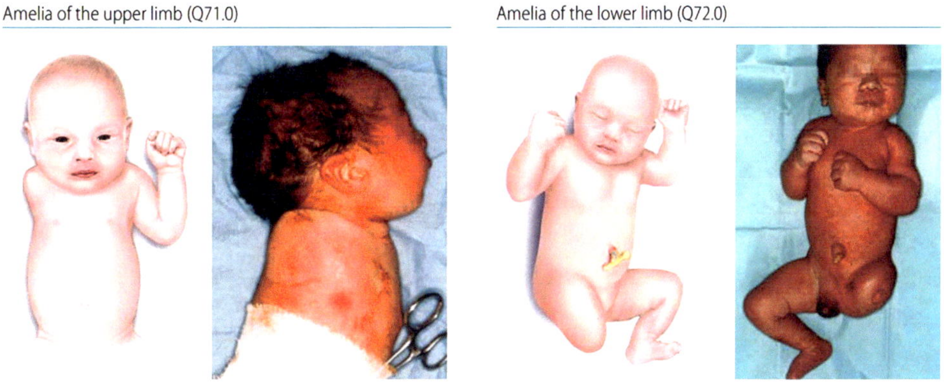

Figure 10.17. Congenital anomalies represent a critical area of study within human osteology.

Source: https://archive.cdc.gov/www_cdc_gov/ncbddd/birthdefects/surveillancemanual/photo-atlas/muscu_html_files/Amelia.jpg.

Test Your Knowledge

1. What are some common pathological conditions affecting the hands and feet, and how do they impact daily activities?
2. How can repetitive stress, injury, or developmental disorders lead to hand and foot pathologies?

SUMMARY

In summary, the study of human osteology, with special emphasis on hands and feet, is worth noting the anatomical significance these extremities provide. The bony structures of the hands and feet support simple motor functions but also aid complex skills reliant on dexterity and strength. This duality is evidence of their role in evolution, as the morphology of these bones has adapted to both locomotion and manipulation. Scientists can learn about human evolution and how particular adaptations have developed to allow for the survival of different societies in different environments by noting the variation in skeletal anatomy across populations. Lastly, the complexity of the hands and feet helps demonstrate the mutual dependency of form and function in human anatomy, providing a strong platform for further research and application in osteology and related fields. Coupled with the pivotal role of the hands and feet in human skeletal anatomy is the important understanding that their research offers regarding broader anthropological issues. Study of these areas not only helps explain individual health and growth but also supplies the background for historical accounts, such as cultural behavior and survival tactics. For example, the study of remains from archaeological burial grounds, such as the recently reassessed execution cemetery at Walkington Wold, teaches us about population patterns, social organization, and the contemporary customs of various periods (Allison et al., 2007). All these findings underscore the significance of osteological research for properly reconstructing past lives and routines, enabling researchers to engage with the intricacies of human existence from a physical perspective. Thus, integrating osteology and anthropological research helps us understand human life in all its aspects throughout time. Finally, what hand and foot studies suggest reverberates to contemporary applications, primarily in medical and educational contexts. Skeletal anatomy is a term that medical professionals need to know because it supports numerous practices, including anatomical education and clinical procedures (Tynes et al., 2014). Incorporating historical data and innovative learning methods, such as constructivist learning, could enhance students' learning and retention of these fundamental concepts. With the increased emphasis on the historical content of anatomy by writers like Vesalius, the establishment of medical knowledge and its continued relevance today are highlighted. By fostering a deeper appreciation of the intersection of osteology, history, and pedagogy, we equip future generations with the tools they need to navigate the complexities of human anatomy and its ongoing relevance in the practice and study of medicine and cultural studies.

The intricate anatomy and function of the hands and feet are fundamental to human osteology, revealing not only the body's structure but also the evolutionary significance of the appendages. A key point in this contention is research on skeletal parts, such as the carpal and metacarpal bones of the hand and the tarsal and metatarsal bones of the foot. Identifying the morphology of these areas unveils a complex interaction between evolutionary adaptation and anatomical function. The evolution of the large bones, including the patella, reveals changes in anatomy over thousands of years, mapping skeletal shape variation across various mammalian species and how it correlates with lifestyle, locomotion, and habitat adaptation. The evolutionary background underscores the significance of human anatomy as a discipline by connecting our current bony structure to its predecessors, thereby highlighting the relevance of comparative examination in osteology (Adams et al., 2017). Forensic anthropology's significant progress is separating human and nonhuman remains, particularly in medical and legal contexts. As researchers construct master databases of skeletal features, they reveal patterns that enable field identification and analysis. For instance, forensic evaluation of nonhuman bones in cases such as those in Kenosha County shows that many nonhuman mammalian species widespread in some geographic regions are commonly misidentified as human by virtue of bone size and shape. This finding underscores the utmost importance of more rigorous training in the differentiation of human and nonhuman skeletal forms, which is critical for ensuring appropriate forensic evaluations. Understanding such fine points not only contributes to improvement in forensic methods but also informs anthropologists about the broader context of osteological research within legal and ethical frameworks (Fourshee et al., 2022). The hands and feet, as complex anatomical structures, not only serve a functional role but also play a crucial role in human evolutionary biology. The evolution of principal features of the bones, such as bone ossification and the adaptability of the skeletal system to different environments, illustrates the dynamic nature of human osteology. As with the evolution of the patella in various lineages of mammals, which occurred multiple times, the growth and involution of bony elements illustrate a rich tapestry of genetic and environmental interplay. This diversity of ossification patterns across mammals illuminates our own evolutionary record, providing a hint of how apes' locomotor capabilities have been adapted over time. The combination of fossils with modern genetic studies is a significant way to understand not only our plan for body inheritance but also the critical functions these structures perform today (Adams et al., 2017).

KEY TERMS FROM THIS CHAPTER

Calcaneus	Capitate
Carpals	Cuboid
Hamate	Intermediate Cuneiform
Lateral Cuneiform	Lunate
Medial Cuneiform	Metacarpals
Metatarsals	Navicular
Phalanges	Pisiform
Scaphoid	Talus
Tarsals	Trapezium

CRITICAL THINKING QUESTIONS

1. **How many bones are there in each hand?**
   a. 27
   b. 28
   c. 30
   d. 26
2. **Which bones form the wrist?**
   a. Tarsals
   b. Metacarpals
   c. Carpals
   d. Phalanges
3. **How many phalanges are present in each hand?**
   a. 12
   b. 14
   c. 16
   d. 18
4. **Which carpal bone articulates with the radius?**
   a. Scaphoid
   b. Capitate
   c. Pisiform
   d. Hamate
5. **What is the anatomical name for the bones in the palm of the hand?**
   a. Metacarpals
   b. Carpals
   c. Phalanges
   d. Tarsals

Short Answer Questions

1. How many bones are present in each hand?
2. Which bone in the hand articulates with the radius?
3. Describe the arches of the hand and their significance.
4. Describe the arrangement of the phalanges in the toes.
5. What is the function of the medial longitudinal arch of the foot?

Answers to Critical Thinking Questions

1. (a); 2. (c); 3. (b); 4. (a); 5. (a)

REFERENCES

1. Bishop, P. J., Hocknull, S. A., Clemente, C. J., Hutchinson, J. R., Farke, A. A., Barrett, R. S., & Lloyd, D. G. (2018). Cancellous bone and theropod dinosaur locomotion. Part III—Inferring posture and locomotor biomechanics in extinct theropods, and its evolution on the line to birds. *PeerJ*, *6*, e5777. https://doi.org/10.7717/peerj.5777Abzhanov, A., Abzhanov, A., Abzhanov, A., Baggiolini, A., Baroffio, A., Beverdam, A., Chevallier, A., et al. (2019). Molecular and cellular mechanisms underlying the evolution of form and function in the amniote jaw. https://core.ac.uk/download/323079229.pdf (accessed on 18th July 2025).
2. Adams, A., Aglietti, A., Ahlberg, A., Alexander, A., Andrews, A., Archibald, A., et al. (2017). Evolution of the patellar sesamoid bone in mammals. https://core.ac.uk/download/82960261.pdf (accessed on 18th July 2025).
3. Adrian, A., Agerholm, A., Aksenov, A., Alvord, A., Bagg, A., Baker, A., et al. (2011). Syndactyly in pigs: A review of previous research and the presentation of eight archaeological specimens. https://core.ac.uk/download/4898961.pdf (accessed on 18th July 2025).
4. Ancrenaz, A., Ashton, P., Cartmill, M., Cartmill, J., Cartmill, A., Curtis, D., et al. (2010). Hand and foot pressures in the aye-aye (*Daubentonia madagascariensis*) reveal novel biomechanical trade-offs required for walking on gracile digits. https://core.ac.uk/download/30704909.pdf (accessed on 18th July 2025).
5. Bailey, G. B., Bartlett, J. E., Boylston, A., Briden, C., Briden, C., Buikstra, J., et al. (2007). An Anglo-Saxon execution cemetery at Walkington Wold, Yorkshire. https://core.ac.uk/download/52301.pdf (accessed on 18th July 2025).
6. Banton, M. E. (2014). Examining reactive arthropathy in military skeletal assemblages: A pilot study using the mass grave assemblage from the Battle of Towton (1461). https://core.ac.uk/download/79496181.pdf (accessed on 18th July 2025).
7. Barrett, A., & Blakey, M. L. (2004). Analysis of two human skeletons from Smith's Fort, Bermuda. https://core.ac.uk/download/235399436.pdf (accessed on 18th July 2025).
8. Barrett, B., Bidmos, M., Bidmos, J., Bilge, A., British Broadcasting Corporation, British Broadcasting Corporation, et al. (2014). The foot in forensic human identification–a review. https://core.ac.uk/download/30660095.pdf (accessed on 18th July 2025).
9. Bayarsaikhan, M., Misheelt, B., & Okazaki, K. (2023). A case of radioulnar synostosis of Mongolia. https://core.ac.uk/download/617921928.pdf (accessed on 18th July 2025).
10. Becker, S. K. (2019). Osteoarthritis, entheses, and long bone cross-sectional geometry in the Andes: Usage, history, and future directions. https://core.ac.uk/download/323311202.pdf (accessed on 18th July 2025).
11. Borrini, M., Eliopoulos, C., & Valoriani, S. (2025). Sharp force trauma death in a young individual from Medieval Gloucester. https://core.ac.uk/download/82957855.pdf (accessed on 18th July 2025).
12. Chamberlain, A. T., Marcé-Nogué, J., Püschel, T. A., & Sellers, W. (2020). The biomechanical importance of the scaphoid-centrale fusion during simulated knuckle-walking and its implications for human locomotor evolution. https://core.ac.uk/download/293754200.pdf (accessed on 18th July 2025).

13. Cunha, E., Fernandes, T., Liberato, M., & Marques, C. (2017). Three cases of feet and hand amputation from Medieval Estremoz, Portugal. https://core.ac.uk/download/92464286.pdf (accessed on 18th July 2025).

14. Dickinson, T. M. (2004). An early Anglo-Saxon cemetery at Quarrington, near Sleaford, Lincolnshire: Report on excavations, 2000–2001. https://core.ac.uk/download/55234.pdf (accessed on 18th July 2025).

15. Dockall, H. D. (1994). Human skeletal remains from the Tyson site (41SY92). https://core.ac.uk/download/215496487.pdf (accessed on 18th July 2025).

16. Eckel, C., Fiallo, M., Mas, J., et al. (2021). Osteology modules for the human structure course. https://core.ac.uk/download/657567126.pdf (accessed on 18th July 2025).

17. Figueirido, B., Janis, C., & Buttrill, K. (2014). Locomotion in extinct giant kangaroos: Were sthenurines hop-less monsters? https://core.ac.uk/download/30673537.pdf (accessed on 18th July 2025).

18. Foster, A. E. (2015). Characterization of a cortical defect of the ulna found in the Fernvale archaeological population (40WM51) of the South Harpeth River Valley in Middle Tennessee. https://core.ac.uk/download/647350885.pdf (accessed on 18th July 2025).

19. Fourshee, J. L. (2022). Differentiating human from nonhuman bone: Insights from a medical examiner's collection, Kenosha, Wisconsin. https://core.ac.uk/download/554010999.pdf (accessed on 18th July 2025).

20. Gamble, J. A., & Gilmour, R. J. (2024). Bones at home supporting haptic learning and universal design beyond the biological anthropology laboratory. https://core.ac.uk/download/644028705.pdf (accessed on 18th July 2025).

21. Hodgin, R. M. (2012). Trauma at Akhetaten (Tell el-Amarna): Interpersonal violence or occupational hazard. https://core.ac.uk/download/84118993.pdf (accessed on 18th July 2025).

22. Inthasan, C., & Mahakkanukrauh, P. (2017). Age estimation from clavicle by histomorphometry method: A review. https://core.ac.uk/download/159613125.pdf (accessed on 18th July 2025).

23. Kelmelis, S., Walden, J., Green Mink, K., Hoggarth, J. A., Ebert, C. E., Freiwald, C., Watkins, T. B., et al. (2025). Biocultural taphonomies and analysis of an emerging terminal classic (750–900 CE) Maya deathway. *Journal of Archaeological Method and Theory, 32.* https://doi.org/10.1007/s10816-024-09689-y (accessed on 18th July 2025).

24. Kivell, T. L., Lemelin, P., Richmond, B. G., & Schmitt, D. (2016). The primate wrist. https://core.ac.uk/download/46164637.pdf (accessed on 18th July 2025).

25. Kress, T. A. (1996). Impact biomechanics of the human body. https://core.ac.uk/download/268768377.pdf (accessed on 18th July 2025).

26. Narayan, E. (2023). Animal science annual volume 2023. *Veterinary Medicine and Science.* https://doi.org/10.5772/intechopen.113979 (accessed on 18th July 2025).

27. Parks, M. A. (2002). Occurrence of degenerative joint disease in the radius: Analysis of skeletal remains from the Poole-Rose ossuary. https://core.ac.uk/download/217391742.pdf (accessed on 18th July 2025).

28. Paulman, L. E., Sargent Jones, L., Terracio, L., Thandani, M. S., et al. (2001). Medical student dissection of cadavers improves performance on practical exams but not on the NBME anatomy subject exam. https://core.ac.uk/download/pdf/85192.pdf (accessed on 18th July 2025).

29. Russeva, V. (2011). Alterations of cervical vertebrae in two individuals from the Late Antiquity Necropolis from the "Big Mound" near Cabyle, Bulgaria. https://core.ac.uk/download/25069090.pdf (accessed on 18th July 2025).

30. Sanders, J. E. (2009). Age estimation of fetal skeletal remains from the forensic context. https://core.ac.uk/download/267571360.pdf (accessed on 18th July 2025).

31. Steele, J., & Uomini, N. (2009). Can the archaeology of manual specialization tell us anything about language evolution? A survey of the state of play. https://core.ac.uk/download/1685151.pdf (accessed on 18th July 2025).

32. Taylor, M. P., & Wedel, M. J. (2012). Why sauropods had long necks; and why giraffes have short necks. https://core.ac.uk/download/29026739.pdf (accessed on 18th July 2025).

33. Tynes, J. F. (2014). A mixed methods investigation of post-secondary students' long bone anatomy knowledge retention through constructivism and the works of Vesalius. https://core.ac.uk/download/217397093.pdf (accessed on 18th July 2025).

34. Venning, G. (2008). A pilot study of the profile of injuries that presented to the student chiropractic sports council at the Pick 'n Pay 94.7 cycle challenge from 2002 to 2004. https://core.ac.uk/download/18215246.pdf (accessed on 18th July 2025).

SKELETAL VARIATION AND IDENTIFICATION IN HUMAN OSTEOLOGY

11

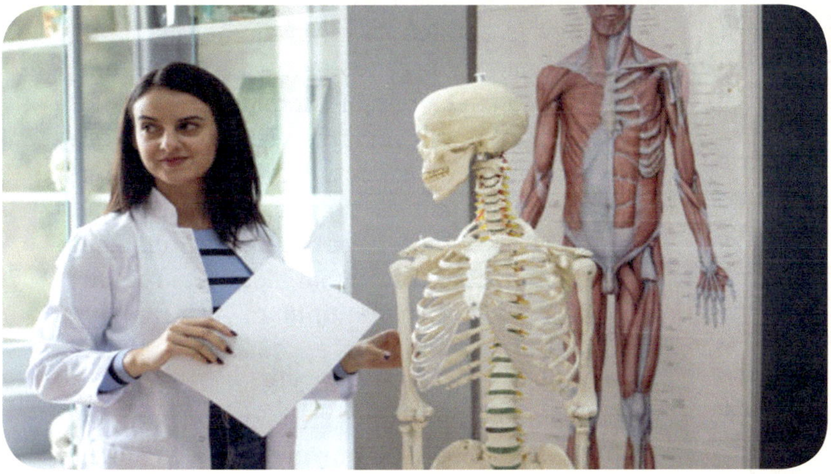

LEARNING OBJECTIVES

After studying this chapter, you will be able to:

1. Discuss the historical context of human osteology
2. Explain the types of skeletal variation
3. Describe the methods of skeletal identification
4. Understand forensic applications of osteology
5. Know skeletal variation across populations
6. Focus on challenges in osteological identification

Introduction

Grasping human biological variety and its role in identification processes is fundamental in studies of human osteology and skeletal variation. Human bones are a primary source of information in scientific disciplines such as forensic science, archaeology, and anthropology. Notably, the accuracy of skeletal identification has the potential to provide meaningful information regarding an individual's biological profile, including age, sex, ancestry, and stature. This information is particularly valuable in forensic cases, where the recognition of decomposed or broken remains poses special challenges. The variability that exists in human skeletal morphology is the result of a multitude of factors, including genetics, environmental factors, and cultural influences, which cumulatively contribute to the challenge of recognizing humans. Understanding these variations enhances the methodologies used in forensic analysis, particularly when remains are incomplete or severely decomposed, requiring a thorough knowledge of skeletal anatomy and variation. One of the critical aspects of skeletal variation is understanding specific anatomical features, which can vary considerably among individuals and groups. For instance, foot anatomy is often overlooked in forensic identification despite its potential to provide critical information regarding the identity of the person. The ongoing research has highlighted how forensic practitioners struggle when attempting to match and identify fragments of the foot bones to their corresponding individuals, necessitating more integrative approaches. As hinted at by an examination of the role of the foot in forensic human identification, a significant gap in the literature points towards the necessity of continued research on the topic. Examination of the bony components of the foot can potentially yield significant information, particularly where cases involve dismembered or fragmented human remains. Hence, taking these skeletal variations into account can significantly influence the efficacy of forensic identification protocols, elevating the science of forensic investigation of human skeletal variation (Barrett et al., 2014). Moreover, the role of training and experience in forensic search has been underscored by a body of studies examining the efficacy of evidence recovery. By determining the recovery rates of skeletal remains from individuals with different levels of expertise and training, researchers are able to determine the impact of human factors on identification success. Such research underscores the need for specialized training in forensic anthropology, as competence in recovery procedures directly affects successful identification of remains. Moreover, awareness of the consequences of variation in searchers' competence will encourage improved methodology in evidence collection, which is particularly crucial when dealing with human skeletal remains. As forensic experts navigate the complexity of skeletal identification, the integration of results of empirical studies into training protocols is needed. This integrated approach will enhance the accuracy and validity of human identification in forensic contexts, ultimately resolving complex cases (Studebaker-Reed et al., 2018).

Definition of Human Osteology

Human osteology is a branch of biological anthropology that focuses on the human skeletal anatomy of remains. This discipline entails a wide range of methods applied to understand the form, function, and variability of bones and to acquire significant information about past human behavior, health, and culture. Osteology is not just the recognition of the bony forms but the interpretation of the biological and anthropological information they express. Human osteology is applied in many areas, including forensic analysis, archaeological investigations, and the advancement of medical science. By analyzing skeletal remains, researchers are able to elucidate aspects of the identity of an individual, such as age, sex, ancestry, and health status, which is particularly important in contexts where traditional historical records may be nonexistent or minimal. As osteology advances, interdisciplinary approaches are being formulated to understand skeletal variation in human populations better. Present studies emphasize the use of employing new techniques, such as isotopic analysis and computer modeling, that can give insights into diets, migration, and the effects of the environment on bone formation. As an illustration, experiments employing isotopic techniques have indicated that diet can significantly influence the chemistry of the bones and, in turn, modify the inference by osteologists concerning subsistence patterns in the past. Also, as seen in recent archaeological digs into Iron Age societies, employing a human-centered framework enables researchers to consider social dynamics and migration as formative factors in skeletal traits (Wilhelmson et al., 2017). This demonstrates how integrating various scientific methods can provide a broader framework for analyzing human osteology. The science of human osteology is further complicated by the clarification of pathological states and their correlation with biomechanical stress endured throughout a lifetime. Entheses and osteoarthritis are examples of pathological states that indicate how the skeletal system adapts to various activities or environmental pressures (Becker et al., 2019). By analyzing such conditions using rigorous methodology, osteologists can establish relationships among health, lifestyle, and skeletal morphology in ancient populations. Emphasizing a "small data" approach allows for close examination of specific population subsets, building a deep understanding of how cultural habits and mechanical loads have influenced aspects of the skeleton in the past. Ultimately, human osteology as an examination is actually not descriptive at all; it is hugely concerned with the nature of how biological information can shed light on historical documents and contribute to broader anthropological debate (Figure 11.1).

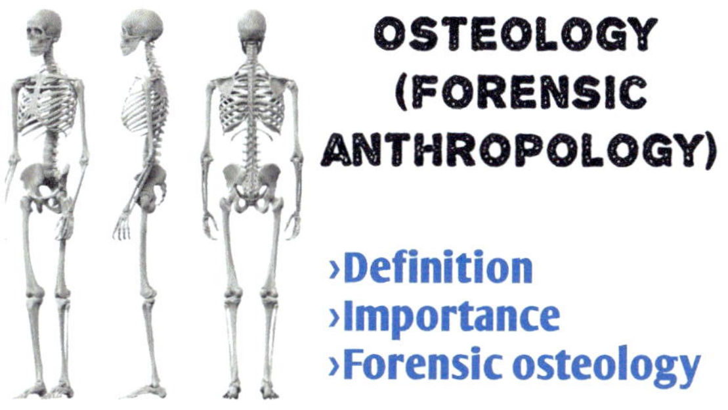

Figure 11.1. Human osteology.

Source: https://external-content.duckduckgo.com/iu/?u=https%3A%2F%2Fi.ytimg.com%2Fvi%2FWoWoo0czMgU%2Fmaxresdefault.jpg&f=1&nofb=1&ipt=c60e4b138f8e2b382ca9d950ea0d5ec19013dfa69fbb32876ea63e0388f1c0e0.

Importance of Skeletal Variation

Variability of the skeleton is at the heart of the science of human osteology, its importance going beyond anatomical variation. It provides a foundation for personal identification, enabling forensic anthropologists to reconstruct biological profiles. Through sensitive examination of remains, size, shape, and form variation enables fundamental information regarding age, sex, ancestry, and health of the individual. As reported in recent forensic studies, these skeletal variations have a high ability to enhance the accuracy of identification processes, especially in cases of fragmented remains, where standard identification methods may fail. Awareness of these variations also facilitates solution-finding regarding issues presented in forensic cases; therefore, the ability to discriminate skeletal variations is paramount in determining identity and, in turn, justice in a courtroom environment (Barrett et al., 2014). This analysis of bone variations also highlights the intersection of biology and culture, demonstrating the active relationship between an individual's genes and environment. Osteological analysis reveals biocultural factors that influence bone structure and informs anthropologists about population patterns and past migrations. The insight that may be gained by analyzing variation in bone structures can be used to understand how various environmental influences, such as diet or physical exercise, contribute to the evolution of bone characteristics. This insight into the complexity of bone variation not only adds value to anthropological studies but also echoes the importance of osteology to epidemiology and public health. With knowledge of the composite nature of human bones, osteologists can provide more detailed, context-dependent profiles, which are essential for forensic examination (Bosnar et al., 2010). Moreover, the increased application of skeletal variation in modern forensic anthropology is a testament to the subject's ongoing development. Technology and innovative methodology now enable scientists to analyze skeletal remains more precisely, revealing subtle differences previously unobserved. These developments offer new opportunities for forensic practitioners to apply osteological findings in criminal investigations and underscore the importance of skeletal variation in crime-solving. As forensic anthropology continues to progress, the application of osteological data into prolonged forensic protocols reinforces the discipline's potential for radical change. The conjunction of past osteological knowledge and present forensic methods underscores the significance of skeletal variation, not only as a means of identification but also as an essential element in exploring the dynamics of human life and death (Barrett et al., 2014; Bosnar et al., 2010) (Figure 11.2).

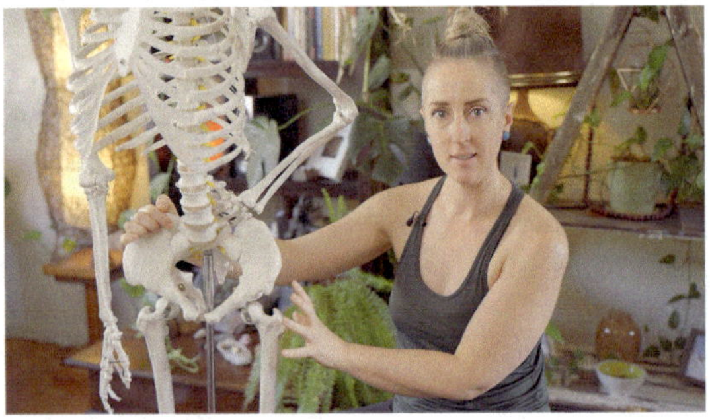

Figure 11.2. Skeletal variation plays a crucial role in the field of human osteology.

Source: https://external-content.duckduckgo.com/iu/?u=https%3A%2F%2Fstatic.wixstatic.com%2Fmedia%2F88e63e_2204ec37b0864a01b7b94710377b88ec~mv2.jpg%2Fv1%2Ffill%2Fw_980%2Ch_551%2Cal_c%2Cq_85%2Cusm_0.66_1.00_0.01%2Cenc_auto%2F88e63e_2204ec37b0864a01b7b94710377b88ec~mv2.jpg&f=1&nofb=1&ipt=1f418a7533deff14bfbe9e0a6e6b9031b7a42a07ad2f75c497bcf424fb769bb2.

Overview of Identification Methods

The identification of skeletal remains is a fundamental component of forensic anthropology and bioarchaeology, supported by several methodologies that provide accurate identification of individuals. A prevalent method in place involves analyzing biological profiles on the basis of skeletal variation, encompassing the assessment of age, sex, ancestry, and stature ascertained on the basis of some osteological indicators. Biological profiling can significantly reduce the number of candidates for identity, particularly in cases of commingled remains. For instance, foot characteristic evaluation, which is typically less well-explored than other skeletal elements, is growing in popularity on the strength of its particular ability to solve identity, especially in more recent studies on fragments of lower limbs and relevance to the identification of individuals, as highlighted in literature related to human remains (Barrett et al., 2014). Another vital method employed in the identification process is DNA testing, particularly when skeletal remains have been destroyed or only minute fragments remain. Mitochondrial and nuclear DNA can provide a powerful means of identification, allowing forensic specialists to compare isolated genetic material with potential relatives or established databases. Such an approach, however, relies on the preservation state of the remains and the availability of reference samples. It also introduces variability associated with environmental factors that can affect DNA degradation. Studies comparing recovery success across various search teams identify the importance of adequate training and the experience level of the searchers in maximizing the collection of evidence, which is paramount for establishing a basis for DNA examination and resulting identification (Studebaker-Reed et al., 2018). Anthropological methods such as cranial analysis and metric assessments are equally important in skeletal identification. These techniques focus on the analysis of some cranial characteristics and measurements that can indicate ancestry and sex, adding more information to the biological profile. Coupled with other methods, such as morphological assessments, these anthropological techniques improve skeletal identification accuracy. The challenge, however, lies in interpreting these differences properly among different populations. The growing recognition of the significance of the foot in forensic identification is an apt illustration of how different skeletal elements can yield valuable information and require further research to expand the scope of identification procedures and consolidate the discipline's existing paradigms (Barrett et al., 2014).

11.1. Historical Context of Human Osteology

Learning Outcome

1. Early work and results
2. Evolution of osteological techniques
3. Contributions of influential figures in the discipline

The history of human osteology is founded on the evolving perception of skeletal remains and their ramifications for anthropology and forensic science. The first osteological activity focused on identifying skeletal features indicative of age, sex, and ancestry. However, the examination of bones was traditionally conducted in three-dimensional space, in accordance with societal beliefs about race and disease. This initial understanding served as the foundation for subsequent advances in osteological techniques, which, in turn, facilitated more advanced means of critically analyzing skeletal variation. Advances in scientific rigor brought techniques into greater systematization and allowed investigation into the implications of skeletal variation to a deeper level within a broader context. The relationships between historical perspectives and modern approaches determine the current status of human osteology, making skeletal analysis a better-understood process, not only as a scientific but also as a cultural artifact reflecting the values of specific periods. Skeletal analysis has also been significantly shaped by specific historical events, underscoring the importance of context in osteological studies. For instance, the excavation of human remains in cemeteries, such as the Acacia Park Cemetery in Minnesota, reveals how histories are constructed from fragments through osteological analysis. From its initial importance to the Dakota, the cemetery site was altered during the 1800s as European settlement expanded, thereby illustrating a fierce intersection of cultural histories. The mixed skeletal remains studied there offered the possibility of reconstructing demographic profiles that illuminate the health conditions and activity patterns of past populations, thereby contributing to knowledge of life in the region during momentous changes. The careful examination of these remains reminds us that human osteology is not just about identifying the individual but is integrated into the larger historical context that affects methodologies and interpretations. Moreover, conflicts over high-profile cases, such as the potential remains of Amelia Earhart, highlight the complexity of osteological evaluations.

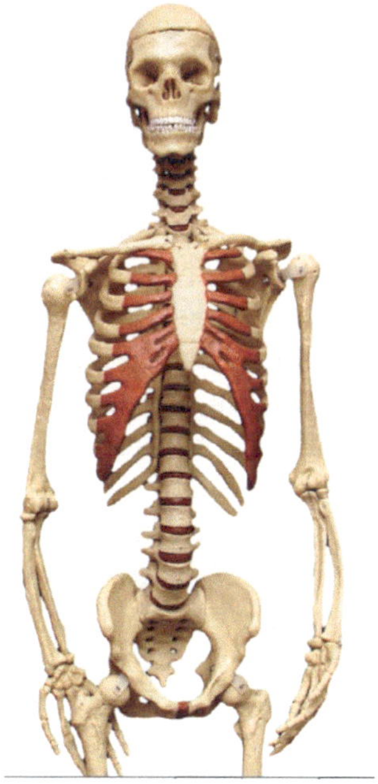

Figure 11.3. The historical context of human osteology.

Source: https://external-content.duckduckgo.com/iu/?u=http%3A%2F%2Fanthropology.iresearchnet.com%2Fwp-content%2Fuploads%2FOsteology-Human-fig.2.jpg&f=1&nofb=1&ipt=704c34bec23d7b6647a0e6f78d7ca6493ad036c29d8ae99bfe813c833e7e835b.

The analyses by British officials in 1940 that concluded the skeleton was male were later challenged by more recent cranial analysis techniques showing the remains could be

Earhart's, an argument supported by additional tests. Close examination of such findings identifies methodological flaws, and the value of scientific stringency in osteological endeavour is brought into focus, as is the impact of historical prejudice that can predetermine interpretations. Such a case highlights the necessity of continued critique and innovation within osteological practice to counteract the impact of past errors. Therefore, knowing the past of human osteology not only enlightens modern practice but also highlights the discipline's adherence to developing scientific norms and an enhanced cultural understanding of human diversity (Figure 11.3).

11.1.1. Early Studies and Discoveries

Early research in human osteology laid the foundation for understanding skeletal variation and identification. A concern of early investigators was the recognition of remains from bones using morphological attributes, such as bone size, shape, and form. As methods improved, the importance of contextualizing skeletal remains within the archaeological and cultural context became increasingly evident. This approach not only enabled greater accuracy in identification but also provided information about the way of life and health of past populations. For instance, variation in long bone morphology was attributed to variations in physical activities, which aimed at how environmental and cultural conditions influence the skeleton's development. As scientists explored these initial findings, more and more came to appreciate the importance of establishing a baseline for skeletal variation, which is pivotal for assessing the health and demography of ancient populations. Osteological science also developed a more sophisticated understanding of skeletal pathologies. Early pathological diagnoses of osteoarthritis and other degenerative bone diseases initiated intense research into the biology of these processes. Investigations, as with techniques described by Verano (1997) in the Andes and by Ortner (2011, 2012) for paleopathological studies, focused on the meticulous documentation of osteoarthritis and the evaluation of the cross-sectional geometry of long bones. By observing such diseases alongside abnormal skeletal changes and biomechanical forces, researchers began to demystify patterns of disease distribution among populations. This interpretation not only directs academic knowledge to health disparities issues today but also enhances the debate about how lifestyle affects skeletal health in the past. Early studies, therefore, established a model to test the relationship between social context and skeletal variation and, in so doing, bridged the gap between past and present within human health studies. Future advancements in the field have since further built on these initial findings, demonstrating the interaction between genetics and environment in skeletal variations. As developments continue to be made in the field, the molecular and cellular processes involved in skeletal development have been brought to the forefront. Specifically, cranial neural crest mesenchyme (NCM) has emerged as a major force in skeletal variation. Researchers investigated how early-life disturbances can create variation and defects, adding another layer of meaning to our understanding of skeletal morphology and its evolutionary importance. These studies paved the way for the inclusion of multidisciplinary approaches, merging osteology with genetics, biomechanics, and paleopathology to formulate an integrated understanding of human skeletal variation. By considering bone morphology's variability and adaptive significance, researchers may lay the foundation for future research in both medical and archaeological contexts.

11.1.2. Evolution of Osteological Techniques

The evolution of osteological techniques has immensely enhanced our understanding of skeletal variation and identification in human osteology. The initial anthropologists began with external morphological assessments dominated by bone structures. However, with advances in technologies such as computed tomography (CT) and digital reconstruction, researchers can now create detailed three-dimensional models that provide enhanced information about skeletal morphology. Such development not only enhances the precision of skeletal analysis but also enables the examination of sophisticated traits that previous methods had concealed. For instance, the application of CT imaging offers a non-destructive approach to analyzing fossilized skeletons, ultimately revolutionizing our capacity to explore the structural development of the skeleton throughout history, particularly through events such as the cynodont–mammaliaform transition, as indicated in the ongoing debate over mammalian origins (Abdala et al., 2016). Technological advances in analytical techniques have also improved the precision with which osteologists can demarcate individual features of skeletal remains, enabling more precise analysis of biological processes. Precisely, cautionary techniques have been developed to address the complexities of differing burial practices, such as cremation. Cremated bodies pose special challenges in osteological analysis due to their fragmentary nature, as noted by researchers assessing bias in bioarchaeological analysis. This fragmentation could result in underrepresentation of demographic groups, such as infants and subadults, and in complications with accurately aging and sexing adults. Comparative paleodemographic questioning has been greatly assisted through the investigation of bias between inhumed and cremated samples to comprehend past populations, allowing for more precise interpretations of reproductive and mortality patterns (Kurila et al., 2015). Furthermore, the history of osteological technique has witnessed increased emphasis on interdisciplinary approaches, fusing classical osteology with genetics, archaeology, and anthropology. Through this interdisciplinary approach, osteologists have been better positioned to understand how various factors—social, environmental, and genetic—interact to shape skeletal variation in human populations. Consequently, contemporary osteologists are better suited to untangle the complexities of human diversity and adaptation through careful analysis of skeletal remains. By incorporating findings from modern imaging techniques and traditional osteological analysis, researchers are continuously refining knowledge of human evolutionary background and skeletal identification. Such multidisciplinary approaches are imperative for advancing a wide, integrative perspective on skeletal variety, which remains at the centre of the science of human osteology and the study of our shared biological heritage (Figure 11.4).

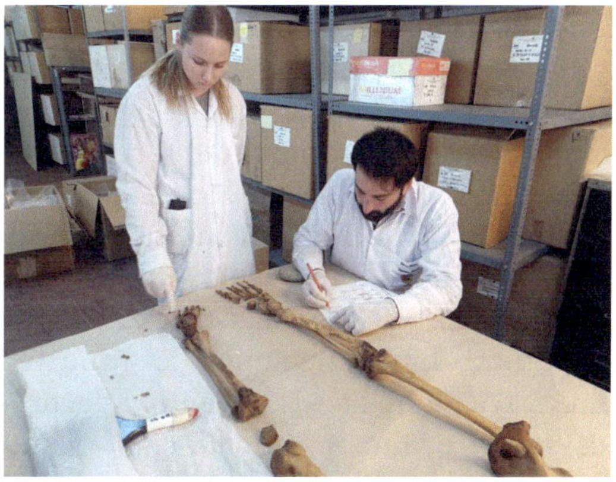

Figure 11.4. The evolution of osteological techniques.

Source: https://external-content.duckduckgo.com/iu/?u=https%3A%2F%2Fwww.archaeological.org%2Fwp-content%2Fuploads%2F2022%2F01%2FWhatsApp-Image-2022-11-16-at-05.09.28-1024x768.jpeg&f=1&nofb=1&ipt=511ab62d6283a33167f728b44f54233ebf2069304357bb89711f057351617c8c.

11.1.3. Contributions of Key Figures in the Field

Human osteology is significantly assisted by the efforts of pioneering figures who laid the foundation for skeletal variation and identification. An example of a pioneering figure is Dr. Robert W. Mann, a well-known practitioner of forensic anthropology whose new school of thought has transformed how skeletal remains are analyzed to determine age, sex, and ancestry. Mann's meticulous study in establishing standards for skeletal identification has been instrumental in formulating standardized procedures that enhance forensic precision. His work highlights the intricate relationship between population genetics and skeletal form, giving rise to greater human diversity. Also, his emphasis on the importance of proper collection and preservation of skeletal material has fostered sensitivity to ethical concerns in the treatment of human remains and caution in osteology as a science. Another significant contributor is Dr. Donn Grayson, whose wide-ranging research in skeletal variation has elucidated the complex interplay between biological and environmental forces in the construction of human bones. Grayson has been interested in how different conditions, such as diet and climate, affect skeletal characteristics in populations. His systematic documentation of variations has done much to educate us on the way the human skeleton is affected by processes of evolution, providing the context that modern identification techniques require. Combining knowledge from the archaeological, anthropological, and biomedical streams, Grayson's work cuts across disciplines and encourages an integrated understanding of human skeletal variation. This integrative method is essential for improving identification techniques, as it enables investigation of a wide range of variables influencing skeletal structure in forensic analysis. Secondly, Dr. T. E. McKern's pioneering techniques in osteometry are also a significant addition to the human osteology science. McKern's establishment of accurate measurement methods for evaluating skeletal remains has allowed researchers to make more confident inferences about demographic characteristics like age and height. His pioneering application of statistical analysis to skeletal research has established a standard for quantitatively oriented research in osteology. As such, professionals in the field adopted his techniques, which have enabled a better understanding of the complexity of skeletal variation within populations. The rigorous standards introduced by McKerr not only strengthened the science of bone measurement but also established a template for subsequent studies, thereby solidifying his position as a leading authority in shaping the identification and analysis of human skeletal remains.

Test Your Knowledge

1. How did early civilizations contribute to the development of human osteology as a scientific discipline?
2. What role did anatomical studies during the Renaissance play in advancing the understanding of the human skeletal system?

11.2. Types of Skeletal Variation

Learning Outcome

1. Genetic determinants of bone shape
2. influences on bone growth
3. Age-related changes in the skeleton

Skeletal variation in human individuals takes many forms, influenced by genetics, environmental factors, and developmental processes. Indeed, variations are categorized in various ways, such as sexual dimorphism, ancestry-related characteristics, and individual differences by age or health. Sexual dimorphism, for example, describes differences between male and female skeletons in morphology, such as pelvic shape, skull morphology, and the strength of limb bones. Having these distinctions at hand is important for forensic purposes to estimate sex accurately since incorrect biological sex identification can result in the making of wrong assumptions about the remains at hand. Furthermore, the osteological features correlated with ancestry underscore the importance of biological background in determining affinities between populations and thus in assisting forensic identification. These differences point to the intricate link between human identification and biological diversity. Another central category of skeletal variation comprises the representation of pathologies and traumas in bone remains. Ailments such as osteoarthritis, fractures, and congenital defects can significantly alter the bone morphology and provide valuable clues about a person's history of health, lifestyle, and potential causes of death. For instance, the presence of specific lesions or deformities might indicate long-standing stressors or trauma endured throughout a person's lifetime. Such skeletal markers may reveal the lives of past populations and serve as compelling evidence in forensic contexts. Further, such pathological markers require a refined understanding of both skeletal biology and the context in which the analyzed remains are found, since they encompass not only intrinsic body changes but also manifestations of environmental stress, diet, and healthcare. The use of advanced methodologies in the study of skeletal variation has continued to improve the efficiency of forensic identification. Advanced techniques such as DNA profiling and radiographic imaging have enhanced the accuracy with which skeletal remains can be examined. For that reason, professionals should be well-grounded in osteological knowledge. Recent research supports the importance of training in the recovery of human skeletal remains; evidence suggests that skill significantly impacts recovery rates and the accuracy of skeletal estimations (Studebaker-Reed et al., 2018).

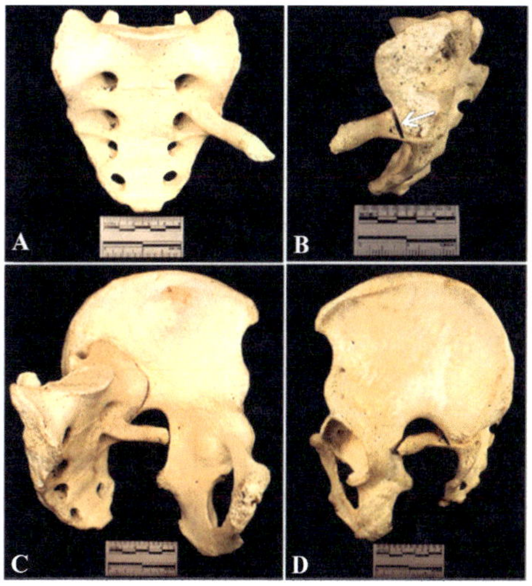

Figure 11.5. Skeletal variation in humans manifests in numerous forms.

Source: https://external-content.duckduckgo.com/iu/?u=https%3A%2F%2Fo.quizlet.com%2F7F15Uxe4mjIZ0ubgF7HTfw.png&f=1&nofb=1&ipt=faecc00f6de5aac2b963e41f9078c157a5952ac77dfe09af287b692bf588cd87.

In addition, this new emphasis on skeletal variability underscores the continued need for better investigation in forensic anthropology; further detailed studies of specific skeletal structures, such as the foot, are essential (Barrett et al., 2014). In general, embracing the complexity of skeletal variations is essential towards advancing identification techniques and expanding our understanding of human osteology (Figure 11.5).

11.2.1. Genetic Factors Influencing Skeletal Structure

Understanding the genetic factors that affect skeletal structure is vital for distinguishing variations among populations. Genetic predispositions dictate underlying characteristics such as bone density, size, and shape, which, in turn, affect skeletal morphology. Such heterogeneity can be a significant consideration in the identification of human skeletons, as evident from recent analyses of morphoscopic traits in skeletal samples. For example, investigations have measured variations in the vertebral column, such as the presence of an abnormal number of thoracic or lumbar vertebrae, underscoring the role of genetic factors in skeletal elements. In addition, these variations must be enumerated based on the known sex and age of subjects, with reference to how internal factors are related to skeletal pathologies and biomechanical loading stresses on the bones over time, thereby enhancing better identification in forensic use. In the context of osteological research, the value of genetic variability extends beyond identifying individuals to include other applications, such as understanding the causes of variation in health across populations. Variations in bone form mirror, in many cases, propensities towards certain diseases or conditions of genetic origin. As a specific example, research on osteoarthritis and long-bone geometry suggests that genetic variation influences the manifestation of these conditions. As mentioned in various studies, the incorporation of a multidisciplinary perspective enables researchers to observe the relationships between variations in the skeleton and its surroundings, and thus, the pathogenesis becomes more specific. This provides scientists with the opportunity to identify how genetic diversity manifests in characteristic bones, providing broader insight into the biology of human diversity and its influence on skeletal health, ultimately enabling identification when remains are discovered. Genetic data integration into skeletal work offers new insights in human variation analysis and its application in forensic identification. Science based on methodologies geared toward accurate documentation and evaluation of morphological characters enhances the ability to differentiate individuals through skeletal analysis. Genetic inheritance-derived differences, as proposed in influential research, tend to have a significant impact on the identification process, enabling improved outcomes in forensic investigations. By drawing on previously constructed anatomical collections, researchers can amass evidence on the prevalence of specific bone traits, contributing to a more accurate understanding of normal and abnormal variation within a population. Increased appreciation for the role of genetic influence on skeletal work not only makes identification of remains easier but also demands continuous methodological improvement to address the needs of human skeletal diversity (Becker et al., 2019; Sanford et al., 2024).

11.2.2. Environmental Impacts on Bone Development

The environment plays a strong role in bone development, both morphologically and in terms of the structural integrity of skeletal remains. Factors such as diet, exercise, and exposure to external stressors also contribute significantly to skeletal differences among populations. Calcium and vitamin D deficiencies can hinder bone development and lead to conditions such as rickets, which can cause deformities visible through skeletal analysis. Physical exercise also plays a significant role in bone strength and density; repeated weight-bearing exercise builds up bone modeling and remodeling. The interaction between such environmental factors puts into the spotlight the necessity of an integrated understanding of how lifestyle and resources affect skeletal health over an individual's life cycle. Moreover, environmental toxins such as heavy metals and endocrine disruptors have become integral factors in determining bone formation. Research indicates that exposure to pollutants can alter bone thickness and cause osteoporosis, a serious condition for those living in industrialized areas or near hazardous waste sites. Additionally, the socio-economic climate under which one finds themselves can regulate exposure to such toxic substances as well as proximity to medical centers, making diagnosis and definition of bone disorders even more complicated. The nuances of these interactions underscore the importance of integrative approaches in forensic anthropology and paleopathology, where an understanding of environmental influences can lead to more accurate interpretations of human skeletal remains. In a broader context, integrating technology and science into the study of environmental impacts on bone development is transforming our understanding of human osteology. Advanced imaging techniques, such as high-resolution X-ray computed tomography (CT), provide tools for non-destructive analysis of bone microstructure and may be capable of providing information on the subtle effects of environmental influences on bone formation. The application of these technologies creates the motivation for interdisciplinary research integrating elements of geosciences, materials science, and forensic science, as seen in efforts such as ToScA North America. With these scientific advances, researchers are better placed to assess the impact of environmental influences and extrinsic stressors on the skeleton, thus providing valuable information to human osteology and forensic science (Ahmed et al., 2017; Studebaker-Reed et al., 2018) (Figure 11.6).

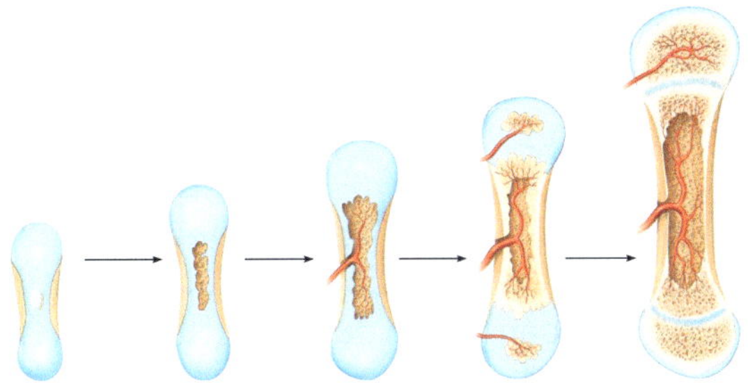

Figure 11.6. The environment exerts a profound influence on bone development.

Source: https://external-content.duckduckgo.com/iu/?u=https%3A%2F%2Fo.quizlet.com%2FGXfKg6U1k6Gvr5--NRufKA_b.jpg&f=1&nofb=1&ipt=01c2df7c1283dcdc51fc1de6fca3bbe328057b7f0ed481b43b32c3956c7893a5.

11.2.3. Age-Related Changes in the Skeleton

With increasing advancement in age estimation methods, as people go through various stages of life, there are definitive age-related alterations in the skeletal system that could prove valuable in both forensic and anthropological applications. During childhood and adolescence, bones develop rapidly, with the ossification of cartilaginous structures and the appearance of growth plates. These alterations are most evident in the knee, as stressed by the continuous improvements in age estimation methods. The Pyle and Hoerr radiographic atlas, for instance, includes a comprehensive model for predicting children's skeletal age, which illustrates the dramatic differential growth rates that develop in the early years of life. Having this information, practitioners can enhance methods for measuring chronological age, leading to improved reliability of skeletal identification in forensic contexts and the provision of data on normative developmental milestones pertinent to various age groups. Beyond the regular changes encountered with growth phases, aging in adulthood also entails significant skeletal changes that may affect identification. As individuals mature, bone mass increases until it reaches a maximum in the late 20s to early 30s. After this, gradual, ongoing bone mass and mineral density loss are recorded, with a tendency towards trabecular bone. This deterioration can lead to a heightened risk of fractures and conditions such as osteoporosis, particularly in the elderly. Furthermore, bone shape can change with cumulative wear and external stress, producing characteristic features that can be recorded and compared in forensic profiles. These changes in morphology, in addition to enabling individuals' age to be determined, can also be used to prove patterns of lifestyle and health impacts over time, adding still further analysis of skeletal remains in forensic and archaeological studies.

The significance of the skeletal age changes is matched by challenges they present to forensic experts, particularly when confronted by fragmented or decomposed human remains. As previous literature indicates, human identification is not always easy, especially when anatomical areas are missing or when skeletal remains are recovered at various stages of decomposition (Barrett et al., 2014). Findings show that some regions, such as the foot, remain comparatively underdeveloped in forensic identification, leaving much scope for reaching complete biological profiles. The use of these gaps with more empirical analyses and studies is crucial to improving the accuracy of identification. For example, the assessment of the methods of skeletal age estimation, such as those shown in the Pyle and Hoerr radiographic atlas, can give important information on normal variations and development timelines that enhance the precision of forensic identifications, leading to more robust methodologies in human osteology (Gallagher et al., 2015) (Figure 11.7).

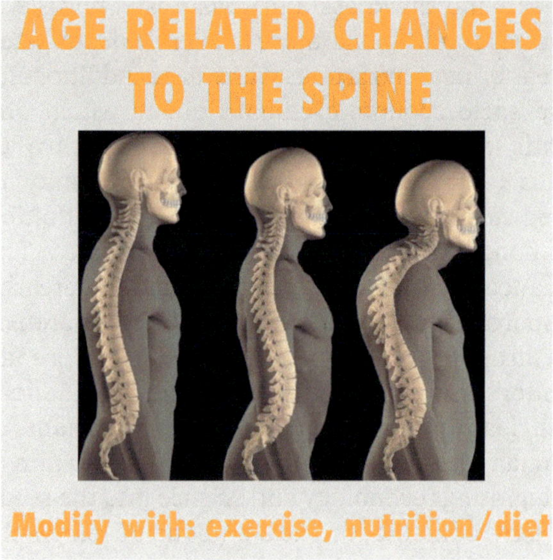

Figure 11.7. Age-related changes in the skeleton.

Source: https://absolutehealthparis.com/wp-content/uploads/2020/03/age-related-change-to-bone.png.

Test Your Knowledge

1. What are the major types of skeletal variation observed in humans, and what factors contribute to these differences?
2. How do age, sex, and environmental influences affect skeletal variation in the human population?

11.3. Methods of Skeletal Identification

Learning Outcome

1. Bone morphological analysis
2. Use of imaging technology
3. DNA analysis in osteology

Methods of skeletal identification vary and use a number of techniques that enable proper identification of human remains. One of the fundamental methods is the conclusion of biological profiles, which involves sex, age, ancestry, and the determination of stature from skeletal features. For instance, the skull and pelvis are particularly effective in sexing since they possess sexually dimorphic characteristics. Age estimation can be more accurate by examining dental development and wear patterns, as well as pubic symphysis morphology. Specific anatomy landmarks and measurements also make it possible to understand population affinities better since this helps reconstruct an individual's identity. This stratified approach emphasizes the complex interdependence of various skeletal features that must be analyzed by forensic anthropologists in order to arrive at a legitimate identification of the remains, the foundation of forensic skeletal analysis. Despite advances in skeletal identification techniques, challenges remain, particularly with disarticulated skeletal remains. Identification of incomplete or disarticulated skeletons involves customized approaches that can accommodate the absence of fundamental anatomical features. The foot, for example, has emerged as a focus of increased attention in forensic environments over the past few years, especially with the recent discoveries of numerous lower limbs along coastlines, which best illustrate the task of correlating individual remains when only partial segments are present. A survey of literature today portrays that there is a considerable deficiency of studies, especially concerning the forensic use of the foot in identifying humans. Therefore, the exploration of the parameters carried by the foot is a valuable subject for further research, offering insights and enhancing current methodology in the analysis of fragmented remains, highlighting the value of an integrative approach in forensic anthropology (Barrett et al., 2014). Training and experience can significantly contribute to successful skeletal identification efforts, particularly in evidence recovery operations. A new study found that searchers of varying backgrounds had different levels of success in recovering evidence, depending on their training and experience. Following mock crime scene searches using line searches, participants located potential evidence, facilitating comparison of recovery rates before and after training. From the evidence in this research, it is evident that professionals with real-world experience and expert training are more competent in evidence recovery, which is crucial when handling skeletal evidence. Investment in full-scale training programs for forensic experts is thus critical in improving identification methods and guaranteeing the success of skeletal recovery (Studebaker-Reed et al., 2018). By emphasizing education and experience in forensic science, this approach ultimately enhances skeletal identification accuracy in most investigative situations.

11.3.1. Morphological Analysis of Bones

Morphology of bones is an essential part of human osteology, particularly when used to understand skeletal variation and aid in the identification of human remains. Bone morphology addresses the examination of bones' size, shape, and internal structure to establish information about an individual's biological profile. Not only does this analysis assist in age estimation, sex, ancestry, and height estimation, but also in forensic analysis, where identification of fragmented remains is challenging. Systematic approaches, such as radiographic techniques, help capture the usual variations in skeletal structures, enabling researchers to establish appropriate standards against which deviations can be quantified. As highlighted in literature, techniques of age estimation based on morphological characteristics, such as those laid out in the Pyle and Hoerr radiographic atlas, are giant leaps in accuracy in age assessments among children, specifically, in breaking the hurdles offered by the nature of the speed of change in development that occurs early in life (Gallagher et al., 2015). Though there has been a leap in morphological analysis, some anatomical regions remain less investigated, particularly in forensic investigations. The foot, as a case in point, has received limited consideration compared to its potential significance in the recognition of remains. This absence of extensive literature makes the need for focused research imperative in order to address knowledge gaps concerning skeletal variations and their relevance to forensic applications. Morphological features of the foot can provide valuable information for identification, especially when remains are dismembered or skeletal elements are missing. Understanding variation in foot morphology can make biological profile estimates more accurate, thereby improving the overall validity of forensic identifications. These types of projects are important, as disarticulated skeletons pose tremendous challenges for practitioners attempting to determine the origin of the body parts unearthed from varied contexts, as is evident in examples from North America (Barrett et al., 2014). With advances in human osteology, continued focus on the morphological examination of bones is essential to developing robust skeletal identification methods. As skeletal remains undergo decomposition, distinct morphological traits tend to endure longer, serving as essential markers for identification. Integrating advanced imaging technologies, statistical analysis, and comparative studies of skeletal populations can further elucidate the complexities of skeletal variation. Researchers are encouraged to collaborate across disciplines, combining expertise in anthropology, forensic science, and biology to enrich the understanding of bone morphology in diverse contexts. This interdisciplinary framework can lead to improved methodologies that not only make better age and sex estimates possible but also improve human identification science in general and elucidate the problems associated with skeletal remains in various states of preservation. This convergence will ultimately enhance the forensic community's ability to cope with the complexities introduced by skeletal variation in human osteology (Figure 11.8).

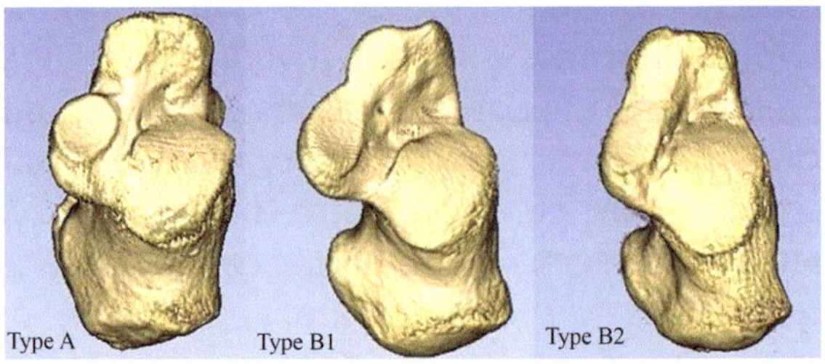

Figure 11.8. Morphological analysis of bones.

Source: https://media.springernature.com/lw685/springer-static/image/art%3A10.1007%2Fs00276-024-03450-6/MediaObjects/276_2024_3450_Fig4_HTML.png.

11.3.2. Use of Imaging Technologies

The application of imaging technology has greatly enhanced the field of human osteology, particularly in the detection and assessment of skeletal remains. Imaging technologies such as X-ray, computed tomography (CT), and magnetic resonance imaging (MRI) provide non-destructive methods of visualizing the inner bone structure and enable comprehensive analysis without destroying the sample's integrity. These modalities allow researchers to identify unique characteristics of the skeleton, thereby enhancing the construction of the biological profile, which is crucial for developing individual identity. Furthermore, visualization of three-dimensional structures improves the accuracy of identifying aspects of skeletal variation; this is particularly critical when dealing with fragmented remains, as outlined in recent studies evaluating the contribution of the foot to forensic identification (Barrett et al., 2014). Thus, the imaging technologies provide scope for more refined forensic techniques, pointing towards their irrepealability in contemporary human osteological research. Secondly, the integration of modern imaging techniques provides scope for investigating the biomechanical properties of skeletal material. For example, CT has facilitated the study of morphological variability in sesamoid bones, such as the patella, and has contributed to our understanding of skeletal variation across populations. Anatomical knowledge derived from imaging not only contributes to baseline data but also serves as the basis for comparative studies across species, as shown in a study on patellar evolution in reptiles (Benjamin et al., 2016). By exposing differences in bone morphology, imaging technology provides an integrative framework for explaining not only human osteology but also evolutionary biology. As a result, these technologies facilitate more informed identifications and classifications, providing information necessary to inform scholarly research as well as forensic applications. Ultimately, imaging technologies are an incentive for interdisciplinarity among anthropology, archaeology, and forensic science. By enabling widespread visualization, these technologies provide an intersubjective understanding of skeletal variation that exceeds that of previous methodologies. In addition, they encourage the creation of databases that compile imaging findings, thereby providing material for future education and research. Due to the discipline's advancing nature, the need for new imaging modalities is increasingly compelling, particularly to address hurdles posed by disintegrating human remains or complex forensic cases. The growing application of imaging technologies in human osteology is not only beneficial; it is essential for advancing identification practice and overall understanding of human skeletal variability across contexts and populations (Figure 11.9).

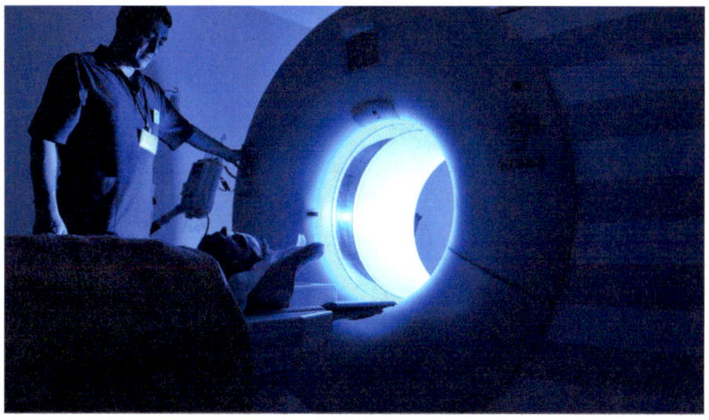

Figure 11.9. The adoption of imaging technologies has markedly enhanced the field of human osteology.

Source: https://www.innovationnewsnetwork.com/wp-content/uploads/2020/08/AI-in-medical-imaging.jpg.

11.3.3. DNA Analysis in Osteological Studies

The integration of DNA analysis into osteology has revolutionized forensic anthropology, particularly in human identification. Using genetic sequencing techniques, forensic specialists can extract DNA from bone and tooth tissues, which are typically more resilient than soft tissues. This enables the production of mitochondrial and nuclear DNA profiles, which are critical for establishing biological relationships and verifying identities. With cases of broken human remains arising, such as those habitually reported in the media, DNA analysis becomes a vital part in determining the biological profile of the remains. The complexity of identifying individuals from broken or incomplete skeletons is reduced by applying genetic evidence, thereby improving the precision of identifications where traditional osteological analysis might prove ineffective (Barrett et al., 2014). Furthermore, DNA testing is not limited to identification alone; it is also used to understand population dynamics and gene flow between human groups.

Genetic markers recovered from bones can reveal patterns indicative of geographic and demographic variation, thereby improving our understanding of human osteology. Such a sophisticated relationship between genetic heritage and skeletal variation is a testament to how biocultural factors have shaped bone morphology over time. The knowledge gained from such analyses also has profound implications for evolutionary research, allowing scientists to track lineages and patterns of migration across different points in history. As a result, the discipline of bioarchaeology has expanded appreciably, with DNA analysis offering greater insight into how cultural habits and environmental conditions have impacted human skeletal characteristics (Bosnar et al., 2010). In forensic examinations specifically, DNA analysis not only identifies people but also significantly aids in the disclosure of information regarding the events surrounding death. Forensic anthropologists can determine family relationships using genetic links, which can reveal valuable information about historical or contemporary events affecting specific populations. Moreover, the combination of DNA data with osteological data can allow for the more complex exploration of patterns of trauma or stress experienced by individuals during life. This interdisciplinary research significantly refines the narrative surrounding human skeletal remains, enabling a better context for interpreting the interactions among biology, culture, and disease in the construction of human identity. The continuous progress in DNA technologies will continue to push the frontiers of forensic anthropology in addressing the complexities of human remains (Bosnar et al., 2010; Barrett et al., 2014) (Figure 11.10).

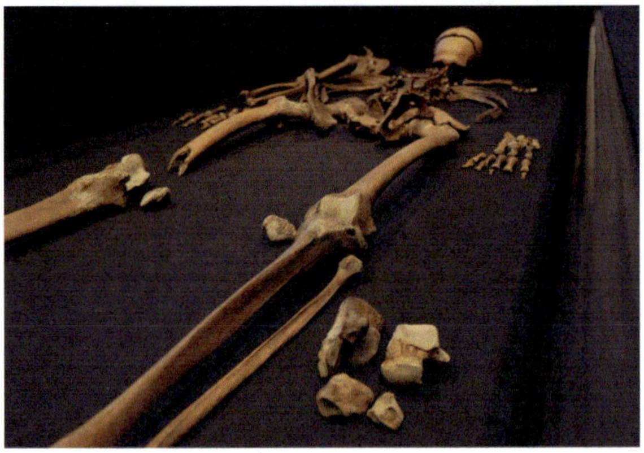

Figure 11.10. The integration of DNA analysis into osteological studies.

Source: https://external-content.duckduckgo.com/iu/?u=https%3A%2F%2Fwww.archaeology.wiki%2Fwp-content%2Fuploads%2F2024%2F10%2FMan_of_the_Well_4.jpg&f=1&nofb=1&ipt=fd637ad1f57e3eba86f980cc2beeb0d96a3bf4381928fd094e75625a9c4af7b3.

Test Your Knowledge

1. What are the key osteological methods used to estimate age, sex, and stature from skeletal remains?
2. How do metric and non-metric traits assist in the identification of unknown skeletal remains?

11.4. Forensic Applications of Osteology

Learning Outcome

1. Its role in crime scene investigations
2. Identification of victims in mass disasters
3. Legal aspects of osteological determination

Osteological methods are widely used in forensic anthropology to provide significant insights into human skeletal remains. experts. Forensic experts apply Osteology to reconstruct a biological profile by identifying significant features such as age, sex, ancestry, and stature from skeletal remains. This analytical tool proves important in cases where identification is otherwise challenging. The ability to identify differences in bone structure allows forensic anthropologists to make informed approximations about the demographic origin of the remains, which can be extremely useful in investigations. Further information regarding the mechanical and morphological properties of bone assists in the explanation of the cause of death. Thus, here, osteology is a valuable tool for explaining not only biological traits but also environmental and lifestyle factors affecting the individuals who left these remains, pointing to historical biocultural forces and their applications to contemporary forensic intent (Bosnar et al., 2010). Another indispensable application of osteology to forensic science is in the assessment of trauma and pathology to skeletal remains. Experts carefully examine bones for evidence of fractures, lesions, or other indications of injury that may contribute to the conditions of the death or survival of an individual. These analyses assist in the determination of the nature of trauma, i.e., is it accidental, self-inflicted, or caused by homicide, and thus become of absolute value to legal verdicts. For instance, the ability to differentiate antemortem and postmortem trauma can clarify injury timing or verify a sequence of events leading to death. Osteological interpretation is not limited to single case analysis but also to macro-level insights regarding societal violence, trauma patterns, and other significant forensic phenomena (Bosnar et al., 2010). While osteological applications have demonstrated their value in forensic investigations, controversies arise from the processes involved in identification, as evidenced in cases such as the Amelia Earhart case. While the initial British analysis indicated that the remains found on Nikumaroro Island belonged to a male, subsequent re-evaluations attempted to shoehorn the findings into Earhart's image using high-level cranial analysis software.

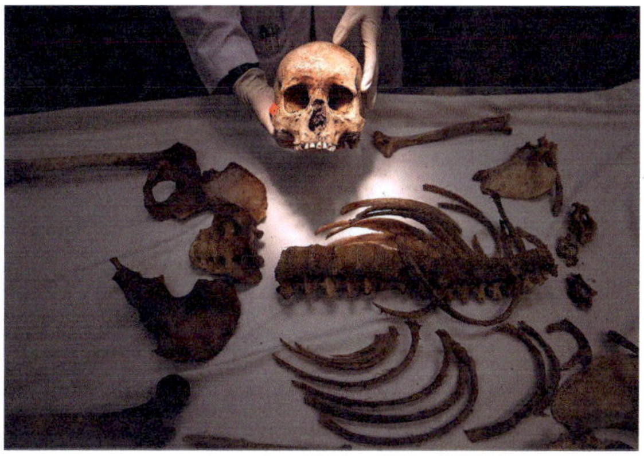

Figure 11.11. The field of forensic anthropology relies heavily on osteological methods to provide critical insights into human skeletal remains.

Source: https://www.thoughtco.com/thmb/9Zekgu7JKFgYudG8xVceed9XEFQ=/1500x0/filters:no_upscale():max_bytes(150000):strip_icc()/forensicanthropologist-5c771363c9e77c0001e98db3.jpg.

The divergent interpretations of these remains underscore the limitations and finiteness in forensic osteology, particularly where information is piecemeal or incomplete. With advancing forensic techniques, the need for interdisciplinary collaboration becomes evident, placing the integration of osteological findings with other scientific techniques into perspective to attain greater accuracy and reliability in bone identification. Finally, these intricacies are a product of ongoing debate among forensic anthropologists regarding best practices in skeletal identification with consideration to the variabilities of human osteology (Figure 11.11).

11.4.1. Role in Crime Scene Investigations

In crime scene investigations, skeletal analysis is particularly important when unidentified remains are discovered. Forensic anthropologists use their knowledge of human osteology to provide critical information about the deceased individual, including age, sex, ancestry, and stature. This information not only helps limit the potential for identification but also enhances the investigation by providing direction for searches for additional evidence related to the victim. As highlighted in recent studies, the effectiveness of these investigations depends significantly on the training and experience of those conducting the searches. Research has indicated that individuals trained in the excavation of human remains had higher recovery rates of evidence than untrained volunteers, further supporting the need for proper training in forensic procedures (Studebaker-Reed et al., 2018). Skeletal analysis not only serves a vital role in the identification of victims but is also a vital aspect in the investigative process of crime scene investigation. The importance of bone variation extends beyond mere identification; it also operates on a parallel trajectory to greater societal issues of race and lineage. Depictions of human variation in popular media oversimplify or misrepresent the complexity of bone features, thereby reinforcing erroneous conceptions of race and biological variation. The popular television drama Bones is a stark representation of the tension between scientific reality and popular portrayal, showing how cultural narratives shape public opinion of forensic science. Studies comparing such representations with actual forensic practice report contradictions that are liable to undermine public knowledge of human variation (Baker et al., 2023). This demonstrates the importance of forensic anthropology not only in case-solving but also in educating the public about the intricacies of human diversity, and in upholding the requirement for accurate scientific descriptions to support an informed public debate. In addition, the incorporation of state-of-the-art methods in skeletal analysis is transforming crime scene investigation. The development of imaging technologies, including computed tomography (CT) scans and 3D modeling, enables forensic anthropologists to examine skeletal remains with unprecedented detail.

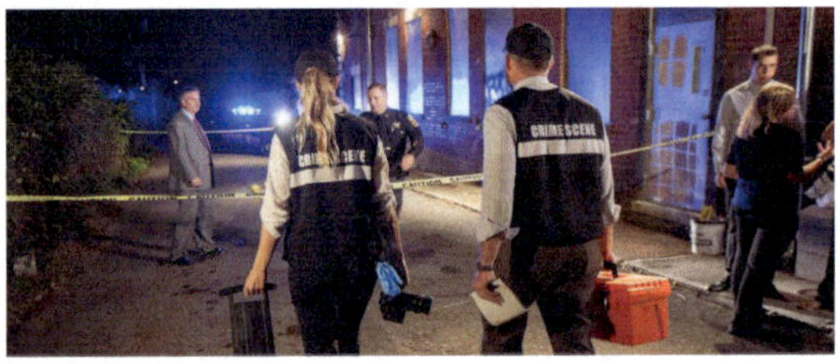

Figure 11.12. Role in crime scene investigations.

Source: https://external-content.duckduckgo.com/iu/?u=https%3A%2F%2Fdcfwfuaf91uza.cloudfront.net%2Fonline%2Fwp-content%2Fuploads%2Fbs-in-criminal-justice-crime-scene-investigation-1024x418.jpg&f=1&nofb=1&ipt=35610a08fe3f9ad91be756a6b5ca0eeeb5bd30268596740414d5d9e4d1f99066.

These advancements enable the virtual reconstruction of skeletal characteristics, which can improve identification and provide vital information about possible circumstances of death. Coupled with traditional anthropological protocols, these emerging procedures demonstrate the value of continuous advancement in the field. As forensic science advances, the ability to adapt to new methodologies characterizes the dynamism of crime scene analysis and the intrinsic role that the diversity of the human skeleton plays in these systems. Lastly, a realization of the intersection of technology, skeletal recognition, and societal understanding can enhance the success of investigations and lead to an enhanced-informed practice of human osteology (Figure 11.12).

11.4.2. Identification of Remains in Mass Disasters

The identification of human remains in mass disaster cases poses specific challenges, underscoring the relevance of skeletal analysis to forensic science. When remains are discovered in such traumatic events, the degree of decomposition can be highly varied, making identification even more challenging. Forensic anthropologists become a key aspect in such cases by analyzing skeletal remains to create a biological profile, including age, sex, and ancestry. Notably, as noted in a recent publication, highlighting features such as the foot enhances identification procedures, particularly when dealing with broken remains, which are prevalent in mass disasters (Barrett et al., 2014). The intricacies of the process illustrate the overlap between forensic anthropology and the emotional imperatives of disaster victim identification, demanding both skilled analysis and expeditious methodologies to afford closure to grieving families. In addition to biological profiling of skeletal remains, osteological changes are also important for information on the death conditions of individuals in mass disasters. Application of osteological techniques allows forensic examiners to detect not only characteristic features but also patterns of injury or trauma, which could assist in determining the cause of death or mechanisms of injury (Bosnar et al., 2010). This kind of analysis is crucial for mass disaster scenarios when victims may exhibit levels of skeletal trauma based on the environment or the collapse of structures. Apart from assisting in identifying the victims, understanding these morphological changes also supports broader forensic investigations, shedding light on potential negligence, crime, or system breakdown that led to the disaster. Hence, the role of osteology extends beyond mere identification, encompassing a broader socio-legal discussion of responsibility and justice. Advancements in forensic methods, particularly those enabled by osteological research, have revolutionized mass disaster identification procedures. The integration of modern technology, such as DNA analysis and three-dimensional reconstruction, with traditional osteological resources enhances the accuracy and efficiency of evaluations (Bosnar et al., 2010). This multi-disciplinary approach allows forensic anthropologists to construct detailed profiles and facilitate comparative analysis with missing persons databases. With mass catastrophes continuing to occur worldwide, ongoing innovation in forensic anthropology techniques and practices is essential for identification and case closure. Such activities not only address the pragmatic needs of forensic science but also highlight the ethical need to provide respectful answers to victims lost in such calamities, emphasizing the paramount significance of osteological studies in contemporary forensic applications.

11.4.3. Legal Implications of Osteological Findings

The legal implications of osteological findings play a crucial part in forensic investigation, particularly in cases of human identification and determining the circumstances surrounding death. Skeletal analysis is exact in establishing legal proceedings since skeletal analysis forms core evidence in criminal cases and civil actions. Forensic anthropologists use many different techniques to assess the biological profile of remains, such as age, sex, ancestry, and stature estimation. These analyses are important not only for the identification of the deceased but also to provide valuable information pertinent to the investigation, including potential instances of homicide or unidentified persons. The complexity of fractured remains, especially decomposed remains, underscores the importance of diligent, systematic examination and highlights the significance of the evidence skeletal remains can provide in forensic settings (Barrett et al., 2014). In examining skeletal variation, the applicability of legal requirements is evident, particularly in courts contesting the admissibility of osteological evidence. Forensic anthropologists must adhere to strict standards to ensure their findings are credible and scientific. Courts are likely to examine the methods used to examine osteological evidence to ensure they meet established standards. The use of radiographic techniques, such as those illustrated in the Pyle and Hoerr radiographic atlas, underscores the need for proper documentation and description of skeletal remains. These techniques facilitate age estimation and identification of individuals to enhance the accuracy in court cases (Gallagher et al., 2015). Complications may arise if osteological evidence is inaccurately interpreted, leading to miscarriages of justice or misidentification, underscoring the central integration of legal implications and osteological outcomes. In addition, legal implications of osteological outcomes extend beyond identification alone; they encompass ethical issues for the disposition of human remains and the legal rights of participants. For instance, the identification process will have to be handled sensitively with respect for the dignity of the deceased and their families. Legal frameworks will usually stipulate what is to be done to remains, particularly in cases of human trafficking or when remains are found in archaeological sites. Legal professionals and forensic anthropologists must operate within these frameworks while maintaining the proper and dignified taking of evidence. By establishing ethical standards and best practices, the legal sector is better placed to help maintain the integrity of skeletal remains as essential evidence in investigations, thereby serving the cause of good osteological practice in pursuit of justice (Barrett et al., 2014) (Figure 11.13).

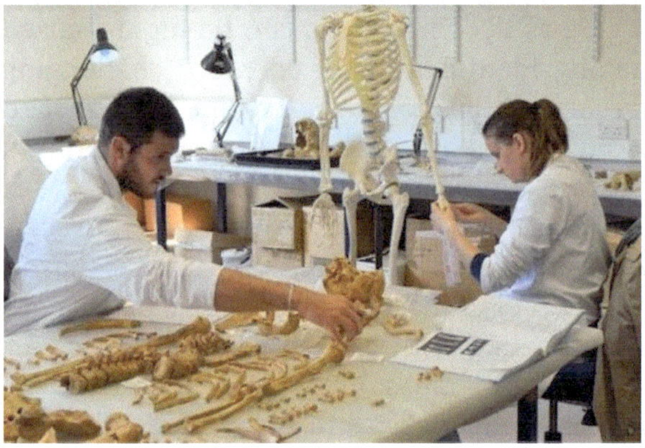

Figure 11.13. The legal implications of osteological findings play a crucial role in forensic investigations.

Source: https://ugc.futurelearn.com/uploads/images/63/77/63777c7b-d289-4d2a-86c0-c9f13182fb91.jpeg.

Test Your Knowledge

1. How is osteology applied in forensic investigations to establish identity and cause of death?
2. What is the importance of skeletal trauma analysis in forensic osteology?

11.5. Skeletal Variation Across Populations

Learning Outcome

1. Comparative study of different ethnic populations
2. Impact of geographical factors on skeletal attributes
3. Cultural practices that affect skeletal structure

Population skeletal variation is an integral part of the study of human osteology, as it provides insight into the broad spectrum of biological and cultural factors that influence human shape. Skeletal attributes are likely to be influenced by factors such as genetic background, environment, dietary practices, and social practices. For instance, populations at lower altitudes may exhibit different skeletal characteristics than those at higher altitudes due to varying physical needs and adaptations to their surroundings. This biomechanical variation reminds anthropologists to consider population-specific contexts in the interpretation of skeletal remains. Lacking this subtle regard, tests may result in sweeping generalizations that are blind to the egregious variation inherent in human populations and may potentially destroy the validity of age estimation and identification techniques applied in bioarchaeological and forensic practice. In constructing methodologies to estimate adult skeletal age, knowledge of the age-mimicry phenomenon, which affects results in population studies, is increasingly recognized. Anthropologists often employ ordinal classes for the categorization of adult age-at-death, yet no categories capture the inbuilt individual variation between these classes. This is particularly pertinent in osteoarchaeology, where many adults are grouped monolithically into the middle adult category, suppressing the fine-grained differentiation that is significant for interpreting skeletal variation. Also, the application of mean ages derived from reference samples is subject to severe biases, especially if the skeletal population under consideration has an age-at-death structure different from that of reference populations. To counter such biases, it is vital that the field realigns itself toward adopting individualized age ranges specific to particular skeletal contexts, as noted in more recent studies (Buckberry et al., 2015). In addition to age determination, the skeletal variability study also involves the analysis of dental enamel microstructure, which can potentially yield significant information on an individual's development and health status during early life. Research has provided evidence that enamel formation differences may reflect both genetic and environmental determinants, thereby contributing to a better understanding of health in populations. As an example, analysis of the enamel of deciduous teeth has allowed archaeologists to reconstruct prenatal development and maternal well-being, and to illustrate the interplay between individual development and overall population trends in health. Integration of this data is the key to skeletal identification and the building of life histories for individuals from various cultures. By incorporating meticulous analyses into osteological practice, researchers can accurately depict the diversity and complexity of human skeletal variation and advance our understanding of past peoples and health trends (Bondioli et al., 2017).

11.5.1. Comparative Analysis of Different Ethnic Groups

The skeletal variations observed within human populations result from a complex interplay among genetic, environmental, and cultural factors. Comparative analysis across different ethnic populations in the field of human osteology is significant for interpreting these variations. Morphological features are often influenced by ethnic variation, which can affect skeletal identification in forensic investigations. These variations are not merely cosmetic;

they have implications related to adaptations developed over generations due to climate, diet, and lifestyle. Such analyses can enable forensic anthropologists to form more precise judgments about ancestry and thus contribute to a richer understanding of human biological variation. Without such a thorough examination of these factors, conclusions about identity based solely on skeletal morphology can be inaccurate and reinforce long-rejected views of race as an essentialized, fixed biological category. Specifically, the difficulties of recognizing skeletal remains from specific ethnic groups, including Native Americans and Asians, highlight the necessity of adapted methodologies in forensic anthropology. Conventional methods tend to fall short in handling the overlapping traits of these populations, which have been lumped into categories such as Mongoloid. This classification by scholars such as Carlton Coon in 1939 has come under fire for its inherent inaccuracies and for perpetuating stereotypes. Recent research emphasizes the application of non-metric cranial features to distinguish Native American from Asian remains to enhance the effectiveness of ancestry identification. Chi-square and logistic regression methods have been used to identify robust features that enable forensic analysts to efficiently compare these groups, positioning skeletal variation analysis at the center of forensic identification procedures (Bodoh et al., 2017). Further, mainstream conceptions of race, formulated by dominant media, are barriers to human variation understanding in public and academic life. Television dramas like Bones provide a platform for discussion about lineage but simplify complex definitions of race and their biological inception. Such representations have consequences that lead to misinterpretations with negative impacts on the public's understanding of biological diversity. Studies by Baker et al. (2023) reveal that while popular culture can raise awareness of racial identity and heritage issues, it can also spread misrepresentations that are detrimental to scientific literacy. By situating popular media accounts alongside scientific protocols, anthropologists can bridge the gap between popular and academic knowledge and enable an accurate discussion of human difference and heritage ancestry in line with the latest research findings (Figure 11.14).

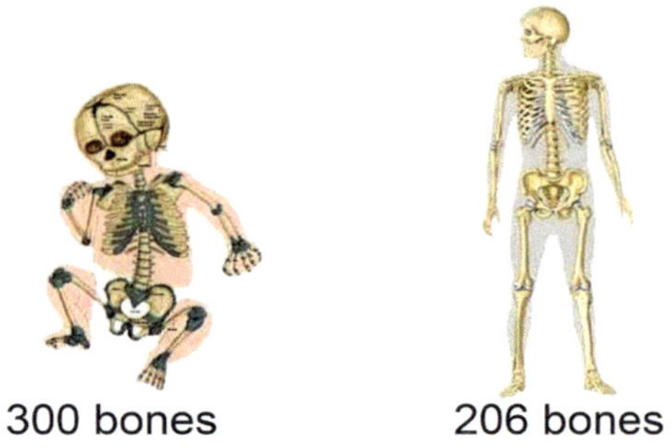

Figure 11.14. The skeletal variations present in human populations reflect a complex interplay of genetic.

Source: https://res.cloudinary.com/jerrick/image/upload/d_642250b563292b35f27461a7.png,f_jpg,fl_progressive,q_auto,w_1024/6583280e31a2e8001d009189.jpg.

11.5.2. Impact of Geographical Factors on Skeletal Traits

A clear understanding of the impact of geographical influences on skeletal features is of utmost importance in anthropological work in human osteology. Human populations exhibit substantial differences in skeletal morphology depending on environmental conditions during development. For example, groups from temperate climates are likely to display prominent skeletal traits that provide insulation and protection for increased body weight. In contrast, individuals from hot climates possess a more gracile skeletal form, which is favorable for enhanced thermoregulation and mobility. These kinds of adaptations are essential to survival as they reflect the body's ability to resist adversity from a range of environments. This morphological plasticity demonstrates the interface between geography and biology, emphasizing that skeletal characteristics are not arbitrary variations but adaptations that may indicate the broader ecological environment of a people's origin. Also, the geographical distribution of populations creates unique skeletal features that serve as identifying marks in forensic anthropology. Forensic anthropologists frequently encounter challenges in identifying skeletal remains, as characteristics shaped by environmental pressures can result in overlapping morphological traits across populations. This is also magnified by the application of traditional racial categories that do not necessarily reflect the intricacies of geographic-based variation within populations. As explained in contemporary forensic literature, the social construct of race makes it difficult to identify individuals, and knowledge of geographic influences can enhance the validity of forensic analysis. The circumvention of racial oversimplification enables forensic practitioners to adopt a more advanced approach that embraces skeletal variation across geography rather than intractable racial bias (Skalic et al., 2018). The need for improved training and methodology in forensic anthropology is also highlighted by the presence of nonhuman skeletal material, which may make identification efforts more challenging. In some geographical regions, there is a high rate of skeletal finds that may include numerous forms of animals, which can be particularly mimetic of human skeletal material. The analysis of bones in forensic facilities, such as the Office of the Chief Medical Examiner in Kenosha County, underscores the need for forensic anthropologists to be able to differentiate between human and nonhuman bones, which can be determined based on regional faunal diversity (Fourshee et al., 2022). Geographical factors not only affect skeletal morphology but also dictate the composition of remains found in forensic contexts. Researchers must emphasize the importance of geographic learning within forensic anthropological training to enhance the precision of identification processes, with human skeletal variation and regional characteristic features appropriately addressed within forensic research.

11.5.3. Cultural Practices Affecting Skeletal Morphology

Cultural practices play a pivotal role in shaping skeletal morphology, as different societies' cultures determine how individuals adapt to their environments and, consequently, to their bodies. Dietary activities through manual labor have the capacity to bring about radical morphological developments that are lifestyle adaptations. For instance, those who engage in hard labor have more advanced muscle attachments and denser bone structures, which are evident in bone remains. This is most evident in societies that engage in farming, where the demands on the body become part of everyday life. The overlap of skeletal morphology and cultural practices emphasizes the importance of considering socio-economic contexts while conducting osteology because the elements together have a definitive bearing on the variation that occurs in human skeletal morphology. It can enhance the precision of skeletal identification and provide information about the modes of life and behavior of ancient populations. Beyond activity levels and work, death and burial cultural funerary practices can have significant effects on skeletal morphology. Specific burial practices, such as inhumation or cremation, can produce various skeletal markers that reflect how populations handle the dead. Research indicates that cremation remains tend to present restrictions and biases in anthropological analysis, as significant demographic data can be distorted due to the nature of recovery and analysis of the material. For instance, the cremation analysis reveals an underestimated juvenile component, which can lead to erroneous conclusions about life expectancy and reproductive life history patterns in a population. Identification and aging of cremation skeletal remains also tend to rely on methodological approaches that disregard important age and sex differential subtleties, thereby making gender and aging estimates potentially inaccurate. Recognition of the importance of these funeral practices enables scientists to paint a wider picture of how cultural influences impact skeletal morphology. Furthermore, body modification practices also leave an indelible mark on skeletal morphology. Various societies engage in cranial shaping, dental modification, or the use of body ornaments, all of which impart unique skeletal features that can be recognized in archaeological contexts. Such modifications can serve numerous purposes, from purely aesthetic to signals of social status or identity. For instance, the classic cranial binding significantly shapes the skull and produces specific morphological patterns that aid in recognizing cultural belonging. However, it is important to interpret such modifications with a refined understanding of the cultural background so that they do not lead to misinterpretation due to modern-day prejudices. Last but not least, the intricate relationship between cultural practices and skeletal morphology underscores the need for a multifaceted research methodology in human osteology, where cultural knowledge augments the story of skeletal variation and identification (Figure 11.15).

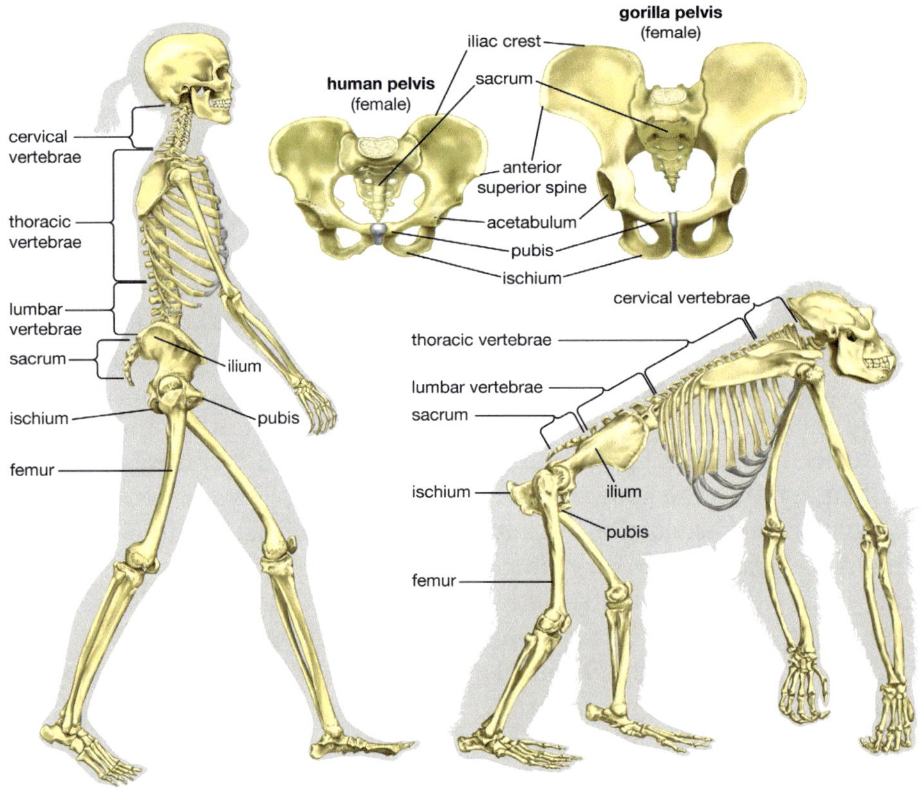

Figure 11.15. Cultural practices play a pivotal role in shaping skeletal morphology.

Source: https://cdn.britannica.com/95/55495-050-EEE4F555/differences-human-being-gorilla-structure-femurs-legs.jpg.

Test Your Knowledge

1. How do genetic and environmental factors influence skeletal variation among different human populations?
2. Why is understanding population-specific skeletal traits important in forensic and anthropological analysis?

11.6. Challenges in Osteological Identification

Learning Outcome

1. Limitations in current-day identification methods
2. Ethical considerations in skeletal examination
3. Impact of preservation conditions on identification

The issues of osteological identification are compounded by a variety of factors, including the physical condition of the skeletal remains and environmental processes of decomposition. Grossly decomposed or fragmented remains are especially challenging to identify, with practitioners having to make an identification from meager anatomical detail to enable the derivation of a biological profile. According to researchers, recent discoveries of fragmented human remains highlight the difficulties forensic anthropologists face when tasked with identifying individuals from partial or disarticulated body parts. The complexity involved in differentiating unique skeletal features, especially where the case involves an extreme fragmentation level, presents it as a challenging undertaking and may hinder precise identifications, which requires more methods and quality research within the field (Barrett et al., 2014). The pedagogic approach to human osteology also plays a significant part in overcoming the challenges of skeletal identification. Hands-on classical learning experience forms the basis of the attainment of practical skills in osteological identification, especially in the identification of the prominent anatomical landmarks and characteristics utilized to distinguish between different individuals. Interruptions, however, such as the COVID-19 pandemic, have compelled a shift to online learning models, which can inadvertently hinder the attainment of essential tactile skills (Barrett et al., 2014). Though take-home models have been implemented at some universities to enhance learning during these unprecedented times, their effectiveness remains questionable. Relying on virtual spaces without direct hands-on experience may impair learners' ability to properly identify and analyze skeletal variations inherent in human populations. Aside from that, the application of conventional osteological methods to a multi-component population is called into question, with a significant impact on identification accuracy. A number of these conventional methods have been developed based on a narrow demographic background, and as such, could potentially have their utility compromised when applied to a broader population base. For example, techniques used to estimate sex and establish age may be successful to varying degrees across ethnic populations, depending on inherent skeletal variations (Gamble et al., 2024). The lack of such studies necessitates a universal re-examination of current methodologies, with the aim of incorporating more representative methods that account for the biological and cultural diversity within human populations. The answer to all of these matters is of great significance not only for enhancing the precision of osteological identification but also for the promotion of fairness in forensic anthropology practice.

11.6.1. Limitations of Current Identification Methods

Current identification methods for human osteology are plagued by a variety of shortcomings, weakening skeletal analysis in terms of both precision and reliability. Among the main issues is disarticulation of remains, which can make the reconstruction of a biological profile extremely complicated. Forensic experts often receive cases in which only a portion of the skeleton is available, e.g., the lower limbs or feet, which can be challenging for identifying the subject from these partial anatomical remains. The existing literature provides evidence of a deficiency in orderly studies that are explicitly focused on identifying skeletal fragments, particularly on less often analyzed bones such as the foot. This research deficiency highlights a critical characteristic of forensic identification methods that warrants further research and development to improve findings in situations involving partial remains (Barrett et al., 2014). Another limitation is the age estimation techniques currently employed in forensic and anthropological contexts. Age development in skeletal and dental morphology is crucial in establishing a biological profile; however, these methods are not always consistent or applicable across all cases. Variation follows from multifarious causes, e.g., intra-individual genetic variation and environmental variables, that can distort age estimates. Additionally, refinement of dental and skeletal age estimation is in progress, but it largely does not address variation across populations. As highlighted in recent specialist forums, there remains a pressing need for advanced techniques capable of accommodating such variation and improving the accuracy of age estimates across different demographic groups. This demand highlights a significant gap in existing identification tools, which have been premised on generic models (Beaumont et al., 2015). Furthermore, the application of morphological characteristics for identification in bones can sometimes yield confusing conclusions. The majority of traditional methods rely heavily on visual inspection and subjective opinion by forensic examiners, which can lead to bias and loss of objectivity in identification. Because of the complexity of human variation, especially regarding ethnicity, sex, and geographic factors, the rigid application of these examination protocols can lead to misidentification. Therefore, the forensic community must encourage the use of analytical tools, such as higher-resolution imaging and genetic analysis, to aid morphological studies. By applying these new methods to existing identification protocols, practitioners can overcome limitations and more effectively carry out identifications, providing a stronger basis for perceiving skeletal variation in human osteology (Barrett et al., 2014).

11.6.2. Ethical Considerations in Skeletal Analysis

Ethical considerations in skeletal analysis are paramount in treating human remains with respect. Anthropologists and osteologists must walk on delicate moral grounds when doing research that deals with the dead. The use of skeletal remains, in this instance, demands a commitment to dignity and respect for the identities and histories of the represented people. Models of consent, particularly where Indigenous people or marginalized communities are concerned, are critical. This encompasses not only asking permission to analyze the skeletal remains but also engaging these groups in the research. By doing so, researchers acknowledge the groups' sovereignty over the ancestral materials and enable mutually collaborative relationships and the establishment of trust. Ethical engagement goes beyond legal compliance; it is an expression of social responsibility and a commitment to ensuring historical records that recognize past mischief and the cultural worth of remains, as exemplified by the growing body of literature that calls for the implementation of ethical standards in anthropology. A critical ethical consideration in skeletal analysis concerns the implications of scientific findings for living descendants and groups. Osteological findings can affect current narratives about race, identity, and cultural heritage. It is a point of worry considering the false history of utilizing skeletal data as a vehicle to propagate racist hypotheses and eugenics theories. It is therefore critical that academics be careful when publishing results so that no further harm is caused by interpretations and that the concerned communities are not misrepresented. Such engagement with descendant communities throughout the process is vital, as it allows for a better understanding of how results are received and applied. This collaborative process not only improves the research but also ensures that ethical guidelines are upheld, enhancing the place of responsible scholarship. The implications extend beyond the academic world and have real-world consequences that can affect community opinions and self-concepts, and hence, there are social responsibilities involved in skeletal analysis. The methods employed in skeletal analysis also raise ethical issues, especially with the advent of advanced technologies like active surface scanning (Errickon et al., 2017). While these technologies are advantageous—e.g., enabling the development of high-resolution 3D models to facilitate preservation and conservation—their limitations have to be taken into account by researchers. The financial costs associated with such technologies may limit accessibility, possibly favoring a limited range of institutions over others. Further, there are ethical considerations in digital archiving that need to be investigated, such as control over data ownership and the misuse of information. Along this line, scientists have an obligation to foster ethical practice, placing great emphasis on transparency and communal involvement in documenting and disseminating skeletal information. By recognizing the ambivalent nature of technological innovations both as a preservation technique and a potential source of inequality, researchers can establish a fairer research scenario respecting both the scientific merit of their research and the communities whose remains are being removed (Figure 11.16).

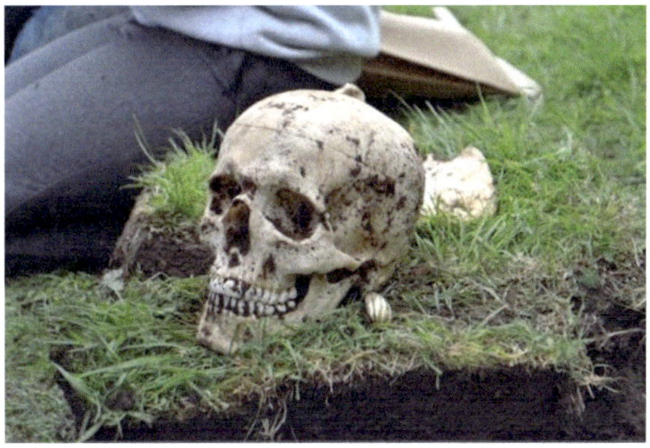

Figure 11.16. The ethical considerations surrounding skeletal analysis.

Source: https://ugc.futurelearn.com/uploads/images/f8/43/f8437827-f55b-4bae-9ee4-7f29425e5b70.jpeg.

11.6.3. The Impact of Preservation Conditions on Identification

Preservation conditions of skeletal remains are of utmost significance for their identification and, by extension, for the quality and completeness of biological data that can be derived from analysis. Insufficient preservation may lead to extensive degradation, hindering the integrity of bone structures that are significant for determining age, sex, and ancestry. For instance, soil pH, moisture levels, and temperature may accelerate decomposition and alter the physical attributes of skeletal remains. A comparative study of cremated and inhumed remains revealed that discrimination between the two burial forms offered varied challenges in skeletal analysis as cremations typically yielded dismembered remains whose identification chances are curbed (Kurila et al., 2015). These circumstances underscore the role of forensic and archaeological experts in objectively assessing preservation before data collection, as biased accounts can arise from incomplete or misclassified remains, ultimately skewing demographic constructions and historical assumptions. Apart from natural conditions, human activities can also significantly impact preservation outcomes. The rearrangement of remains, for example, from historical cemeteries, makes identification problematic. For instance, commingled remains at Acacia Park Cemetery demonstrate the issue disturbance of past burials creates, as they typically result in mixed contexts that obscure individual identities (Winter et al., 2016). When remains are disturbed or relocated, follow-up analysis is susceptible to issues surrounding loss of contextual information, which is crucial for effective identification. The difficulty in demarcating a distinctive narrative for each individual may hamper researchers' ability to place findings within broader demographic contexts. The consequences of preservation conditions for human intervention are thus important for clear identification assessments and for compensating for biases that arise from such intricacies. Generally, the impact of preservation circumstances on identification in human osteology encompasses natural and anthropogenic processes that affect the state of skeletal remains. The impact of environmental degradation and previous practices underscores the importance of meticulous archaeological practice. Confronted with undesirable preservation scenarios, for instance, those observed in cremated versus inhumed contexts or in commingled samples, osteological analysis must be adapted to provide sound interpretations. This entails the application of various techniques for estimating biological profiles, even under challenging preservation conditions (Kurila et al., 2015; Winter et al., 2016). By acknowledging and resolving such discrepancies, scientists can gain a better understanding of skeletal variation and improve identification precision. Thus, a multifaceted approach to preservation conditions remains paramount for advancing human osteology and facilitating accurate reconstructions of historic populations.

Test Your Knowledge

1. What are the major challenges faced when identifying individuals from fragmentary or damaged skeletal remains?
2. How do taphonomic processes and post-mortem changes complicate osteological identification?

SUMMARY

In Conclusion, the field of skeletal variation and identification in human osteology underscores the subtlety and relevance of human skeletal remains to contextualizing human identity. This understanding is crucial to forensic experts, particularly where decomposed or fractured remains are present, where accurate identification can challenge even the best-performing experts. The subtleties of bone variation driven by genetic, environmental, and lifestyle factors underscore the need for forensic anthropologists to handle each case using a specialized method that recognizes the unique attributes embedded in the skeletal record. This is then aggravated by societal issues, such as the fascination the public has with very fragmented remains like the found lower limbs on beaches, which present a captivating tale and a challenging investigation for authorities to come up with their identification (Barrett et al., 2014). Moreover, ongoing studies of human osteology are still required, especially regarding the methodologies employed in skeletal identification. Research indicates a key disparity in understanding cranial and postcranial elements, and this is an area ripe for examination. The identification of these skeletal markers has the capacity to enable forensic anthropologists better to reconstruct biological profiles and close cases with unidentifiable remains. Moreover, the use of technological innovation coupled with a multi-disciplinary approach can increase the effectiveness of these techniques. Ultimately, as science is ever-evolving, the embracement of new approaches to human skeletal analysis will serve to advance the accuracy of identifications and contribute to the evolving nature of forensic practice (Studebaker-Reed et al., 2018). Wherefore skeletal variation, identification, and forensic science ultimately characterize the topic of human osteology in the domain of forensic science. As demand for reliable identification methods increases, driven by the growing number of unidentified remains, there is substantial motivation for improved training and education for practitioners. Incentives to education, such as multivariate analysis of search success and recovery rates of evidence, recognize the role of training in improving the competence of practitioners responsible for human remains identification (Studebaker-Reed et al., 2018). Hence, professional development programs aimed at building expertise and fostering cooperation between forensic disciplines are called for. Not only do they promise to eliminate existing knowledge gaps, but they also enhance the practice of forensic anthropology, ultimately contributing to better results in human identification work overall.

The analysis of skeletal variation is the backbone of human osteology, particularly in identification methods. One of the most important problems that comes up in the field is discrimination between different skeletal material, particularly when working with partial or cremated remains. Analysis can be challenging due to the paucity of morphological data in incomplete specimens. This lack can lead to diagnostic bias, as highlighted by studies on the validity of skeletal analysis. For instance, analysis of skeletal remains claimed to be Amelia Earhart's and initially identified as those of a male was redone with the aid of sophisticated techniques and provided alternative explanations for the same evidence. This situation highlights the complexity of skeletal identification, in which different methods may yield varied outcomes from a single set of remains (Cross et al., 2015). In exploring osteological analysis of cremated remains, researchers have identified key limitations to be addressed to render bioarchaeological findings more credible. The disarticulation character of cremated bone poses intrinsic complications, which compound potential biases of demographic analysis, as in comparative examination of cremation and inhumation. Variations in subadult representation between these two forms of burial, for instance, distort life expectancy assessments and reproductive profiles. By employing rigorous methods, e.g., paleodemographic issues, such studies try to produce more accurate mortality profiles, which indicate infant mortality underestimation and misassignment of adolescents. These results emphasize the need for the development of more sophisticated analytical techniques to reduce bias and improve the accuracy of skeletal interpretation in past and living populations (Kurila et al., 2015). The general synthesis of skeletal variation and identification demonstrates the need for immediate methodological development and interdisciplinary collaboration in human osteology. Diverse analytical strategies and vigilant attention to context are essential in shaping the accuracy of skeletal identification. Examples such as Earhart's both underscore the potential for reevaluating long-held conclusions and the usefulness of modern technologies to complement earlier approaches. Similarly, recent research on the cremation bias underscores a broader movement within the discipline of osteology, emphasizing greater sensitivity in how skeletal material is analyzed, aged, and sexed. Hence, the most significant implications that follow from contemporary osteological investigations call for an integrated understanding of skeletal variation and how this relates to identification techniques, paving the way for more accurate and informed interpretations of human skeletal remains in archaeological and forensic contexts (Cross et al., 2015; Kurila et al., 2015).

KEY TERMS FROM THIS CHAPTER

- Age Estimation
- Anthropometry
- Asymmetry
- Biological Profile
- Bone Density
- Bone Remodeling
- Cranial Sutures
- Craniofacial Features
- Dental Morphology
- Dimorphism (Sexual Dimorphism)
- Epiphyseal Fusion
- Ethnic Markers
- Metric Variation
- Non-Metric Traits

CRITICAL THINKING QUESTIONS

1. **What is the primary factor causing skeletal variation among individuals?**
   a. Environmental influences
   b. Genetics
   c. Age
   d. All of the above
2. **Which skeletal feature is most commonly used for sex determination?**
   a. Femur length
   b. Pelvic morphology
   c. Skull size
   d. Rib curvature
3. **What characteristic of the skull is typically more pronounced in males than females?**
   a. Rounder eye orbits
   b. Smaller mastoid process
   c. Larger brow ridge
   d. Narrower nasal aperture
4. **Which bone is the most reliable for determining age at death in adults?**
   a. Humerus
   b. Pelvis
   c. Skull
   d. Vertebrae
5. **Epiphyseal fusion is used to estimate what characteristic in skeletal remains?**
   a. Sex
   b. Stature
   c. Age
   d. Ancestry

Short Answer Questions

1. What are the leading causes of skeletal variation in humans?
2. Which bones are most commonly used for sex determination?
3. How does the pelvis differ between males and females?
4. What features of the skull are helpful in determining sex?
5. How can epiphyseal fusion help estimate an individual's age?

Answers to Critical Thinking Questions

1. (d); 2. (b); 3. (c); 4. (b); 5. (c)

REFERENCES

1. Abdala, A., Abdala, A., Adams, A., Allin, E. F., Allin, C., Anthwal, N., Barghusen, H., et al. (2016). Morphological evolution of the mammalian jaw adductor complex. https://core.ac.uk/download/151161615.pdf (accessed on 18th July 2025).
2. Woronowicz, K.C., Schneider, R.A. Molecular and cellular mechanisms underlying the evolution of form and function in the amniote jaw. *EvoDevo* **10**, 17 (2019). https://doi.org/10.1186/s13227-019-0131-8Ahmed, F., & Maisano, J. (2017). ToScA North America (6–8 June 2017, The University of Texas, Austin, TX) Program. https://core.ac.uk/download/211334283.pdf (accessed on 18th July 2025).
3. Baker, A. L. (2023). Science literacy and popular culture: Forensic anthropology in application and fiction. https://core.ac.uk/download/592759495.pdf (accessed on 18th July 2025).
4. Barrett, A., Bidmos, M., Bidmos, J., Bidmos, A., Bilge, A., British Broadcasting Corporation, British Broadcasting Corporation, et al. (2014). The foot in forensic human identification–a review. https://core.ac.uk/download/30660095.pdf (accessed on 18th July 2025).
5. Beaumont, J., Buckberry, J., Dean, M. C., Liversidge, H. M., Buckberry, J., Konigsberg, L., Marquez-Grant, N., et al. (2015). Age estimation [editorial]. https://core.ac.uk/download/76945364.pdf (accessed on 18th July 2025).
6. Becker, S. K. (2019). Osteoarthritis, entheses, and long bone cross-sectional geometry in the Andes: Usage, history, and future directions. https://core.ac.uk/download/323311202.pdf (accessed on 18th July 2025).
7. Benjamin, M., Camp, C. L., Castanet, J., Cope, E. D., Gauthier, J. A., Haines, R. W., Haines, R. W., et al. (2016). Anatomy, morphology and evolution of the patella in squamate lizards and tuatara (*Sphenodon punctatus*). https://core.ac.uk/download/36779107.pdf (accessed on 18th July 2025).
8. Bodoh, D. M. (2017). Non-metric cranial differentiation between Asian and Native American populations for ancestry assessment. https://core.ac.uk/download/217412243.pdf (accessed on 18th July 2025).
9. Bondioli, L., Coppa, A., Dean, C., et al. (2017). New regression formula to estimate the prenatal crown formation time of human deciduous central incisors derived from a Roman imperial sample (Velia, Salerno, Italy, I-II cent. CE). https://core.ac.uk/download/98348292.pdf (accessed on 18th July 2025).
10. Bosnar, A., Petaros, A., & Čengija, M. (2010). When osteology is put into practice: Forensic anthropology. https://core.ac.uk/download/14420112.pdf (accessed on 18th July 2025).
11. Buckberry, J. (2015). The (mis)use of adult age estimates in osteology. https://core.ac.uk/download/76945106.pdf (accessed on 18th July 2025).
12. Christian, A., Hultgren, B. D., Emerson, C. L., Holliday, C. M., Gilmore, C. W., Schwarz, D., Frey, E., et al. (2013). The effect of intervertebral cartilage on neutral posture and range of motion in the necks of sauropod dinosaurs. https://core.ac.uk/download/29026918.pdf (accessed on 18th July 2025).
13. Cross, P. J., & Wright, R. (2015). The Nikumaroro bones identification controversy: First-hand examination versus evaluation by proxy–Amelia Earhart found or still missing? https://core.ac.uk/download/76945212.pdf (accessed on 18th July 2025).

14. Errickson, D., Gowland, R. L., Griffith, S. J., et al. (2017). Towards a best practice for the use of active non-contact surface scanning to record human skeletal remains from archaeological contexts. https://core.ac.uk/download/322328997.pdf (accessed on 18th July 2025).
15. Fourshee, J. L. (2022). Differentiating human from nonhuman bone: Insights from a medical examiner's collection, Kenosha, Wisconsin. https://core.ac.uk/download/554010999.pdf (accessed on 18th July 2025).
16. Gamble, J. A., & Gilmour, R. J. (2024). Bones at home supporting haptic learning and universal design beyond the biological anthropology laboratory. https://core.ac.uk/download/644028705.pdf (accessed on 18th July 2025).
17. Kurila, L. (2015). Cremation as limitation? A paleo demographic inquiry into the accuracy of macroscopic analysis of cremated human remains based on an East Lithuanian sample. https://core.ac.uk/download/43658404.pdf (accessed on 18th July 2025).
18. Sanford, L. A. (2024). Numerical variations in the thoracic and lumbar vertebrae within the John A. Williams Skeletal Collection, Western Carolina University, Cullowhee, NC (USA). https://core.ac.uk/download/610528747.pdf (accessed on 18th July 2025).
19. Skalic, C. B. (2018). A critical approach to ancestry in forensic anthropology: An assessment of Fordisc 3.1 and AncesTrees. https://core.ac.uk/download/215530254.pdf (accessed on 18th July 2025).
20. Studebaker-Reed, M. S. E. (2018). The impact of training and experience on the recovery of evidence in outdoor forensic scenes: Implications for human remains recovery. https://open.bu.edu/bitstream/2144/31280/5/StudebakerReed_bu_0017N_13567.pdf (accessed on 18th July 2025).
21. Taylor, M. P., & Wedel, M. J. (2013). Caudal pneumaticity and pneumatic hiatuses in the sauropod dinosaurs *Giraffatitan* and *Apatosaurus*. https://core.ac.uk/download/29026919.pdf (accessed on 18th July 2025).
22. Wilhelmson, H. (2017). Perspectives from a human-centered archaeology: Iron Age people and society on Öland. https://core.ac.uk/download/83658101.pdf (accessed on 18th July 2025).
23. Winter, R. M. (2016). Analysis of a commingled skeletal sample from Acacia Park Memorial Cemetery. https://core.ac.uk/download/230810544.pdf (accessed on 18th July 2025).

LABORATORY AND FIELD METHODS IN OSTEOLOGY

12

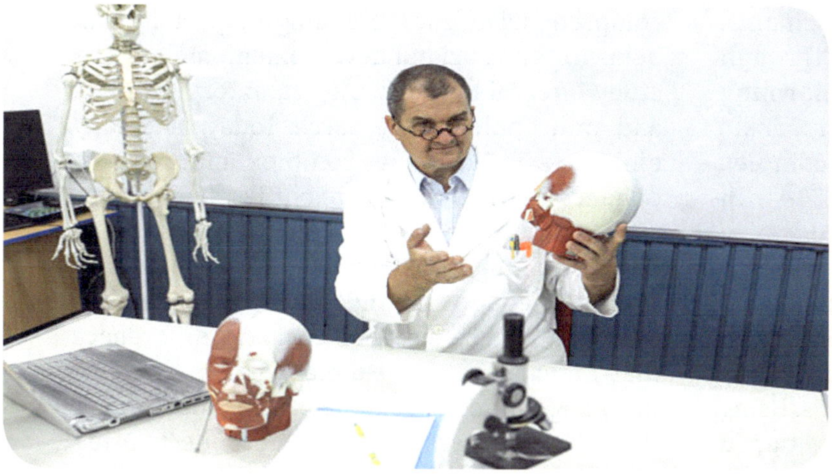

LEARNING OBJECTIVES

After studying this chapter, you will be able to:

1. Discuss the historical context of osteology
2. Explain the laboratory methods in osteology
3. Understand field methods in osteology
4. Know comparative osteology
5. Focus on ethical considerations in osteological research
6. Learn about technological advances in osteology

Introduction

The scientific analysis of osteology, both forensic and biological, of human skeletons is of the utmost importance across a broad range of scientific fields, including archaeology, bioarchaeology, and forensic anthropology. By analyzing skeletons, scientists can reveal rich details about an individual's identity, health, and way of life. This method not only helps create demographic profiles such as age, sex, and ancestry, but also supports inferences about pathological conditions. The intricacy and variability of human skeletons require the application of a combination of laboratory and field techniques for analysis. Examining such methods creates a background for appreciating the strengths and limitations inherent in osteological analysis to determine significance in both scientific and applied contexts. Further, as technology improves and is integrated into conventional practices, skeletal analysis can be enhanced in terms of effectiveness and efficiency. Field osteology techniques comprise various methods used during recovery and preliminary screening of skeletal remains. Forensic experts usually find it hard to make identifications in the process, particularly when handling decomposed or fragmented remains. The investigation of individual cases, such as recent discoveries of lower legs and feet on beaches, underscores the need for specialization in field recovery techniques. While interest can be provoked among the general public by such horrific finds, they reveal widespread issues with forensic identification. As noted in the literature, the research gap regarding the role of the foot in forensic identification necessitates a focused effort to recover and examine such remains. Expansion of research in this area through concerted efforts is essential to informing holistic protocols that will help forensic anthropologists effectively address complex identification cases (Barrett et al., 2014). In the laboratory setting, analytical methods play a central role in interpreting evidence gathered using skeletal analysis. Analytical methods such as Generalized Estimating Equations (GEE) have been widely used to address scalar problems in osteoarthritis studies of human skeletons. Using such approaches, scientists are better positioned to evaluate joint condition complexity, thereby developing more robust conclusions about the individuals under study. Notably, studies have demonstrated the efficacy of GEE in analyzing elbow joint pathology variation across populations and in identifying sex- and age-related differences that may reflect specific cultural practices or environmental influences (Bass et al., 2019). Thus, integrating systematic laboratory techniques with field processes not only improves the overall quality of osteological research but also broadens the range of outcomes amenable to bioarchaeological and forensic analysis, thereby enriching our understanding of human variation through time.

Definition of Osteology

Osteology, or the scientific study of bones, is an important field within the broader disciplines of anthropology and archaeology. It entails the study and analysis of bones to gain insight into many facets of life in the past, including those of human beings and animals. As an interdisciplinary science, osteology crosses boundaries such as biology, paleontology, and forensic science and utilizes a wide variety of laboratory and field methods to gather data. By examining skeletal morphology, pathology, and chemical composition, researchers can infer diet, health, social structure, and even the migrations of ancient populations. This blending of osteological data enables a more comprehensive understanding of past human behavior and societal development, making the study integral to archaeological interpretations and anthropological research. Today, osteology employs increasingly complex methods to enhance its analytical capabilities. Techniques such as isotopic analysis have enhanced the understanding of diet and migration within prehistoric populations. Isotopic signatures in bones can be used to examine differences that indicate not only dietary habits but also the geographic movement of individuals over time. The success of these methods has led to breakthroughs, establishing connections between skeletal data and broader archaeological narratives. The most fascinating in this regard is the human-centered approach, which points toward the need to understand the lived experiences of humans by their remains. With the integration of osteological observations into archaeological contexts with caution, scholars are increasingly gaining insight into the complexities of the dynamics of ancient societies, moving away from taxonomic classifications to a more intricate understanding of human existence and culture (Wilhelmson et al., 2017). In addition, osteology has been forced to adapt to the need for interdisciplinarity and innovative technological advancements. With the integration of digital aids such as 3D imaging and graph-based network analysis, scientists are better positioned to observe and comprehend complex data. These methods enhance the study of dependencies between skeletal remains, environmental trends, and archaeological contexts. The continued evolution of traditional morphometric techniques and modern analytical methods signifies a milestone within the discipline. Osteology not only sheds light on biological and cultural human history but also on the broader study of the human experience across varied environments. Consequently, the role of osteology in archaeology has become an integral part of deciphering the complexities of human society and its evolution over time (Bartosiewicz et al., 2020) (Figure 12.1).

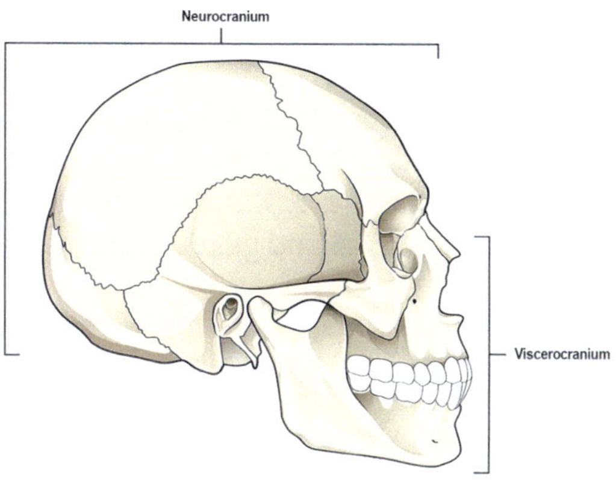

Figure 12.1. The scientific study of bones.

Source: https://pressbooks-dev.oer.hawaii.edu/explorationsbioanth/wp-content/uploads/sites/139/2020/07/A.11.png.

Importance of Studying Bones

The study of bones, osteology, is critical to many areas of research, from anthropology to medicine, because it provides information about the biology and evolution of animals and humans, as well as their health. The study of the skeleton explains differences at the individual and species levels in biology. In anthropology, skeletal remains are examined to draw conclusions about ancient populations' diets, health, and social structures. Moreover, the identification of skeletal traits enhances forensic science by aiding the investigation and proper identification of remains. Since osteology relates to numerous other fields, it has become a central support for understanding a wide array of biological and cultural phenomena, influencing our view of life on Earth. Moreover, technological advancements have greatly enhanced the processes employed in osteological studies. Techniques such as high-resolution X-ray computed tomography (CT) provide non-destructive methods for examining bone structure, enabling the examination of previously inaccessible details. The application of multimodal imaging technologies enables more in-depth investigations, bridging gaps between traditional anthropological practices and contemporary medical and material science practices. Collaborations among institutions, such as the University of Texas High-Resolution X-ray CT Facility and natural history museums, are indicative of an emerging emphasis on cross-disciplinary work. As technologies advance, they will radically improve the validity of skeletal assessments, enabling researchers and practitioners to more accurately conclude about the past and present through analyses of bones (Ahmed et al., 2017). Also, the significance of haptic (hands-on) learning experience in osteological training cannot be overstated. Recent studies indicate that tactile interaction highly facilitates learning in human osteology courses, enhancing basic skills such as bone identification and age and sex estimation. For instance, during the COVID-19 pandemic, remote learning students used plastic model skeletons, which were effective in bridging the hands-on gap that would normally be offered in lab settings. The study found that remotely educated undergraduates excelled in bone identification but had limitations when it came to sex and age estimation methods. Such reports highlight the importance of having efficient education plans, particularly in a field that relies on the physical manipulation of specimens. Facilitation of accessible educational plans can thus lead to improved learning and a more solid grasp of human osteology (Gamble et al., 2024) (Figure 12.2).

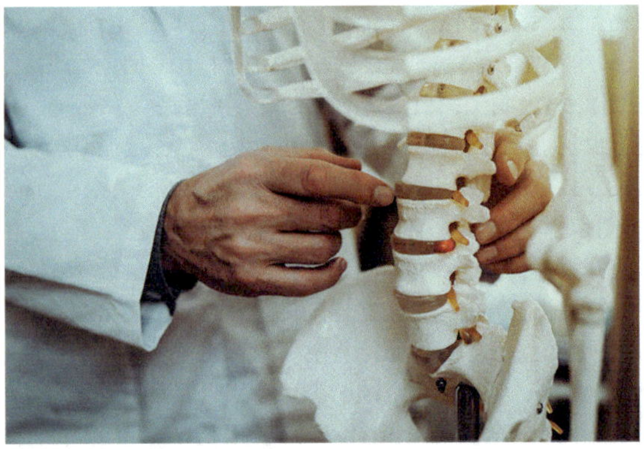

Figure 12.2. The study of bones, known as osteology.

Source: https://www.northshore.org/globalassets/healthy-you/blog/2020/bone-facts.jpg.

Overview of Laboratory and Field Methods

The methods applied in osteology can be broadly categorized into laboratory and fieldwork, each with unique information and challenges. Laboratory methods are typically those in laboratory settings where specimens can be examined with precision. Methods such as morphometric analysis, histology, and molecular genetics form the basis of understanding the structure and function of bones at macroscopic and microscopic scales. Advanced imaging technologies, such as X-ray computed tomography (CT), enable non-destructive testing of internal parts, providing more information about skeletal irregularities and phylogenetic relationships. These technologies are of immense value in identifying species and understanding phylogenetics, greatly contributing to advancing the field by enabling complete tests without compromising the integrity of the sample. Conversely, field methods play an important role in the initial stage of osteological research, namely excavation and specimen collection. They entail cautious planning and execution, often involving surveys, systematic sampling, and stratigraphic exploration in order to preserve contextual information. Fieldwork provides context in which bone assemblages can be seen in association with their contexts, and such modifying phenomena as sedimentology and taphonomy can be quantified. Furthermore, the use of geographical information systems (GIS) broadens field data collection by mapping grave sites and studying environmental conditions, thereby providing information about past ecosystems and human use of those ecosystems. These methods are crucial in constructing an overall image of the fossil record and human evolution, with a focus on the requirements for interdisciplinary practice in osteology. The integration of laboratory and field techniques offers a general context for the study of osteology. For instance, field specimens can undergo intense laboratory analysis to uncover detailed morphological and genetic information.

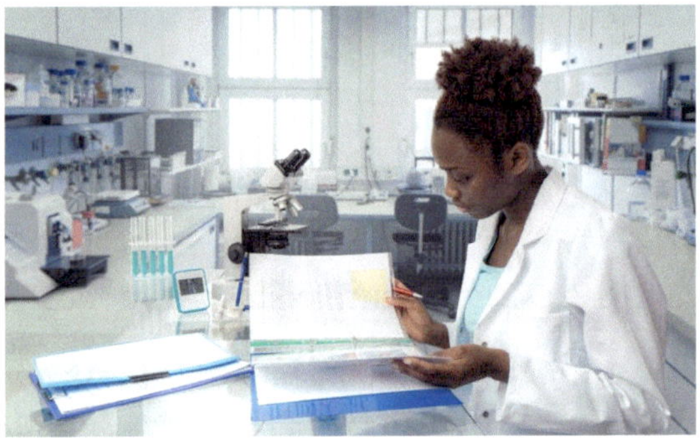

Figure 12.3. The methodologies employed in osteology can be broadly categorized into laboratory and field methods.

Source: https://external-content.duckduckgo.com/iu/?u=https%3A%2F%2Fsnco.com%2Fwp-content%2Fuploads%2F2021%2F12%2F0g81FJeLauyQ7I0udlbmv7M84uKH0Rb01640009035.jpg&f=1&nofb=1&ipt=bcbe558c0022db2354c9a9fbad597044f961846692593884e5011865ec536c06.

The integration has promoted innovation in multimodal imaging techniques, which combine information from multiple imaging platforms to offer a more comprehensive understanding of bone structure and function. Facilities like the University of Texas High-Resolution X-ray CT Facility (UTCT) have led the way with such techniques, demonstrating how multidisciplinary work has optimized the study of skeletal biology in both modern and paleontological contexts. Moreover, resources have been placed in motion, like ToScA North America, that are pushing the boundaries of innovation in materials science and biological imaging, ensuring that osteological approaches remain at the vanguard of scientific discovery and research, ultimately enhancing our insight into skeletal remains in the different areas of study (Figure 12.3).

12.1. Historical Context of Osteology

Learning Outcome

1. Early practices in bone analysis
2. Progress in methods over time
3. Key figures in osteological development

The history of osteology reflects significant progress guided by evolving archaeological methodologies and socio-cultural understandings of human bones. From the early days of human skeletal examination, which were anatomically focused, to current practices involving genetic and proteomic analyses, osteological methodology has evolved in step with broader cultural shifts. Early studies of skeletons were simple, aimed at basic sex and age determination, and primarily employed for burial reconstruction. However, as cemetery excavation methods became more refined, so did the appreciation for the detailed tales these skeletons could reveal. For instance, the analysis of the Acacia Park Cemetery skeletons illustrates how osteological technique has conditioned our understanding of colonial and pre-colonial Minnesota demographics and health (Winter et al., 2016). This shift reflects a greater appreciation for the social and cultural context embedded in human remains. Refinement in laboratory technique has further enriched skeletal analysis. The application of genomic analysis allows for a more nuanced interpretation of biological sex estimation, which can refine earlier doubts about inherent osteological techniques. As has already been observed in the analysis of the Panoría megalithic cemetery, fresh analytical techniques have been able to examine sex ratios and social structure more accurately and to reveal profound insights into previously under-rated aspects of funerary practice and social structure (Jiménez et al., 2024). The balance of sex ratio, or more precisely the surprising superiority of females, contradicts accepted accounts of past cultures and prompts reconsideration of the roles of gender in past civilizations. Thus, contemporary field and laboratory techniques in osteology not only build up body profiles but also challenge preconceived cultural assumptions, refining our knowledge of ancient populations. The applicability of these techniques extends beyond mere anatomical inquiry, for they permit researchers to reconstruct broader historical settings and cultural traditions. By uniting ancient osteological techniques with novel technological advancements, researchers can link together physical health, social distinction, and cultural symbolism. This multidisciplinary method, evident in the research of both Acacia Park and Panoría, underscores the critical role of osteology within the tapestry of archaeology and anthropology as a whole. Through each analysis of the skeleton, new tales begin to emerge, where the complex narratives of individuals and peoples over time are woven together. The commitment to a stringent method within the field and laboratory settings showcases the enduring relevance of osteology in enabling us to enhance our appreciation of human experience, bridging the past with contemporary cultural interpretations within a confusing and complex world (Winter et al., 2016; Jiménez et al., 2024) (Figure 12.4).

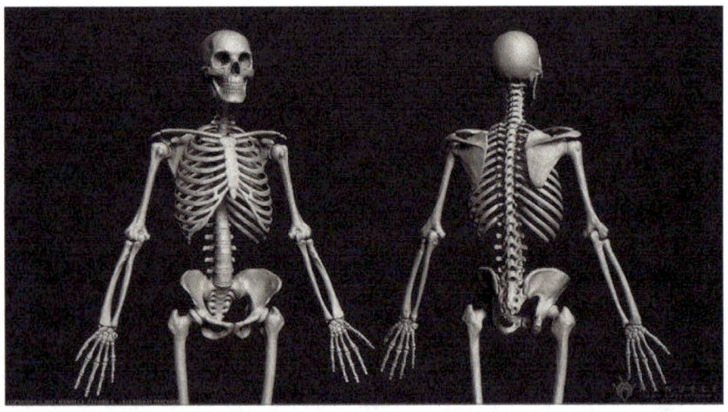

Figure 12.4. The historical context of osteology.

Source: https://i.ytimg.com/vi/6OhAA2LwoMw/hq720.jpg?sqp=-oaymwEhCK4FEIIDSFryq4qpAxMIARUAAAAAGAElAADIQj0AgKJD&rs=AOn4CLCSA7WTp8t3O7y-M54pFw-etaNzQw.

12.1.1. Early Practices in Bone Analysis

An investigation of ancient bone analysis techniques identifies a transition from primitive observation techniques to more sophisticated methods that changed our understanding of skeletal remains. Bone examination in the past relied primarily on morphological observations, where scientists identified differences in size, shape, and structural details. These behaviors were, however, prone to constraints of subjectivity in the observer and the difficulty of species differentiation, particularly where domestic animals were involved. By incorporating technological advances, such as ancient DNA sequencing, researchers were able to distinguish among various canid species, as evidenced by excavations of prehistoric Native Californians, whose results supported the common presence of domesticated dogs in graves (Byrd et al., 2013). Not only did this shift from qualitative to quantitative analysis make it more accurate, but it also helped provide a better understanding of human-animal relationships in past societies. The paleopathology role further illustrates the history of bone analysis methods, which have provided insights into people's past health, diet, and social circumstances. In early paleopathology, investigations were primarily aimed at detecting overt lesions or traumatic injuries—more advanced methodology developed over time, with the introduction of refined imaging technology and biochemical processes. For instance, the application of stable isotope analysis in skeletal studies provides valuable information on diet and nutrition, enabling researchers to reconstruct past subsistence practices. In one such notable investigation of medieval Livonian skeletons, findings indicated that children were as capable as adults of accessing food sources, offering valuable data on social dynamics and health during the period (Morrone et al., 2022). Hence, these advancements in bone analysis enhance not only our understanding of individual health but also enable longer socio-cultural interpretation.

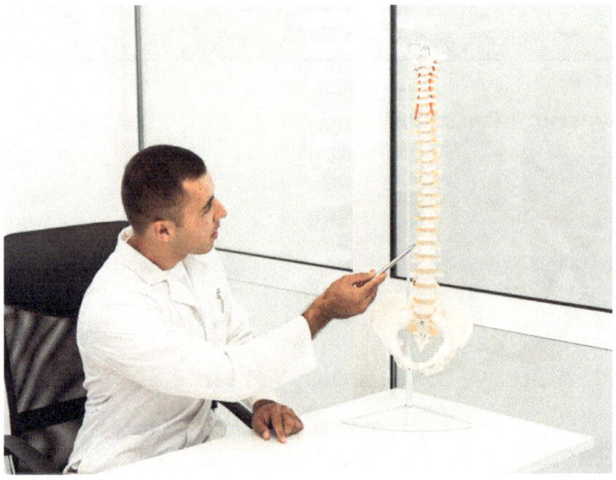

Figure 12.5. The study of early practices in bone analysis.

Source: https://www.voltadiagno.com/img/bone%20quality.jpg.

Moreover, early advances in bone analysis have also assisted in interpreting funerary behavior and societal roles as attested in burial evidence. Analysis of skeletal remains can provide information about an individual's gender, age, and health, revealing their status and roles within their society. Ethnographic and archaeological information are often added to osteological evidence, creating a more detailed image of ancient social structure. The one that comes to mind is the analysis of burial contexts with canid burials, which allowed researchers to explore the relationship of ritual and utilitarian uses of animals (Byrd et al., 2013). Alongside recent advances in technique, early advances in the analysis of bone form a solid basis for understanding the complexities of prehistoric societies and reinforce the interdisciplinary nature of osteological research and its role in comprehending human history (Figure 12.5).

12.1.2. Evolution of Techniques Over Time

Progress in osteological techniques represents a dramatic transition from traditional methods to more advanced, technology-driven solutions. Early research on bones relied on visual inspection and simple equipment, with scientists studying skeletal morphology through direct observation and rudimentary measuring instruments. With the passage of time, radiographic methods enabled better imaging of bony structures, greatly increasing the ability to diagnose and evaluate bone pathology. This change not only enhanced the accuracy of osteological evaluations but also accelerated subsequent improvements in imaging technologies, including computed tomography (CT) and magnetic resonance imaging (MRI). Consequently, as these technologies became more accessible, they offered new opportunities to investigate the mechanical properties of bones and to discover the underlying biological processes, enabling scientists to develop more advanced models of skeletal function in living and extinct animals. As osteology emerged, interdisciplinary collaboration became a driving force in research innovations. Techniques from disciplines such as materials science, biomechanics, and computer modeling began to intersect with osteological studies, increasing knowledge of bone structures and their mechanical implications. For instance, the application of finite element modeling to bone load-bearing capacity provided invaluable data on skeletal adaptations over evolutionary time. The intersection of these diverse methodologies enabled scientists to investigate complex questions regarding locomotor biomechanics, particularly for extinct animals. By analyzing cancellous bone structure using highly advanced imaging, as seen in studies of theropod dinosaurs, osteologists were able to infer locomotor aspects and postural strategies indicative of specific adaptations related to evolutionary pressures (Abourachid et al., 2018). This multi-disciplinary procedure ultimately enhanced the completeness of osteological research. Moreover, high-resolution imaging technology has advanced the field further by enabling non-destructive testing of bone structure. A case in point is the University of Texas High-Resolution X-ray CT Facility that enables internal, detailed examination of bone tissue without damage to fragile samples (Ahmed et al., 2017). Developments like these are critical in osteology science where protection of archeological and paleontological finds is of prime importance. Moreover, visualization of minute variations in bone structure also enables better understanding of evolutionary relationships among species. Such ongoing evolution in technique not only establishes the methodological foundations of osteology but also promotes the scientific ethos in which prevailing hypotheses are regularly challenged in light of new information. With advancing technology, the possibility of groundbreaking discoveries in bone biology and its evolution becomes brighter.

12.1.3. Key Figures in the Development of Osteology

The development of osteology has been shaped by numerous key players whose contributions have significantly altered our understanding of bone biology and application. Among the key players is Giovanni Battista Morgagni, better known as the father of modern pathology. His meticulous studies of the 18th century laid the foundation for understanding the links between disease and anatomy, as a basis for explaining bone anomalies. Morgagni's methodical approach towards viewing the human cadaver laid the foundation for anatomical sciences, influencing generations of osteologists. His contributions emphasized the requirement to combine laboratory practices with fieldwork, a process that remains essential in contemporary osteological research. This integration of laboratory tests with field observation is significant for the overall appreciation of osteological phenomena and, therefore, for the enduring impact of his work on what is currently done in the field. In addition to Morgagni, Thomas Bell played an important role in advancing the study of osteology in the 19th century. His detailed illustrations and scholarly treatment of numerous vertebrate skeletons were highly informative sources of data to scholars and students. Bell's systematic classification of bones provided the foundation of modern ichthyology and comparative osteology, which not only emphasized structural details but also functional details of the skeletal systems of various species. His insistence on marrying rigorous laboratory procedures with empirical fieldwork underscored the necessity of researching actual contexts in skeletal morphology. The methodology has been central in modern osteological practice, where bone structure and adaptations are studied in an all-round manner from both laboratory and field data, thus establishing the importance of Bell's contribution to establishing contemporary osteology. The work of early 20th-century scholars like George Gaylord Simpson further expanded the scope of osteology by incorporating evolutionary biology into the subject of skeletal structures. His foundational work on how bone formation relates to evolutionary forces opened the door to applying biomechanical principles to osteological studies. Simpson's observation that the evolutionary significance of cancellous bone, as described in comparative anatomy research, outlined how skeletal forms have been shaped by environmental forces as well as the mechanics of locomotion. This convergence is particularly relevant in ongoing studies of extinct animals, including ongoing studies using cancellous bone architecture to infer the biomechanics of theropod locomotion and thereby bridge lab results to paleontological work. Work done by early pioneers continues to inform contemporary research paradigms, driving an even-handed understanding of how skeletal systems change and adapt over time, as exemplified through pathbreaking studies on extinct non-avian theropods like Daspletosaurus and Troodon, linking bone loading mechanics to evolutionary directions (Abourachid et al., 2018) (Figure 12.6).

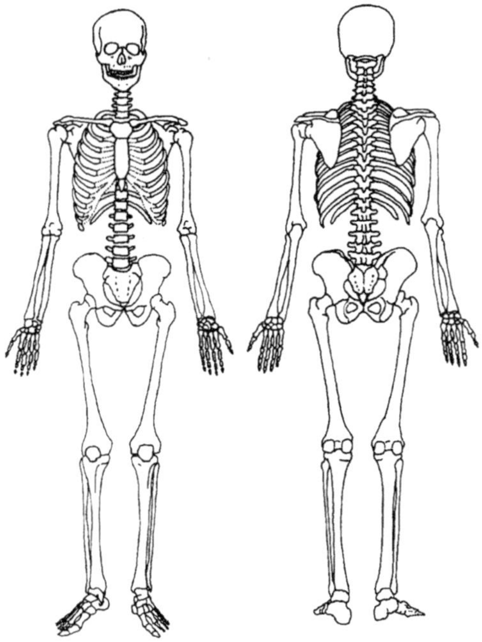

Figure 12.6. The field of osteology has been shaped by numerous pivotal figures.

Source: https://external-content.duckduckgo.com/iu/?u=https%3A%2F%2Fo.quizlet.com%2F6LEYzCMvD6NrD2r-uLvOfA_b.jpg&f=1&nofb=1&ipt=864c0f9ccf362c33d63933ea3f65424f99abdd15b824bd70dc5673a76eadfc3a.

Test Your Knowledge

1. What were the early practices used in bone analysis in the historical development of osteology?
2. Who are the key figures that contributed to the development of osteology, and what were their major contributions?

12.2. Laboratory Methods in Osteology

Learning Outcome

1. Radiographic methods
2. Histological analysis
3. Biochemical analyses

Laboratory methods in osteology play a crucial role in the analysis and interpretation of human remains, providing valuable information across various fields, e.g., anthropology, archaeology, and forensic science. The primary role of such laboratory methods is to establish the biological profile of unknown remains, which entails estimating age, sex, ancestry, and stature. Techniques such as osteometric analysis and morphological assessment are used consistently to determine these characteristics from bones. Furthermore, advances in molecular techniques, including DNA analysis, have greatly enhanced the ability to identify individuals and determine genetic relationships. By integrating traditional anthropological practices with modern molecular biology, forensic experts can build a full profile of skeletal remains, thereby cracking cases that would otherwise remain unsolved. It is only in contemporary osteological laboratories that a range of analytical tools and techniques is employed in the structured examination of bone remains. As a case in point, imaging tools such as X-ray and CT scans can provide three-dimensional images of bones and thus assess inner details that are crucial for identification and analysis. Additionally, histological processes, involving microscopic assessment of bone structure, can reveal information on health and age at death. These lab techniques are complemented by statistical analysis, placing skeletal data in the context of general populations, thereby increasing the validity of the findings. The combination of qualitative and quantitative methods provides a rich framework for understanding skeletal evidence's biological and demographic inferences, thereby enhancing the field of osteology.

Furthermore, the study of skeletal remains is highly useful in forensic investigations, particularly in decomposed or fragmented body cases. One pressing issue in this regard is the identification of incomplete and severely disturbed remains, as often signified by the recovery of dismembered human remains in forensic cases. The literature shows that the role of the foot in forensic identification is less researched, but it presents specific challenges and benefits for understanding one's biological makeup (Barrett et al., 2014). As with the discipline of archaeology, ranging from the study of post-war skeletal remains, which illustrates the need for a precise anthropological approach to gain estimates of biological sex and age (Allmäe et al., 2015). These examples underscore the necessity of continuous research and methodological refinement in laboratory practices to address the complexity of skeletal analysis, ultimately enhancing investigation success in forensic and archaeological contexts (Figure 12.7).

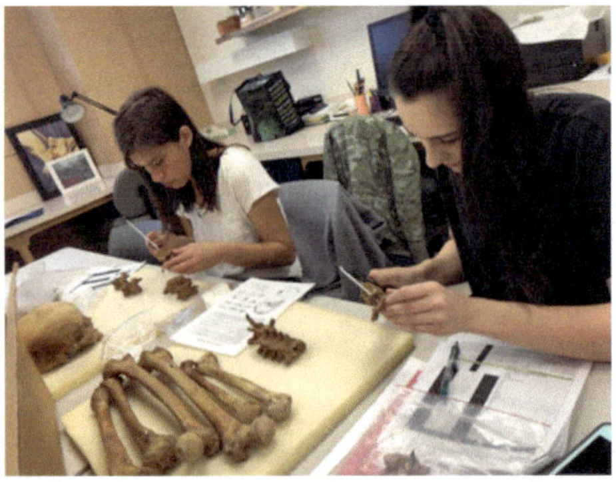

Figure 12.7. Laboratory methods in osteology.

Source: https://anthgr.colostate.edu/wp-content/uploads/sites/69/2019/02/Human-Osteo-Lab-Students-400.jpg.

12.2.1. Radiographic Techniques

Radiographic techniques are a core part of osteology, as they enable skeletal elements to be imaged without subjecting specimens to invasive procedures. Among these, sophisticated imaging modalities such as X-ray and computed tomography (CT) yield high-quality information on both normal and pathologic bone conditions. X-rays remain a fundamental tool for precise skeletal assessment in early diagnosis, providing baseline radiographs that can be utilized to differentiate fractures from degenerative alterations. CT scans, by virtue of their ability to create cross-sectional images, enable more accurate evaluation of complex structures, discrimination between tissue types, and identification of minor abnormalities. These imaging devices are not only utilized in research but also play a crucial role in the clinical setting, where proper diagnosis and treatment depend on their successful application. The integration of 3D imaging techniques is a significant advancement in radiographic practice. These methods combine traditional imaging with sophisticated computational methods to reconstruct comprehensive 3D models from skulls. One technique developed at University College London specifically emphasizes the potential of 3D imaging to reconstruct faces, using laser imaging to capture a skull's features onto a rotating disc. The methods' effectiveness is enhanced when photographs of a living individual, selected for demographic similarity, are used alongside measurements from the skull, seemingly producing a lifelike image of the person who died. Such progress is, however, countered by detracting testing and verification problems because the application of historic remains tends to complicate the validity assessments of the images produced, which is an issue that is expressed in ongoing debate within the field (Addyman et al., 1994). Despite the promise of radiographic techniques, ongoing research must continue to simplify these methodologies and extend their application in osteology. The questioning of the validity of combining data from living subjects and bone remains also underscores the need for rigorous testing procedures to validate these approaches. Preliminary findings indicate that variations in the anatomical features of living models and bone remains result in variations in reconstructed images. Social and ethical considerations of utilizing living subjects for this type of modeling should also be noted as the discipline evolves. Future research must aim at the production of standard protocols for generating and improving images so that they are enriched by both scientific accuracy and practical utility in applications ranging from forensic science to historical scholarship (Thornton et al., 2019) (Figure 12.8).

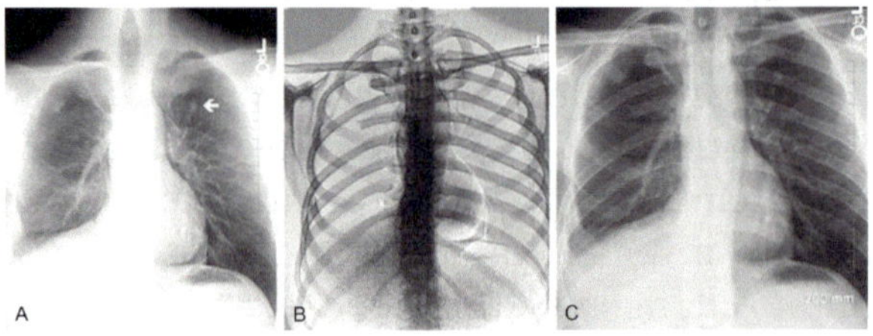

Figure 12.8. Radiographic techniques.

Source: https://radiologykey.com/wp-content/uploads/2020/10/f005-010-9780323041324.jpg.

12.2.2. Histological Analysis

Histological analysis is a key methodology within the broader umbrella of laboratory and field methods in osteology. This technique involves microscopic examination of bone tissue, enabling researchers to observe numerous histological characteristics that can assist in demonstrating age, species, and physiological condition of the skeletons. Histological study of past and forensic specimens can reveal characteristics of bone structure, including mineralization, as well as the composition of specific tissues. By creating a photomicrograph catalogue of burnt and unburnt bone characteristics, researchers lay the groundwork for sound qualitative analyses. Such systematic approaches not only enhance our understanding of osteological material but also increase confidence when applied to forensic analysis, effectively bridging laboratory findings and field use. The significance of histological examination is heightened by its use in distinguishing human from non-human bone, as shown in recent studies. A systematic decision-tree analysis based on histological features achieved exceptional accuracy, with human bone identification achieving 100% success. This precision is remarkable even under specific circumstances, e.g., burning damage rendering the sample hard to assess, as seen in 96% precision when unidentified-burning samples are to be identified. Through a methodical classification process that considers various variables, scientists can make remarkable advances in bioarchaeology and forensic science. Such methodological exactness demonstrates the power of histological analysis, in which the nuances of bone anatomy are salient to both scientific research and forensic inquiry. As imaging and analytical technology evolve increasingly rapidly, the uses of histological methods in osteology become increasingly varied. Facilities like the University of Texas High-Resolution X-ray CT Facility and the Natural History Museum are at the forefront of advancing ways to enhance multimodal imaging techniques relevant to histology. The technology holds potential for increased integration of histological information with other fields of science, like materials science and medical biology. Through interdisciplinary cooperation, researchers can sharpen their methodological skills, making osteological research not only comprehensive but also adaptable to evolving social demands, such as forensic analysis and training. As highlighted by advancements in imaging and data integration methodologies, histological investigation has remained at the forefront of modern scientific research, bearing witness to its relevance in demystifying the dynamics of ancient and modern skeletal material and informing critical forensic processes.

12.2.3. Biochemical Assays

Biochemical assays play a critical role in osteology, where bone metabolism and composition are examined. These tests enable scientists to quantify a variety of biochemical markers to provide insight into bone function and the development of disease. The quantitation of specific proteins, enzymes, and minerals, for instance, can be used to interpret disorders such as osteoporosis and osteomalacia. By using biochemical tests, scientists are able to detect changes at the molecular level, giving valuable information to complement traditional morphological assessment of bone tissue. This fusion of biochemical data with osteological data further solidifies the overall understanding of bone health and delivers essential data for diagnostic and therapeutic purposes. Additionally, biochemical assays are used to evaluate therapies for bone disease and other treatments. For example, significant advancements have been made in the development and evaluation of recombinant proteins, i.e., transgenic recombinant human Factor IX. One may subject such proteins to biochemical assays to assess their efficacy and safety for coagulopathy treatment, as in some research goals of product formulation and hemophilia model assessment (Dernell et al., 2005). These studies provide useful information for guiding clinical practices and developing regulatory filings necessary for trial approval, underscoring the relevance of biochemical assays to translational medicine. Biochemical assays are not confined to medical use; they can also be used in research related to paleobiology and anthropology. By applying such techniques to bone samples excavated from archaeological sites, researchers can obtain information about ancient populations' diets, health, and way of life. Such assays that probe isotopic signatures, for example, help reconstruct dietary habits and determine the prevalence of diseases in the past. This blend of biochemistry and osteology illustrates the flexibility and usefulness of biochemical assays beyond contemporary clinical settings (Thornton et al., 2019). Thus, not only are these assays diagnostic in practice, but they are also instrumental in uncovering past biological processes, thereby enriching our understanding of human evolution and adaptation (Figure 12.9).

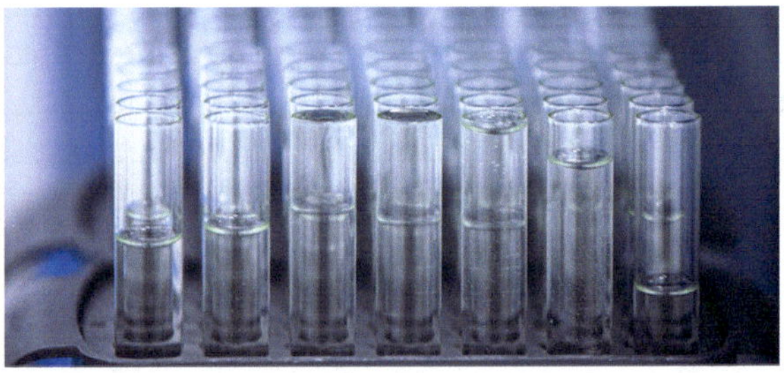

Figure 12.9. Biochemical assays.

Source: https://external-content.duckduckgo.com/iu/?u=https%3A%2F%2Fwww.irbm.com%2Fwp-content%2Fuploads%2FIRBM_biochemical_assays.jpg&f=1&nofb=1&ipt=2c9c9254b329404d4df9e261aec929be949e59519d20e8f197664c9268703252.

Test Your Knowledge

1. How are radiographic methods used in the laboratory analysis of bones in osteology?
2. What is the role of biochemical analyses in studying bone composition and health?

12.3. Field Methods in Osteology

Learning Outcome

1. Excavation techniques
2. Site documentation and mapping
3. Collection and preservation of specimens

Field techniques of osteology serve as the foundation for collecting information on skeletons to achieve accuracy and rigor in bone research. Systematic surveys and excavation techniques are the first course of action, which might involve recovering remains in varying states of preservation. When fragmented human remains are encountered, professionals face specific challenges, most notably identification and the creation of a biological profile. The challenge posed by such fragmented remains highlights the importance of careful fieldwork that considers the finds' context, the environment, and possible forensic consequences. Given the paucity of literature on certain of the anatomical structures, for instance, the foot in forensic identification, it is thus critical that osteologists become involved in wide-ranging field techniques that bridge gaps in knowledge and enhance the credibility of findings (Barrett et al., 2014). Moreover, the incorporation of new technologies into field techniques can significantly complement the traditional methods used by osteologists. Digital data collection tools, including Geographic Information Systems (GIS) and 3D scanning, enable precise documentation and spatial analysis of bones. These tools enable scientists to visually examine patterns and correlations among anatomical structures, thereby improving understanding of locomotor biomechanics and evolutionary patterns. For instance, scientists have employed various methodologies to infer the biomechanical properties of cancellous bone architecture in extinct animals. By correlating such observations with contemporary models, osteologists can reconstruct postures and movement patterns that span the evolutionary range between extinct and extant species (Abourachid et al., 2018). Such a combination of technology not only amplifies field practices but also improves interdisciplinary work, supporting osteology as a course of study. In summary, the success of field practices in osteology lies in the blend of age-old excavation techniques and recent technological innovations. These methods not only produce accurate recovery and identification of skeletal remains but also close significant knowledge gaps, particularly in understanding complex anatomical structures and evolutionary processes. While scientists continue to grapple with the challenge posed by fragmented remains and varying preservation conditions, the requirement for holistic approaches becomes all the more imperative. Lastly, the evolution of field methodology in osteology demonstrates a commitment to quality and rigor in the scientific investigation of human and non-human bone. As the discipline evolves further, ongoing refinement and adjustment of field practice will ensure osteologists are well set to make significant contributions to both forensic science and understanding of biomechanical evolution (Barrett et al., 2014; Abourachid et al., 2018) (Figure 12.10).

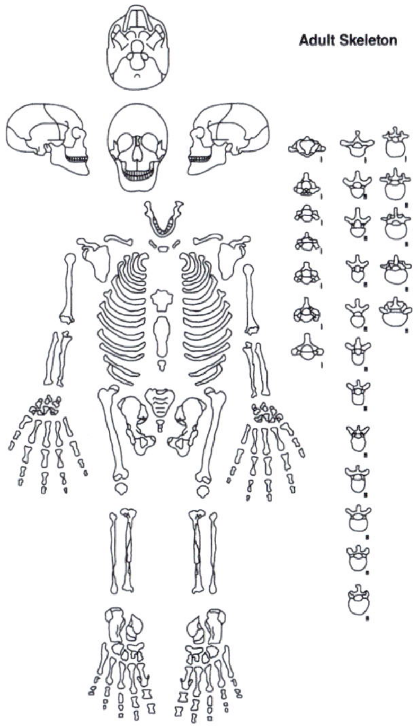

Figure 12.10. The field methods serve as the foundation for collecting skeletal data.

Source: https://static.cambridge.org/binary/version/id/urn:cambridge.org:id:binary:20191127061401508-0579:9781139013826:19522fig7_1.png?pub-status=live.

12.3.1. Excavation Techniques

Osteological excavation techniques are crucial for recovering and analyzing skeletal evidence, enabling us to understand more about human behavior in the past and cultural practices. Using both outdated and modern methods, archaeologists meticulously plan excavation activities so that the spatial context of the findings is not disrupted. Of note is the integration of Geographic Information Systems (GIS), which has revolutionized excavation processes through complex data mapping and spatial analysis. For instance, the UAE's Tell Abraq excavation shows that merging modern technology with traditional methods yields more information about mortuary practices. The ability to superimpose artifacts and remains onto digital maps makes it much easier to analyze, allowing more sophisticated archaeological interpretations, but at the same time, acknowledging the value of hand-drawn records that preceded these advances, while remaining useful for site context and history of practices related to burial rites (Calleja et al., 2016). With technological advancement, excavation techniques must also adapt to the specific challenges posed by different environments. For example, while excavating significant sites like early Neolithic graves, archaeologists encounter peculiar conditions like soil and climatic conditions that could jeopardize the preservation of artifacts. The Coldrum burial chamber excavation demonstrates the importance of careful treatment in such situations. *In situ* analysis of the remains, e.g., osteological analysis and isotopic analysis, provides data on the social structure and diet of the time. The careful documentation of stratigraphy from such excavations makes possible the reconstruction of temporal sequence, and thus furnishes valuable information regarding funeral rites and ritual practices. Such detailed stratigraphic records are not only valuable in the local context of the excavation but also for broader historical accounts of cultural development in prehistoric Britain (Alexander et al., 2013). Finally, the combination of excavation technique and bioanalysis commends the multi-disciplinary investigation that analysis in bioarchaeology warrants. As the only way excavations yield skeletal remains, the application of osteological analysis in the field interprets demographic and health trends among ancient populations. From the observation of cut-marked bones and the application of radiocarbon dating, researchers can infer data about practices in societies, such as ritual cannibalism or treatment of the dead. The combination of excavation data and osteological analysis not only promotes a holistic comprehension of human behaviors but also increases the identification of regional and temporal patterns in burial practices. Such a collaborative approach in excavations provides a multidimensional view of past human life, underscoring that the excavation method plays a vital role in the development of the disciplines of osteology and bioarchaeology in the study of human history.

12.3.2. Site Documentation and Mapping

Documentation and mapping of sites is a critical function in osteology and serves as the foundation for the scientific investigation of skeletons and their associated contexts. Accurate documentation enables researchers to maintain a clear record of excavation, environmental contexts, and spatial associations between finds. Detailed mapping assists in analyzing site organization and, by extension, in understanding burial and habitation patterns. By documenting each layer of sediment and each location of artifacts in detail, archaeologists can also establish connections between bone remains and their temporal or cultural significance. Precise documentation lays the groundwork for future research, enabling the field of osteology to build a cumulative body of knowledge. Documentation, therefore, is not an exercise in administrative procedure; it is a scientific requirement that provides interpretative rigor to osteological study. Moreover, the significance of mapping is highlighted in real-life applications in archaeological research. For instance, during large-scale site surveys of the Island of Barbuda by multidisciplinary research teams, mapping has been of utmost significance to respond to the impacts of climate change and human intervention on archaeological contexts. As detailed in the accounts of the Saladoid site at Seaview and the Troumassoid site at Indian Town Trail, mapping not only documents present conditions but also captures the threat these sites currently pose due to sea level rise and erosion (Klemm et al., 2024). Preemptively doing so preserves significant data concerning skeletal remains and their contexts in the context of active environmental change. Mapping thus becomes an essential tool for site protection and analysis of archaeological sites, further enriching our understanding of ancient societies. Site documentation and mapping coupled with osteological analysis play a pivotal role in reconstructing past human behavior and health. For example, careful excavation and documentation at sites like La Milpa in Belize provide valuable insights into the biological profiles of those buried there. The structuring of structures with burial contexts allows researchers to infer cultural practices from skeletal attributes, thereby gaining better insights into the people and communities portrayed in the archaeological record (Trachman et al., 2009). Moreover, contemporary research using such holistic methods enables the application of radiocarbon dating to obtain ages for skeletal samples, providing a chronological framework that can shed light on discussions of mortality, pathologies, and social structures in past communities. In this sense, field recording and mapping are crucial components of holistic osteology, linking fieldwork to interpretive research.

12.3.3. Collection and Preservation of Specimens

The collection and preservation of specimens in osteology is an essential process that forms the foundation for subsequent study and interpretation. Properly collected specimens allow scientists to build informed biological profiles, providing insights into the sex, age, and health of ancient populations. The choice of method for specimen collection should consider the context and condition of skeletal remains. For instance, employing techniques that minimize damage to delicate structures but assure sample integrity is of utmost importance. Effective collection typically involves field sampling methods that take environmental conditions and the potential for contamination into account, factors that could significantly affect accuracy in future analysis. Therefore, standard working procedures are typically established to support osteologists in the labor-intensive field of specimen collection, documentation, and appropriate care. Preservation techniques also have an equally significant function to fulfill in osteology, determining the future usability of specimens collected.

Preservation techniques that span from chemical treatments that prevent rot, right through to physical methods employed to stabilize fragile bones, are employed. The selection of preservation techniques is greatly dependent on the condition of the specimens and the resources available to researchers. For example, while some might use freeze-drying to remove moisture and inhibit microbial growth, others might use chemical preservatives to maintain structural integrity. Additionally, cross-contamination and environmental exposure must be strictly controlled to ensure the authenticity of specimens is not compromised. Ultimately, the conservation process has an immense impact on the validity of osteological information and increases the value to our understanding of skeletal remains over time. Moreover, the processing of samples gathered can be heavily influenced by quantitative methods, for example, the calculation of the Minimum Number of Individuals (MNI) and the Minimum Number of Elements (MNE). Such estimates play an important role in demographic dimensions of a population estimated from skeletal assemblages and consequently influence interpretations in both archaeological and forensic contexts. The validity of such estimates can vary significantly depending on the methods employed. As is evident from studies comparing different methods of estimation, including those presented in Bonthorne et al. (2016), inconsistencies in MNI estimates may result from methodological biases. Insight into such differences is significant because they can alter perceived demographic composition and ultimately inform anthropological conclusions. This focus on careful methodology is thus at the heart of proper analysis of skeletal remains, allowing analysts to sound conclusions from robust evidence.

Test Your Knowledge

1. Why is accurate site documentation and mapping important in field osteology?
2. What methods are used for the proper collection and preservation of osteological specimens in the field?

12.4. Comparative Osteology

Learning Outcome

1. Significance of comparative analysis
2. Comparison techniques for skeletal remains
3. Uses in discerning evolutionary relationships

In comparative osteology, emphasis lies on understanding the differences in bone structure across different species. Comparative osteology plays a significant role in identifying evolutionary connections and biomechanical specializations of particular organisms. By studying skeletal traits, researchers can identify phylogenetic relationships that describe how locomotion, habitat, and lifestyle have shaped bone form. Such analyses can significantly contribute to our understanding of functional anatomy and allow us to infer the behavioral tendencies of both extinct and current species. It highlights the importance of precise measurement and sophisticated analysis in the laboratory, as it equips scientists with the tools to make reasonable inferences about skeletal adaptations and evolutionary divergence. As a result, comparative analysis of osteological characteristics not only enhances our understanding of biology but also has practical uses in forensic science and paleontology. Careful attention to cancellous bone architecture is specifically significant in comparative osteology because it can provide information about locomotor biomechanics. Cancellous bone is a dynamic structure that changes to accommodate the mechanical load that is exerted on it, thus reflecting the locomotion habits of the organism. Recent research, such as that contained in Abourachid et al. (2018), confirms that cancellous bone architectural patterns may qualitatively reflect the distinctive postures and biomechanics of extinct organisms, such as theropod dinosaurs. Through sophisticated modeling, it is feasible to illustrate how cancellous bone structure adapts to varying locomotor modes and loads, and to provide clues about how these species have evolved over time. Such data emphasize the value of combining sophisticated biomechanical analysis with laboratory and field methods in osteology and provide a rich insight into skeletal function and evolutionary modification. It is of utmost importance in forensic use for human remains identification and determination of their biological composition. The intricacy of variation in the human skeleton poses challenging questions, particularly when dealing with decomposing or fragmentary bodies, as noted by Barrett et al. (2014). This would typically require reconciling comparative techniques to infer gender, age, and ancestry from limited anatomical fragments. The emerging understanding of foot anatomy, as documented in the literature, reflects the lacunae in existing research and underscores the need to continue research in this area. By means of comparative osteology principles, forensic practitioners can design more effective identification procedures whereby even most fragmentary remains can be adequately examined. With the development of forensic sciences and the integration of comparative osteology, human identification practices will become more accurate and efficient, demonstrating the broad influence of this research discipline on applied uses (Figure 12.11).

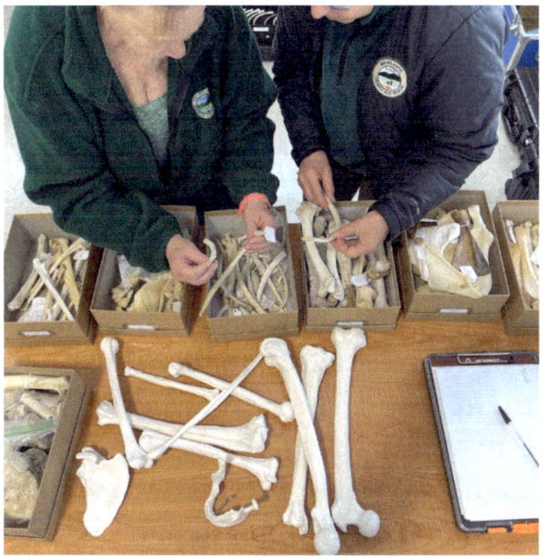

Figure 12.11. The comparative osteology.

Source: https://wildtraining.org/wp-content/uploads/2025/01/comparative-osteology.webp.

12.4.1. Importance of Comparative Analysis

Comparative analysis plays a key role in osteology in enabling us to understand skeletal morphology between species and habitats better. By systematically examining morphological variation in skeletal remains, scientists can draw valuable conclusions about the evolutionary and functional shifts of species. For instance, comparative analysis can help establish how different external factors, such as locomotion or environment, influence bone structure and density. This is crucial in the study of fragmented remains, particularly in forensic science, as it can help establish the biological profile of human beings from fragmentary specimens. As the literature reaffirms, a lack of in-depth studies in some areas, such as the foot in forensic human identification, underscores the need for comparative research to address existing knowledge gaps (Barrett et al., 2014). Comparative analysis is not only important for the purposes of identification but also for the determination of the biomechanical implications inherent in skeletal architecture. Through comparative investigations, scientists can analyze cancellous bone architecture across species and how it correlates with locomotion and behavior. For example, analysis of the architectural patterns of cancellous bone in theropod dinosaurs allows us to understand their locomotor biomechanics and how their bones are structured by evolutionary forces over time. This methodology not only helps to make sense of extinct species but also better to comprehend the mechanics and functional adaptation of extant organisms. The findings from these comparative analyses are invaluable to evolutionary biology, helping reconstruct ecological interactions and evolutionary processes (Abourachid et al., 2018). Finally, the importance of comparative analysis in osteology is highlighted by its power to synthesize laboratory techniques and field observation. Standardized protocols can be utilized within the laboratory for morphometric analysis, whereas fieldwork permits access to contextual data by which the ecological significance of conclusions can be comprehended. Such a concatenation strengthens osteological work, enabling improved analysis of bones in forensic and paleontological cases. Secondly, by evaluating skeletal characteristics based on comparative approaches, researchers can make more reasonable correlations between functional morphology and environmental adaptations. This analysis is key to advancing the field, as it paves the way for further research and enables the formulation of improved identification strategies, eventually allowing for a better understanding of extinct and extant vertebrate species (Figure 12.12).

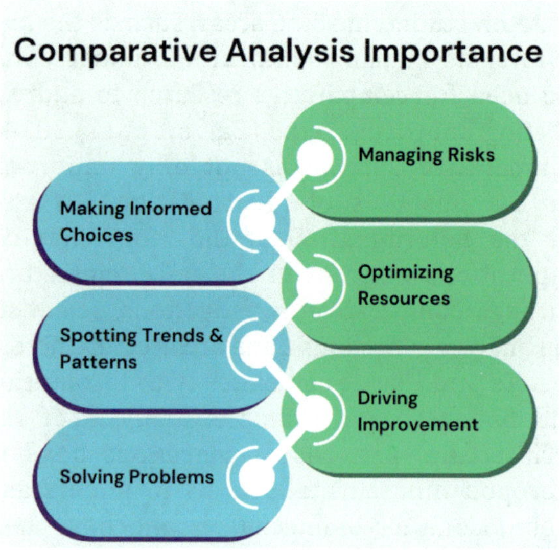

Figure 12.12. Importance of comparative analysis.

Source: https://static.surveysparrow.com/site/strapi-content/uploads/2024/09/importance_of_using_Comparative_Analysis_9d278d64b7.png.

12.4.2. Methods for Comparing Skeletal Remains

Various techniques applied in the comparison of skeletal remains are crucial in identifying demographic and health-related trends in populations in osteology. A key technique that is very useful is Generalized Estimating Equations (GEE), a statistical method used to address scalar problems common in bioarchaeological investigations. For instance, when analyzing osteoarthritis (OA) across multiple articular surfaces, traditional techniques can yield biased estimates due to correlated data points within subjects. GEE permits the investigator to assess the elbow joint in a population without weakening the dataset's validity by accounting for interdependencies among articular surfaces. This methodological development enhances understanding of OA frequency and highlights significant differences between demographic groups, such as the core and colony Tiwanaku populations, as reported in recent studies (Bass et al., 2019). The use of GEE has profound implications since it facilitates more precise evaluations in bioarchaeological and osteological analysis. A further crucial aspect in comparing remains is age estimation, which has significant implications for archaeological interpretation. Traditional older procedures tend to categorize adults into broad ordinal ranks, such as young adult or middle adult, without considering the individual variations in aging processes. The practice, referred to as age mimicry, brings in biases that may skew demographic analysis. Recent studies emphasize the need for improved age-estimation techniques, with anthropologists advised to move towards individual age ranges or probability distributions rather than mean ages from the reference sample. These advances in methodology allow for accurate estimates of age-at-death structures across diverse populations, enabling scientists to draw more prudent conclusions about demographic trends and measures of health over time (Buckberry et al., 2015). Finally, the marriage of statistical techniques and advanced age-estimation methods requires an integrated analysis of skeletal populations. By combining these methods, researchers not only refine the accuracy of individual tests but also improve generalizability across wider datasets. Multi-pronged methods foster a stronger understanding of ancient populations, such as variables of socioeconomic status, health disparities, and interactions between populations. The application of advanced statistical models and individual-age estimation models in conjunction promotes the field of osteology by introducing more nuanced, richer contexts for understanding bone remains. Moreover, such methods are easily applied in both laboratory and field settings, thereby demonstrating their adaptability and applicability in disseminating osteological research across various research areas.

12.4.3. Applications in Understanding Evolutionary Relationships

Applications of evolutionary analysis are necessary in osteology, particularly as they relate to the methodologies used in laboratory and field settings. The addition of imaging technologies, such as high-resolution X-ray computed tomography (CT), has radically changed how scientists examine skeletal material. The technology allows visualization of a specimen's interior in high detail without damaging it, which is important for analyzing fossils. Technologies such as the University of Texas High-Resolution X-ray CT Facility provide researchers with access to state-of-the-art hardware that enables the exploration of morphological divergence across species. With multi-modal imaging approaches, researchers can have a better understanding of evolutionary processes and functional adaptation, and hence a more sophisticated perspective on biological diversity through time (Ahmed et al., 2017). Moreover, genetic analysis is used as a cornerstone in establishing phylogenetic relationships among organisms. For instance, studies using molecular data and supported by morphological evidence enhance the distinctiveness of evolutionary lineages. A case in point is research on cricket frogs, where genetic sequencing revealed distinct phylogeographic groups within *Acris crepitans* and *Acris gryllus*. These morphological classifications in the traditional sense did not agree with evolutionary associations drawn from genetic data, exposing discrepancies among those features that were easily visible and the deeper genetic reality. This challenge is itself a testament to the necessity of integrative methods within taxonomy to allow reconsideration of accepted subspecies and to uncover new species based on genetic evidence, thereby informing conservation strategies (Berendzen et al., 2008). The implications of the knowledge of these evolutionary relationships extend beyond taxonomy to bigger ecological and conservation endeavors. By tracing the evolutionary tracks of species, scientists can identify patterns of biodiversity that are vital for ecological research. Establishing various evolutionary lineages allows for targeted conservation methods, particularly for species under threat of extinction by habitat loss or climate change. As seen in the case of *Acris blanchardi*, reclassified as a separate species due to drastic declines, it is essential to understand evolutionary relationships when prioritizing conservation strategies. Therefore, integrating laboratory methods and field data not only defines the field of osteology but also promotes the intelligent actions necessary for the conservation of biological heritage (Berendzen et al., 2008).

Test Your Knowledge

1. What is the significance of comparative analysis in the study of osteology?
2. What techniques are commonly used to compare skeletal remains in comparative osteology?

12.5. Ethical Considerations in Osteological Research

Learning Outcome

1. Handling human remains
2. Cultural sensitivity during fieldwork
3. Legal codes governing osteological research

The ethics of osteological work entail a diversity of considerations that researchers must address during the study, particularly in relation to how human remains are handled. Osteologists must appreciate the cultural and historical significance of the skeletal materials they excavate and analyze. Such acknowledgment not only highlights the importance of respectful treatment but also demands a commitment to obtaining proper permissions and ensuring that any research conducted is respectful of the values of the communities from which the remains may be derived. Stakeholder consultation, including with descendant communities, is an important step that can facilitate trust generation and accountability within the research process. Ethical development enables more nuanced, knowledge-informed interpretations of the biological and cultural backgrounds of remains, enhancing the scientific rigor of osteological investigations without dishonoring personal narratives. Over the past several years, the integration of advanced methodologies into osteological investigation has prompted a rethinking of ethical standards for both laboratory- and field-based investigations. Particularly during the COVID-19 pandemic, shifting online instruction in biological anthropology to incorporate more haptic and tactile learning opportunities, and addressing the ethics of education policies, matters. Through the observation of the Mount Royal University and University of Manitoba research, the use of plastic model skeletons to help instruct through remote learning allowed students to work through critical learning outcomes. However, critical evaluation reveals that while these models aided early bone identification proficiency, they also highlighted deficiencies in other areas of need, such as age and sex estimation methods and the identification of incomplete elements. Hence, though innovative teaching strategies can benefit students, balanced ethical training remains core to strong osteological training and research standards (Gamble et al., 2024). Ethical standards need to go further into analysis and display of human remains, particularly cremated remains, which are now more frequently occurring in osteological studies over the past decades. More studies of cremated human remains have shown a lack of literature on the ethical side of their excavation, analysis, and display. Researchers are encouraged to adopt best practices that include appropriate ethics training for students and professionals when handling sensitive materials such as cremated bones. Ethical practice guidelines emphasize the need for standardized procedures that acknowledge specific challenges to working with cremated remains and require coordination with field experts. This wide-ranging ethical stance on osteology not only encourages respect for the past but also promotes a broader discussion of archaeological practice (N/A, 2025) (Figure 12.13).

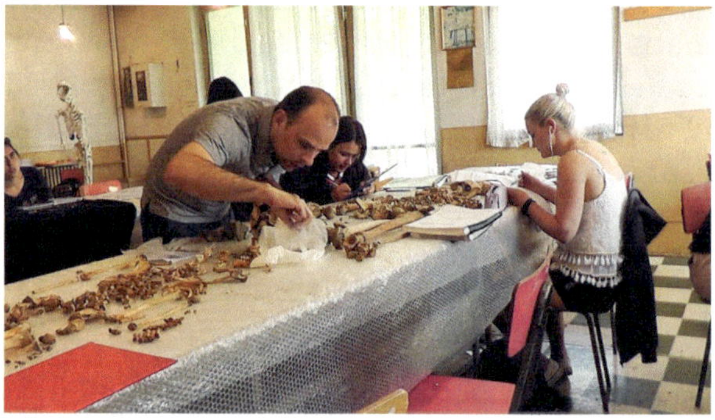

Figure 12.13. Ethical considerations in osteological research.

Source: https://www.archaeological.org/wp-content/uploads/2019/03/Lab-work-1-1024x576.jpg.

12.5.1. Treatment of Human Remains

Treatment of human remains in osteology comprises a series of techniques that are key to dealing with the biological, cultural, and historical context of skeletal collections. Depending on the objectives of a study, researchers may employ laboratory and field methods to analyze human remains. Field methods typically involve the application of accurate excavation methods intended to maintain the integrity of the burial context. They involve thorough documentation of the remains' orientation and location, facilitating an integrated understanding of burial practices and meaning. These are the key factors, as evidenced at Coldrum, where osteological analysis revealed cut-marked human remains indicating practiced funerary rituals with care, emphasizing the significance of handling remains with care to convey complex rituals associated with identity and heritage (Alexander et al., 2013). Laboratory methods complement field methods by using advanced analytical techniques that enable thorough investigations of human remains. For instance, osteologists can use radiographic imaging and isotopic analysis to provide information on the age, sex, health, and diet of individuals recovered from skeletal assemblages. These methods provide information on the bioarchaeological context of the remains, which supports the reconstruction of the lifestyles and health of past populations. The Coldrum site demonstrates this through isotopic analysis, which provides an image of the subtlety of subsistence practice, differentiating the elevated levels of nitrogen that indicate a diet heavy in aquatic foods (Alexander et al., 2013). This new knowledge is not only being introduced to the science of osteology but is also added to wider anthropological histories that link the human remains to broader societal transformation through time. The ethical problems surrounding the work on human remains are paramount in both field and laboratory settings. The researcher must tiptoe around the law, cultural sensitivities, and the probable effect of the findings on descendant communities. It is key to successful research partnerships with local people and stakeholders to ensure respectful relationships and that research protocols comply with the community's values. For example, exhumation of historical figures such as Gaspare Pacchierotti has raised ethical issues regarding consent, intent, and the potential effect of revealing sensitive information through scientific analysis. As methods of analyzing human remains advance in osteology, ethical guidelines must come first to honor the dignity of individuals whose remains constitute skeletal collections, preserving their histories and extending scientific understanding (Figure 12.14).

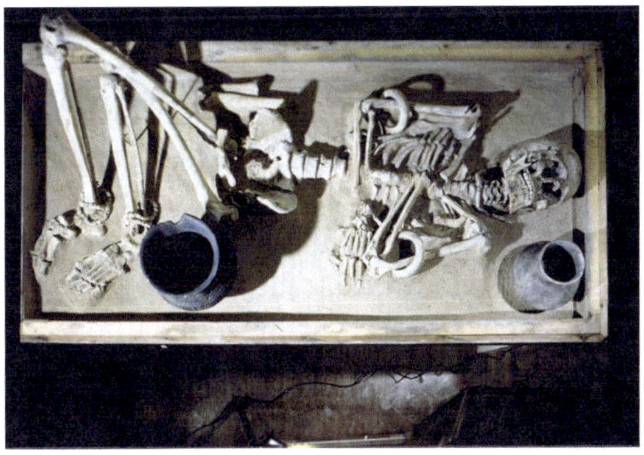

Figure 12.14. The treatment of human remains in osteology.

Source: https://www.preussischer-kulturbesitz.de/fileadmin/user_upload_SPK/images/schwerpunkte/provenienz_eigentum/rp/h_00027012_grab_lb.jpg.

12.5.2. Cultural Sensitivity in Fieldwork

Cultural sensitivity in fieldwork is a critical factor in osteological research, particularly when dealing with human remains of cultural significance to descendant peoples. The ethical handling of skeletal remains requires sensitive consideration of local context and history. Researchers must find ways to develop an appreciation for the cultural narratives surrounding the remains they handle. For instance, engaging with Indigenous people and recognizing their spiritual connection to ancestors' remains is significant for developing cooperation and trust. From the examination of various methods for sex estimation of human skeletal remains, collaboration with local communities can certainly enhance the validity of results and respect their heritage, integrating scientific investigation with cultural values (Arellano et al., 2020). This approach not only enhances research integrity but also empowers local communities by engaging their voices in the archaeological discourse. In addition, field practices can greatly affect social interactions among researchers and the community. Cultural sensitivity must do more than formally acknowledge beliefs; it must actively engage in conversation and decision-making. For example, the Belize Archaeological Project is concerned with how relationships with the people should be initiated through mutual field exploration and excavation rather than imposing external methods upon them (Cortes-Rincon et al., 2014). Interdisciplinary approaches involve a mutual process of learning whereby researchers learn about indigenous methods and transfer scientific knowledge. This cooperative partnership not only deepens the archaeological narrative but also generates a sense of ownership and pride among people. By prioritizing inclusivity and respect, scientists are better able to traverse complex cultural landscapes and conduct their work responsibly and ethically. Finally, the impacts of cultural sensitivity echo far beyond the particular fieldwork context itself, into broader discourses within osteology and anthropology. Ethical systems with respect for culture are needed to guide future archaeological policy and practice. The dissemination of results from culturally sensitive research can educate the wider academic community regarding the benefits of ethical methods in the study of human remains. By investigating how proteomics and osteology have been appropriately incorporated into sex estimation, researchers are demonstrating methodology attention and respect for cultural value (Arellano et al., 2020). Finally, increasing cultural sensitivity in fieldwork cultivates an ethic of reflection that benefits not just the scientific community but also the cultural heritage of multicultural societies, leading to more responsible and inclusive research outputs.

12.5.3. Legal Regulations Governing Osteological Studies

The legal regime governing osteological research largely depends on legislation aimed at safeguarding human remains and cultural heritage. In the majority of regions, the law acts to mediate scientific investigation and ethical issues regarding the treatment of human remains. These legal provisions are particularly significant in bioarchaeology, where the study of human remains may intersect with sensitive cultural and spiritual issues. The requirement for ethical guidelines stems from previous misconduct in the field, prompting a growing consensus on treating the dead with respect. Researchers are thus faced with the twin mandate of advancing scientific knowledge while maintaining legal standards governing the respectful treatment of remains. The United States' Native American Graves Protection and Repatriation Act (NAGPRA) is a paradigm in this regard, restructuring the relationship between bioarchaeologists and indigenous people. Signed into law in 1990, NAGPRA mandates the repatriation of culturally affiliated human remains and funerary objects to Native American tribes. The law initiated an on-going debate about the ethical components of osteological research that has led scientists to re-emerge earlier methodologies, particularly while using indigenous skeletal material. The evolving interpretation of Section 106 of the National Historic Preservation Act further complicates this landscape, as federally recognized tribes are becoming more assertive in exercising sovereignty over their ancestral remains. Such regimes need to adopt an interagency, collaborative approach to osteological research. The involvement of indigenous communities makes the research environment evenhanded, forcing bioarchaeologists to incorporate tribal insights and knowledge into their work. The delicate dance between contemporary indigenous cultures and archaeological practice emphasizes collaboration rather than independent action. Study here becomes a means not just of discovery but of restitution, laying the foundation for the need for scientifically rigorous as well as culturally sensitive methodology. As bioarchaeology navigates these legal and ethical waters, the need for reform in research practice highlights the role of legal controls in shaping the direction of osteological research (Ezzo et al., 2021; Hamilton et al., 2004).

Test Your Knowledge

1. Why is ethical handling of human remains essential in osteological research?
2. What legal codes or regulations govern the practice of osteological research?

12.6. Technological Advances in Osteology

Learning Outcome

1. Application of 3D imaging and modeling
2. Application of DNA analysis
3. Integration of data analysis software

The incorporation of technological advances into osteology has revolutionized the means at researchers' disposal, significantly enhancing laboratory and field work. Technologies such as computed tomography (CT) scanning and three-dimensional (3D) printing enable non-destructive examination of skeletal material, allowing accurate imaging of internal detail without compromising the integrity of the specimen. In addition, these technologies allow for the visualization of pathological states, which is crucial in the understanding of past populations' lifestyles and health. The application of 3D modeling not only aids in the recording of human variation in bones but also in the production of replicas for educational purposes and for archives. As a result, osteological studies now have access to an increased number of interdisciplinary techniques, drawing from anthropology, archaeology, and even medicine to create more detailed histories of people's lives in the past, for example, in works that analyze crania at sites such as Verteba Cave (Lillie et al., 2025). In the field itself, advances in portable technology have changed how osteologists dig and analyze human remains. Handheld X-ray fluorescence (XRF) spectrometers, for instance, enable on-site, instant chemical analysis of bone chemistry to obtain dietary and environmental exposure information without the need for laboratory processing. The use of drones with high-definition cameras also provides improved aerial coverage of digs, enabling mapping of burial contexts and identifying potential anomalies that may indicate human presence. By integrating such technologies into field methods, researchers can streamline data collection and make it more effective, thereby gaining a clearer picture of archaeological contexts. Such integration of technology allows for better visualization of ancient populations, which, in conjunction with state-of-the-art imaging technologies and field surveys, unearths information about their social interactions and health status (Boyd et al., 2003). The ethical use of advanced technologies in osteology cannot be overlooked, particularly where human remains are involved and the issues are sensitive. While researchers access these innovations, care must be taken to consider the cultural symbolism of the remains being examined, particularly in cases concerning marginalized populations. The application of technologies such as virtual reconstructions and bioarchaeological analysis must be done with sensitivity, ensuring that the narratives produced are respectful and representative of the sociocultural contexts from which the remains are drawn. Collaboration with descendant communities then becomes necessary. These engagements also foster a deeper understanding of the cultural beliefs associated with the deceased and help researchers make sound decisions about how to treat and interpret human skeletal material. The emphasis on ethical obligation, in conjunction with the technical capabilities enabled by advanced technology, creates a more ethical approach to osteological research that considers scientific inquiry and cultural heritage (Lillie et al., 2025).

12.6.1. Use of 3D Imaging and Modeling

The integration of 3D modeling and imaging in osteology has dramatically changed the analysis and interpretation of skeletal populations. Traditional methods largely relied on manual measurements and physical models, which were not only time-consuming but also prone to human error. The development of technology, particularly in X-ray microcomputed tomography (micro-CT), enables rapid, non-destructive visualization of complex morphological features in contemporary and fossilized bones. This shift to digital approaches permits scientists to build large data sets, hence enabling more accurate comparisons and analyses. With increased resolution and detail, elements of the skeleton can be examined at finer levels, permitting greater appreciation of anatomical diversity and patterns of evolution within groups. The growing prevalence of 3D imaging techniques has begun to de-emphasize distinctions, making it easier for more institutions, e.g., universities and museums, to undertake advanced osteological research (Ahmed et al., 2017). In addition, 3D modeling is not merely visualization; it makes collaborative study independent of geography. Researchers can share 3D images and information with peers worldwide, fostering an open science culture in which research can be criticized and validated. Research done using micro-CT, such as research on amphibians, is the best way to show this collaborative potential. For instance, comparisons between established bone-cartilage staining techniques and micro-CT have demonstrated the efficiency and precision of the latter, with both techniques having no profound difference in vertebral numbers (Jiang et al., 2018). Observations such as these not only speed up data collection but also expand research tools by combining computational techniques into vertebrate development and phylogenies. The interactive capabilities of 3D modeling also help augment educational outreach and engagement by making sophisticated osteological concepts more widely accessible. Additionally, the implications of 3D imaging technology also echo in conservation and cultural heritage initiatives. By creating accurate digital models of skeletal tissues and artifacts, researchers can preserve valuable data when original specimens are damaged or destroyed. The ability to generate accurate 3D models ensures that morphological structures can be retained, even as they might be lost over time or through environmental exposure. These models can also serve as a significant source for both scientific investigation and educational purposes in the form of interactive platforms, whereby users can examine the anatomy of osteological specimens without actually coming into physical contact with them. As the field of osteology becomes more technology-oriented, ongoing developments and enhancements in 3D imaging technologies can further revolutionize laboratory and field methods and offer a sound foundation for future research (Ahmed et al., 2017) (Figure 12.15).

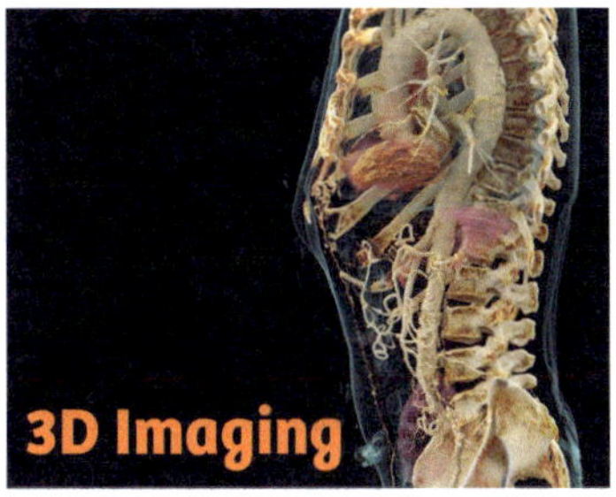

Figure 12.15. The integration of 3D imaging and modeling into the field of os.

Source: https://external-content.duckduckgo.com/iu/?u=https%3A%2F%2Fmarketing.webassets.siemens-healthineers.com%2F027eb26d0dd1fbf6%2Fea8f83071b64%2Fv%2Fcd356e8114d6%2F8406_cc_ns_125jahre_roentgen_1920x1080px_april4.jpg&f=1&nofb=1&ipt=2d123d88a63e4d4dd017d766b96a7bbc750404734ebc3f2a277a8b9ed59f23b2.

12.6.2. Application of DNA Analysis

The application of DNA analysis has greatly benefited osteology, particularly in the interpretation of bone age and genetic ancestry. With advanced techniques such as peptide nucleic acid (PNA) and DNA sequencing, researchers can identify aging-related mutations in bone samples. A study identified an A189G point mutation in bone and reported a systematic disparity among the elderly. Interestingly, the mutation was found in 20% of individuals aged over 60, but in only 1% of individuals aged 38 years and above, thus graphically illustrating the potential of DNA analysis to improve age estimates in living and fossil populations. This intersection of osteology and molecular genetics enhances the precision of identification in forensic analysis and in the anthropological research of ancient populations (Brandstätter et al., 2008). The more significant use of DNA analysis in archaeological and forensic research has also transformed the method used in exhumation cases. Exhumation, as defined as the excavation of remains from legally sanctioned burial sites, allows the use of DNA analysis to address forensic queries, especially where unidentified remains or mass graves are concerned. By matching DNA profiles recovered from skeletal remains to individuals known in that context, forensic anthropologists can establish kinship relationships, which help identify individuals. Particularly in regions whose political and historical contexts are complex, such as the investigations of Brazil's civil-military dictatorship killings, DNA analysis serves not only a scientific purpose but also a crucial role in the determination of human rights violations (Arrabaça Francisco et al., 2017).

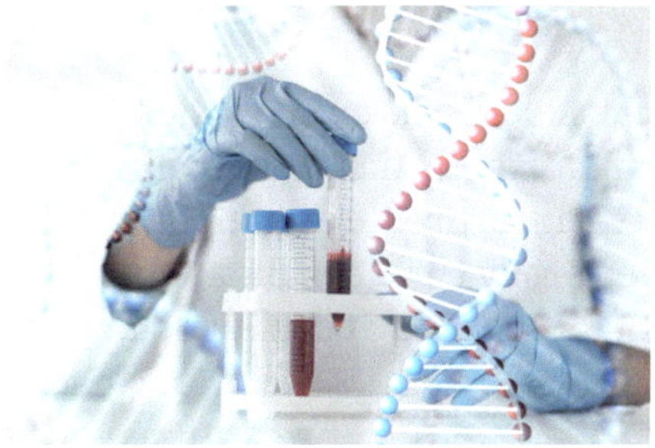

Figure 12.16. The application of DNA analysis in osteology.

Source: https://external-content.duckduckgo.com/iu/?u=https%3A%2F%2Fknowyourdna.com%2Fwp-content%2Fuploads%2F2024%2F01%2F58801386_m_normal_none-2048x1344.jpg&f=1&nofb=1&ipt=0af12b65e36c4cded728fc73fc43b0eaa34f8c927bce404c3556779b7dcd8892.

Such applications demonstrate the interconnectedness between molecular biology and osteological methods. The use of DNA analysis does not end with straightforward identification, as it also contributes to broader understanding of population genetics and human migration trends. In osteology, the study of ancient DNA isolated from bones allows researchers to rebuild demographic histories, shedding light on population dynamics over the passing millennia. Differences in genetic markers can reveal how migration, interbreeding, and disease transmission have occurred, piecing together a history of human evolution and adaptation. This DNA-based perspective complements traditional osteological examination by offering a deeper interpretation of past human presence and social structure. With the evolution of osteology as a science, applications of DNA analysis remain central to explaining complex aspects of human history and heritage, establishing it as an integral part of both laboratory and field methods of investigation (Figure 12.16).

12.6.3. Integration of Software for Data Analysis

Data analysis software integration in osteology has transformed the paradigms by which scientists interpret skeletal data. With the utilization of advanced computational techniques, researchers are able to deal with large datasets produced from experiments performed in a laboratory as well as observations in the field, and as such, their results become more valid and credible. For instance, software packages can model the geometry of the skeleton and its biomechanical properties. This approach not only facilitates visualizing complex bone structures but also provides insights into functional changes in fossil species. Such analysis software has a close association with research aimed at understanding non-avian theropod locomotor biomechanics, as it can simulate a range of scenarios based on observed cancellous architecture and ultimately yield more advanced re-evaluations of their evolution (Abourachid et al., 2018). The use of software in the analysis of skeletal data is more than mere chi-squared tests or linear regressions; it involves sophisticated techniques such as finite element analysis (FEA) and three-dimensional modeling. Such a shift in methodology is most useful for osteological analysis, allowing researchers to create dynamic models that consider the mechanical environments influencing bone structure. For example, researchers may relate cancellous bone architectural designs to three-dimensional musculoskeletal models to gain important insights into the postures and locomotion of extinct animals such as Daspletosaurus and Troodon. Simulation visualization of these interactions improves knowledge of evolutionary biomechanics by enabling a direct relationship between physical adaptations and the biomechanical stressors that such organisms underwent over time (Abourachid et al., 2018). With the advancement of software integration, its application in the field of osteological study is sure to grow, particularly in the domain of interdisciplinary collaboration. Software used to process the skeletal data can be developed further through more advancements in imaging technology along with data management. Institutional collaborations, such as projects undertaken by the University of Texas High-Resolution X-ray CT Facility, can amplify the volume of data to be processed in osteology. In addition, networks for comparative investigation, educational dissemination, and data exchange offer larger research potential. By facilitating this kind of interdisciplinarity, the addition of software will not only facilitate data analysis but also enhance the level of scientificity in discussions related to skeletal studies to further enable a more comprehensive understanding of both present and fossilized organisms in paleontology and biomechanics.

Test Your Knowledge

1. How is 3D imaging and modeling applied in modern osteological studies?
2. How does data analysis software enhance research and interpretation in osteology?

SUMMARY

The complementary nature of these environments is of utmost significance in human remains studies. Laboratory methods are required for precision and control in analyzing skeletal material, conducting painstaking analyses that yield valuable information about age, sex, ancestry, and height. Field procedures are required for the recovery and documentation of remains, as they lay the groundwork for the subsequent laboratory analysis. The interaction of these two methods underscores the richness of forensic anthropology, particularly in cases of public interest, for example, cases with fragmented remains found along coastlines, which have been a trend in recent literature (Barrett et al., 2014). An integrated method, therefore, which initiates the application of laboratory and field methods, is pivotal to our development of knowledge regarding osteological remains. In addition, the development of osteological research underscores the need for continued methodological improvement. Identification and analysis of human remains depend not only on current practice but also on the integration of novel technologies and multidisciplinary approaches. As discussed recently in the anthropology community, considerable progress has been made in age estimation techniques that unite biological anthropology and forensic science (Beaumont et al., 2015). These developments enhance the accuracy of identifications and improve the quality of data accessible to research. As such, constant interaction between academic and forensic circles is essential to enhance techniques, promote innovation, and in the end, the capacity of the disciplines to address challenges of the times. Lastly, the conclusion drawn from this discussion emphasizes the importance of interdisciplinary cooperation and methodological rigor in osteological investigations. As forensic scientists increasingly face difficult cases, the integration of laboratory and field methodologies is vital to achieving accurate identifications and advancing overall awareness of human biology. The composition of fragmented remains cases reveals an urgent need for additional research and development in this class (Barrett et al., 2014). In the future, the field of osteology will need to focus not only on improving existing techniques but also on developing new methods to keep pace with the ever-evolving features of forensic analysis. Merging these procedures will not only help identify human bones but also contribute to the broader field of forensic anthropology and its sociological implications.

To understand the methodologies applied in osteology, one needs a detailed understanding of lab and field methods. Lab methods primarily focus on studying bone remains using techniques such as radiographic imaging, isotopic analysis, and histological investigation. These allow scholars to examine bone growth patterns, diet, and health status over time. In addition, lab settings provide environmentally controlled conditions where experiments can be repeated to yield good-quality data. For instance, how larval development in fish populations applies has been realized through controlled studies, where it was demonstrated how developmental characteristics may lead to systemic evolutionary theories in osteology (Kendall et al., 1984). By focusing on skeletal forms across different eras, researchers can identify patterns related to species adaptation and survival. Field methods, while different, are as vital to osteology as they are to providing context and real-world usefulness to laboratory findings. Fieldwork most often involves excavation, site survey, and systematic sampling, all necessary for the recovery of large amounts of information about the environmental setting of skeletal remains. That environmental influences play a role in the preservation and breakdown of bones is especially useful to recognize. For example, fisheries productivity can be significantly affected by ecological processes and thus makes the contribution of healthy ecosystems to both aquatic and terrestrial organisms all the more important (Kolb et al., 1953). Field data incorporation is thus bound to complement laboratory testing and help sharpen our understanding of species interaction with the environment over time. This lab-to-field interface provides a holistic understanding of osteological studies. In addition, comparative incorporation of outcomes from field and laboratory methods can significantly advance osteological research, particularly in animal behavior and human evolution. Merging of the interpretation obtained from analysis of skeletons in the lab with contextual data obtained from investigation in the field enables scientists to create more comprehensive accounts of biological and ecological transformations. The critical evaluation of such methods enables a greater understanding of skeletal morphology and population dynamics. Such as the evaluation of commercial fish decline in the context of ecological study and skeletal analysis enables illuminating conclusions toward species resilience and adaptation processes through time (Kolb et al., 1953). Therefore, an interdisciplinary approach that draws on both laboratory and field methods is critical to advancing our knowledge and addressing contemporary problems in osteology.

KEY TERMS FROM THIS CHAPTER

- 3D Imaging
- Age Estimation
- Artifact Association
- Bone Cleaning
- Bone Preservation
- Calipers
- CT Scanning
- DNA Extraction
- Excavation Techniques
- Isotope Analysis
- Measurement Standards
- Osteometric Board
- Pathology Assessment
- Photography

CRITICAL THINKING QUESTIONS

1. **What is the first step in analyzing skeletal remains in the laboratory?**
   a. Age estimation
   b. Cleaning and preparation
   c. Sex determination
   d. Stature estimation
2. **Which tool is commonly used for measuring bones in osteology?**
   a. Calipers
   b. Microscope
   c. Tape measure
   d. X-ray machine
3. **What does a skeletal inventory involve?**
   a. Determining age and sex
   b. Cataloging and identifying all skeletal elements
   c. Measuring bone density
   d. Extracting DNA from bones
4. **Which part of the skeleton is most commonly used to estimate biological sex?**
   a. Skull
   b. Femur
   c. Pelvis
   d. Radius
5. **What method is commonly used to estimate age in subadult skeletons?**
   a. Cranial sutures
   b. Dental eruption
   c. Pubic symphysis
   d. Long bone measurements

Short Answer Questions

1. What are the primary objectives of osteological analysis in the laboratory?
2. What equipment is essential for cleaning and preparing skeletal remains?
3. How is skeletal inventory conducted in a laboratory setting?
4. What techniques are used to estimate age from skeletal remains?
5. How is biological sex determined using osteological methods?
6. What is the process for identifying pathological conditions in bones?

Answers to Critical Thinking Questions

1. (b); 2. (a); 3. (b); 4. (c); 5. (b)

REFERENCES

1. Bishop, P. J., Hocknull, S. A., Clemente, C. J., Hutchinson, J. R., Farke, A. A., Barrett, R. S., & Lloyd, D. G. (2018b). Cancellous bone and theropod dinosaur locomotion. Part III—Inferring posture and locomotor biomechanics in extinct theropods, and its evolution on the line to birds. *PeerJ*, *6*, e5777. https://doi.org/10.7717/peerj.5777Addyman, S. M. (1994). The use of three-dimensional laser imaging for facial reconstruction. https://core.ac.uk/download/268808652.pdf (accessed on 18th July 2025).
2. Ahmed, F., & Maisano, J. (2017). ToScA North America (6–8 June 2017, The University of Texas, Austin, TX) Program. https://core.ac.uk/download/211334283.pdf (accessed on 18th July 2025).
3. Alexander, A., Ashbee, A., Ashbee, A., Ashbee, A., et al. (2013). Dates, diet, and dismemberment: Evidence from the Coldrum megalithic monument, Kent. https://core.ac.uk/download/20544701.pdf (accessed on 18th July 2025).
4. Allmäe, R., & Limbo-Simovart, J. (2015). Conventional ageing and sexing methods based on teeth and dry bone morphology in the person's identification (victims of red terror in 1946). https://core.ac.uk/download/43658427.pdf (accessed on 18th July 2025).
5. Aranda Jiménez, G., Becerra Fuello, P., Díaz-Zorita Bonilla, M., Fregel, et al. (2024). Female sex bias in Iberian megalithic societies through bioarcheology, aDNA, and proteomics. https://core.ac.uk/download/620801197.pdf (accessed on 18th July 2025).
6. Arellano, M., Buonasera, T., Byrd, B. F., et al. (2020). A comparison of proteomic, genomic, and osteological methods of archaeological sex estimation. https://core.ac.uk/download/534394688.pdf (accessed on 18th July 2025).
7. Arrabaça, F., Castro Pinheiro, M. E., da Silva, R., et al. (2017). Procedural and political aspects of forensic exhumation in Brazil. https://core.ac.uk/download/80693793.pdf (accessed on 18th July 2025).
8. Barrett, A., Bidmos, M., Bidmos, J., Bidmos, A., Bilge, A., British Broadcasting Corporation, British Broadcasting Corporation, et al. (2014). The foot in forensic human identification–a review. https://core.ac.uk/download/30660095.pdf (accessed on 18th July 2025).
9. Bartosiewicz, L. (2020). Nesutarimai dėl kaulų. Pamąstymai apie osteoarcheologiją ir Baltijos regioną. https://core.ac.uk/download/401879900.pdf (accessed on 18th July 2025).
10. Bass, W. M., Brothwell, D. R., Buikstra, J. E., Dieppe, P., Felson, D., Gagnon, C. M., Gagnon, C. M., et al. (2019). Evaluating elbow osteoarthritis within the prehistoric Tiwanaku state using generalized estimating equations (GEE). https://core.ac.uk/download/323311271.pdf (accessed on 18th July 2025).
11. Basso, N. G., Bunge, M. M., Martinazzo Giménez, L. B., et al. (2011). A new genus of neobatrachian frog from southern Patagonian forests, Argentina and Chile. https://core.ac.uk/download/223030536.pdf (accessed on 18th July 2025).
12. Beaumont, J., Buckberry, J., Dean, M. C., Liversidge, H. M., Buckberry, J., Konigsberg, L., Marquez-Grant, N., et al. (2015). Age estimation [editorial]. https://core.ac.uk/download/76945364.pdf (accessed on 18th July 2025).
13. Berendzen, P. B., Gamble, T., Shaffer, H. B., et al. (2008). Species limits and phylogeography

of North American cricket frogs (*Acris*: Hylidae). https://core.ac.uk/download/286544054.pdf (accessed on 18th July 2025).

14. Bonthorne, E., Gerdau-Radonic, K., Lambacher, N., et al. (2016). Evaluating three methods to estimate the number of individuals from a commingled context. https://core.ac.uk/download/46571822.pdf (accessed on 18th July 2025).
15. Borrini, M., Cole, C., Eliopoulos, C., et al. (2017). An anthropometric method for sex determination from the mandible: Test on British Medieval skeletal collections. https://core.ac.uk/download/131226347.pdf (accessed on 18th July 2025).
16. Boyd, D. K., & Tiné, A. L. (2003). Archaeological excavation and reburial of unmarked historic graves in the Pioneer Cemetery (41BO202), Brazoria County, Texas. https://core.ac.uk/download/72740111.pdf (accessed on 18th July 2025).
17. Brandstätter, A., Brandstätter, A., Chomyn, A., Cormio, A., Schmitt, A., Kadenbach, B., Ludes, B., et al. (2008). Detection of the A189G mtDNA heteroplasmic mutation in relation to age in modern and ancient bones. https://core.ac.uk/download/50543720.pdf (accessed on 18th July 2025).
18. Buckberry, J. (2015). The (mis)use of adult age estimates in osteology. https://core.ac.uk/download/76945106.pdf (accessed on 18th July 2025).
19. Byrd, B. F., Carpenter, T. R., Cornellas, A., et al. (2013). The role of canids in ritual and domestic contexts: New ancient DNA insights from complex hunter-gatherer sites in prehistoric central California. https://core.ac.uk/download/70425670.pdf (accessed on 18th July 2025).
20. Calleja, M. (2016). Commingled tombs and ArcGIS: Analyzing the mortuary context and taphonomy at Bronze Age Tell Abraq. http://digitalscholarship.unlv.edu/cgi/viewcontent.cgi?article=3649&context=thesesdissertations (accessed on 18th July 2025).
21. Cortes-Rincon, M., Hyde, D. M., & Valdez, F. (2014). Research reports from the Programme for Belize Archaeological Project, Volume Six. https://core.ac.uk/download/211339237.pdf (accessed on 18th July 2025).
22. Crawley, M., Forbes, G., Mulhern, D. M., Nelson, R., & Stout, S. (2016). Decision tree analysis as a supplementary tool to enhance histomorphological differentiation when distinguishing human from non-human cranial bone in both burnt and unburnt states: A feasibility study. https://core.ac.uk/download/42137084.pdf (accessed on 18th July 2025).
23. Dernell, W., Key Person, J., Cooper, L. E., Lead Investigator, M., et al. (2005). cGMP recombinant FIX for IV and oral hemophilia B therapy. https://core.ac.uk/download/17214933.pdf (accessed on 18th July 2025).
24. Ezzo, A. R. (2021). When the voices of children are heard: Evaluating the biological effects of socioeconomic status on children in postmedieval London. https://core.ac.uk/download/519866948.pdf (accessed on 18th July 2025).
25. Gamble, J. A., & Gilmour, R. J. (2024). Bones at home supporting haptic learning and universal design beyond the biological anthropology laboratory. https://core.ac.uk/download/644028705.pdf (accessed on 18th July 2025).
26. Hamilton, M. D. (2004). Seeking after empire: Bioarcheologists and American Indians in the new millennium. https://core.ac.uk/download/268795320.pdf (accessed on 18th July 2025).

27. Jiang, J., Li, C., Shu, G., et al. (2018). A rapid, non-invasive method for anatomical observations of tadpole vertebrae *in vivo*. https://core.ac.uk/download/199410535.pdf (accessed on 18th July 2025).
28. Kendall, A. W., & Vinter, B. (1984). Development of hexagrammids (Pisces: Scorpaeniformes) in the northeastern Pacific Ocean. https://core.ac.uk/download/11018531.pdf (accessed on 18th July 2025).
29. Klemm, M. M. (2024). The osteobiography of human remains from the Seaview and Indian Town Trail archaeological sites. https://core.ac.uk/download/610528749.pdf (accessed on 18th July 2025).
30. Kolb, H., & Mansueti, R. (1953). A historical review of the shad fisheries of North America. https://core.ac.uk/download/11025329.pdf (accessed on 18th July 2025).
31. Lillie, M., Nikitin, A., Potiekhina, I. D., et al. (2025). First evidence for interpersonal violence in Ukraine's Trypillian farming culture: Individual 3 from Verteba Cave, Bilche Zolote. https://core.ac.uk/download/151159376.pdf (accessed on 18th July 2025).
32. Morrone, A. (2022). Vaikuse lapsed: Lõuna-Eesti kesk- ja varauusaegsete laste toitumise ja tervise multidistsiplinaarsed uuringud arheolooglise ainese põhjal. https://core.ac.uk/download/541335832.pdf (accessed on 18th July 2025).
33. N/A. (2025). Cremated bone in archaeology: Ethical considerations in the excavation, analysis, storage, and display of cremated bone in the United Kingdom. https://core.ac.uk/download/635797915.pdf (accessed on 18th July 2025).
34. Rippa Bonati, M., Scattolin, G., Zampieri, F., et al. (2016). Occupational markers and pathology of the castrato singer Gaspare Pacchierotti (1740–1821). https://core.ac.uk/download/53529342.pdf (accessed on 18th July 2025).
35. Thornton, R. (2019). Towards a biological profile for South African perinatal remains: Osteological and genetic perspectives. https://core.ac.uk/download/161128473.pdf (accessed on 18th July 2025).
36. Trachman, R. M., & Valdez, F. (2009). Research reports from the Programmed for Belize Archaeological Project, Volume Three. https://core.ac.uk/download/211349318.pdf (accessed on 18th July 2025).
37. Wilhelmson, H. (2017). Perspectives from a human-centered archaeology: Iron Age people and society on Öland. https://core.ac.uk/download/83658101.pdf (accessed on 18th July 2025).
38. Winter, R. M. (2016). Analysis of a commingled skeletal sample from Acacia Park Memorial Cemetery. https://core.ac.uk/download/230810544.pdf (accessed on 18th July 2025).

INDEX

N

O

P

R

S